The Harmonic Mind

The Harmonic Mind

From Neural Computation to Optimality-Theoretic Grammar

Volume 2. Linguistic and Philosophical Implications

Paul Smolensky and Géraldine Legendre

A Bradford Book
The MIT Press
Cambridge, Massachusetts
London, England

MIT Press books may be purchased at special quantity discounts for business or sales promotional use. For information, please e-mail special_sales@mitpress.mit.edu or write to Special Sales Department, The MIT Press, 55 Hayward Street, Cambridge, MA 02142-1315.

This book was set in Book Antiqua, Bernhard Modern BT, and Garamond by the authors.

Printed and bound in the United States of America.

Library of Congress Cataloging-in-Publication Data

Smolensky, Paul, 1955–
     The harmonic mind: from neural computation to optimality-theoretic grammar / Paul Smolensky and Géraldine Legendre.
          p.   cm.
     "A Bradford book."
     Contents: Vol. 2. Linguistic and philosophical implications.
     Includes bibliographical references and index.
     ISBN 0-262-19527-5 (alk. paper) — ISBN 0-262-19528-3 (set : alk. paper)
     1. Neural networks (Computer science) 2. Natural language processing (Computer science) 3. Artificial intelligence. I. Legendre, Géraldine, 1953– II. Title.

QA76.87.S623 2006
006.3'2 — dc22
                                                            2005054385

10   9   8   7   6   5   4   3   2   1

To Natalie Rabinowitz Smolensky, Eugene Smolensky,
and Joshua Legendre Smolensky

for all you have given us

Contents

Volume 1. Cognitive Architecture

Part I
Toward a Calculus of the Mind/Brain: An Overview

Part II
Principles of the Integrated Connectionist/Symbolic Cognitive Architecture

Volume 2. Linguistic and Philosophical Implications

Part III
Optimality Theory: The Cognitive Science of Language

Part IV
Philosophical Foundations of Cognitive Architecture

Contributors

Lisa Davidson
Department of Linguistics
New York University

Paul Hagstrom
Department of Modern Foreign
    Languages & Literatures
Boston University

John Hale
Department of Linguistics
Michigan State University

Kristin Homer
Aurora, Colorado

Peter Jusczyk
deceased

Géraldine Legendre
Department of Cognitive Science
Johns Hopkins University

Donald W. Mathis
Department of Cognitive Science
Johns Hopkins University

Yoshiro Miyata
Department of Media Arts and
    Sciences
Chukyo University

Alan Prince
Department of Linguistics
Rutgers University

William Raymond
Department of Psychology
University of Colorado at Boulder

Paul Smolensky
Department of Cognitive Science
Johns Hopkins University

Melanie Soderstrom
Cognitive and Linguistic Sciences
Brown University

Antonella Sorace
Theoretical and Applied Linguistics
University of Edinburgh

Suzanne Stevenson
Department of Computer Science
University of Toronto

Bruce Tesar
Department of Linguistics
Rutgers University

Marina Todorova
Department of Cognitive Science
Johns Hopkins University

Anne Vainikka
Department of Cognitive Science
Johns Hopkins University

Colin Wilson
Department of Linguistics
UCLA

Preface

The goal of this book is twofold: to present a proposal for a cognitive architecture—with particular attention to the language faculty—and to instantiate a formal, aggressively interdisciplinary conception of cognitive science. The cognitive architecture centrally involves mathematics that will be unfamiliar to many in an interdisciplinary audience. To maximize accessibility, the ideas are presented at multiple levels of formal elaboration: the introductory chapters should be accessible to all, with elaborations for specialists relegated to later chapters. Also to promote ease of access, numerous expository boxes offer concise but substantial summaries of relevant background material from several disciplines.

At many colleges and universities, interdisciplinary groups of faculty, postdocs, and students meet to learn about and discuss work in cognitive science outside their own disciplines. Such a group provides a good model for this book's intended audience. The more introductory chapters and background boxes are written to be accessible to those with little training in the relevant field. Other chapters are written to provide experts with substantial results. The same examples are used in many chapters to facilitate the progression from more basic to more sophisticated treatments.

To maximize usability, this book is constructed to function when only a subset of the chapters are read. Increasing the extent to which chapters are self-contained introduces an unavoidable but hopefully acceptable degree of recapitulation, especially of the basic ideas that play a major role in multiple chapters.

Chapter 1 (Section 7) presents the specifics concerning the expository boxes, the interdependence of the chapters, the various disciplines they draw upon, and their inherent accessibility; it also gives a chapter-by-chapter summary of the entire book. The interrelatedness of the chapters is recalled in the introductions to the four parts of the book and in the abstracts to individual chapters; the abstracts attempt in particular to situate the content of each chapter in the big picture, sketched in the final section of Chapter 2: the ICS map. A table of contents for each chapter also identifies the topics discussed in that chapter.

To aid in navigating the book, the footers at the bottom of each page contain information concerning the location of the chapter's figures, tables, boxes, sections, and numbered items. The page on which, say, Figure 5 appears has 'Figure 5' at its foot; this label persists in the footers of subsequent pages until the appearance of Figure 6. The item numbered '(55)' in Chapter 5 is referred to in other chapters as 'Chapter 5 (55)'; 'Section 5:5.5' refers to Section 5.5 of Chapter 5. In our use of cross-references, we have done our best to optimize the conflicting demands of (1) readability and (2) precision in the use of terminology and reference to explicit principles.

In preparing these volumes, we have received much inspiration from the new generation of students who are training to become genuine cognitive scientists. For them, we offer this book as one conception of their emerging field.

Acknowledgments

Our deepest appreciation goes to our coauthors, especially Alan Prince, for all we have learned from them, for the great satisfaction we have derived from working with them, for their permission to include some of our joint research here, and for their patience with the excruciatingly long process of completing this book. Most of this joint work was already complete in the December 2000, prior to the subsequent additions which expanded the work by 50%.

For many helpful comments on a large part of the manuscript, we are grateful to Mark Johnson and especially to Matt Goldrick. We have benefited from the detailed feedback of students in seminars devoted to earlier drafts, at Johns Hopkins University in 2001 and 2002 and at Stanford University in spring 2002. We are extremely grateful to Tom Wasow, who not only gave us his own detailed critiques of nearly every chapter, but also painstakingly transmitted copious comments from the participants in his Stanford seminar. It was largely in response to this input that we undertook major revisions that culminated in the final draft of February 2004.

The multidisciplinary research discussed in these volumes connects with a vast heterogeneous literature of which the nearly 1,000 references included here barely scratch the surface. We regret that we were not able to do better, but the care and feeding of the manuscript became overwhelming; since we prepared camera-ready copy ourselves, managing the figures, formatting, typesetting, and copyediting became all-consuming. The erratic citation profile is one of the side effects of the intricate derivational history of a work built by folding together and attempting to homogenize materials written over a span of two decades.

For crucial help in preparing the manuscript, we thank Rebecca Hanna, Victoria Chan, Rachel Gawron, Emily Mosdell, and Joshua Legendre Smolensky. We are also extremely grateful to Josh for the original cover artwork, inspired by several trips as a threesome to the Vancouver area where we discovered a common love for and a desire to understand this unique form of native American art.

The manuscript benefited greatly from the painstaking copyediting of Anne Mark, whose heroic efforts extending over a year displayed her legendary skill at finding errors of every conceivable sort, from arrows in figures to typos in French to dates of references. Any remaining errors—and departures from perfect editorial consistency—are our own responsibility, and likely the result of oversights in implementing Anne's corrections.

At MIT Press we thank Tom Stone for sharing our vision for this work. For their help in bringing the book to press, we thank Sandra Minkkinen, Yasuyo Iguchi, and especially Margy Avery. We owe the index to the strenuous efforts of Holman Tse. For their encouragement and help with publication early on (starting in 1992), we warmly thank Amy Pierce Brand and Tammy Kaplan.

We are most grateful to our faculty and student colleagues in the uniquely stimulating environment of the Department of Cognitive Science at Johns Hopkins. The untimely loss in 2001 of our friend and collaborator Peter Jusczyk has been a terrible blow to us, as to so many others; we are thankful for the time we had to learn from him.

For partial support of the research reported here, we gratefully acknowledge NSF grants IRI-8609599, ECE-8617947, IST-8609599, BS-9209265, IRI-9596120, IIS-9720412, DGE-9972807, and BCS-0446954.

A work of this size has a large impact on family life. We might not have survived the experience with sane minds were it not for all the family members who supported us throughout this endeavor.

For allowing us to forget about the book and for providing much-needed relief with noisy gatherings à la française, fine food, and wine galore, we thank the faraway Legendre family.

For sharing our hopes and travails during the endless gestation of these two volumes, we thank Natalie and Gene Smolensky.

We reserve our most heartfelt thanks for Josh, a real mensch, who made this book possible by allowing it to intrude on our family from the day he moved to Baltimore as a seven-year-old (1994) to the day he left for college (2005).

Part III

Optimality Theory:
The Cognitive Science
of Language

The most well-developed component of the Integrated Connectionist/Symbolic Cognitive Architecture (ICS) is Optimality Theory (OT), which was laid out in detail in Chapter 12. In this part, we examine OT's prospects as the theoretical foundation for an integrated cognitive science of language. Chapters 13–16 address contributions to theoretical linguistics. Chapter 13 reprints a key chapter from the original OT book manuscript (Prince and Smolensky 1993/2004); like Chapter 14, it concerns theoretical phonology, while Chapters 15 and 16 address theoretical syntax. Potential contributions of OT to the study of language acquisition are the topics of Chapters 17 and 18. Chapter 17 reports experimental tests, with infants and adults, of OT-derived predictions concerning the initial and final states of the phonological grammar. Chapter 18 uses OT syntax to analyze the first productions of French-learning children. Chapter 19 concerns language processing: it applies OT syntax to the explanation of empirical patterns of difficulty experienced by the human sentence processor. Chapters 20 and 21 examine the relation between OT and lower-level analysis of ICS. Chapter 20 considers the relation between OT and Harmonic Grammar, discussed in Part II. Chapter 21 closes Part III with a rather speculative exploration of whether—indeed, how—the type of universal grammar proposed by OT could be realized in connectionist networks and encoded in an 'abstract genome'.

13

Optimality in Phonology I: Syllable Structure

Alan Prince and Paul Smolensky

How well does the explanatory program of Optimality Theory, detailed in Chapter 12, fare when confronting the universal patterns at play in the languages of the world? This chapter and the next three provide case studies addressing the data of theoretical linguistics: this chapter and Chapter 14 concern the phonological component of the grammar; Chapters 15 and 16, the syntactic component. All contribute to ② of Figure 6 in the Integrated Connectionist/Symbolic Cognitive Architecture (ICS) map of Chapter 2.

This chapter reprints a crucial portion (Chapter 6) of the original OT manuscript, Prince and Smolensky 1993/2004. The work reported here was the first demonstration that reranking of simple universal constraints could explain a central, well-known linguistic typology: basic syllable structure (Prince and Smolensky 1991). The Basic CV Syllable Theory defined here is the basis of examples in Chapters 4, 12, 14, 17, 20, 22, and especially 21, which explores its realization at the subsymbolic levels of abstract neural networks and an abstract genome.

For consistency with this book, certain typographical modifications have been made; notably, the original names 'ONS' and '–COD' have been replaced with the 'ONSET' and 'NOCODA' of McCarthy and Prince 1993. Section k here reprints Section 6.k of the original; the paragraphs preceding Section 1 reprint the original's introduction to Part II: Syllable Theory. To compute the numbering of items in the original, add 112 to the item numbers here (e.g., (1) here is (113) in the original). Likewise, add 49 to compute original footnote numbers. See Box 12:2 of this book for introduction to the phonological concepts and terms presumed. Box 1 reprints the introductory section of Chapter 8 of Prince and Smolensky 1993/2004.

Contents

The typology of syllable structure systems has been the object of a successful research effort over the last century and is fairly well understood empirically.[1] Basic theoretical questions remain open or undecided, of course, despite (or because of) the body of modern work in the area. Here we aim to show that the fundamental typological generalizations receive principled explication through the notion of **factorial typology**. The idea is that universal grammar (UG) provides a set of violable constraints on syllable structure, and individual grammars fix the relative ranking of these constraints. The typology of possible languages is then given by the set of all possible rankings.

Because of the considerable complexity that inheres in this domain, it is appropriate to approach it via the strategies of Galilean science, sometimes referred to as 'rational inquiry' in the linguistic literature. Our discussion will therefore proceed through three degrees of decreasing idealization. In this chapter, we examine a kind of CV theory: the key simplifying assumption being that the terminal nodes (segments) are presorted binarily as to their suitability for peak (V) and margin (C) positions (McCarthy 1979; Clements and Keyser 1983). Further, we consider only syllables with at most *one* symbol C or V in any syllabic position. Under these restrictions, the basic structural constraints are introduced and the ranking-induced typology is explored. Then, still within CV theory, we examine the finer grain of interactions between the structural constraints and various methods of enforcing them upon recalcitrant inputs.

In Chapter 7 of Prince and Smolensky 1993/2004, we show how the theory allows a rich set of alternations in the Australian language Lardil to be explicated strictly in terms of the interactions of constraints on prosodic structure. In Chapter 8 of that book (see Box 1 below), we extend the CV theory, taking up the more ambitious task of constructing syllables from segments classified into a multidegree sonority scale. We show how simple assumptions in UG explain a universal typology of inventories of onset, nucleus, and coda segments. A licensing asymmetry between onsets and codas is derived from the structural asymmetry in the basic theory: well-structured syllables *possess* onsets but *lack* codas. In the course of extracting these typological consequences, a number of general analytical techniques are developed.

Syllable Structure Typology: The CV Theory

1 THE JAKOBSON TYPOLOGY

It is well known that every language admits consonant-initial syllables .CV~., and that some languages allow no others; that every language admits open syllables .~V. and that some admit only those. Jakobson puts it this way:

---

[1] We do not pretend to cite this veritably oceanic body of work. The interested reader should refer to such works as Bell and Hooper 1978 and, say, the references in the references of Goldsmith 1990.

There are languages lacking syllables with initial vowels and/or syllables with final consonants, but there are no languages devoid of syllables with initial consonants or of syllables with final vowels. (Jakobson 1962, 526; Clements and Keyser 1983, 29)

As noted in the fundamental work of Clements and Keyser (1983), whence the quotation was cadged, these observations yield exactly four possible inventories. Using Σ^{XYZ} to denote the language whose syllables fit the pattern XYZ, the Jakobson typology can be laid out as follows, in terms of whether onsets and codas are obligatory, forbidden, or neither:

(1)   CV syllable structure typology

		Onsets	
		Required	Not required
Codas	Forbidden	Σ^{CV}	$\Sigma^{(C)V}$
	Allowed	$\Sigma^{CV(C)}$	$\Sigma^{(C)V(C)}$

There are two independent dimensions of choice: whether onsets are required (first column) or not (second column); whether codas are forbidden (row one) or allowed (row two).

The **basic syllable structure constraints**, which generate this typology, divide notionally into two groups. First, the structural or **markedness** constraints — those that enforce the universally unmarked characteristics of the structures involved:

(2)   ONSET

A syllable must have an onset.

(3)   NOCODA

A syllable must *not* have a coda.

Second, those that constrain the relation between output structure and input:

(4)   PARSE

Underlying segments must be parsed into syllable structure.

(5)   FILL

Syllable positions must be filled with underlying segments.

PARSE and FILL are **faithfulness** constraints, collectively denoted **FAITHFULNESS**: they declare that perfectly well-formed syllable structures are those in which input segments are in one-to-one correspondence with syllable positions.[2] Given an interpre-

---

[2] Both FILL and PARSE are representative of families of constraints that govern the proper treatment of child nodes and mother nodes, given the representational assumptions made here. As the Basic CV Syllable Theory develops, FILL will be articulated into a pair of constraints:

tive phonetic component that omits unparsed material and supplies segmental values for empty nodes, the ultimate force of PARSE is to forbid deletion; of FILL, to forbid insertion.

It is relatively straightforward to show that the factorial typology on the basic syllable structure constraints produces just the Jakobson typology. Suppose FAITHFULNESS dominates *both* structural constraints. Then the primacy of respecting the input will be able to force violations of both ONSET and NOCODA. The string /V/ will be parsed as an onsetless syllable, violating ONSET; the string /CVC/ will be parsed as a closed syllable, violating NOCODA: this gives the language $\Sigma^{(C)V(C)}$.

When a member of the faithfulness family is dominated by one or the other or both of the structural constraints, a more aggressive parsing of the input will result. In those rankings where ONSET dominates a faithfulness constraint, every syllable must absolutely have an onset. Input /V/ cannot be given its faithful parse as an onsetless syllable; it can either remain completely unsyllabified, violating PARSE, or it can be parsed as .□V., where '□' represents an empty structural position, violating FILL.

Those rankings in which NOCODA dominates a faithfulness constraint correspond to languages in which codas are forbidden. The imperative to avoid codas must be honored, even at the cost of expanding upon the input (*FILL) or leaving part of it outside of prosodic structure (*PARSE).

In the next section, we will explore these observations in detail. The resulting factorial construal of the Jakobson typology looks like this (with 'FAITH' denoting the faithfulness set and 'F_i' a member of it):

(6)   Factorial Jakobson typology

		Onsets	
		ONSET ≫ F_j	FAITH ≫ ONSET
Codas	NOCODA ≫ F_i	Σ^{CV}	$\Sigma^{(C)V}$
	FAITH ≫ NOCODA	$\Sigma^{CV(C)}$	$\Sigma^{(C)V(C)}$

At this point, it is reasonable to ask whether there is any interesting difference between our claim that constraints like ONSET and NOCODA can be violated under domination and the more familiar claim that constraints can be *turned off*—simply omitted from consideration. The factorial Jakobson typology, as simple as it is, contains a clear case that highlights the distinction. Consider the language $\Sigma^{(C)V(C)}$. Since onsets are not required and codas are not forbidden, the Boolean temptation would be to hold that both ONSET and NOCODA are merely absent. Even in such a language, however, one can find certain circumstances in which the force of the supposedly

---

FILL^{Nuc}:   Nucleus positions must be filled with underlying segments.
FILL^{Mar}:   Margin positions (Ons and Cod) must be filled with underlying segments.
Since unfilled codas are never optimal under syllable theory alone, shown below in Section 2.3 (29), FILL^{Mar} will often be replaced by FILL^{Ons} for perspicuity.

nonexistent structural constraints is felt. The string CVCV, for example, would always be parsed .CV.CV. and never .CVC.V. Yet both parses consist of licit syllables; both are entirely faithful to the input. The difference is that .CV.CV. satisfies ONSET and NOCODA while .CVC.V. violates both of them. We are forced to conclude that (at least) one of them is still active in the language, even though roundly violated in many circumstances. This is the basic prediction of ranking theory: when all else is equal, a subordinate constraint can emerge decisively. In the end, summary global statements about *inventory*, like Jakobson's, emerge through the cumulative effects of the actual parsing of individual items.

2 THE FAITHFULNESS INTERACTIONS

Faithfulness involves more than one type of constraint. Ranking members of the faithfulness family with respect to each other and with respect to the structural constraints ONSET and NOCODA yields a typology of the ways that languages can enforce (and fail to enforce) those constraints. We will consider only the faithfulness constraints PARSE and FILL (the latter to be distinguished by sensitivity to nucleus or onset); these are the bare minimum required to obtain a contentful, usable theory, and we will accordingly abstract away from distinctions that they do not make, such as between deleting the first or second element of a cluster, or between forms involving metathesis, vocalization of consonants, devocalization of vowels, and so on, all of which involve further faithfulness constraints, whose interactions with each other and with the markedness constraints will be entirely parallel to those discussed here.

2.1 Groundwork

To make clear the content of the basic syllable structure constraints ONSET, NOCODA, PARSE, and FILL, it is useful to lay out the Galilean arena in which they play. The inputs we will be considering are CV sequences like CVVCC; that is, any and all strings of the language {C,V}*. The grammar must be able to contend with any input from this set: we do not assume an additional component of language-particular input-defining conditions; the universal constraints and their ranking must do all the work (for further discussion, see Prince and Smolensky 1993/2004, Sec. 9.3; also Section 12:1.6 of this book). The possible structures that may be assigned to an input are all those that parse it into syllables--more precisely, into zero or more syllables. There is no insertion or deletion of *segments* C, V.

What is a syllable? To avoid irrelevant distractions, we adopt the simple analysis that the **syllable node** σ must have a daughter **Nuc** and *may* have as leftmost and rightmost daughters respectively the nodes **Ons** and **Cod**.[3] The nodes Ons, Nuc, and Cod, in turn, may each dominate Cs and Vs, or they may be empty. Each Ons, Nuc,

---

[3] For versions of the structural constraints within the perhaps more plausible moraic theory of syllable structure see Hung 1992; Kirchner 1992a, c; Samek-Lodovici 1992, 1993; Zoll 1992, 1993; McCarthy and Prince 1993.

or Cod node may dominate at most one terminal element C or V.

These assumptions delimit the set of candidate analyses. Here we list and name some of the more salient of the mentioned constraints. By our simplifying assumptions, they will stand at the top of the hierarchy and will be therefore unviolated in every system under discussion:

Syllable form:

(7)   **Nuc**

        Syllables must have nuclei.

(8)   ***Complex**

        No more than one C or V may associate to any syllable position node.[4]

Definition of C and V, using M(argin) for Ons and Cod and P(eak) for Nuc:

(9)   ***M/V**

        V may not associate to Margin nodes (Ons and Cod).

(10)   ***P/C**

        C may not associate to Peak (Nuc) nodes.

The theory we examine is this:

(11)   **Basic CV Syllable Theory**

        • Syllable structure is governed by the basic syllable structure constraints:
           Onset, NoCoda, Nuc; *Complex, *M/V, *P/C; Parse, and Fill.

        • Of these, Onset, NoCoda, Parse, and Fill may be relatively ranked in any domination order in a particular language, while the others are fixed in superordinate position.

        • The basic syllable structure constraints, ranked in a language-particular hierarchy, will assign to each input its optimal structure, which is the output of the phonology.

The output of the phonology is subject to phonetic interpretation, about which we will here make two assumptions, following familiar proposals in the literature:

(12)   Underparsing phonetically realized as deletion

        An input segment unassociated to a syllable position (**underparsing**) is not phonetically realized.

This amounts to 'Stray Erasure' (McCarthy 1979; Steriade 1982; Itô 1986, 1989). Epenthesis is handled in the inverse fashion:

---

[4] On *complex* margins, see Bell 1971, a valuable typological study. Clements 1990 develops a promising quantitative theory of crosslinguistic margin-cluster generalizations in what can be seen as harmonic terms (see Section 14:6). The constraint *Complex is intended as no more than a cover term for the interacting factors that determine the structure of syllable margins. For a demonstration of how a conceptually similar complex versus simple distinction derives from constraint interaction, see Prince and Smolensky 1993/2004, Secs. 9.1–2.

(13)   Overparsing phonetically realized as epenthesis

A syllable position node unassociated to an input segment (**overparsing**) is phonetically realized through some process of filling in default featural values.

This is the treatment of epenthesis established in such works as Selkirk 1981; Lapointe and Feinstein 1982; Broselow 1982; Archangeli 1984; Kaye and Lowenstamm 1984; Piggott and Singh 1985; and Itô 1986, 1989 (cf. Anderson 1982 on empty syllabic positions in underlying forms).

The terms 'underparsing' and 'overparsing' are convenient for referring to parses that violate FAITHFULNESS. If an input segment is not parsed in a given structure (not associated to any syllable position nodes) , we will often describe this as 'underparsing' rather than 'deletion' to emphasize the character of our assumptions. For the same reason, if a structure contains an empty syllable structure node (one not associated to an input segment), we will usually speak of 'overparsing' the input rather than 'epenthesis'.

Suppose the phonology assigns to the input /CVVCC/ the following bisyllabic structure, which we write in three equivalent notations:

(14)   Transcription of syllabic constituency relations, from /CVVCC/

a.
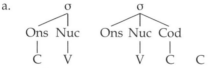

b. $[_\sigma [_{Ons} C] [_{Nuc} V]]$ $[_\sigma [_{Ons}] [_{Nuc} V] [_{Cod} C]]$ C

c.   .CV́.□V́C.⟨C⟩

Phonetic interpretation ignores the final C, and supplies featural structure for a consonant to fill the onset of the second syllable.

The dot notation (14c) is the most concise and readable; we will use it throughout. The interpretation is as follows:

(15)   Notation

a.   .X.   The string X *is a* syllable.

b.   ⟨x⟩   The element x has no parent node; is free (unparsed).

c.   □   .A node Ons, Nuc, or Cod is empty.

d.   x́   The element x is a Nuc.

In the CV theory, we will drop the redundant nucleus-marking accent on V́, writing only V. Observe that this is a 'notation' in the most inert and de-ontologized sense of the term: a set of typographical conventions used to refer to well-defined formal objects. The objects of linguistic theory—syllables here—are not to be confused with the literal characters that depict them. Linguistic operations and assessments apply to structure, not to typography.

We will say a syllable 'has an onset' if, like both syllables in the example (14), it has an Ons node, regardless of whether that node is associated to an underlying C; similarly with nuclei and codas.

The technical content of the basic syllable structure constraints (2)–(5) above can now be specified. The constraint ONSET (2) requires that a syllable node σ have as its left-most child an Ons node; the presence of the Ons node satisfies ONSET whether empty or filled. The constraint NOCODA (3) requires that syllable nodes have no Cod child; the presence of a Cod node violates NOCODA whether or not that node is filled. Equivalently, any syllable that does not contain an onset in this sense earns its structure a mark of violation *ONSET; a syllable that does contain a coda earns the mark *NOCODA.

The PARSE constraint (4) is met by structures in which all underlying segments are associated to syllable positions; *each* unassociated or free segment earns a mark *PARSE. This is the penalty for deletion. FILL (5) provides the penalty for epenthesis: each unfilled syllable position node earns a mark *FILL, penalizing insertion. Together, PARSE and FILL urge that the assigned syllable structure be faithful to the input string, in the sense of a one-to-one correspondence between syllable positions and segments. This is FAITHFULNESS in the basic theory.

2.2 Basic CV Syllable Theory

We now pursue the consequences of our assumptions. One important aspect of the Jakobson typology (1) follows immediately:

(16)   *Theorem.* Universally optimal syllables

No language may prohibit the syllable .CV. Thus, no language prohibits onsets or requires codas.

To see this, consider the input /CV/. The obvious analysis .CV. (i.e., $[_\sigma [_\text{Ons} C] [_\text{Nuc} V]]$) is **universally optimal** in that it violates *none* of the universal constraints of the Basic CV Syllable Theory (11). No alternative analysis, therefore, can be more harmonic. At worst, another analysis can be equally good, but inspection of the alternatives quickly rules out this possibility.

For example, the analysis .CV□. violates NOCODA and FILL. The analysis .C□.V. violates ONSET in the second syllable and FILL in the first. And so on, through the infinite set of possible analyses ([.⟨C⟩V.], [.C□⟨V⟩.], [.□.C□.□V.], etc. ad inf.). No matter what the ranking of constraints is, a form that violates even one of them can never be better than a form, like .CV., with no violations at all.

Because every language has /CV/ input, according to our assumption that every language has the same set of possible inputs, it follows that .CV. can never be prohibited under the Basic CV Syllable Theory.

2.2.1 Onsets

Our major goal is to explicate the interaction of the structural constraints ONSET and NOCODA with faithfulness. We begin with onsets, studying the interaction of ONSET with PARSE and FILL, ignoring NOCODA for the moment. The simplest interesting input is /V/. All analyses will contain violations; there are three possible one-mark analyses:

(17)   /V/ →

    a.   .V.   i.e., $[_\sigma [_{Nuc} V]]$

    b.   ⟨V⟩   i.e., no syllable structure

    c.   .□V.   i.e., $[_\sigma [_{Ons}] [_{Nuc} V]]$

Each of these alternatives violates exactly one of the basic syllable structure constraints (2)–(5).

(18)   Best analyses of /V/

Analysis	Interpretation	Violation	Remarks
.V.	σ lacks Ons	*ONSET	satisfies FILL, PARSE
⟨V⟩	null parse	*PARSE	satisfies ONSET, FILL
.□V.	Ons is empty	*FILL	satisfies ONSET, PARSE

Every language must evaluate all three analyses. Since the three candidates violate one constraint each, any comparison between them will involve weighing the importance of different violations. The optimal analysis for a given language is determined precisely by whichever of the constraints ONSET, PARSE, and FILL is *lowest* in the constraint hierarchy of that language. The lowest constraint incurs the least important violation.

Suppose .V. is the optimal parse of /V/. We have the following tableau:

(19)   Onset not required

/V/	FILL	PARSE	ONSET
☞ .V.			*
⟨V⟩		*!	
.□V.	*!		

The relative ranking of FILL and PARSE has no effect on the outcome. The violations of PARSE and FILL are fatal because the alternative candidate .V. satisfies both constraints.

Of interest here is the fact that the analysis .V. involves an onsetless syllable. When this analysis is optimal, then the language at hand, by this very fact, does not absolutely require onsets. The other two inferior analyses do succeed in satisfying ONSET: ⟨V⟩ achieves this vacuously, creating no syllable at all; .□V. creates an onsetful syllable by positing an empty Ons node, leading to epenthesis. So if .V. is best, it is because ONSET is the lowest of the three constraints, and we conclude that the language does not require onsets. We already know from Theorem (16) that onsets can never be forbidden. This means the following condition holds:

(20)   If PARSE, FILL ≫ ONSET, then onsets are not required.

(The comma'd grouping indicates that PARSE and FILL each dominate ONSET, but that there is no implication about their own relative ranking.)

On the other hand, if ONSET is not the lowest-ranking constraint—if either PARSE or FILL is lowest—then the structure assigned to /V/ will be consistent with the language requiring onsets. The following two tableaux lay this out:

(21)   Enforcement by overparsing (epenthesis)

/V/	ONSET	PARSE	FILL
.V.	*!		
⟨V⟩		*!	
☞ .□V.			*

(22)   Enforcement by underparsing (deletion)

/V/	FILL	ONSET	PARSE
.V.		*!	
☞ ⟨V⟩			*
.□V.	*!		

These lucubrations lead to the converse of (20):

(23)   If ONSET dominates either PARSE or FILL, then onsets are required.

There is an important difference in status between the two ONSET-related implications. To prove that something is *optional*, in the sense of 'not forbidden' or 'not required' in the inventory, one need merely exhibit one case in which it is observed and one in which it isn't. To prove that something is *required*, one must show that everything in the universe observes it. Thus, formal proof of (23) requires considering not just one trial input, as we have done, but the whole (infinite) class of strings on {C,V}* that we are taking to define the universal set of possible inputs for the Basic CV Syllable Theory. For this exercise, see the appendix of Prince and Smolensky 1993/2004; in Chapter 8 of that book (see Box 1 below), we develop general techniques that enable us to extend the above analysis to arbitrary strings, showing that what is true of /V/ and /CV/ is true of all inputs.

The results of this discussion can be summarized as follows:

(24)   **Onset Theorem**

Onsets are not required in a language if ONSET is dominated by both PARSE and FILL.

Otherwise, onsets are required in all syllables of optimal outputs.

In the latter case, ONSET is enforced by underparsing (phonetic deletion) if PARSE is the lowest ranking of the three constraints; and by overparsing (phonetic epenthesis) if FILL is lowest.

If FILL is to be articulated into a family of node-specific constraints, then the version of FILL that is relevant here is FILL^{Ons}. With this in mind, the onset finding may be recorded as follows:

Lowest constraint	Onsets are ...	Enforced by ...
ONSET	not required	N/A
PARSE	required	V 'deletion'
FILL^{Ons}	required	C 'epenthesis'

2.2.2 Codas

The analysis of onsets has a direct parallel for codas. We consider the input /CVC/ this time; the initial CV provides an onset and nucleus to meet the ONSET and NUC constraints, thereby avoiding any extraneous constraint violations. The final C induces the conflict between NOCODA, which prohibits the Cod node, and faithfulness, which has the effect of requiring just such a node. As in the corresponding onset situation (18), the parses that violate only one of the basic syllable structure constraints are three in number:

(25) Best analyses of /CVC/

Analysis	Interpretation	Violation	Remarks
.CVC.	σ has Cod	*NOCODA	satisfies FILL, PARSE
.CV⟨C⟩.	no parse of 2nd C	*PARSE	satisfies NOCODA, FILL
.CV.Cǔ.	2nd Nuc is empty	*FILL	satisfies NOCODA, PARSE

The optimal analysis of /CVC/ in a given language depends on which of the three constraints is lowest in the domination hierarchy. If .CVC. wins, then the language must allow codas; NOCODA ranks lowest and violation can be compelled. If .CVC. loses, the optimal analysis must involve open (codaless) syllables; in this case, NOCODA is enforced through empty nuclear structure (phonetic V-epenthesis) if FILL is lowest, and through nonparsing (phonetic deletion of C) if PARSE is the lowest, most violable constraint. In either case, the result is that open syllables are *required*. This is a claim about the optimal parse in the language of every string, and not just about /CVC/, and formal proof is necessary (see the appendix to Prince and Smolensky 1993/2004).

The conclusion, parallel to (24), is this:

(26) **Coda Theorem**

Codas are allowed in a language if NOCODA is dominated by both PARSE and FILL^{Nuc}.

Otherwise, codas are forbidden in all syllables of optimal outputs.

In the latter case, NOCODA is enforced by underparsing (phonetic deletion) if PARSE is the lowest ranking of the three constraints; and by overparsing (epenthesis) if FILL^{Nuc} is the lowest.

The result can be tabulated like this:

Lowest constraint	Codas are ...	Enforced by ...
NOCODA	allowed	N/A
PARSE	forbidden	C 'deletion'
FILL^{Nuc}	forbidden	V 'epenthesis'

Motivation for distinguishing the constraints FILL^{Ons} and FILL^{Nuc} is now available. Consider the languages Σ^{CV} in which only CV syllables are allowed. Here ONSET and NOCODA each dominate a member of faithfulness group. Enforcement of the dominant constraints will be required. Suppose there is only one FILL constraint, holding over all kinds of nodes. If FILL is the lowest ranked of the three constraints, we have the following situation:

(27)   Triumph of epenthesis

Input	Optimal analysis	Phonetic
/V/	.□V.	.CV.
/CVC/	.CV.C□́.	.CV.CV̇.

The single uniform FILL constraint yokes together the methods of enforcing the onset requirement ('C-epenthesis') and the coda prohibition ('V-epenthesis'). There is no reason to believe that languages Σ^{CV} are obligated to behave in this way; nothing that we know of in the linguistic literature suggests that the appearance of epenthetic onsets requires the appearance of epenthetic nuclei in other circumstances. This infelicitous yoking is avoided by the natural assumption that FILL takes individual node-classes as an argument, yielding FILL^{Nuc} and FILL^{Ons} as the actual constraints. In this way, the priority assigned to filling Ons nodes may be different from that for filling Nuc nodes.[5]

It is important to note that onset and coda distributions are completely independent in this theory. Any ranking of the onset-governing constraints {ONSET, FILL^{Ons}, PARSE} may coexist with any ranking of the coda-governing constraints {NOCODA, FILL^{Nuc}, PARSE}, because they have only one constraint, PARSE, in common. The universal factorial typology allows all nine combinations of the three onset patterns given in (24) and the three coda patterns in (26). The full typology of interactions is portrayed in table (28). We use subscripted *del* and *ep* to indicate the

---

[5] It would also be possible to break this yoke by having two separate PARSE constraints, one that applies to C and another to V. Basic syllable structure constraints that presuppose a C/V distinction, however, would not support the further development of the theory in Prince and Smolensky 1993/2004, Chap. 8 (see Box 1), where the segment classes are derived from constraint interactions.

phonetic consequences of enforcement; when both are involved, the onset-relevant mode comes first.

(28)   Extended CV syllable structure typology

			Onsets		
			Required		**Not required**
			ONSET, FILL^{Ons} $\gg$ PARSE	ONSET, PARSE $\gg$ FILL^{Ons}	PARSE, FILL^{Ons} $\gg$ ONSET
Codas	**Forbidden**	NOCODA, FILL^{Nuc} $\gg$ PARSE	$\Sigma^{CV}_{del,del}$	$\Sigma^{CV}_{ep,del}$	$\Sigma^{(C)V}_{del}$
		NOCODA, PARSE $\gg$ FILL^{Nuc}	$\Sigma^{CV}_{del,ep}$	$\Sigma^{CV}_{ep,ep}$	$\Sigma^{(C)V}_{ep}$
	Allowed	PARSE, FILL^{Nuc} $\gg$ NOCODA	$\Sigma^{CV(C)}_{del}$	$\Sigma^{CV(C)}_{ep}$	$\Sigma^{(C)V(C)}$

If we decline to distinguish between the faithfulness constraint rankings, this simplifies to the Jakobson typology of (6).

2.3 The theory of epenthesis sites

The chief goal of syllabification-driven theories of epenthesis is to provide a principled account of the location of epenthetic elements (Selkirk 1981; Broselow 1982; Lapointe and Feinstein 1982; Itô 1986, 1989). Theories based on manipulation of the segmental string are capable of little more than summary stipulation on this point (e.g., Levin [Blevins] 1985, 331; see Itô 1986, 159, and 1989 for discussion). The theory developed here entails tight restrictions on the distribution of empty nodes in optimal syllabic parses and therefore meets this goal. We confine attention to the premises of the Basic CV Syllable Theory, which serves as the foundation for investigating the theory of epenthesis, which ultimately involves segmental and prosodic factors as well.

There are a few fundamental observations to make, from which a full positive characterization of syllabically motivated epenthesis emerges straightaway.

(29)   *Proposition 1.* *[ ]$_{Cod}$
     Coda nodes are never empty in any optimal parse.

Structures with unfilled Cod can never be optimal; there is always something better. To see this, take a candidate with an unfilled Cod and simply remove that one node. This gives another candidate which has one less violation of NOCODA and one less violation of FILL. Since removing the node has no other effects on the evaluation, the second candidate must be superior to the first. (To show that something is *non-optimal*, we need merely find something better: we don't have to display the best. This method of demonstration is **harmonic bounding**: the structure with unfilled Cod is **harmonically bounded** by the Cod-less competitor. See Prince and Smolensky 1993/2004, Sec. 9.1.1, for general discussion.)

We know from the earlier discussion that Ons and Nuc must be optimally unfilled in certain parses under certain grammars. So the remaining task is to determine the conditions under which these nodes must be posited and left empty.

(30) *Proposition 2.* $*.(\square)\dot\square$.

A whole syllable is never empty in any optimal parse.

The same style of argument applies. Consider a parse that has an entirely empty syllable. Remove that syllable. The alternative candidate thereby generated is superior to the original because it has (at least) one less FILL^{Nuc} violation and no new marks. The empty syllable parse can always be bested and is therefore never optimal.

Of course, in the larger scheme of things, whole syllables can be epenthesized, the canonical examples being Lardil and Axininca Campa (Hale 1973; Klokeid 1976; Payne 1981; Payne, Payne, and Santos 1982; Itô 1986; Wilkinson 1988; Spring 1990; Black 1991; Kirchner 1992b; McCarthy and Prince 1993). In all such cases, it is the impact of additional constraints that forces whole-syllable epenthesis. In particular, when the prosody-morphology interface constraints are taken into account, prosodic minimality requirements can force syllabic epenthesis (see the discussion of Lardil in Prince and Smolensky 1993/2004, Chap. 7).

(31) *Proposition 3.* $*.(\square)\dot\square C$.

No syllable can have Cod as its only filled position.

Any analysis containing such a syllable is bested by the alternative in which the content of this one syllable (namely, 'C') is parsed instead as .C$\dot\square$. This alternative incurs only the single mark $*$FILL^{Nuc}, but the closed-syllable parse .$(\square)\dot\square C$. shares this mark and violates NOCODA as well. (In addition, the closed-syllable parse must also violate either ONSET or FILL^{Ons}.)

Such epentheses are not unknown: think of Spanish /slavo/ $\rightarrow$ *eslavo* and Arabic /ħmarar/ $\rightarrow$ *ʔiħmarar*. We must argue, as indeed must all syllable theorists, that other constraints are involved (for Arabic, see McCarthy and Prince 1990).

(32) *Proposition 4.* $*[\ ][\ ]$

Adjacent empty nodes cannot occur in an optimal parse.

Propositions 1, 2, and 3 entail that [ ][ ] cannot occur inside a syllable. This leaves only the intersyllabic environment .C$\dot\square$.$\square$V~. This bisyllabic string incurs two marks, $*$FILL^{Nuc} and $*$FILL^{Ons}. Consider the alternative parse in which the substring /CV/ is analyzed as tautosyllabic .CV~. This eliminates both marks and incurs no others. It follows that two adjacent epentheses are impossible.

We now pull these results together into an omnibus characterization of where empty nodes can be found in optimal parses.

(33) FILL **Violation Theorem**. Location of possible epenthesis sites

Under the basic syllable structure constraints, epenthesis is limited to the following environments:

a. Ons, when Nuc is filled:

  .□V.

  .□VC.

b. Nuc, when Ons is filled:

  .C□.

  .C□C.

Furthermore, two adjacent epentheses are impossible, even across syllable boundaries.

We note that this result carries through in the more complex theory developed in Prince and Smolensky 1993/2004, Chap. 8, in which the primitive CV distinction is replaced by a graded sonority-dependent scale (see Box 1).

Box 1. Universal syllable theory:

Ordinal construction of C/V and onset/coda licensing asymmetry

Syllabification must reconcile two conflicting sources of constraint: from the bottom up, each segment's inherent featural suitability for syllable peak or margin; and from the top down, the requirements that syllables have certain structures and not others. The core conflict can be addressed in its most naked form through the idealization provided by CV theory. Input Cs need to be parsed as margins; input Vs need to be parsed as peaks. Syllables need to be structured as onset-peak-coda—ideally, with an onset present and a coda absent. In the Basic CV Syllable Theory, only one input segment is allowed per syllable position. Problematic inputs like /CCVV/ are ones that bring the bottom-up and top-down pressures into conflict. These conflicts are resolved differently in different languages, the possible resolutions forming the typology explored in the text of this chapter.

   The CV theory gives some articulation to the top-down pressures: syllable shapes deviate from the ideal onset-peak in the face of bottom-up pressure to parse the input. By contrast, the bottom-up is construed relatively rigidly: C and V either go into their determined positions, or they remain unparsed. In real syllabification, of course, a richer set of possibilities exists. A segment ideally parsed as a peak may actually be parsed as a margin, or vice versa, in response to top-down constraints on syllable shape. One of the most striking examples of the role of optimality principles in syl-

---

Box 1

labification, Tashlhiyt Berber (Prince and Smolensky 1993/2004, Chap. 2; see Section 20:3 of this book), exploits this possibility with maximal thoroughness. Berber syllabification on the one hand and CV syllabification on the other constitute extremes in the flexibility with which input segments may be parsed into different syllable positions in response to top-down pressure. In between the extremes lies the majority of languages, in which some segments can appear only as margins (like C in the CV theory), other segments only as peaks (like V), and the remaining segments, while ideally parsed into just one of the structural positions, can under sufficient top-down pressure be parsed into others.

This box provides an overview of Chapter 8 of Prince and Smolensky 1993/2004, which seeks to unify the treatments of the two extremes of syllabification, Berber and the CV theory. Like the CV theory, the theory developed there deals with an abstract inventory of input segments, but instead of just two abstract segments, each committed to a structural position, the inventory consists of abstract elements distinguished solely by the property of **sonority**, taken to define a strict order on the set of elements. For mnemonic value we denote these elements *a, i, …, d, t*; but it should be remembered that all dimensions other than sonority are idealized away. In the CV theory, the universally superordinate constraints *M/V and *P/C prohibit parsing V as a margin or C as a peak. In the more realistic theory of Chapter 8, the corresponding constraints are not universally superordinate: the constraints against parsing any segment α as a margin (*M/α) or as a peak (*P/α) may vary crosslinguistically in their rankings. What UG requires is only that more sonorous segments make more harmonic peaks and less harmonic margins.

From these simple assumptions there emerges a universal typology of inventories of possible onsets, peaks, and codas. The inventories turn out to be describable in terms of derived parameters π_{Ons}, π_{Nuc}, and π_{Cod}, each with values ranging over the sonority order. The margin inventories are the sets of segments *less* sonorous than the corresponding parameter values π_{Ons} or π_{Cod}, and the peak inventory is the set of segments *more* sonorous than the value of π_{Nuc}. Languages in which $\pi_{\text{Ons}} > \pi_{\text{Nuc}}$ are therefore languages with ambidextrous segments, which can be parsed as either onset or nucleus. The following diagram pictures the situation; the double line marks the zone of overlap.

(1)   Languages with ambidextrous segments

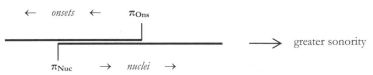

The theory entails a universal licensing asymmetry between onsets and codas: codas can contain only a subset, possibly strict, of the segments appearing in onsets. This fundamental licensing asymmetry follows from the asymmetry between onset and coda in the basic syllable structure constraints. From the fact that onsets should be present and codas absent, it follows in the theory that coda is a weaker licenser.[6] To our knowledge, no other approach has been able to connect the structural propensities of syllables with the licensing properties of syllabic positions, much less to derive one from the other. This is surely a significant result, one that indicates that the theory is on the right track in a fundamental way. The exact nature of the obtained licensing asymmetry has some empirical imperfections that can be traced to the oversimplified analysis of codas in the internal structure of the syllable, and Prince and Smolensky 1993/2004 suggests possible refinements.

Chapter 8 constitutes a larger-scale exploration of our general line of attack on the problem of universal typology. UG provides constraints, which individual languages rank differently in domination hierarchies; it also provides certain universal conditions on these hierarchies, which all languages must respect. The results obtained involve a further development of the basic idea: **parameterization by ranking**. The parameters π_{Ons}, π_{Nuc}, and π_{Cod} are epiphenomenal, in that they do not appear at all in UG, or indeed, in particular grammars: they are not, for example, mentioned in any constraint. These parameters are not explicitly set by individual languages. Rather, individual languages simply rank the universal constraints, and it is a *consequence* of this ranking that the (derived, descriptive) parameters have the values they do in that language. The procedures for reading off these parameter values from a language's constraint dominance hierarchy are not, in fact, entirely obvious.

The analysis developed in Chapter 8 introduces or elaborates several general concepts of the theory:

(2)   Push/pull parsing

       The parsing problem is analyzed in terms of the direct conflict between two sets of constraints:

       a.   ASSOCIATE constraints: PARSE, FILL, ONSET, and the like, which penalize parses in which input segments or structural nodes *lack* structural associations to a parent or child.

       b.   DON'T-ASSOCIATE constraints: *M/V, *P/C, NOCODA and the like, which penalize parses that *contain* structural associations of various kinds.

(3)   Universal constraint subhierarchies

       The DON'T-ASSOCIATE constraints *M/V, *P/C, superordinate in the CV theory, are replaced by an articulated set of anti-association constraints *M/a, *M/i, ..., *M/d, *M/t; *P/a, *P/i, ..., *P/d, *P/t that penalize associations between margin or peak nodes on the one hand and particular input segments on the other. UG requires that the domination hierarchy of each language rank these constraints *M/α, *P/α relative to one another in conformity with the following universal domination conditions:

---

[6] The demonstration will require some work, however; perhaps this is not surprising, given the simplicity of the assumptions.

Box 1

$$*M/a \gg *M/i \gg \cdots \gg *M/d \gg *M/t \quad \text{(margin hierarchy)}$$
$$*P/t \gg *P/d \gg \cdots \gg *P/i \gg *P/a \quad \text{(peak hierarchy)}$$

The margin hierarchy states that it's less harmonic to parse a as a margin than to parse i as margin, less harmonic to parse i as a margin than r, and so on down the sonority ordering. The peak hierarchy states that it's less harmonic to parse t as a peak than d, and so on up the sonority order.

(4)   Associational Harmony

The universal margin and peak hierarchies ensure the following universal ordering of the Harmony of possible associations:

$$M/t \succ M/d \succ \cdots \succ M/i \succ M/a$$
$$P/a \succ P/i \succ \cdots \succ P/d \succ P/t$$

These represent the basic assumption that the less sonorous an element is, the more harmonic it is as a margin; the more sonorous, the more harmonic it is as a peak.

(5)   Prominence Alignment

These universal rankings of constraints (3) and ordering of associational Harmonies (4) exemplify a general operation, **Prominence Alignment**, in which scales of prominence along two phonological dimensions are **harmonically aligned**. In this case, the first scale concerns prominence of structural positions within the syllable,

Peak > Margin,

while the second concerns inherent prominence of the segments as registered by sonority:

$$a > i > \cdots > d > t.$$

(6)   Encapsulation

It is possible to greatly reduce the number of constraints in the theory by **encapsulating** sets of associational constraints $*M/\alpha$, $*P/\alpha$ into defined constraints that explicitly refer to *ranges* of sonority. This corresponds to using a coarse-grained sonority scale, obtained by collapsing distinctions. This must be done on a language-specific basis, however, in a way sensitive to the language's total constraint hierarchy: which sets of associational constraints can be successfully encapsulated into composite constraints depends on how the language inserts other constraints such as PARSE, FILL, ONSET, and so on, into the margin and peak hierarchies, and how these two hierarchies are interdigitated in the language. Encapsulation opens the way to developing a substantive theory of the sonority classes operative in syllable structure phenomena.

Along with these conceptual developments, Chapter 8 introduces a collection of useful techniques for reasoning about constraint domination hierarchies in complex arenas such as that defined by the segmental syllable theory. A few of these techniques are:

(7)   Harmonic bounding for inventory analysis

In order to show that a particular kind of structure φ is not part of a universal or language-particular inventory, we consider any possible parse containing φ and show constructively that there is some competing parse (of the same input) that is more harmonic; thus, no structure containing φ can ever be optimal, as it is always bounded above by at least one more-harmonic competitor. (This form of argument was used to establish the distribution of epenthesis sites in Section 2.3 of this chapter.)

(8)   Cancellation/Domination Lemma

In order to show that one parse B is more harmonic than a competitor A that does not incur an identical set of marks, it suffices to show that every mark incurred by B is either (i) canceled by an identical mark incurred by A, or (ii) dominated by a higher-ranking mark incurred by A. That is, for every constraint violated by the more harmonic form B, the losing competitor A either (i) matches the violation exactly, or (ii) violates a constraint ranked higher.

(9)   The method of universal constraint tableaux

A generalization of the method of language-specific constraint tableaux, this yields a systematic means for using the Cancellation/Domination Lemma to determine which parse is optimal, not in a specific language with a given constraint hierarchy, but in a typological class of languages whose hierarchies meet certain domination conditions but are otherwise unspecified.

Chapter 8 contains a considerable amount of analysis. That extended analysis is necessary to establish the results can be appreciated as follows. The most complex result of Chapter 8 is the onset/coda licensing asymmetry:

(10)   Crosslinguistically, the inventory of possible codas is a subset of the inventory of possible onsets, but not vice versa.

To show just what is necessary to establish this result, (11) gives a step-by-step reduction of (10) to the elements in terms of which it must actually be demonstrated:

(11)   Onset/coda licensing asymmetry dissected

a.   For all languages admitted by UG, the inventory of possible codas is a subset of the inventory of possible onsets, but not vice versa.

b.   For all constraint hierarchies $\mathcal{H}$ formed by ranking the universal syllable structure constraints as allowed by UG, the inventory of possible codas is a subset of the inventory of possible onsets, but not vice versa.

c.   For all rankings $\mathcal{H}$ of the universal syllable structure constraints allowed by UG, and

for all segments λ,

if λ is a possible coda in the language given by $\mathcal{H}$

then λ is a possible onset in $\mathcal{H}$,

but not vice versa.

Box 1

    d. For all rankings $\mathcal{H}$ of the universal syllable structure constraints allowed by UG, and

        for all segments λ,

            if there is an input string I_λ

                containing λ

                for which the optimal parse (with respect to $\mathcal{H}$) is one in which

                    λ is associated to Cod,

            then there is an input string $I_\lambda{}'$

                containing λ

                for which the optimal parse (with respect to $\mathcal{H}$) is one in which

                    λ is associated to Ons;

    but not vice versa.

    e. **For all** rankings $\mathcal{H}$ of the universal syllable structure constraints allowed by UG, and

        for all segments λ,

            if there exists an input string I_λ

                containing λ

                for which **there is** a parse $B_{Cod/\lambda}$ in which λ is associated to Cod

                such that

                    if C is any other candidate parse of I_λ,

                    then $B_{Cod/\lambda}$ is more harmonic than C with respect to the ranking $\mathcal{H}$ ($B_{Cod/\lambda} \succ_{\mathcal{H}} C$),

            then there exists an input string $I_\lambda{}'$

                containing λ

                for which **there is** a parse $B_{Ons/\lambda}{}'$ in which λ is associated to Ons

                such that

                    if C$'$ is any other candidate parse of $I_\lambda{}'$,

                    then $B_{Ons/\lambda}{}'$ is more harmonic than C$'$ with respect to the ranking $\mathcal{H}$ ($B_{Ons/\lambda}{}' \succ_{\mathcal{H}} C'$);

    but **not** vice versa.

In the final formulation, as in all the others, the phrase 'but not vice versa' means that if 'Cod' and 'Ons' are interchanged in the proposition that precedes, then the resulting proposition is false. The logical quantifiers and connectives in this assertion have been set in boldface in order to indicate the logical structure of the proposition without resorting to predicate calculus. The innermost embedded propositions ($B_{Cod/\lambda} \succ_{\mathcal{H}} C$, and likewise for the primed parses) are themselves somewhat complex propositions that involve comparisons of the hosts of marks incurred by parses of entire strings.

References

ROA = Rutgers Optimality Archive, http://roa.rutgers.edu

Anderson, S. R. 1982. The analysis of French schwa, or how to get something for nothing. *Language* 58, 534–73.

Archangeli, D. 1984. Underspecification in Yawelmani phonology and morphology. Ph.D. diss., MIT.

Bell, A. 1971. Some patterns of occurrence and formation of syllable structures. *Working Papers on Language Universals* 6, 23–137.

Bell, A., and J. B. Hooper. 1978. *Syllables and segments.* Elsevier–North Holland.

Black, H. A. 1991. The optimal iambic foot and reduplication in Axininca Campa. *Phonology at Santa Cruz* 2, 1–18.

Broselow, E. 1982. On the interaction of stress and epenthesis. *Glossa* 16, 115–32.

Clements, G. N. 1990. The role of the sonority cycle in core syllabification. In *Papers in laboratory phonology I: Between the grammar and the physics of speech,* eds. J. Kingston and M. Beckman. Cambridge University Press.

Clements, G. N., and S. J. Keyser. 1983. *CV phonology: A generative theory of the syllable.* MIT Press.

Goldsmith, J. A. 1990. *Autosegmental and metrical phonology.* Blackwell.

Hale, K. 1973. Deep-surface canonical disparities in relation to analysis and change: An Australian example. *Current Trends in Linguistics* 11, 401–58.

Hung, H. 1992. Relativized suffixation in Choctaw: A constraint-based analysis of the verb grade system. Ms., Brandeis University.

Itô, J. 1986. Syllable theory in prosodic phonology. Ph.D. diss., University of Massachusetts at Amherst.

Itô, J. 1989. A prosodic theory of epenthesis. *Natural Language and Linguistic Theory* 7, 217–60.

Jakobson, R. 1962. *Selected writings I: Phonological studies.* Mouton.

Kaye, J., and J. Lowenstamm. 1984. De la syllabicité. In *Forme sonore du langage,* eds. D. H. F. Dell and J.-R. Vergnaud. Hermann.

Kirchner, R. 1992a. Harmonic Phonology within one language: An analysis of Yidiny. MA thesis, University of Maryland at College Park.

Kirchner, R. 1992b. Lardil truncation and augmentation: A morphological account. Ms., University of Maryland at College Park.

Kirchner, R. 1992c. Yidiny prosody in Harmony Theoretic Phonology. Ms., UCLA.

Klokeid, T. J. 1976. Topics in Lardil grammar. Ph.D. diss., MIT.

Lapointe, S., and M. Feinstein. 1982. The role of vowel deletion and epenthesis in the assignment of syllable structure. In *The structure of phonological representations, part II,* eds. H. van der Hulst and N. Smith. Foris.

Legendre, G., P. Smolensky, and C. Wilson. 1998. When is less more? Faithfulness and minimal links in *wh*-chains. In *Is the best good enough? Optimality and competition in syntax,* eds. P. Barbosa, D. Fox, P. Hagstrom, M. McGinnis, and D. Pesetsky. MIT Press and MIT Working Papers in Linguistics. ROA 117.

Levin [Blevins], J. 1985. A metrical theory of syllabicity. Ph.D. diss., MIT.

McCarthy, J. J. 1979. Formal problems in Semitic phonology and morphology. Ph.D. diss., MIT.

McCarthy, J. J., and A. Prince. 1990. Prosodic morphology and templatic morphology. In *Perspectives on Arabic linguistics: Papers from the Annual Symposium on Arabic Linguistics.* Vol. 2, *Salt Lake City, Utah 1988,* ed. M. Eid and J. J. McCarthy. Benjamins.

McCarthy, J. J., and A. Prince. 1993. Prosodic Morphology I: Constraint interaction and satisfaction. Technical report RuCCS-TR-3, Rutgers Center for Cognitive Science, Rutgers University, and University of Massachusetts at Amherst. ROA 482, 2001.

Payne, D. 1981. *The phonology and morphology of Axininca Campa.* Summer Institute of Linguistics.

Payne, D., J. Payne, and J. Santos. 1982. *Morfología, fonología y fonética del Ashéninca del Apurucayali (campa-arawak preandino).* Ministerio de Educación and Instituto Lingüístico de Verano.

Piggott, G., and R. Singh. 1985. The phonology of epenthetic segments. *Canadian Journal of Linguistics* 30, 415–53.

Prince, A., and P. Smolensky. 1991. Notes on connectionism and Harmony Theory in linguistics. Technical report CU-CS-533-91, Computer Science Department, University of Colorado at Boulder.

Prince, A., and P. Smolensky. 1993/2004. *Optimality Theory: Constraint interaction in generative grammar.* Technical report, Rutgers University and University of Colorado at Boulder, 1993. ROA 537, 2002. Revised version published by Blackwell, 2004.

Samek-Lodovici, V. 1992. Universal constraints and morphological gemination: A cross-linguistic study. Ms., Brandeis University.

Samek-Lodovici, V. 1993. A unified analysis of cross-linguistic morphological gemination. In *Proceedings of Console 1.*

Selkirk, E. 1981. Epenthesis and degenerate syllables in Cairene Arabic. In *Theoretical issues in the grammar of the Semitic languages,* eds. H. Borer and J. Aoun. MIT Working Papers in Linguistics.

Spring, C. 1990. Implications of Axininca Campa for prosodic morphology and reduplication. Ph.D. diss., University of Arizona.

Steriade, D. 1982. Greek prosodies and the nature of syllabification. Ph.D. diss., MIT.

Wilkinson, K. 1988. Prosodic structure and Lardil phonology. *Linguistic Inquiry* 19, 325–34.

Zoll, C. 1992. When syllables collide: A theory of alternating quantity. Ms., Brandeis University.

Zoll, C. 1993. Ghost consonants and optimality. In *Proceedings of West Coast Conference on Formal Linguistics 12.*

14

Optimality in Phonology II: Harmonic Completeness, Local Constraint Conjunction, and Feature Domain Markedness

Paul Smolensky

To what extent can Optimality Theory (Prince and Smolensky 1993/2004) provide theoretical phonology a satisfactory formalization of markedness theory? This is a central question for linking OT and actual empirical patterns: ② of Figure 6 in Chapter 2's Integrated Connectionist/Symbolic Cognitive Architecture (ICS) map.

Through several case studies, it is argued here that OT makes possible formal markedness-based explanations of both broad universal generalizations and complex language-particular patterns—provided the theory incorporates conjunctive constraint interaction. The nonderivational character of OT drives the development of a nonstandard type of constituent in phonological representations: the headed feature domain. The empirical realms investigated are place markedness, vowel harmony, and the sonority structure of syllables.

Contents

The whole problem of vowel harmony will have to be reconsidered in the light of the theory of markedness,
which undoubtedly in some version will form a chapter of generative phonology.
— *Paul Kiparsky 1973, 33*

The core of the formalization of markedness laid out in Chapter 9 of Prince and Smolensky 1993/2004 is extremely simple (see Chapter 12 (41)).[1] Let a dimension of variation of linguistic representations be encoded by a binary feature φ with values $[\pm\varphi]$. If the universally marked (dispreferred, lower-Harmony) pole is, say, $[+\varphi]$, then the universal ranking (1a) holds.

(1)   Universal markedness hierarchy. Marked pole: $[+\varphi]$

   a. $*[+\varphi] \gg_{UG} *[-\varphi]$
   b. $*[+\varphi] \in Con$, $*[-\varphi] \notin Con$

(1a) states that, whereas universal grammar (UG) by default allows all possible rankings of its constraints, in the case of the particular constraints $*[+\varphi]$ and $*[-\varphi]$, only the ranking of (1a) is permitted in a possible human grammar.[2] This typological restriction is denoted by the subscript in the symbol '$\gg_{UG}$'. $*[+\varphi]$ is a constraint in the markedness family, violated by each occurrence of the feature value $[+\varphi]$ in a representation. Sometimes it is convenient to work with a simplification of (1a), according to which the universal constraint set *Con* contains the constraint $*[+\varphi]$ but simply does not contain any constraint $*[-\varphi]$: (1b).

As one means of evaluating the adequacy of Optimality Theory's approach to formalizing markedness, in Section 1 OT is compared with an approach to markedness that plays an important role in rule-based phonology, **Underspecification Theory**. The case of **coronal place unmarkedness** is analyzed to show how the general types of language-internal markedness effects achieved through Underspecification Theory are inevitable consequences of OT's computational architecture, eliminating the additional stipulation of underspecified representations (and the problems they entail). In Section 2, it is shown that the typologies produced by OT respect markedness, and that the theory therefore successfully unifies language-internal and crosslinguistic generalizations, a fundamental job of a theory of markedness.

In Section 2, it is also shown that OT's success in capturing markedness-based typology is only partial. While all OT inventories respect markedness, a class of markedness-respecting inventories is not generable within OT. This represents a shortcoming of basic OT if such problematic inventories are indeed empirically attested, as claimed in Section 4. A general formal device (introduced in Chapter 12 (43))—**local conjunction of constraints**—is developed in Section 3 and shown to enable OT to generate the problematic inventories. The formal analysis in the Appendix

---

[1] The concept of markedness was introduced in Section 4:2; for the markedness family of OT constraints, see Section 12:1.4. For general introduction to markedness theory, see Battistella 1990, 1996.
[2] See de Lacy 2002 for arguments that such markedness rankings can be "ignored, but never reversed" by grammars.

demonstrates the adequacy of this device as a general solution, with respect to a highly simplified idealization of the fundamental character of inventories.

The sections discussed above all derive their empirical content from extremely broad generalizations that underlie markedness theory. In Section 4, the empirical content comes from very specific facts of particular languages that instantiate broad language-internal markedness generalizations. This level of specificity is necessary to empirically evaluate whether basic OT's inability to generate certain inventories is a virtue or a deficiency. This research addresses vowel harmony (Box 1), where markedness effects are often quite evident. These studies provide evidence that the problematic inventories do indeed exist; this work also shows how local conjunction provides an empirically adequate means of generating them. They show further how the general arguments of Section 1 concerning OT and Underspecification Theory play out concretely in a phonological area where underspecification has previously played an important role in explaining markedness effects.

Local conjunction combines simple constraints to make a more complex constraint. Normally, the simple constraints are standard OT constraints, while the conjoined constraint is more complex. But local conjunction can be used in the other direction as well: a standard OT constraint can be regarded as the 'complex' constraint resulting from the local conjunction of still more elementary constraints. Used in this way, local conjunction can perform another conceptually quite different function: increasing the depth of explanation provided by certain standard OT constraints, by reducing them to conjunctions of even more basic constraints. This is pursued in Section 6, which addresses the role of sonority in syllable structure; familiar constraints like ONSET are reduced to conjunctions of more elementary constraints. This section returns to the mode of empirical evaluation via broad generalizations rather than detailed language-specific analysis.

To make contact with the empirical facts of vowel harmony and syllable structure, it is necessary to commit to specific phonological representations. These representations must allow OT to achieve many of the results of Autosegmental Phonology, which has played a central role in the analysis of vowel harmony. Inspired by Autosegmental Phonology, I propose in Section 2 a general representational system for phonological features: **headed feature domains**. The particular phonological analyses of Sections 4–6 depend crucially on this representational system, and thus these analyses pertain not only to the empirical status of local conjunction, but also to that of headed feature domains. The analyses of Sections 4–6 illustrate the consequences expected to arise from fully specified representations with headed feature domains interacting via local conjunction.

As a preview of the more substantive claims of this chapter, let us consider two major formal devices that were the focus of much work in phonological theory during the last quarter of the twentieth century: underspecified representations, and autosegmental rules and representations. These two devices relate to OT in interesting ways.

The direct mapping from underlying to surface form characteristic of most OT work does not provide the derivational architecture needed for these devices. Autosegmental representations support rules of creation, deletion, linking, delinking, and spreading of feature values (autosegments) on their respective tiers (Goldsmith 1976, 1990; Williams 1976; see Box 12:2); in the absence of derivations, OT must employ other devices, implementable in direct input-output phonology, to provide the functionality of the autosegmental apparatus. These devices will be representational, not processual: feature domains that correspond essentially to the span of a single feature value along its tier. It is a main goal of this chapter to develop the notion of feature domains. I will focus on the role of the **head** of a feature domain: developing this concept is a major component of the work presented here. The concept is inspired by the distinguished status of the source of a spreading feature in Autosegmental Phonology; but as it develops, the feature domain head takes on a character of its own, only loosely related to its autosegmental progenitor.

While not so obviously as Autosegmental Phonology, Underspecification Theory also depends upon a derivational computational architecture. Our interest in underspecification here is as a means of formalizing aspects of the notion of markedness; thus, it is the **radical** version of Underspecification Theory that is most relevant (Kiparsky 1982; Archangeli 1984). In this theory, the preferred or unmarked value of a feature (in a given context) is unspecified in the underlying form—underlying representations are literally not 'marked' with this feature value. In the course of the derivation, this absent feature value typically gets inserted. After its value is inserted, the feature behaves essentially like any other feature, but prior to insertion it clearly cannot: it is phonologically **inert**, neither undergoing nor triggering phonological processes.

Input underspecification is a problematic device in OT; I will mention only two of the reasons here. First, OT's fundamental principle, Richness of the Base (Section 12:1.6), bans any systematic restrictions on the input: work done previously by special input properties (such as lack of specification for unmarked values) must in OT be done by the grammar itself. Second, even if inputs could be guaranteed to be unspecified for certain features, these features typically must be present in the output, so these features' distinguishing status—absence—could not obtain at the one point where such special status could be phonologically relevant in OT: the output. The input is only visible to faithfulness constraints, which demand only that it be matched by the output. It is of course markedness constraints that distinguish marked from unmarked feature values, and these constraints 'see' only the output.

But the markedness constraints of OT provide a formalization of markedness directly; the general architecture of OT should provide the power to capture markedness generalizations, and no additional device—in particular, input underspecification—should be needed. As a markedness device, underspecification would be at best conceptually redundant in OT. So a second goal of this chapter is to understand how OT's inherent markedness theory accounts for the inertness of unmarked features, previously analyzed in terms of their absence at early stages of derivation.

The third goal is to use OT to sharpen the formal characterization of a central aspect of the crosslinguistic component of markedness theory: implicational universals (Greenberg 1978). Such a universal asserts that if a language's inventory includes some type of element *X*, it will also include another type of element *X'*; this is diagnostic of a markedness relationship, where *X'* is less marked than *X*. In OT, an inventory with this property is said to be **harmonically complete** (Prince and Smolensky 1993/2004, Chaps. 8, 9). A typology is said to have the **strong harmonic completeness (SHARC)** property if it consists of all and only the harmonically complete inventories. In this chapter, the SHARC property is explored both theoretically and empirically. Theoretically, basic OT typologies will be shown to have this property — with local conjunction, but not without it. Empirically, vowel harmony systems will be analyzed as complex, harmonically complete inventories. For the OT analysis of these inventories, local conjunction is necessary and sufficient. The explanatory power of OT with local conjunction is illustrated by showing how even vowel harmony systems requiring many complex spreading rules under Autosegmental Phonology can be understood as the consequence of the interaction of simple universal violable constraints encoding fundamental markedness relationships. In a more speculative mode, I will sketch a typological theory unifying vowel harmony with other seemingly unrelated phenomena, a direct consequence of the interaction, under OT with local conjunction, of headed feature domains.

A goal of the type of research reported here is to explain major empirical generalizations from principles that are as simple and irreducible as possible. The explanations sought are therefore necessarily complex: the simpler the basic principles, the more extended the argumentation required to deduce major results. The explanatory objectives here include constructing, from more basic notions, concepts that otherwise would be taken as primitives subject to stipulated principles. Thus, it should be entirely expected that the explanations developed in this chapter are generally analytically more complex than their antecedents: the hope is that the results offer a compensating increase in the depth of understanding of the empirical phenomena.

Box 1. Vowel harmony

In its pure form, vowel harmony is a phonological system in which all the vowels in a single word must have the same value of the harmonizing feature. Consider the classic case of Finnish, illustrated in (1) (all Finnish data from Välimaa-Blum 1986). To a first approximation, all vowels in a Finnish word have the same value of the feature [±back] (the values of [±high], [±low], and [±round] are also indicated).[3]

(1)   Finnish harmonizing vowels

    a.   [+back] vowels: u, o, a ([+hi, −lo, +rd], [−hi, −lo, +rd], [−hi, +lo, −rd])

[3] The following feature abbreviations will be used through the chapter: [back] = [bk] or B; [front] = [fr] or F; [low] = [lo] or L; [round] = [rd] or R; ATR (advanced tongue root) = A.

Box 1

          i.   pouda+lla   'in sunny summer weather'
          ii. kuoka+lla   'with a hoe'
          iii. kuka+ssa   'in the flower'
    b. [−back] vowels: ü, ö, ä ([+hi, −lo, +rd], [−hi, −lo, +rd], [−hi, +lo, −rd])
          i.   südän-tä   'of the heart'
          ii. pöüdä+llä   'on the table'
          iii. höürü+ssä   'in the steam'

The suffix -*ssa* in (1a) becomes -*ssä* in (1b), the suffix vowel agreeing with the stem vowels in backness.

The next order of approximation brings in the remaining two Finnish vowels, *i* and *e*. These are [−back] vowels, but they can appear with [+back] vowels, as shown in (2a).

(2)   Transparent vowels: i, e ([+hi, −lo, −rd], [−hi, −lo, −rd])
    a. With [+back] vowels
          i.   sotilas+ta   'of the soldier'
          ii. Suome+ssa   'in Finland'
          iii. kusiaise+lla   'on the ant'
    b. With [−back] vowels
          i.   äidi-ltä   'from mother'
          ii. pimeä+ssä   'in the dark'
          iii. ilkeä stä   'from the naughty'
    c. Alone
          i.   neiti+ä   'of the miss'
          ii. tie+llä   'of the round'
          iii. eines+tä   'of prepared food'

The suffix vowels are [+back] if there is a [+back] vowel in the stem; otherwise, they are [−back]. Importantly, there are no [+back] counterparts to the [−back] vowels *i*, *e* in the Finnish inventory—hence, they cannot participate in the [±back] alternation. These vowels are **transparent** to harmony: they are invisible to the principles determining the [±back] values of suffix vowels. In (2a.ii), the [+back] values of the first two vowels 'spread through' the transparent third [−back] vowel to determine the [+back] value of the suffix vowel (Kiparsky 1981; Gafos 1996; Walker 1998; Section 1.5.3).

Another behavior sometimes exhibited by nonalternating vowels in harmony systems is **opacity**. Were *e* opaque in Finnish, the suffix vowel in (2a.ii) would be [−back], *ä*, in agreement with *e* itself. An opaque vowel blocks harmonic spread across it, instead triggering harmony with its own feature value. A vowel may be opaque throughout the language, or individual occurrences of the vowel in particular morphemes may be opaque (Vago 1980).

Finnish illustrates a **root-controlled** harmony system: suffix vowels alternate but stem vowels do not. The other main type of harmony system is **dominant-recessive**: in this case, certain 'dominant' feature values, or the feature values of certain vowels, do not alternate, even in affixes; they force 'recessive' vowels to harmonize with them, even in stems (Bakovic 2000).

One of the most complex vowel harmony systems is that of Lango, discussed at length in Section 4.1. In Lango, when two vowels with disagreeing features come together, whether vowel harmony occurs, and if so, which vowel alters its feature, depends in a highly complex way on the precise identity of the two vowels in question, their linear order, and their syllabic environments—in sum, on the relative markedness of the alternatives.

The final degree of approximation to the intricacies of vowel harmony taken up here concerns **disharmony**. Exceptions within vowel harmony systems are rather common, and are interesting because there is typically a phonological pattern to the exceptions. The case of Turkish is considered in Section 1.5.4.

1 Markedness, Harmony, and phonological invisibility

1.1 The problem

In most languages, all nasal consonants in the inventory are voiced. In such languages, it is thus reasonable to ask whether a segment specified [+nasal] must in addition be specified [+voice]. Since [+voice] is the unmarked value of voicing in the context of the feature [+nasal], this question can be generalized: must a feature be specified in a representation if it bears the unmarked value (in its context)?

There is a profound motivation for regarding unmarked values as unspecified. As Itô, Mester, and Padgett (1995, 571) put it:

(2)   Inertness of the unmarked

"It is a common observation that redundant phonological features are mostly inert, neither triggering phonological rules nor interfering with the workings of contrastive features. ... This distinction between 'active' contrastive and 'inactive' redundant features is expressed in the theory through the notion of (under)specification of features in phonology."

Redundant features, and unmarked feature values more generally, tend to be phonologically inert, as if invisible to the phonology; this follows with perspicuous elegance from the assumption that such features are simply not present in the representations on which phonology acts. This assumption is the basis of Radical Underspecification Theory (Kiparsky 1982, 53ff.; Archangeli 1984, 1988; Mester and Itô 1989). Underspecification Theory is a formalization of markedness theory: it interprets 'un-

Box 1

marked' as a literal description of linguistic representations, which are not marked so as to indicate the value of the unspecified feature.[4]

Thus, the very loose generalization I seek to explain in this section is (3).

(3) Activity Generalization (absolute version): Unmarked ⇒ Inactive
     Unmarked elements are phonologically inactive.

If OT's notion of Harmony provides an adequate formalization of markedness, such a generalization should follow from OT principles without the need for further assumptions. Underspecification in OT would be a second way of encoding unmarkedness; such a redundant device should not be needed to derive the Activity Generalization (3). If underspecification were necessary to derive (3), it would be possible to have an OT phonology without underspecification in which the Activity Generalization would be violated.

But we will see that this is impossible: there is no way in OT to formulate a grammatical theory that violates the Activity Generalization, even if all representations are fully specified. In this sense, the Activity Generalization is an integral, inevitable property of OT. In contrast, it is only by stipulating underspecification that a rule-based theory can derive the Activity Generalization; it is logically possible to have a rule-based theory lacking underspecification that would as a result violate the Activity Generalization.

As mentioned earlier, there are several reasons internal to OT for avoiding (dependence upon) underspecified representations. Outputs underspecified for φ cannot truly be evaluated by OT constraints sensitive to the value of φ. And depending upon inputs being systematically unspecified for φ is ruled out by Richness of the Base: in OT, it is not possible to restrict inputs in this way. Inputs specified for φ cannot be prevented from entering the grammar; the grammar must enforce the Activity Generalization, and so this result cannot be a consequence of input underspecification.

---

[4] This conception was explicit in Trubetzkoy 1939/1969 (emphasis original):

The signifier of the system of language consists of a number of elements whose essential function it is to distinguish themselves from each other. Each word must distinguish itself by some element from all other words of the same system of language. The system of language, however, possesses only a limited number of such differential means, and since their number is smaller than the number of words, the words must consist of combinations of discriminative elements ("marks" in K. Bühler's terminology). (p. 10)

Privative oppositions are oppositions in which one member is characterized by the presence, the other by the absence, of a mark. For example: "voiced"/"voiceless", "nasalized"/"nonnasalized", "rounded"/"unrounded". The opposition member that is characterized by the presence of the mark is called "marked", the member characterized by its absence "unmarked". This type of opposition is extremely important for phonology. (p. 75)

In cases of this type one of the opposition members occurs in the position of neutralization, and its choice is in no way related to the nature of the position of neutralization. However, due to the fact that one of the opposition members occurs in that position as the representative of the respective archiphoneme, its specific features become nonrelevant, while the specific features of its partner receive full phonological relevance: the former opposition member that is permitted in the position of neutralization is *unmarked* from the standpoint of the respective phonemic system, while the opposing member is *marked*. (p. 81)

Independent of OT, there are several reasons to seek alternatives to underspecification (e.g., Mohanan 1991; McCarthy and Taub 1992; Steriade 1995; Bakovic 2000). As McCarthy and Taub put it, underspecification analyses rely on a "now you see it, now you don't" shell game with unmarked features. With respect to certain processes, these features are inactive, so at the stage of derivation when the relevant rules apply, the unmarked feature must be unspecified. With respect to other processes, these same features may be active, so they must be present when these other rules apply. Orchestrating the appearance of unmarked values to achieve this poses significant descriptive and explanatory problems.[5]

A second problem McCarthy and Taub raise is that, while unmarked features could conceivably be inactive because they don't exist, this distinguishing property of unmarked values is not consistent with another hallmark of unmarkedness: greater diversity. Specifically with respect to the markedness of oral places of articulation, the unmarked place suggested by inactivity is [coronal]; but it is precisely here that the greatest diversity of other featural contrasts is to be found. As formalized in feature geometry, this diversity means that the [coronal] node has many dependents relative to the nodes for marked places of articulation, exactly the opposite of what would be expected if the distinguishing property of [coronal] is its nonexistence. Independent of feature geometry, it remains a problem that nonexistence does not seem to be a formal property that can unify two central characteristics of the unmarkedness of [coronal]: that it is inactive, and that it licenses a diversity of other features.

The problems associated with underspecification, both those that are internal to OT and those that are not, disappear if unmarked elements (e.g., [coronal]) are present in representations, and if their higher Harmony, relative to their more marked counterparts, accounts for both their inactivity and their enhanced licensing power.

1.2 The proposed solution

The main claim of Section 1 is this.

(4)   More harmonic ⇒ Less active

The working hypothesis is that "less marked" can be formalized in OT as **more harmonic** according to markedness constraints, and that universal markedness relationships such as "[−φ] is less marked than [+φ]" are encoded in UG via universally fixed

---

[5] McCarthy and Taub (1992) point out that the English processes to which coronals seem "invisible" range from the derivationally very early to the derivationally very late. The same is true of English processes to which coronals must be "visible." A diagnostic used (see the next point in the text) is whether plain coronals (simple alveolars) pattern differently from complex coronals (like θ and ʃ); the former are unspecified in radical Underspecification Theory, but the latter cannot be, since they have features that are dependents of the [coronal] node. Processes to which plain but not complex coronals are invisible must be ordered before the default rule filling in [coronal], while processes to which all coronals are visible must of course be ordered after the default rule. McCarthy and Taub observe that it is quite unlikely that such an ordering of processes is possible given the other ordering requirements imposed by English phonology, and that in any event "such an ordering will sometimes be quite arbitrary" (p. 365).

Box 1

rankings, as in (5)

(5) $*[+\varphi] \gg_{UG} *[-\varphi]$

(or by the presence of $*[+\varphi]$ and the absence of $*[-\varphi]$ in the universal constraint set *Con*, as discussed below (1)).

Let an input element x be said to "undergo a process" if it has no faithful output correspondent, and to "trigger a process" if its presence entails that constraints will force other input elements to undergo the process. Let x be phonologically "active" if it undergoes or triggers a process. Then the claim is:

(6)   Less marked elements are less active.

>   If a more harmonic element surfaces unfaithfully or induces another element to surface unfaithfully, then a less harmonic element will also.[6]

This must be understood in a very broad, liberal sense, commensurate with the empirical generalization (3) that it is intended to explain. It is too broadly stated to be a literal theorem, and indeed it is far from a crisp result. Rather than attempting to substantiate this broad claim as such, I will instead consider several classes of "phonological processes" for which the generalization holds. In many of these cases, underspecification can also provide an account.

The essence of the argument is encapsulated in (7).

(7)   Key idea (absolute version): No marks $\Rightarrow$ Invisible

>   In OT, outputs are evaluated and selected solely on the basis of the constraints they violate, or the **marks** ($*$s) they are assessed by these constraints. Hence, a phonological element can be "invisible" to the phonology even when present, *if it does not incur any marks*—that is, if it is literally 'unmarked'.

Underspecification Theory takes "unmarked" literally, "marked" being understood in the sense of 'specified'. OT takes "unmarked" literally too; but here, "marked" is understood as 'bearing the $*$ marking a constraint violation'. The constraints relevant in (7) are markedness constraints, naturally.

The absolute version of the main idea states that an element that incurs no mark is phonologically invisible; an element that incurs a mark is potentially visible. The idea also applies in a more subtle way that fully exploits the Harmony scale of OT.

---

[6] To illustrate the triggering case: consider a language E (like English; see Section 1.4.3) in which consonant clusters can only have one noncoronal consonant. Suppose the grammar imposes this by deleting segments: if an input contains, say, /pv/, then p is deleted; /ps/ surfaces faithfully, however, since only p is noncoronal. Thus, v "triggers the deletion of /p/" but s does not. Now consider another language, M (like the Polynesian language Maori; e.g., Hale 1973, 417), lacking clusters altogether, and suppose again that repair is effected by deletion. Then in M, /pv/ $\rightarrow$ v, as in E. But in M, /ps/ $\rightarrow$ s: even the presence of s triggers deletion of p. The less place-marked s is sufficiently "visible" to the cluster simplification "process" to trigger it; and so certainly is the more-marked v. In E, however, v but not s is visible to the process. In both languages, the more-marked v is more visible to the process than the less-marked s; in E, s is sufficiently invisible to prevent deletion, while in M it is not. For the proposed analysis of this type of pattern, see Section 1.4.3.

(8)   Key idea (relative version): Lower marks $\Rightarrow$ Less active

In OT, the lower a constraint is ranked, the less *active* it is in the phonology. A mark assessed by a low-ranking constraint functions almost like no mark at all. Thus, if structure u incurs lower-ranked marks than structure m, then u will interact with fewer constraints than m, and hence be less phonologically active.

The sense of 'active constraint' used here is formally defined in Prince and Smolensky 1993/2004, (110): a constraint is active in a grammar if it actually rules out candidates during the Harmony evaluation process defining optimality.

1.3 The challenge: The coronal syndrome

In the remainder of Section 1, I will focus on particular types of phonological processes relevant to the markedness of oral places of articulation. The unmarked status of [cor] place is documented in the important collection Paradis and Prunet 1991. In their argument for Underspecification Theory, Paradis and Prunet (p. 21) issue the challenge (9); the current project may be seen in part as an attempt to provide an OT response to this challenge. I have inserted the numbers of the subsections below that address the particular phenomena listed by Paradis and Prunet.

(9)   The challenge

"Mohanan 1989, in an overview of underspecification theories, suggests that (at least some of) the phenomena attributed to underspecification could be handled by a theory of markedness. ... It is not clear how such an approach would handle any of the various arguments presented here for the special status of coronals:

the coda and cluster conditions [Sections 1.4.3, 1.4.4],

assimilation [Section 1.4.5],

neutralization [Section 1.4.4],

transparency [Section 1.5.3],

deletion [Section 1.4.2],

epenthesis [Section 1.4],

substitution, the frequency of coronal harmonies, etc.

It is even less clear how it could connect all of these properties together."

So our first question is, which of these effects can be explained (and thereby 'connected') via the key idea (8): 'Lower marks $\Rightarrow$ Less active'? Second, is it possible to go further and connect the effects listed in (9) with other markedness phenomena, such as those listed in (10)?

(10)   Further markedness phenomena

a.   Coronal diversity [Section 1.5.2]

b.   Universal markedness patterns delimiting segmental inventories (presence/absence) [Section 1.5]

Box 1

c. Contrastiveness of features in segmental inventories [Section 1.5.1]

d. Markedness effects within segmental inventories (e.g., markedness conditions on targets of feature spread) [Section 1.5.4]

At the root of all the OT explanations is the single universal fixed ranking expressing the unmarked status of coronal (henceforth, [cor]) relative to other oral places, such as labial ([lab]):

(11) Universal place markedness hierarchy

$$*[lab] \gg_{UG} *[cor]$$

This is to be seen as an instance of the general schema (1). It was proposed in Prince and Smolensky 1993/2004, Chap. 9 (see also Chapter 12 (41) of the present book). As in that work, here [lab] will stand in for [dorsal], as well as denoting labial place; [dorsal] is treated formally just like [lab] in the theory.[7]

1.4 Invisibility phenomena

1.4.1 Epenthesis

Paradis and Prunet claim (Paradis and Prunet 1991, 21) that coronal underspecification correctly predicts that oral epenthetic consonants will have coronal place. (Concerning the empirical status of this generalization, see Lombardi 2002.)

Consider a simple hypothetical input such as /an/. As shown in Chapter 13, the ranking shown in tableau (12) leads to epenthesis of an onset consonant. Because ONSET dominates a faithfulness constraint, it will be enforced by some kind of unfaithfulness; thus, candidate (12a) is not optimal. Because PARSE dominates FILL, the optimal type of unfaithfulness is a FILL violation, that is, overparsing or "epenthesis"; the maximally underparsed null parse (12b), denoted ⟨an⟩ in the notation of Chapter 13, is nonoptimal. This leaves only overparsed candidates like (12c) and (12d) containing an epenthetic onset segment (boxed). FILL^{Ons} is violated by the epenthesized onset.

(12) Epenthesis of coronals

/an/ →	Epenthesize onset				Place markedness	
	ONSET	PARSE	FILL^{Ons}	FILL^{Pl}	*[lab]	*[cor]
a. an	*!					
b. ⟨an⟩		*! *				
c. p̄an			*	*	*!	
d. ☞ t̄an			*	*		*

---

[7] Lombardi (2002) argues that the hierarchy should be further extended to include *[cor] $\gg_{UG}$ *[pharyngeal].

Chapter 13 operated at a level of abstraction that failed to distinguish among consonants, so no internal structure was needed for the onset segment. Now I assume that candidate outputs include completely specified segments, including a value for place. This place is not filled by underlying material, so it violates FILL^{Pl}. The two places under consideration are [cor] and [lab], so in addition to the FILL violations, the epenthetic segment will violate either *[lab] or *[cor], the relevant *STRUCTURE constraints (Chapter 12 (40a)). By the coronal unmarkedness condition (11), the latter violation is universally more harmonic than the former; thus, labial candidates like (12c) are suboptimal, and the optimal candidate will have an epenthesized coronal, like candidate (12d). (Other constraints, encoding the unmarked values of other features, will determine just which coronal consonant is optimal.)

In tableau (12), where the place markedness constraints are ranked relative to the other constraints influences whether epenthesis occurs (e.g., if both are ranked higher than PARSE, the null parse (12c) will be optimal). But it is only the ranking of the place constraints relative to each other—universally fixed—that influences the choice among epenthetic segments. All marks of candidates (12c) and (12d) cancel except those assessed by the place constraints (highlighted with the heavy boxes); so wherever they are ranked, the place markedness constraints ensure that the coronal (12d) is more harmonic than the labial (12c).

The conclusion is that the universal markedness subhierarchy *[lab] $\gg_{UG}$ *[cor] entails that, ceteris paribus, epenthetic consonants are coronals. Epenthetic material should be as 'invisible' as possible: not in the sense of having an absent place value, but in having an absent place *mark*—or, since this is impossible, coming as close as possible to no place mark, by having the lowest-ranked place mark possible: *[cor].

1.4.2 Deletion

Paradis and Prunet claim that coronal underspecification explains the invisibility of coronals to deletion in Japanese (1991, 2; citing Grignon 1984, 324). An idealization of the intended situation might be the behavior of *s* in the following verbal paradigm:[8]

(13)   Coronal invisibility to deletion

      a. /~VC$_1$+C$_2$V~/ → ~V.⟨C$_1$⟩C$_2$V~ if C$_1$ = [lab]

      b. → ~V.C$_1$□.C$_2$V~ if C$_1$ = [cor]

      c. /~VC$_1$+V~/ → ~V.C$_1$V~ if C$_1$ = [cor] or [lab]

Tableau (16) shows how the markedness hierarchy *[lab] $\gg_{UG}$ *[cor] can explain

---

[8] Thanks to Junko Itô and Armin Mester (personal communication) for suggesting this piece of the Japanese grammar; they are in no way responsible for my idealization or use of it, of course. With the gerundive suffix /-te/, the *noncoronal* place of stem-final consonants does not surface in /tob/ → *tonde* 'fly', /kaw/ → *katte* 'buy', /tok/ → *toite* 'solve'. The *coronal* place of stem-final /s/ is however preserved by epenthesis of *i*, /hanas/ → *hanasite* 'speak'. (Itô and Mester suggest that the special status of /s/ results from its sibilance, not shared by other coronals, which do not trigger epenthesis: /tor/ → *totte* 'take', /sin/ → *sinde* 'die'; Itô and Mester 1986, 58–9; cf. Iwasaki 2002, 61ff.)

Box 1

why an unsyllabifiable labial consonant will delete, but a coronal will not (its survival requires V-epenthesis, however).

The "deletion process" pertains to the first two inputs in (16), when the initial C is unsyllabifiable (owing to restrictions on coda consonants). Ignoring place markedness, the basic syllable structure constraints are ranked so that such a stranded C is parsed by epenthesizing a following V rather than by deleting the C: FILL^{Nuc} is lower ranked than PARSE. Application of deletion corresponds to outputs with *PARSE marks. The labial consonant undergoes this process—is visible to it—because

(14)   *[lab] ≫ PARSE.

In contrast, the coronal consonant is invisible to this process because

(15)   PARSE ≫ *[cor].

(16)   Coronal invisibility to deletion

Inputs	Outputs	Σ^{CV} NoCoda,Onset, Fill^{Ons}; Fill^{Pl}	C[lab] → Ø *[lab]	C[lab] → Ø Parse	C[cor] → C[cor]◌́ *[cor]	C[cor] → C[cor]◌́ Fill^{Nuc}
C[lab]+C₂V	☞ .C₂V.			*		
	.C[lab]◌́.C₂V.		*!			*
	C[cor]◌́.C₂V.	*Fill^{Pl} !				
C[cor]+C₂V	.C₂V.			*!		
	☞ .C[cor]◌́.C₂V.				*	*
C[lab]+V	☞ .C[lab]V.		*			
	.V.	*Onset !	*			
	C[cor]V.	*Fill^{Ons} *Fill^{Pl}!	*		*	
C[cor]+V	☞ .C[cor]V.				*	
	.V.	*Onset !	*			

The mark assessed by the *[lab] constraint, denoted '*[lab]', is what makes the labial visible; the mark *[cor] is low ranked (i.e., assessed by a low-ranked constraint)—it might as well not be there at all. The PARSE violation incurred by "deleting" segment X can be optimal if the faithful structure (containing X) incurs a mark worse than *PARSE: otherwise, X is "invisible to the deletion process." Since *[lab] ≫$_{UG}$ *[cor], it is possible for *[lab] to be "visible" without *[cor] being visible, but not vice versa.[9]

The crucial contrast between [lab] and [cor] place is the difference between (14)

---

[9] Note that if PARSE and FILL^{Nuc} are interchanged, it is still not the case that [cor] is more visible than [lab] to deletion: both types of consonants delete. It is the relative ranking of *[lab] and *[cor] that is critical to their contrast, not the ranking of PARSE and FILL^{Nuc}. The generalization is that if coronals delete, so must labials.

and (15); this particular contrast is possible because

(17)   *[lab] $\gg_{\text{UG}}$ *[cor].

1.4.3 Cluster conditions and local conjunction

In addition to the relative invisibility of coronals to phonological processes, under-specification of [cor] can account for the relative invisibility of coronals to certain **conditions** (inviolable constraints) of the sort that have often been overlaid on rule-based architectures. The instance Paradis and Prunet refer to in (9) is the following type of cluster condition (see also Prince 1984 concerning such constraints on melodic sequences, independent of syllable structure):

(18)   Coronal invisibility to cluster conditions

"In monomorphemic words, English clusters never include more than one non-coronal...

CLUSTER CONDITION: Adjacent consonants are limited to at most one place specification." (Yip 1991, 63)

To handle multiple segments, the universal place hierarchy must be scaled up to achieve something like Clements's (1990, 313) Sequential Markedness Principle, which asserts essentially that if A is more marked than B, then the sequence XAY is more marked than the sequence XBY. Using the 'less harmonic than' symbol ≺ to de-note "more marked than,"[10] this principle takes the form (19).

(19)   Sequential Markedness Principle

A ≺ B ⇒ XAY ≺ XBY

For example, if the place of A is less harmonic (more marked) than the place of B, then a cluster containing A is less harmonic (more marked) than one con-taining B, all else equal.

To achieve this, it is necessary to combine separate instances of the place hierar-chy for each consonant in the cluster. Consider first clusters with two consonants. The required hierarchy is shown in (20).

(20)   Cluster place markedness hierarchy (for two-segment clusters)

*[lab] $\&_{\text{cl}}$ *[lab] $\gg_{\text{UG}}$ *[lab] $\&_{\text{cl}}$ *[cor] $\gg_{\text{UG}}$ *[cor] $\&_{\text{cl}}$ *[cor]

The constraint *[lab] $\&_{\text{cl}}$ *[lab] is violated if the two consonants in the cluster are both labial. Crucially, it is *not* violated by two separated labial consonants in a word (✓ *puff*), as they are not in a single cluster. That is, the constraint *[lab] $\&_{\text{cl}}$ *[lab] is violated if there are two violations of *[lab] in a common **domain**, defined here as a cluster (**afp*). This is an instance of the general operation of **local conjunction** of con-straints (Chapter 12 (43)), a central topic of this chapter.

---

[10] Harmony crucially combines MARKEDNESS and FAITHFULNESS (Chapter 12 (45k)); but here FAITH-FULNESS does not apply.

Box 1

(21) Local conjunction within a domain $\mathcal{D}$

*A &$_\mathcal{D}$ *B is violated if and only if a violation of *A and a (distinct) violation of *B both occur within a single domain of type $\mathcal{D}$.

If we are conjoining a constraint with itself, so that *A = *B, then the **self-conjunction** *A &$_\mathcal{D}$ *A is violated if (and only if) there are two distinct violations of *A in a single domain $\mathcal{D}$ (formal details in Box 3 below, page 123). This is instantiated in (20) in the constraint *[lab] &$_{cl}$ *[lab]. (*A &$_\mathcal{D}$ *A is often written more simply as *A^2.)

Now we can see the cluster place markedness hierarchy (20) as the result of locally conjoining the single-segment place markedness hierarchy with each of the two constraints in that hierarchy.

(22) Deriving the cluster place markedness hierarchy by local conjunction

a. For single segments:

*[lab] $\gg$ *[cor].

b. Locally conjoin this hierarchy with the constraint *[lab], where the domain of locality is the cluster:

*[lab] &$_{cl}$ *[lab] $\gg$ *[lab] &$_{cl}$ *[cor].

c. Do the same with *[cor]:

*[cor] &$_{cl}$ *[lab] $\gg$ *[cor] &$_{cl}$ *[cor].

d. Since conjunction is symmetric, *[cor] &$_{cl}$ *[lab] = *[lab] &$_{cl}$ *[cor], combining the above two hierarchies gives

*[lab] &$_{cl}$ *[lab] $\gg$ *[lab] &$_{cl}$ *[cor] $\gg$ *[cor] &$_{cl}$ *[cor].

e. All domination relations here are universal.

Clearly, the principle formalizing Clements's Sequential Markedness Principle (19) that has been used in (22b) is (23); this was introduced in Chapter 12 (44).

(23) Preservation of universal markedness hierarchies under local conjunction

*A $\gg_{UG}$ *B $\Rightarrow$ *X &$_\mathcal{D}$ *A $\gg_{UG}$ *X &$_\mathcal{D}$ *B

Now we are prepared to deal with the Cluster Condition (18). Restricting attention for the moment to two-consonant clusters, the effect of this condition is to define a cluster inventory that includes [cor][cor] and [lab][cor], but excludes [lab][lab]. This inventory "bans only the worst of the worst" (Prince and Smolensky 1993/2004, Chap. 9); this important property will be designated **BOWOW** and will be a recurring theme throughout the entire chapter.[11] BOWOW inventories are common, and they are the hallmark of local conjunctive constraint interaction.

The particular case of two-consonant clusters is treated in tableau (24). Here, the PARSE/FILL version of FAITHFULNESS due to Prince and Smolensky 1993/2004, used in Chapter 13, has been upgraded to the Correspondence Theory version due to

---

[11] Padgett (2002a) also addresses what he dubs 'WOW inventories'.

McCarthy and Prince 1995, introduced in Section 12:1.4. (Input and output segments bearing the same superscript are in correspondence.)

In (24), the first input, a labial-coronal cluster, surfaces faithfully (candidate (24a)). The markedness of this cluster, registered by its mark from the constraint *[lab] &$_{cl}$ *[cor], is less than the penalty incurred for any unfaithfulness, whether it be change of place (candidate (24b), violating the constraint IDENT[Pl] requiring corresponding segments to have the same place), or consonant deletion (candidate (24c), violating the constraint MAX requiring all input segments to have output correspondents), or vowel epenthesis (candidate (24d), violating the constraint DEP prohibiting output segments with no input correspondent).

(24)   Cluster Condition

	MAX DEP	*[lab]&$_{cl}$ *[lab]	IDENT[Pl]	*[lab]&$_{cl}$ *[cor]	*[cor]&$_{cl}$ *[cor]
/C$^1_{[lab]}$C$^2_{[cor]}$/ →					
a. ☞ C$^1_{[lab]}$C$^2_{[cor]}$				*	
b. C$^1_{[cor]}$C$^2_{[cor]}$			*!		*
c. C$^2_{[cor]}$	*MAX!				
d. C$^1_{[lab]}$V.C$^2_{[cor]}$	*DEP!				
/C$^1_{[lab]}$C$^2_{[lab]}$/ →					
a'. C$^1_{[lab]}$C$^2_{[lab]}$		*!		*	
b'. ☞ C$^1_{[cor]}$C$^2_{[lab]}$			*	*	

An input containing an even less marked coronal-coronal cluster would also surface faithfully.

But an input with a labial-labial cluster cannot surface faithfully because it is sufficiently highly marked that eliminating this markedness is optimal even though a FAITHFULNESS violation is necessary. The unfaithfulness (or "repair") exhibited in the optimal candidate is of the type that violates the lowest-ranking faithfulness constraint below *[lab] &$_{cl}$ *[lab]; in the ranking shown here, this is IDENT[Pl], so the optimal unfaithful candidate (24b) changes a labial to a coronal. The result is that surface clusters can have no more than one noncoronal place.

The inputs relevant to Yip's Cluster Condition (18) are monomorphemic, so the type of input-output disparity evident in the mapping /C$^1_{[lab]}$C$^2_{[lab]}$/ → C$^1_{[cor]}$C$^2_{[lab]}$ would never be observed as an alternation; there is (presumably) no morphological environment in which the putative underlying C$^1_{[lab]}$ would ever reveal its labiality. According to the OT principle of Richness of the Base, it is exactly a grammar with this property that corresponds to a language obeying the Cluster Condition: *even if there were* underlying forms containing labial-labial sequences, they would surface with only a single labial. There is no input that can produce an output cluster with

Box 1

more than one noncoronal place; hence, the cluster inventory of the language is the one specified by the Cluster Condition.

Only a cluster with two labials is sufficiently "visible" to be targeted by the de-labialization "process" in this grammar. It is as though the place of coronals were absent, for the marks incurred by coronal-containing clusters are too low ranked to matter; they might as well not exist.

Of course, the universality of the cluster place markedness hierarchy (20) ensures that there can be no language in which the roles of coronal and labial place are exchanged. Labial-labial clusters are universally the most marked — the worst of the worst — so if an inventory excludes a single type of cluster on the basis of place, it must be labial-labial clusters. (But see Footnote 13.)

The preceding analysis can be scaled up to clusters with more than two consonants. The lowest-ranked conjunctive constraints will necessarily be those violated by clusters with at most one noncoronal; just as in (24), these are ranked below a relevant faithfulness constraint F while the more highly ranked constraints are ranked above F.

For an application of markedness conjunction to explain consonant cluster inventories revealed in performance data, see Section 17:3.

1.4.4 Neutralization and coda conditions

Paradis and Prunet claim that coronal underspecification explains why coronals meet coda conditions that prohibit codas from having their own place specification (Paradis and Prunet 1991, 9, 13) and why place contrasts are neutralized in coda position, with only coronals surfacing (e.g., Steriade 1982; Itô 1986, 21; Yip 1991, 62).

Effects of the Coda Condition, like those of the Cluster Condition, can be understood in present terms as producing a kind of BOWOW inventory. Here, the "worst of the worst" refers to consonants that not only occupy the "worst" syllable position (coda, marked by NOCODA) but also have the "worst" place, noncoronal (represented here, as before, by labial). These consonants are those that violate the local conjunction NOCODA $\&_{seg}$ *[lab], where the locality domain is the segment, taken as the locus of the violation of NOCODA as well as the locus of the *[lab] violation. (Again, co-locality of violation is crucial: we need to ban forms that have a labial in coda position, not forms that have both a labial onset and a coronal coda.)

Conjoining the basic place markedness hierarchy (11) with NOCODA yields (25) (Smolensky 1993; Zoll 1998; Itô and Mester 2002; Morris 2002).

(25)   Coda place markedness hierarchy

NOCODA $\&_{seg}$ *[lab] $\gg_{UG}$ NOCODA $\&_{seg}$ *[cor]

Now the same sort of argument we have seen in the other cases applies, as tableau (26) illustrates.

The first input in (26) features a word-final labial consonant. The faithful candidate (26a) has a labial coda that violates NOCODA $\&_{seg}$ *[lab], whereas changing the place to coronal (26b) instead violates only lower-ranked NoCoda &$_{seg}$ *[cor], as well as the faithfulness constraint Ident[Pl]. This is optimal, because the ranking has been chosen so that eliminating the coda altogether by deletion (26c) or by V-epenthesis (26d) violates highest-ranked Max or Dep, respectively.

(26)   Coda place neutralization to [cor]

	Max Dep	NoCoda &$_{seg}$ *[lab]	Ident[Pl]	NoCoda &$_{seg}$ *[cor]
/VC$_{[lab]}$/ →				
a. VC$_{[lab]}$		*!		
b. ☞ VC$_{[cor]}$			*	*
c. V	*Max!			
d. V.C$_{[lab]}$V	*Dep!			
/VC$_{[cor]}$/ →				
a'. ☞ VC$_{[cor]}$				*
c'. V	*Max!			

On the other hand, a final consonant with coronal place surfaces faithfully (26a'), violating only low-ranked NoCoda &$_{seg}$ *[cor]. Since [cor] is already the least marked place, the only way to improve upon this violation is to eliminate the coda altogether; but as before, the ranking makes this impossible (e.g., the deletion option, candidate (26c'), fatally violates Max).

With this sort of ranking, the only possible coda consonant is one with unmarked place. Conjoining the place hierarchy with NoCoda allows neutralization to coronal place only in coda position; the unconjoined constraint *[lab] must be lower ranked than the lowest relevant faithfulness constraint, Ident[Pl], because otherwise labials could not surface even in onset position, it being more harmonic to change underlying [lab] to surface [cor]. Thus, the elevation of *[lab] through conjunction with NoCoda allows an inventory permitting codas and labials, but banning the worst of the worst: a segment that is *both* a coda *and* a labial.

1.4.5 Assimilation

Paradis and Prunet assert that underspecification of coronal place explains a generalization that in place assimilation, it is the *marked* place that spreads; /C$_{[lab]}$C$_{[cor]}$/ surfaces as C$_{[lab]}$C$_{[lab]}$ rather than C$_{[cor]}$C$_{[cor]}$ (Kiparsky 1985, 100). This is one pattern that *cannot* be explained from the present OT perspective, since clearly place Harmony is greater with two coronals than with two labials. This is an open problem for the present approach, and to my knowledge it is the only general markedness-related

Box 1

phenomenon that can be accounted for by underspecification but not by the OT analysis presented here.[12]

While it is certainly premature to claim a solution to this problem, there is reason to believe that an OT theory of recoverability may explain this assimilation generalization (Boersma 1998, 181–3). Assimilation prevents an underlying feature specification, such as [cor], from being expressed; it must be recovered in comprehension though absent from the surface expression. If place markedness constraints are active during comprehension, imputing an underlying [cor] feature without surface evidence will be less marked than imputing an underlying [lab] feature without surface evidence. Such a recoverability-based account of the assimilation generalization subsumes it under a higher generalization according to which material absent in surface expressions is preferably unmarked material that can be filled in during comprehension—the same overarching generalization under which the effect of the syntactic constraint DROPTOPIC (Chapter 12 (18e)) is subsumed by a theory of recoverability (see Footnote 12:13).

The remaining phenomenon Paradis and Prunet cite as explicable via underspecification of [cor] involves the transparency of coronals to vowel feature spread. Discussion of this last facet of invisibility is deferred until Section 1.5.3.

1.5 Markedness phenomena in segmental inventories

Section 1.4 considered the six principal challenges Paradis and Prunet placed before any theory of markedness (9). These are six phenomena in which unmarked elements appear invisible to the phonology. But there are other important phenomena that a theory of markedness must explain, and that it must unify with the invisibility phenomena considered above.

We will next briefly consider three such phenomena, all relating to segmental inventories. The first are universal implications concerning these inventories, where presence of a marked element in the inventory (say, a noncoronal) entails the presence of related, less-marked (coronal) elements. This is the topic of Section 1.5.1, which introduces the notion of **harmonic completeness**, the subject of Section 2.

The second markedness phenomenon is the greater diversity of coronals in consonant inventories of the world; more generally, the generalization states that less-marked contexts license a greater variety of contrasts, another facet of which—coda markedness—was discussed in Section 1.4.4 (and, less obviously, Section 1.4.3). This topic is taken up in Section 1.5.2. The results of Sections 1.5.1 and 1.5.2 were derived in Prince and Smolensky 1993/2004, Chap. 9; in the latter case, because it better illustrates the general themes of this chapter, I present an analysis employing local conjunction that is a variant of the original analysis.

---

[12] Extending a proposal made by Kiparsky (1994), de Lacy (2002) develops an approach to constraint construction in which the pressure to faithfully express underlying material is greater for marked elements; this allows straightforward treatment of the assimilation generalization.

The third makredness phenomenon involves the connection between inventories and the Paradis and Prunet invisibility phenomenon postponed from Section 1.4: transparency of unmarked elements to the featural spread characterizing harmony phenomena. This is taken up in Section 1.5.3, which serves as a brief prelude to the much more extensive discussion of vowel harmony in Section 4. The full harmony analysis requires the feature-domain representational device introduced in Section 2.

1.5.1 Implicational universals

The coronal-unmarkedness ranking (11) was in fact proposed in Prince and Smolensky 1993/2004, Secs. 9.1–9.2, as a means of deriving universal inventory implications (Greenberg 1978; see Chapter 12 (45h)). I will just quickly review this as a simple instance of harmonic completeness.

First a qualification. There may be special environments (say, a nasal preceding a labial stop) where there exists a markedness constraint M (Nasal Place Agreement; Box 12:2) that becomes active and favors [lab] over [cor]. Call this a 'nonneutral' environment, the other environments being 'neutral'. In a nonneutral environment, [lab] can be less marked than [cor], thanks to M; in a neutral environment, [cor] is unmarked. The implication we seek is that when an inventory contains a more marked segment, it must contain a less marked one as well, and we are assuming that [cor] is the unmarked place for this purpose—so the relevant type of environment is a neutral one. The goal is to show that, in a neutral environment, if the inventory of a language includes a labial, then that inventory must also include a coronal.[13]

Now recall how an inventory is defined in OT (see Sections 12:1.6–1.7). A structure x is present in the inventory of a language if and only if for some input I, the optimal parse of I contains x. According to Richness of the Base, if a labial segment such as p is *absent* from a language L's inventory, then this means not that p is an impossible *input*, but rather that it is an impossible *output*. No matter what the input, the grammar of L ensures that an optimal output will never contain p. If the input contains p, the grammar assigns an unfaithful parse that lacks p.

On the other hand, when p is *present* in the segmental inventory of L, a p in an input I_p surfaces as a p in the optimal output O_p—in the case of interest, in a neutral environment. When does this happen? Consider any unfaithful competitor X to output O_p where in X the [lab] of p does not surface; this violates some faithfulness constraints $\{F_k\}$. The markedness constraint *[lab] prefers X; so, since O_p is optimal, there

---

[13] The specification of a neutral environment is but one of several technical assumptions needed to rigorously prove '[lab] $\Rightarrow$ [cor]'. That level of rigor is relegated to the Appendix. In a nonneutral environment E, it is [lab] that is unmarked. For example, before a [lab] stop, a [lab] nasal is less marked than a coronal nasal with respect to the Nasal Place Agreement constraint NPA (see Chapter 17); if NPA is sufficiently high ranked, the overall markedness of a [lab] segment in E may be less than that of the corresponding [cor] segment. To derive implicational universals concerning E, [lab] would replace [cor] as the least marked place. The same analysis used in the text could be applied to E, with the role of the general constraints *[lab] $\gg$ *[cor] being played by more specialized constraints— effectively, *[cor in E] $\gg$ *[lab in E].

Box 1

must be an active constraint $\mathbb{C}$, dominating *[lab], which prefers that [lab] surface. In a neutral environment, by definition, no active markedness constraint favors [lab] over [cor], so $\mathbb{C}$ must be one of the faithfulness constraints $\{F_k\}$: for some j, $F_j \gg$ *[lab]. But since necessarily *[lab] $\gg$ *[cor], this means $F_j \gg$ *[cor] (domination is transitive). So if in the input I_p we replace [lab] with [cor], getting an input I_t, the faithful candidate O_t must still be better than an unfaithful candidate in which [cor] does not surface; if eliminating an underlying place feature is too costly to avoid the mark *[lab], it must surely be too costly to avoid the lower-ranked mark *[cor].[14] It follows that an underlying coronal t must surface faithfully, as labial p does. Thus, $\mathcal{L}$'s inventory admits the coronal counterpart of any admitted labial.

In other words, in a neutral environment, if a language has labials, then it must have coronals.

The segmental inventory of a language $\mathcal{L}$ is **harmonically complete** with respect to some structural dimension d (e.g., place) if and only if the following holds: if x is a legal segment in $\mathcal{L}$, and y differs from x only in that it is more harmonic (less marked) with respect to d, then y is also a legal segment in $\mathcal{L}$. (Harmonic completeness is the topic of Section 3.)

The argument above shows that under the treatment of coronal unmarkedness in Prince and Smolensky 1993/2004, segmental inventories must be harmonically complete with respect to place. The argument can clearly be immediately generalized to any other dimension d, with [lab] being replaced by the marked pole of d, and [cor] by the unmarked pole.

Making the above argument rigorously correct actually requires a bit of work, as we will see in Section 3 and the Appendix (see also Box 2). Implicit above are assumptions that, although reasonable, must ultimately be rendered explicit.

1.5.2 Coronal diversity

The greater diversity of segments with coronal place can be understood as an instance of the general tendency for less-marked structures to "license" more contrasts. Consider the contrast [±cont] between obstruents that are continuants (fricatives, more marked) and those that are not (stops, less marked). Will this contrast be preserved at [cor] or [lab] places?

Suppose the relevant markedness constraints include, in addition to those pertaining to individual features, conjunctions of single-feature constraints. Then, analo-

---

[14] The plausible but unstated assumption here is that the operation on [lab] yielding X can be applied to [cor] and that the same (or higher) degree of faithfulness violation results. If this assumption fails, however, a different outcome is possible. For example, if the operation is segmental deletion, violating MAX, and there are constraints MAX$_{Pl}(x)$ requiring that a specific place specification [x] in the input have an identical correspondent in the output (violated by segmental deletion), an inventory could admit [lab] while rejecting [cor]: with MAX$_{Pl}$(lab) $\gg$ *[lab] $\gg$ *[cor] $\gg$ MAX$_{Pl}$(cor) $\gg$ MAX, an underlying coronal gets deleted but an underlying labial does not. This is possible because the faithfulness cost of eliminating [cor] is lower than that of eliminating [lab]. The formal analysis of the Appendix makes explicit assumptions ruling out this sort of situation.

gously to (22), the universal place constraint hierarchy (11) entails (27), by Chapter 12 (44).

(27)   *[lab] & *[+cont] $\gg_{UG}$ *[cor] & *[+cont]

Now consider the ranking in (28).

(28)   *[lab] & *[+cont] $\gg$ IDENT[Pl] $\gg$ {*[cor] & *[+cont], *[lab]} $\gg$ {*[cor], *[+cont]}

This generates an inventory, like that of Tagalog (Schachter 1987, 938), in which coronal place hosts both [+cont] and [–cont] segments (e.g., *t/s*), but there is less diversity at labial place, where only the less-marked noncontinuant segment is allowed (e.g., *p/*f, *ɸ*).

This argument can clearly be generalized from [±cont] to a large number of other contrasts, including the contrast among *secondary* places of articulation distinguishing complex segments, the case treated in the original analysis in Prince and Smolensky 1993/2004, Sec. 9.1.2. The general considerations of this subsection will figure prominently in Section 3.

1.5.3 Transparency and the Harmony/Inventory Theorem

Here, I will depart from the example of context-free coronal unmarkedness and shift to a case of contextual featural markedness, or the markedness of certain feature combinations. The relevant case will be the markedness of [+back] in the context of a vowel also bearing the features [–low, –round] (see, e.g., Archangeli and Pulleyblank 1994 and the references therein). This markedness is captured by the **feature co-occurrence constraint** (29).

(29)   *[+bk, –lo, –rd]

The markedness of [+back] here is relative to [–back]; the relevant universal markedness hierarchy is thus (30).

(30)   Backness markedness hierarchy in context [–low, –round]

$\qquad$ *[**+bk**, –lo, –rd] $\gg_{UG}$ *[**–bk**, –lo, –rd]

This entails two markedness relations on segments, (31a) for [+high] and (31b) for [–high].

(31)   Markedness of [±back] in the context [–low, –round]

$\qquad$ a.   i $\succ$ ï

$\qquad$ b.   e $\succ$ ë

Here [+back, –low, –round, +high], IPA *ɯ*, is represented *ï* (or sometimes *ɨ* as customary for Turkic); [+back, –low, –round, –high], IPA *ɤ* (or *ʌ*), is represented *ë*. According to Section 1.5.1, such markedness relations predict two implicational universals: *ï* $\Rightarrow$ *i* (if a language's inventory contains *ï*, then it will contain *i*) and *ë* $\Rightarrow$ *e*.

Our question is whether the fundamental proposal, 'Lower marks $\Rightarrow$ Less active' (8), can explain the "invisibility" of redundant features in vowel harmony systems,

Box 1

invisibility that is implemented literally in Radical Underspecification Theory. The relevant sense in which such a feature [–φ] is invisible in a segment is that this feature does not trigger the spread of [–φ], or block the spread of [+φ], the way it does in segments in which it is not redundant. To say here that a feature [–φ] is redundant in a segment that also bears other features [... ψ ...] is to say that while [–φ ... ψ ...] is in the language's segmental inventory, [+φ ... ψ ...] is not. A goal of the following analysis is to show how this potential consequence of inventory shape—invisibility to spread—is made possible by the very constraint rankings which are responsible for producing that inventory in the first place.

In the Finnish vowel inventory (*ü/u, ö/o, ä/a, i, e*), the two [–low, –round] front vowels *i* and *e* lack back counterparts: the missing vowels are exactly the two segments *ï* and *ë* identified as marked in (31). Thus, the feature [–back] is redundant in *i* and *e*. Moreover, these vowels are invisible to the backness harmony system of Finnish: the vowels are **transparent** in that [+back] spreads right through them (Kiparsky 1973; see Box 1).

As we saw in Section 1.5.1, the presence in the inventory of *i* and *e*, and the absence of *ï* and *ë*, is a consequence of the rankings in (32), where F_{max} and F_{min} are respectively the highest- and lowest-ranked faithfulness constraints relevant to the markedness constraints *[±**bk**, –lo, –rd].*[15]

(32)   Finnish inventory

    a.   i, e present; ï, ë absent

        *[+**bk**, –lo, –rd] $\gg F_{max}$

        $F_{min} \gg$ *[–**bk**, –lo, –rd]

    b.   ü/u, ö/o present

        $F_{min} \gg$ *[±**bk**, +rd]

For concreteness, let us take F_{min} to be IDENT[back]; this means that the input segments /ï, ë/ will surface as *i, e.*

Since an extended discussion of vowel harmony and feature domains consumes much of the rest of this chapter, for brevity here I will simply present two tableaux illustrating harmony and briefly explain the critical elements.

The input in (33) is a word with final stem vowel *e* and a suffixal vowel that is underlyingly /o/. As shown in the optimal output (33a), these vowels surface as *e ö* (e.g., /heret+koon/ → *heretköön* 'let him/her quit'; /keret+koon/ → *keretköön* 'let him/her make it on time'; Jussi Valtonen, personal communication). The suffixal vowel has harmonized with the final stem vowel: *e* spreads [–back] to *o*, forming *ö.* This shows that even if a suffix vowel is underlyingly specified with the 'wrong' value of [±back], it will surface with the correct, harmonized value. The representation in candidate (33a) consists of a [–back] **feature domain**, including both vowels;

---

[15] A faithfulness constraint F is **relevant** to a markedness constraint M if and only if a violation of M can be avoided by incurring a violation of F.

---

this means both vowels express this feature value. Clearly, faithfulness to backness, IDENT[back] (IDENTᴮ ≡ IDᴮ), is violated at the output *ö*; this is indicated by a violation mark '*ö'. In addition, the surface vowels *e* and *ö* violate the feature co-occurrence constraints *[−bk, −lo, −rd] ≡ *−B,−L,−R and *[−bk, +rd] ≡ *−B,+R, respectively.

(33)   Harmonic feature domains under Richness of the Base

...e...+...o...	Inventory gap		Transparency					No gap	
−B +B	*+B,−L,−R	IDᴮ_stem	*−B,−L,−R	AL⁺ᴮ	*EMBᴮ	AL⁻ᴮ	IDᴮ	*−B,+R	*+B,+R
a. ☞ [−B e ö]			*e				*ö	*ö	
b. [−B e][+B o]			*e			*o!			*o
c. [+B ë o]	*ë!	*ë					*ë		*o
d. [−B e [+B o]]			*e		*o!				*o

   The unfaithful mapping of underlying /o/ to surface *ö*, violating IDENTᴮ and increasing the back-markedness to *[−bk, +rd] from lower-ranked *[+bk, +rd], is compelled by the harmony-inducing constraint ALIGN-R($\mathcal{D}_{-B}$, Wd) ≡ ALIGN⁻ᴮ ≡AL⁻ᴮ: this requires that the right edge of each [−back] domain $\mathcal{D}_{-B}$ coincide with the right edge of the word. This constraint is violated by the faithful candidate (33b), as shown by the ALIGN⁻ᴮ mark '*o' (labeled by the alignment-violating vowel separating the right edge of $\mathcal{D}_{-B}$ from the right word-edge: *o*). This violation renders (33b) suboptimal because of the ranking (34).

(34)   [−back] Harmony: ALIGN⁻ᴮ ≫ *[−bk, +rd]

Since Finnish also has [+back] harmony, the corresponding ranking also holds for ALIGN⁺ᴮ.

   Candidate (33c) satisfies the harmony constraint ALIGN⁺ᴮ (and ALIGN⁻ᴮ, vacuously); it represents regressive harmony from the suffix to the stem. This is suboptimal because its unfaithfulness, at the stem vowel, is more marked than the optimal candidate's unfaithfulness at the affix vowel. Employing a standard OT method of expressing this, positional faithfulness (Chapter 12 (45k); Beckman 1997; Smith 2002; cf. Bakovic 2000), a constraint IDENTᴮ_stem specialized to stems is violated by stem unfaithfulness, but not by affixal unfaithfulness; its high rank ensures that stem-controlled harmony, as in (33a), is always more harmonic than affix-controlled harmony, as in (33c). Consideration of the final candidate (33d) will be momentarily deferred.

   Underspecification theories often take harmonizing vowels, like the affixal one here, to be unspecified underlyingly for the harmonizing feature (e.g., Clements 1976; Pulleyblank 1983). In OT, Richness of the Base requires that the grammar accept *any* input and produce a grammatical output, so whether or not underspecified inputs are included in an OT account, we cannot *count on* harmonizing segments to be unspecified. The input we have just considered is a worst case since the affixal vowel is underlying given the 'wrong' specification for this stem, and it must change from the less- to the more-marked vowel, from *o* to *ö*.

Box 1

The input of tableau (35) is relevant to the transparency of less-marked vowels. This input contains a stem vowel *o* followed by two vowels taken to be underlyingly *ë ü*. In the optimal output, candidate (33a), these three vowels surface as *o e u*: the [+back] of stem *o* has 'spread through' stem *e* to change the underlying suffixal *ü* to *u*. (The surface form is exemplified by *totellut*, 'the one having obeyed'; Olli 1958, 181.) The intermediate vowel surfaces as *e*, even though it is underlyingly *ë* and *ë* has the value [+back] in harmony with the surrounding vowels. We must relate this to the fact that *ë* is not in the Finnish vowel inventory. (Again, Richness of the Base forces the grammar to produce the correct output even for the worst-case input considered here, where the vowel that must surface as *e* is underlyingly 'mis'-specified as [+back].)

(35) Transparency of redundant features

...o...ë...+... ü ... +B +B −B	Inventory gap			Transparency			No gap		
	*+B, −L,−R	ID^B_{stem}	***−B, −L,−R**	AL^{+B}	$*Emb^B$	$AL^{−B}$	ID^B	***−B, +R**	***+B, +R**
a. ☞ [₊B o [−B e] u]		*e	*e		*e	*u	*e *u		*o *u
b. [₊B o ë u]	*ë!						*u		*o *u
c. [₊B o ë][−B ü]	*ë!				*ü		*ü		*o
d. [₊B o [−B e ü]]		*e	*e		*e *ü!		*e	*ü	*o
e. [₊B o][−B e ü]		*e	*e	*e *ü!			*e	*ü	*o
f. [−B ö e ü]		*ö! *e	*e				*e	*ö *ü	
g. [₊B o [−B e [₊B u]]]		*e	*e			*e *u! [*u]	*e *u		*o *u

Before tackling this imposing tableau, let's consider an underspecification account, where the vowel *e* would be unspecified underlyingly for [back], and the [+back] feature of the stem vowel would spread to the right edge of the word, producing the desired final *u* as well as a medial *ë*. At this intermediate stage of derivation, the entire word shares [+back]. Then a rule inserts the value [−back] for the [−low, −round] medial segment, changing it from *ë* to *e*, and breaking up the span of [+back] so that now the [+back] value on the final *u* is no longer connected to its source in the stem by a contiguous span of [+back] vowels (Vago 1973; Clements 1977). Alternatively, *i* and *e* are assumed not to be [±back]-bearing units; feature spread ignores them, as it does consonants (Clements 1976; Kiparsky 1981). Again the result is that a [+back] domain extends throughout the whole word.

The representation in candidate (35a) has an outer [+back] domain including all vowels; it corresponds to the intermediate derivational stage in the underspecification account. Candidate (35a) also has a [−back] domain (bold) *embedded within* the larger [+back] domain. It is the innermost feature value that determines a segment's phonetic interpretation, so the medial vowel surfaces [−back], as *e* not *ë*.

Suffixal /ü/ surfaces unfaithfully here for the same reasons that suffixal /o/ surfaced unfaithfully in (33). What is new in the optimal candidate (35a) is the embedded feature domain, which violates a constraint *EMBED^B ≡ *EMB^B. This violation is avoided in the nonembedded candidate (35b), which is suboptimal because without the embedded domain, the medial vowel surfaces as *ë*, violating undominated *[+bk, −lo, −rd]. For the same reason, the faithful candidate (35c) is suboptimal.

There are several ways the medial vowel can surface as *e*, which requires that the deepest domain containing this vowel be [−back]. This [−back] domain could extend to the right edge of the word, as in candidates (35d) and (35e). This has the virtue of satisfying ALIGN^{-B}, but as this is ranked below *EMBED^B, candidate (35d) is suboptimal. It is assumed here that *EMBED is violated once for each segment in an embedded domain; this constraint provides a pressure to minimize the extent of embedded domains, which favors the optimal candidate (35a) over (35d). Candidate (35e) satisfies ALIGN^{-B}, and avoids *EMBED^B violations altogether, but it violates the higher-ranked ALIGN^{+B}.

In candidate (35f), the [−back] domain including medial *e*, extends to cover the entire word, avoiding violations of *EMBED^B and ALIGN^{+B} (vacuously). But it is suboptimal since it is unfaithful to a stem vowel, fatal in this stem-controlled harmony ranking.

The final candidate, (35g), has the same phonetic interpretation as the optimal candidate (35a). But there is no motivation for the most embedded [+back] domain; this candidate can never be more harmonic than (35a) because (35a)'s marks are a proper subset of (35g)'s marks: no matter the ranking, (35a) must be more harmonic than (35g). Candidate (35a) harmonically bounds candidate (35g) (see Section 12:1.6). Segments transparent to vowel harmony must surface in the simplest form exhibiting transparency, the single embedding of candidate (35e).

That *e* is transparent, rather than opaque, to backness harmony is determined by the ranking ALIGN^{+B} ≫ *EMBED^B ≫ ALIGN^{-B}. Under other rankings of these constraints, *e* will continue to not participate in backness harmony, but vowels following *e* will share its [−back] domain. For example, if *EMBED^B dominates the alignment constraints, embedding will not be optimal, so there is no way for [±back] values of vowels preceding *e* to influence vowels following it. [+back] domains will extend rightward until they reach an *e*, at which point a [−back] domain will begin and continue rightward. It is thus not the transparency of *e*, but more generally its nonparticipation in harmony that will prove crucial; this is what is linked to feature redundancy.

The task at hand is to relate the transparency of [−back] in the segment *e* to its redundancy, that is, to the shape of the segmental inventory, which is what makes this feature redundant in this segment. The ranking shown in tableau (33) determines that [±back] is redundant in *e*, but not in *o*, as follows. The most directly relevant environment is the stem-internal one, where harmony does not complicate the mapping of [back]. In stems, the key constraint is IDENT$^B_{stem}$. Since it dominates both *[−bk, +rd] and *[+bk, +rd], both underlying vowels /o, ö/ will surface faithfully. [back] is

Box 1

contrastive, not redundant, in the context [+round]. But IDENT^B$_{stem}$ is ranked *between* the constraints of the backness markedness hierarchy in [−low, −round] segments. Thus, only the unmarked value of [back] can surface in these segments: *e*, but not *ë*, is in the inventory — [back] is redundant in *e*.

The general argument exemplified in tableaux (33)–(35) culminates in the Harmony/Inventory Theorem (36). The analysis considers some vowel feature denoted φ, with marked pole [+φ].

(36)   **Harmony/Inventory Theorem**

Suppose a language has an A$^{+φ}$-process in an environment *E* and that some [−φ] segment *s*$_−$ fails to undergo it. Then, in *E*, *s*$_+$ is not in the underlying inventory.

Here, *s*$_+$ is the segment identical to *s*$_−$ except with value [+φ]. To say that in *E*, *s* is in the **underlying inventory** is to say that in *E*, underlying *s* surfaces as *s*.

Informally, the theorem's proof amounts to this. The nonharmonization of *s*$_−$ can only be due to either highly ranked φ faithfulness or highly ranked markedness of the harmony result, *s*$_+$. The former is not possible because it would prevent harmony for *any* segment. The latter means that the markedness of *s*$_+$ must exceed that of disharmony, which in turn must exceed that of unfaithfulness if there is to be any harmony at all; thus, the markedness of *s*$_+$ must exceed that of unfaithfulness, which eliminates *s*$_+$ from the underlying inventory.

Suppose some segment *s*$_−$ is invisible to [+φ] harmony in the way that transparent vowels are. Among other things, this entails that *s*$_−$ fails to undergo harmony. According to the Harmony/Inventory Theorem, this can only happen if *s*$_+$ is outside the underlying inventory. This is possible only if *s*$_+$ is the marked, and *s*$_−$ the unmarked, member of the opposition (by Section 1.5.1). Thus, the invisibility of the [−φ] value is directly tied to its unmarkedness.

The rest of this subsection provides the formal statement and proof of the Harmony/Inventory Theorem (36). The reader uninterested in such formalities can continue directly to Section 1.5.4.

The definitions assumed for this theorem are given in (37).

(37)   *Definitions*

a.   A segment *x* is in the **underlying *E*-inventory** if in environment *E*, /x/ → *x*.

b.   Let A be a markedness constraint. A segment *x* **undergoes an A-process** if, when A is applicable in environment *E*,

i.   x violates A,

ii.   /x/ → *y*, where *y* violates A to a lesser degree than does *x*, and

iii.   *y* has lower Harmony than *x* with respect to the hierarchy of markedness constraints other than A.

c.   A language **has an A-process** if some segment undergoes it.

d.   Let φ be a vowel feature. A **[+φ] vowel harmony constraint**, when it applies, requires all vowels in some domain 𝒟 to bear the feature [+φ]. In the

standard case, such a constraint will apply when [+φ] is borne by some
controlling vowel, typically at one edge of $\mathcal{D}$. Let such a constraint be de-
noted $A^{+\varphi}$, and such a domain be denoted $\mathcal{D}^{+\varphi}$. $A^{-\varphi}$ and $\mathcal{D}^{-\varphi}$ are defined
analogously.

e. A language **has [+φ] vowel harmony** if it has an $A^{+\varphi}$-process.

f. A **minimal φ-pair** are two segments x_- and x_+ that are featurally identical
except that x_- is [−φ] and x_+ is [+φ]. The notation x_-/x_+ will always denote
a minimal φ-pair.

These are straightforward except perhaps for (37b.iii). The point is simply that if /x/
→ y and y has lower Harmony than x even without considering the constraint A, then
there is no reason to believe it is A that is responsible for this mapping of /x/ to y;
just as possibly, it is merely a coincidence that A also favors y over x, while it is in fact
some other, higher-ranked constraint that renders this unfaithful mapping optimal.

The proof of the Harmony/Inventory Theorem (36) will be given in (42) below;
first, two simple lemmas are established, (38) and (41). Assume throughout that in
the relevant environment, harmony is the only relevant process: other constraints are
ranked so that for /y_-/, all outputs other than y_- and y_+ must be suboptimal (e.g., deletion of /y_-/, or changing a feature other than φ, cannot be optimal).

The first lemma simply asserts the intuitively obvious fact that there can be no
harmony unless the harmony-driving constraint dominates the faithfulness constraint that must be violated when a segment undergoes harmony.

(38) Harmony Lemma

If a language has [+φ] harmony in an environment E, then in that environment,

$$A^{+\varphi} \gg F^{+\varphi},$$

where $A^{+\varphi}$ is the harmony constraint and $F^{+\varphi}$ is the highest-ranked faithfulness
constraint violated in E when an underlying [−φ] segment x_- surfaces as a corresponding [+φ] output segment x_+.

Proof. (Abbreviate $A^{+\varphi}$ simply by A. Also, everything in this proof is implicitly relativized to E.) Since the language has an A-process, there is some domain $\mathcal{D}^{+\varphi}$ in which A
applies and some segment y_- that undergoes it; that is, /y_-/ → y_+, where y_- violates A
and y_+ satisfies it, and where in E, y_+ has lower Harmony than y_- ($y_+ \prec y_-$) with respect
to the markedness constraints excluding A. This optimal mapping violates the markedness constraints violated by y_1 in environment E, $M(y_+)$, as well as faithfulness constraints, the highest of which can be called F. The suboptimal identity mapping
/y_-/ → y_- violates the harmony constraint A and the other markedness constraints
violated in E by y_-, $M(y_-)$. Then harmony — the mapping /y_-/ → y_+ — can be optimal
only if the marks it incurs have higher Harmony than the marks incurred by the faithful mapping /y_-/ → y_-:

(39) $\{M(y_-), *A\} \prec \{M(y_+), *F\}$.

That is, each mark in the right-hand set must be dominated by a mark in the left-hand
set — the Cancellation/Domination Lemma (Chapter 12 (21)). Since y_+ is more marked
(excluding A) than y_-, the marks in $M(y_+)$ cannot be dominated by those in $M(y_-)$, so

---

Box 1

they must be dominated by *A: *A $\prec$ M(y_+). *F must be dominated by *A, or by a mark in M(y_-). In the latter case, *F is dominated also by *A, since M(y_-) is dominated by M(y_+) which we have just seen is dominated by *A. The conclusion then is that *A $\prec$ *F—that is,

(40)   A $\gg$ F.

(41)   Uphill Harmony Lemma

Suppose a language has [+φ] harmony in an environment *E*. Let $x_\pm$ be a minimal pair such that x_+ has higher Harmony (is less marked) than x_- with respect to a language's ranked markedness constraints, excluding $A^{+\varphi}$. Then x_- undergoes harmony (i.e., in a domain $\mathcal{D}^{+\varphi}$, /x_-/ $\to x_+$).

Proof. The notation used here will be the same as in the proof of (38); everything pertains to environment *E*. The harmonizing mapping $x_- \to x_+$ will be optimal if and only if each of its marks {M(x_+), *F} is canceled or dominated by a mark of the faithful mapping $x_- \to x_-$, {M(x_-), *A}. Since the language in question has [+φ] harmony, by the Harmony Lemma (38), A $\gg$ F, so the mark *F is dominated by *A. Since x_+ is less marked than x_-, the marks M(x_+) not canceled by marks in M(x_-) are each dominated by the highest uncanceled mark in M(x_-).

(42)   Proof of the Harmony/Inventory Theorem (36)

(Everything is relativized to the environment *E*.) The segment s_- of the theorem fails to undergo harmony in the relevant environment, so by the Uphill Harmony Lemma (41) s_+ must be more marked than s_- relative to the markedness constraints excluding $A^{+\varphi}$:

(43)   M(s_+) $\prec$ M(s_-).

In a harmonic domain $\mathcal{D}^{+\varphi}$, consider the mapping $s_- \to s_+$ comprising [+φ] harmony; it incurs marks {M(s_+), *F}. The faithful alternative $s_- \to s_-$ incurs {M(s_-), *A}. By the hypothesis of the theorem, s_- does not undergo harmony, so we must have

(44)   {M(s_+), *F} $\prec$ {M(s_-), *A}.

Each mark on the right side of (44) must be dominated by a mark on the left side. The marks M(s_-) are dominated by M(s_+), according to (43). The mark *A must be dominated by either *F or M(s_+). Now since the language has [+φ] harmony, by the Harmony Lemma (38), A $\gg$ F, or

(45)   *A $\prec$ *F,

so *A cannot be dominated by *F; it must be dominated by a mark in M(s_+):

(46)   M(s_+) $\prec$ *A.

By transitivity of Harmony, (45) and (46) imply

(47)   M(s_+) $\prec$ *F.

Now consider a segment *not* in a harmonic domain $\mathcal{D}^{+\varphi}$. An underlying /s_+/ may surface faithfully, incurring M(s_+), or unfaithfully as s_-, incurring *F and M(s_-). By (47) and (43), the unfaithful mapping is optimal. Thus, s_+ is not in the underlying inventory.

A summary of the possible harmonic behaviors is given in the theorem (48).

(48)   *Theorem.* Typology of Harmonic Behavior

Consider a language with [+φ] harmony. Then the following are the only possibilities for the harmonic behavior of x_-.

a. If undergoing harmony would decrease markedness, x_- must undergo harmony ($x_- \prec x_+ \Rightarrow x_- \rightarrow x_+$ in $\mathcal{D}^{+\varphi}$).

b. If undergoing harmony would increase markedness ($x_- \succ x_+$), then

i. x_- may undergo harmony ($x_- \rightarrow x_+$ in $\mathcal{D}^{+\varphi}$), with either

✦ x_+ in the underlying inventory (outside $\mathcal{D}^{+\varphi}$, $x_+ \rightarrow x_+$), or

✦ x_+ not in the underlying inventory: possible only under compulsion by harmony (outside $\mathcal{D}^{+\varphi}$, $x_+ \rightarrow x_-$),

ii. x_- may fail to undergo harmony ($x_- \rightarrow x_-$ in $\mathcal{D}^{+\varphi}$), in which case x_+ is not in the underlying inventory (outside $\mathcal{D}^{+\varphi}$, $x_+ \rightarrow x_-$).

Proof. The theorem follows from the following table.

	$x_+ \prec x_-$ ($\exists$ *x_+)	$x_- \prec x_+$ ($\exists$ *x_-)
Inside harmonic domain $\mathcal{D}^{+\varphi}$ (where $x_- \Rightarrow$ *A)		
x_- accepts [+φ]:	*A $\prec$ {*F, *x_+} $\Leftrightarrow$	{*A, *x_-} $\prec$ *F $\Leftrightarrow$
$x_- \rightarrow x_- \prec x_- \rightarrow x_+$ {*A (*x_-)} $\prec$ {*F (*x_+)}	[A ≫ ~~F and~~ A ≫ *x_+] ①	[*x_- ≫ F or A ≫ F] ✓②
x_- rejects [+φ]:	{*F, *x_+} $\prec$ *A $\Leftrightarrow$	*F $\prec$ {*A, *x_-} $\Leftrightarrow$
$x_- \rightarrow x_+ \prec x_- \rightarrow x_-$ {*F (*x_+)} $\prec$ {*A (*x_-)}	[~~F ≫ A or~~ *x_+ ≫ A] ④	[F ≫ A and F ≫ *x_-] ✗③
Outside harmonic domain $\mathcal{D}^{+\varphi}$ (A does not apply; is vacuously satisfied)		
x_+ in underlying inventory:	*F $\prec$ *x_+ $\Leftrightarrow$	{*F *x_-} $\prec$ { } $\Leftrightarrow$
$x_+ \rightarrow x_- \prec x_+ \rightarrow x_+$ {*F (*x_-)} $\prec$ { (*x_+)}	F ≫ *x_+ ⑦	✓ (always true) ⑤
x_+ not in underlying inventory:	*x_+ $\prec$ *F $\Leftrightarrow$	{ } $\prec$ {*F *x_-} $\Leftrightarrow$
$x_+ \rightarrow x_+ \prec x_+ \rightarrow x_-$ { (*x_+)} $\prec$ {*F (*x_-)}	*x_+ ≫ F ⑧	✗ (always false) ⑥

If $x_+ \prec x_-$, then let *x_+ be the highest-ranked constraint preferring x_- to x_+; if $x_- \prec x_+$, then let *x_- be the highest-ranked constraint preferring x_+. The table shows (in boldface) the necessary and sufficient rankings for achieving the behavior of x_- and x_+ shown in each row, given the two relative markedness situations in the two columns. The only consistent combinations are those listed in the theorem.

In the leftmost column, sets of marks for competing mappings are shown, including '(*x_+)', which means 'the mark *x_+ assessed by *x_+, if it exists'; this constraint *x_+ exists in the middle column (x_+ more marked) but not in the rightmost column (x_- more marked). The reverse is true for '(*x_-)'. Ignore the ~~strike-through~~ and other marking for the moment.

Since harmony exists, there must be some y that accepts [+φ] inside $\mathcal{D}^{+\varphi}$; so by

---

Box 1

cell ① it must be that A ≫ F. This is the Harmony Lemma (38). Then in ① the first conjunct holds, so it can be ignored; it is struck through. Also, A ≫ F entails that the condition in cell ② must hold; it is annotated '✓'. Likewise, the condition in cell ③ must always be false; it is marked '✗'. The truth of ② and falsity of ③ result from the Uphill Harmony Lemma (41). In cell ④, the first disjunct 'F ≫ A' is false: it is struck through and can be ignored.

Cells ⑤ and ⑥ assert that x_+ must be in the underlying inventory when it is less marked than x_-. That is because here the only process/unfaithfulness under consideration is changing the feature [±φ]: that is what is at issue in harmony. In the larger scheme of things, it could be that both x_+ and x_- are sufficiently marked that it is optimal to simply delete them. But then both these segments $x_±$ are not in the inventory and hence not relevant to the relation of harmony to inventory.

The interesting column of the typology is the one for x_+ more marked than x_-. The cells in this column, ① ④ ⑦ ⑧, are plotted differently in the following table. All four combinations of accept/reject [+φ] harmony and in/not in the underlying inventory are possible, except one: rejecting harmony ④ and being in the inventory ⑦. This requires F ≫ $*x_+$ ⑦ and $*x_+$ ≫ A ④, so by transitivity of domination, F ≫ A; but this contradicts the ranking A ≫ F already established from ①. The impossibility of this typological cell is the Harmony/Inventory Theorem (36).

			x_-'s behavior with respect to [+φ] harmony	
			accepts	rejects
			① A ≫ $*x_+$	④ $*x_+$ ≫ A
x_+ in the under-	yes	⑦ F ≫ $*x_+$	✓	✗ [F ≫ $*x_+$ ≫ A]
lying inventory?	no	⑧ $*x_+$ ≫ F	✓	✓

1.5.4 Effects of target markedness in vowel harmony

In Finnish, the feature co-occurrence condition *[+bk, –lo, –rd] eliminated *i* = *i* from the vowel inventory. The more subtle status of feature co-occurrence conditions in OT — violable rather than inviolable constraints — predicts that such conditions should produce more subtle markedness effects in languages where they are not unviolated. In such a language, *i* would be present in the inventory, but its markedness relative to *i*, due to *[+bk, –lo, –rd], should limit its distribution.

Such a language is Turkish. Like Finnish, Turkish displays [back] harmony, but unlike Finnish, the Turkish inventory includes *i*. The *e/ä* distinction of Finnish is absent in Turkish, where *e* plays the role of *ä* as the [–back] harmonic alternate of *a*.

Within Turkish roots, exceptions to vowel harmony are common. However, within morphemes, (49) holds.

(49)   "The vowels /ü, ö, i/ do not occur disharmonically in VC₀V sequences, except that /i, ü/ may occur in either order." (Clements and Sezer 1982, 228)

Here, we consider only one facet of this behavior: within a root, a disharmonic sequence *ati* may occur, but disharmonic *eti* may not. This will be explained as resulting from the markedness of *ɨ* relative to *i*, with the disharmonic environment admitting only the less-marked segment. Despite its markedness, however, *ɨ* surfaces in roots and affixes under [+back] harmony, and as a sole root vowel.

(50)   Markedness and Turkish root disharmony
        Ranked below the constraints shown: IDᴮ, *[−B,−L,−R], *[−B,+L], *[+B,+L]

	*EMBᴮ	IDᴮ°	*B°_aff	*+B,−L,−R	IDᴮ_stem	ALᴮ
/a ɨ + a/ →						
a. $[_{+B}\,a°][_{−B}\,ɨ°] + [_{+B}\,a°]$			*a°!			
b. $[_{+B}\,a°\,[_{−B}\,ɨ° + e]]$	*ɨ *e!					
c. ☞ $[_{+B}\,a°][_{−B}\,ɨ° + e]$						*ɨ *e
d. $[_{+B}\,a°\,ɨ + a]$				*ɨ!	*ɨ	
e. $[_{−B}\,e\,ɨ° + e]$					*e!	
/e ɨ + e/ →						
c'. $[_{−B}\,e°][_{+B}\,ɨ° + a]$				*ɨ!		*ɨ *a
d'. ☞ $[_{−B}\,e°\,i + e]$					*i	
e'. $[_{+B}\,a\,ɨ° + a]$				*ɨ!	*a	
/a ɨ + e/ →						
a''. $[_{+B}\,a°][_{−B}\,ɨ + e°]$			*e°!		*ɨ	*ɨ *a
c''. ☞ $[_{+B}\,a°\,ɨ + a]$				*ɨ		
d''. $[_{−B}\,e\,ɨ° + e]$		*ɨ!			*e *ɨ	
e''. $[_{+B}\,a°][_{−B}\,ɨ° + e]$		*ɨ!			*a	*ɨ *a

The tableaux in (50) exhibit the *i/ɨ* contrast. The new element introduced here is the feature domain **head**, a major topic of Section 2. Each φ domain has exactly one head, marked φ°. The constraint IDENT°[φ] ≡ IDᵠ° requires that the head of a φ domain be faithful in φ. The constraint *φ°_aff prohibits a φ head from appearing in an affix; this is key to the stem-controlled nature of Turkish [back] harmony in this analysis. (These two constraints are actually derived by local conjunction from a fundamental constraint of headed-domain theory: *HD[φ], the member of the *STRUCTURE family penalizing the additional structure identifying the head of a φ domain. IDENT°[φ] is IDENT[φ] &_seg *HD[φ]; *φ°_aff is *AFFIX &_seg *HD[φ], where *AFFIX is the constraint assessing the segments of affixes as marked relative to those in stems.)

The first input of tableau (50) is a word containing the vowel sequence *a ɨ* in the root, with a suffix containing the vowel *a*, as in /tarih+sal/ → *tarihsel* 'historic'.[16] The faithful candidate (50a) violates undominated *B°_aff, because the suffixal vowel heads

---

[16] Turkish examples are from Lewis 1967, 65, 65, 83, 63, and 60, respectively.

Box 1

its own domain. Because this constraint outranks IDENT^B and all feature co-occurrence constraints, it is more harmonic to include suffixal vowels in root-headed [back] domains, even if this requires being unfaithful to underlying affixal [back] values. Thus, suffixal vowels are not heads in all remaining candidates. Candidates (50b–c) include the affix vowel in a [back] domain headed by the root-final vowel; this is embedded within, or follows, a domain headed by the root-initial vowel. Because *EMBED^B outranks *ALIGN^B, all embedded-domain candidates are less harmonic than their nonembedded counterparts; thus, candidate (50b) is less harmonic than candidate (50c). Candidate (50c) is in fact optimal. Its highest-ranked mark is *ALIGN^B. This is eliminated in candidates (50d–e), but these are suboptimal because each violates higher-ranked IDENT$^B_{stem}$. The optimal output *a i + e* displays harmony of the affixal vowel to the stem-final vowel, but disharmony within the root.

The second input reverses the roles of [±back] (e.g., /cebir+sal/ → *cebirsel* 'algebraic'). Candidate (50c′) is the counterpart of optimal (50c), but now its faithful stem-final vowel violates the high-ranking feature co-occurrence constraint marking *ɨ*, *[+bk, –lo, –rd]. Because this outranks IDENT$^B_{stem}$, it is more harmonic to include /ɨ/ in the [–back] domain headed by the initial vowel: candidate (50d′), the counterpart of (50d). Clearly, this is more harmonic than a single domain headed by *ɨ*, candidate (50e′). The resulting output *e i + e* is fully harmonic.

The point is that the markedness of *ɨ* relative to *i* makes possible a ranking in which faithfulness to stem [±back] values generates disharmonic stems, except when there is a chance to eliminate /ɨ/ by inclusion in a [–back] domain headed by a stem vowel.

As the third input in tableau (50) shows, it is suboptimal to eliminate /ɨ/ by including it in an affix-headed [–back] domain, or in a [–back] domain that it heads as a surface *i*, unfaithfully to its underlying [+back] value (incurring *IDENT$^{B°}$). Underlying /a ɨ + e/ surfaces as *a ɨ + a*, fully harmonic despite the resulting surface *ɨ* (as in /altɨ + şer/ → *altɨşar* 'six each').

The first input in tableau (51) makes a similar point, showing that a single root /ɨ/ surfaces as *ɨ* and initiates a [+back] harmony domain (/yɨl + lik/ → *yɨllɨk* 'yearling'). The second input in this tableau shows that a disharmonic *ɨ* in a root is impossible not only when it follows *e* (50), but also when it precedes *e* (this input surfaces like *liseli* ← /lise + lɨ/ 'lycée student', given a hypothetical disharmonic stem /lɨse/).

Notice that ALIGN^B does no work here; disharmonic affix vowels are suboptimal because they require a head in an affix, which is more marked than unfaithfulness in affixes. In many harmony situations, domain heads eliminate the need for alignment constraints. The simplest φ-harmony-inducing constraint is *HD[φ]: 'No heads φ°'. Minimizing φ head structure requires having a single φ domain (in the relevant context where MAX prevents total segment deletion).

(51)   Markedness and Turkish root disharmony, continued

	*EMB^B	ID^B°	*B°_aff	*+B,−L,−R	ID^B_stem	AL^B
/ɨ + i/ →						
a. ☞ [+B ɨ° + i]				*ɨ *ɨ		
b. [+B ɨ°] + [−B ɨ°]			*ɨ°!	*ɨ		
c. [−B ɨ° + i]		*ɨ°!			*ɨ	
d. [−B ɨ + ɨ°]			*ɨ°!		*ɨ	
/ɨ e + ɨ/ →						
q. [+B ɨ° [−B e° + i]]	*e*i!			*ɨ		
r. [+B ɨ°][−B e° + i]				*ɨ!		*ɨ *e
s. [+B ɨ° [−B e°] + i]	*e!			*ɨ *ɨ		*a
t. [+B ɨ° [−B e° + [+B ɨ°]]]	*e *a *a!		*ɨ	*ɨ *ɨ		
u. [+B ɨ° a + ɨ]				*ɨ *ɨ!	*a	
v. ☞ [−B i e° + i]					*ɨ	

1.6 Summary

The point I have tried to make in Section 1 is simply this. A wide range of phenomena that have been attributed to underspecification can be accounted for in a simple, uniform way, using only the central grammatical apparatus of OT, without stipulating a separate representational device for unmarkedness: invisibility. "Invisibility" is a *derived* property. (53) summarizes the examples discussed in this section. Note that all these explanations are merely various consequences of the elementary defining property of coronal unmarkedness, (52).

(52)   *[lab] $\gg_{\text{UG}}$ *[cor]

Rather than structural absence, what may ultimately explain the invisibility of the unmarked is quite simply the invisibility to the optimizing grammar of nonexistent or low-ranked marks—inactive constraint violations. This property of the unmarked is integral to the grammatical architecture of OT; there is no need—and indeed no opportunity—to manipulate the visibility of phonological material with special representational stipulations controlling the inputs to the grammar. The OT perspective connects the invisibility properties of unmarked elements with their role in inventories, including the implications of inventory shape for vowel harmony systems. Also inherent in this unified theory of markedness is an explanation of an important property quite at odds with structural absence: the strong licensing capabilities of the unmarked, as manifest for example in the relative diversity of coronals in segmental inventories.

Box 1

(53) Process marks ≫ Element marks ⇒ Element is invisible to process

Sec.	*Visible element* Constraint	≫	*Condition/Process* Constraint	≫	*Invisible element* Constraint
1.4	*Epenthetic labial* *[lab]	≫	**Epenthesis**	≫	*Epenthetic coronal* *[cor]
1.4.2	*Labial segment* *[lab]	≫	**Deletion** PARSE	≫	*Coronal segment* *[cor]
1.4.3	*Lab-lab cluster* *[lab] &$_{cl}$ *[lab]	≫	**Cluster Condition** IDENT[Pl]	≫	*Lab-cor, cor-cor clusters* *[lab] &$_{cl}$ *[cor] ≫ *[cor] &$_{cl}$ *[cor]
1.4.4	*Labial coda* *[lab] & NOCODA	≫	**Coda neutralization** IDENT[Pl]	≫	*Coronal coda* *[cor] & NOCODA
1.4.5	*[Lab]??*		**Assimilation??**		*[Cor]??*
1.5.3	*Banned +B* *[+B,−L,−R] ≈ *ë	≫	**Nonharmonizing −B** *ID^{B}$_{stem}$	≫	*Redundant −B* *[−B,−L,−R] ≈ *e
1.5.4	*Highly marked +B* *[+B,−L,−R] ≈ *i	≫	**Delete disharmonic +B** *ID^{B}$_{stem}$	≫	*Unmarked +B* *[+B,+L] ≈ *a

2 FEATURE DOMAINS AND THEIR HEADS

This section develops the notion **headed feature domain**. We saw already in Section 1 some of the work this notion can do within OT—in particular, in the realm of vowel harmony, a primary concern of this chapter. Feature domains are a response to the formal challenge for OT posed by Autosegmental Phonology. In nonderivational OT, how are we to do the work of the autosegmental rules for linking, delinking, relinking, and spreading? How are we to understand a principle such as the **Obligatory Contour Principle** (OCP) that depends on the subtle distinction in autosegmental representations between two vowels sharing a feature (good) and those two vowels each independently bearing that feature (bad)?

A simple illustration of the rough relation between autosegmental and feature domain representations is shown in (54). Autosegmentally, regressive [+ATR] harmony (leftward spread of the advanced tongue root (ATR) feature) is a rule that spreads left from the final vowel a [+ATR] feature (or autosegment), delinking the initial vowel's underlying [−ATR] specification. The result is that underlying /ɔ/ surfaces as *o*, agreeing with *i* in [+ATR] .

The OT counterpart developed here has as input a stem and a suffix vowel, each a collection of features, and as output a set of feature domains. Feature domains were first introduced within OT by Kirchner (1993) and Smolensky (1993). Cole and Kisseberth (1994a, b, 1995a, b, c, 1997) develop the concept within what they call 'Optimal Domains Theory'. Cassimjee (1998) and Cassimjee and Kisseberth (1998) extend this theory to incorporate domain heads.

Feature domains fall in the class of **suprasegmental** structures. Such structures were conceptualized as entities in their own right in several phonological theories current around 1950; these were among the historical sources of Autosegmental Phonology (Goldsmith 1976, 5–15; 1990, 3–4). In Prosodic Theory (Firth 1948; Palmer 1970), the suprasegmental entities were known as **prosodies**. Indeed, Trubetzkoy (1939/1969) also discusses suprasegmental 'prosodic' properties at some length (pp. 92, 170–207, esp. 184–8).

(54)   From autosegmental derivations to feature domain representations

gɔ̀‑ₐt 'mountain' ~ gò₊ₐd‑í 'mountains'   (Lango; A ≡ ATR)

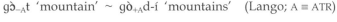

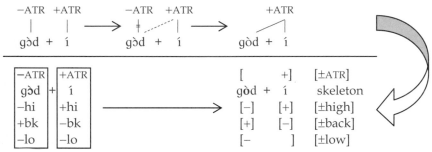

In this section, I will begin the characterization of feature domains by quickly identifying several key characteristics. It is the analyses of particular vowel harmony systems in Section 4, the typology of conjunctive domain interactions in Section 5, and the derivation of the sonority profile of syllable onsets in Section 6 that best bring out the important properties of feature domains.

First, the relation between domains and expressed feature values.

(55)   Feature domains

   a.   Inputs and outputs contain segments with feature values. Outputs are fully specified. I leave it open here whether inputs may contain only partially specified segments; on underspecification, see Section 1.

   b.   The feature values of output segments *determine* the feature domains.

   c.   A maximal contiguous span of φ‑bearers with a common value [±φ] is a **[±φ] domain 𝒟[±φ]**.
        Convention: Any statement containing '[±φ]' abbreviates two statements, one with [+φ], the other with [−φ].

   d.   Thus, by definition, contiguous domains of the same φ value are impossible.

   e.   All output segments are specified for all their features; every segment in

Box 1

the output is a member of either a domain $\mathcal{D}[+\varphi]$ or a domain $\mathcal{D}[-\varphi]$.

The [low] tier in (54) illustrates the case of adjacent identical feature values, which must lie in a common domain.

The characterization in (55) ignores the possibility that feature domains may be embedded one within another: in Section 1.5.3, embedded feature domains were used to treat the challenging case of segments transparent to harmony, with the phonetically realized feature value determined by the innermost domain. In the remainder of this chapter, we will not be concerned with transparency, and so will ignore all candidates with embedded domains. The constraint *EMBED can be viewed as undominated in all the cases we consider.

The next characteristic of feature domains will figure prominently in Section 6.

(56)   Feature domains have edges

   a.   The edges of domains support a spreading imperative: ALIGN-L/R($\mathcal{D}[\pm\varphi]$, Wd), requiring the left or right edge of a [+φ] or [–φ] feature domain to align with the left or right edge of the word (or other harmony domain; Kirchner 1993; Smolensky 1993; Cole and Kisseberth 1994b). This constraint was used in the analyses of harmony in Section 1, until the final Section 1.5.4, which relied instead on domain head markedness; the latter is the approach used in the remainder of the chapter, as discussed in (58).

   b.   Faithfulness to edges may be at the heart of the OCP – but this will not be pursued here.[17]

Perhaps the conceptually most important – yet also the most subtle – property of feature domains is their representational status.

---

[17] A sketch of the basic idea goes as follows. A featural contrast [±φ] may be marked on every segment; or it may be marked only once in an entire word; or it may be contrastive at an intermediate level, where, for example, a melody of at most two tones may be realized over more than two vowels. When a contrast is not marked on every segment, recoverability of underlying specifications is direct if only one segment expresses each feature; but if the feature spreads over multiple segments, perhaps to facilitate its perception or production, then the expression of a feature value by a segment becomes a weaker cue to the location of the underlying feature value. If spreading is directional – say, rightward – then it is the *left edge* of the domain of the spread feature that carries the information that an underlying feature value is specified. Specifying a high tone H on an underlying vowel may be viewed as specifying, not an absolute segmental property, but the location of an *edge* of a pitch value, or a *contour* of pitch. Preserving this edge or contour is what faithfulness should require, if it serves to support recovery of underlying specifications. The edge marked H may by default be marked by a pitch rise. But if already preceded by a high pitch, the existence of the underlying H specification may be indicated by a pitch *drop*, either a major change characteristic of a HL contour, or a minor change characteristic of downstep H!. Thus, recoverability under feature spread may be the heart of the problem with adjacent identical feature specifications, which the OCP prohibits. If a morpheme marked H, spreading right, meets a following morpheme marked H, and all vowels realize the same high pitch, then the specification of the second vowel is lost. If the second H blocks spreading of the first, and is then "deleted to satisfy the OCP," the second H is now recoverable, realized in the *low* tone of the second morpheme. What has been preserved is the *tonal edge* where H is specified; it is faithfulness to this edge, rather than to an absolute segmental pitch value, that is optimized.

---

(57) Feature domains are entities

a. A language is defined in part by an inventory of legal feature domains.

b. Such inventories often demand local conjunction: the conjunctive domain is the feature domain $\mathcal{D}[\pm\varphi]$.

This facet of feature domains will be used in Sections 4.1.7 and 4.1.8 to explain Lango source-conditioned ATR harmony.

As previewed in Section 1.5.4, feature domain heads correspond roughly to the source of a spreading autosegmental feature.

(58) Feature domains have heads

a. The edges of feature domains are determined by the feature values of segments.

b. *Gen* adds an element of structure not present in underlying forms: exactly one segment per domain is marked as the domain **head**.

c. A head is represented by additional structure — for example, a head node projected on a given tier from a given segment.

d. Notation

i. The head segment is denoted $\varphi°$.

ii. When a feature domain is represented as [+], as in (54), the location of $\pm$ identifies the head; this is equivalent to $[+ + +°]$.

e. Heads are in part a representationalization of "directionality of spread."

i. Heads are typically aligned left or right in their domain (corresponding to progressive/regressive spread).

ii. HD-L/R$[\pm\varphi]$: A $[\pm\varphi]$ domain's head must fall at its left/right edge

$\equiv$ ALIGN-L/R $(Hd(\mathcal{D}[\pm\varphi]), \mathcal{D}[\pm\varphi])$.

Once heads are part of the representations produced by *Gen*, the general structure of OT entails the existence of certain constraints.

(59) Heads are marked

a. Since the head involves additional structure, it is marked on general principles by a markedness constraint of the *STRUCTURE or 'structural economy' family (Chapter 12 (40a)):

*HD$[\pm\varphi]$: No domain head.[18]

b. Since *Gen* produces only candidates in which each feature domain has exactly one head, minimal violation of *HD$[\pm\varphi]$ requires a single domain — in other words, a domain that spans the entire form.

c. *HD$[\pm\varphi]$ is a spreading imperative (also denoted AGREE$[\varphi]$).

d. The *location* of a *HD violation is crucial: it identifies the segment that heads a domain.

---

[18] Thanks to Colin Wilson for initially identifying the importance of this constraint.

Box 1

e. Thus, *HD[φ] & ℂ *is a positional version of* ℂ *applying at* φ *domain heads.*

  i. ℂ ∈ MARKEDNESS: positional markedness (in Sections 4.1.7 and 4.1.8, this is used to explain Lango source-conditioned ATR harmony; Smolensky 1993, 1997; Zoll 1998).

  ii. ℂ ∈ FAITHFULNESS: positional faithfulness (in Section 4.2.4, this is used to explain Javanese parasitic ATR harmony; Beckman 1997).

The local conjunction operation in (59e) was defined in (21); it is the primary topic of Section 3. Here, and everywhere else in the chapter where not specified otherwise, the domain of conjunction is the segment: *HD[φ] & ℂ is violated if and only if one and the same segment violates ℂ and *HD[φ] (i.e., if and only if a φ domain head violates ℂ). (59e) is a type of conjunction that plays a major role in the analysis of vowel harmony systems presented in the next section.

Because a segment can not only fall in a feature domain, but in fact head one, there are two grades of faithfulness that will prove important.

(60) Faithfulness to φ

  a. F[±φ] An input segment bearing [±φ] must correspond to an output segment *in* a $\mathcal{D}$[±φ] (like MAX[±φ]).

  b. F°[±φ] An input segment bearing [±φ] must correspond to an output segment *heading* a $\mathcal{D}$[±φ] (something like a "super-MAX[±φ]" constraint[19]).

These constraints show different violations under different harmony configurations.

(61) Faithfulness in harmony

  a. Nonvacuous spreading of φ violates both F[φ] and F°[φ]:

$$•_1 \quad •_2 \quad \rightarrow \quad •_1 \quad •_2 \quad progressive \sim$$
φ: +   −   [+   ] *left-headed*
                    ⇑ violation of F[−φ] and F°[−φ]

  b. Vacuous "spreading" of φ violates only F°[φ]:

$$•_1 \quad •_2 \quad \rightarrow \quad •_1 \quad •_2$$
φ: +   +   [+   ]
                    ⇑ violation of F°[+φ] only

  c. Thus, F[φ] & ℂ is a positional version of ℂ applying at targets of nonvacuous spreading of φ. For example:

    ℂ = M[φ]: Can prevent spreading of φ when this would *create* an M[φ]-marked segment (used in Sections 4.1.7 and 4.1.8 to explain Lango target-conditioned ATR harmony).

  d. F°[φ] & ℂ is a positional version of ℂ applying at *all* non-φ heads. For example:

---

[19] This term is due to Laura Benua, a collaborator in part of the work summarized in Section 4.2.

    i. $\mathbb{C}$ = M[φ]: Can ban an M[φ]-marked segment except at a φ head (used in Section 4.2.2 to treat Kirghiz target-conditioned round harmony).

   ii. $\mathbb{C}$ = *HD[ψ]: Nonobviously, can make ψ harmony parasitic on φ agreement (used in Section 4.2.4 for Javanese ATR harmony under height agreement).

3 TYPOLOGIES RESPECT MARKEDNESS: STRONG HARMONIC COMPLETENESS AND LOCAL CONJUNCTION

A key consequence of OT is that a configuration X can only be ungrammatical in a language if it is marked. This seems intuitively obvious, but a formal proof is not trivial. Appropriate assumptions concerning *Gen*, *Con*, and X must first be made explicit, and this is itself not entirely straightforward. Box 2 illustrates the point with this simple example: if ungrammatical, then marked. Later results will require formal machinery of similar type, but more extensive; this is discussed in the Appendix.

If ungrammaticality arises in OT from markedness, it stands to reason that if X is ungrammatical, and Y is more marked than X, then Y too must be ungrammatical: X is already too marked to be permitted, so surely Y is even more so. Indeed, just this sort of inference is what motivates the typological diagnosis of markedness: if it is observed that any language that bans X also bans Y, this is to be explained by the postulate that Y is more marked than X.

This property of OT was introduced in Prince and Smolensky 1993/2004 under the name **harmonic completeness**. Inventories are complete with respect to Harmony in the sense of (62b).

(62) *Definition.* Harmonic completeness (Prince and Smolensky 1993/2004, Chap. 9)

Let I be an inventory of elements of some type $\mathcal{T}$ in a language $\mathcal{L}$. Elements in I are **legal** or **grammatical**. Let $\mathbb{C}$ be a markedness constraint evaluating elements of type $\mathcal{T}$ along some structural dimension d. I is harmonically complete with respect to d if and only if it satisfies the following requirement:

  a. If X is ungrammatical, then any configuration more marked than X (with respect to $\mathbb{C}$) must also be ungrammatical. Equivalently:

  b. If Y is grammatical, then any element more harmonic than Y (with respect to $\mathbb{C}$) must also be grammatical.

Intuitively, a harmonically complete inventory "respects markedness" — if x is legal, then y can only be illegal if it is more marked than y with respect to some markedness constraint.

Formulating and proving a formally correct version of the harmonic completeness property is nontrivial, and largely relegated to the Appendix; a summary is presented at the end of this section. At this point, I would like to introduce several empirical instances of the harmonic completeness property pertaining to vowel harmony.

Box 1

The first markedness-related vowel harmony pattern is the one most clearly predicted by OT; it will be analyzed for Lango ATR harmony in Section 4.2.1.

(63) *Definition.* Target-markedness-conditioned harmony

Harmony spreads feature φ

 a. *except when* doing so would *create* an especially *marked* segment, or

 b. *only when* doing so would *create* an especially *unmarked* segment.

This is expected because whether φ spreads to a segment will be determined in OT by whether the candidate with spreading is more harmonic than the one without spreading: a competition among the constraint compelling spread, faithfulness to the target segment—and the target's markedness with/without undergoing harmony.

More subtle is the second type of pattern, also exhibited in Lango; it is analyzed in Section 4.2.3.

(64) *Definition.* Source-markedness-conditioned harmony

Harmony spreads feature φ

 a. *except when* the *source* is especially *marked*, or

 b. *only when* the *source* is especially *unmarked*.

Most subtle is the final pattern, 'parasitic' harmony; it is illustrated in Section 4.2.4 by Javanese ATR harmony.

(65) *Definition.* Sharing-conditioned (parasitic) harmony (Javanese)

Harmony spreads feature φ *only when* **source and target share** *the value of another feature* ψ ('φ harmony is parasitic on ψ').

Because it does not explicitly refer to the markedness of segments, this pattern seems to be quite outside the scope of the OT analyses provided for the first two patterns. We will see in Section 4.2.4, however, that headed feature domains allow all three patterns to be treated in a unified fashion. Source-markedness-conditioned harmony will be analyzed using the principle (66).

(66) Head Markedness Propagation

A more marked head yields a more marked feature domain.

The parasitic case will be analyzed with a closely related principle, (67).

(67) Head Markedness Principle

 a. Initiating a new feature value is marked; that is,

 b. a feature domain head is a marked position.

All these markedness-related harmony patterns correspond to certain restrictions on a language's **inventory of feature domains**. The markedness-based restrictions will correspond to harmonic completeness. An example from the analysis of Lango ATR harmony in Section 4.1 is shown in (68); the constraints and structures will be fully explained there.

(68)   Lango harmonic ATR domains

     a.   The inventory of single vowels is $I_{seg} = \{i, e, ə, o, u, ɪ, ɛ, a, ɔ, ʊ\}$.

     b.   A **harmonic [+ATR] domain** is the output domain in one of the mappings:

         i.   Left-headed: $/CV_{+A}(C)CV_{-A}/ \rightarrow C[_{+A}\, V°(C).CV]$

         ii.   Right-headed: $/CV_{-A}(C)CV_{+A}/ \rightarrow C[_{+A}\, V(C).CV°]$

         (V_{+A} denotes a [+ATR] vowel.)

     c.   Specialize to the case where V_{+A} is [−fr] and V_{-A} is [+fr]. (Here, [±front] ≡ [∓back].)

     d.   The inventory of such harmonic [+ATR] domains is shown in the white rows of the following table: the shaded rows correspond to excluded domains, also marked '*' to their left.

	Structural dimension:	V_{-A}: [±hi] [+fr]	(C).C	V_{+A}: [±hi] [−fr]	L/R-headed
	Markedness constraint:	*[+ATR, −hi] *at nonhead*	*V_{+A}C.	*[+ATR, −hi] *at head*	ALIGN-L
	[u°.Ci]				
	[u°.Ce]	*			
	[u°C.Ci]		*		
	[u°C.Ce]	*	*		
	[o°.Ci]			*	
	[o°.Ce]	*		*	
*	[o°C.Ci]		*	*	
*	[o°C.Ce]	*	*	*	
	[i.Cu°]				*
	[e.Cu°]	*			*
*	[iC.Cu°]		*		*
*	[eC.Cu°]	*	*		*
*	[i.Co°]			*	*
*	[e.Co°]	*		*	*
*	[iC.Co°]		*	*	*
*	[eC.Co°]	*	*	*	*

This inventory is harmonically complete with respect to the structural dimensions identified in the top row of the table. This means that if one domain is illegal, a more marked domain must be as well. The arrows show this explicitly. Consider the row for the illegal domain *[o°C.Ci] (a shaded row). As indicated by the two marks '*' in this row, this [+ATR] domain is marked with respect to two dimensions, syllable structure and head height: *V_{+A}C. asserts that [+ATR] vowels are marked in closed syllables, and *[+ATR, −hi] says that [+ATR], the feature value for the domain in question, is marked in [−high] vowels. The domain is unmarked in the remaining two dimen-

Box 1

sions, however: nonhead height and head polarity. So this domain could be made more marked by becoming marked on these dimensions as well. To become marked with respect to nonhead height would be to become the domain [o°C.Ce]: now *e* not *i* is the nonhead ("target of [+ATR] spread"). The transition from unmarked to marked on this dimension is indicated by the leftmost descending arrow from the *[o°C.Ci] row. The arrow leads to another shaded row, that is, to another illegal domain, as it must in a harmonically complete inventory. The same is true if *[o°C.Ci] becomes more marked instead on the head polarity dimension, changing from a left (un-marked) to a right (marked) head (yielding domain *[iC.Co°]). As all the arrows show, starting with any illegal domain and making it more marked on any dimension leads to another illegal domain. The reader may directly verify the contrapositive: starting with a legal (unshaded) domain and making it *less* marked on any dimension leads again to another legal domain. (This slice of the Lango ATR domain inventory is displayed graphically in (110), p. 98.)

The theoretical and empirical work in this chapter provides bits of evidence for the first pair of main claims, (69).

(69) The good news

    a. *Broad empirical claim 1.* Inventories in natural languages are harmonically complete.

    b. *Informal theoretical claim 1.* An inventory defined in OT is harmonically complete.

We have already previewed the theoretical claim (69b). It counts as good news for OT to the extent that the empirical claim (69a) holds. I take the validity of this very broad claim to explain why the Prague School linguists invented the concept of markedness in the first place, and why it has proved so generally useful. Section 4 discusses three specific instances of complex yet harmonically complete vowel-tier inventories in languages with vowel harmony.

    The central challenge addressed in this chapter is expressed in the second pair of main claims, (70).

(70) The not-so-good news

    a. *Informal theoretical claim 2.* Only a small subset of all harmonically complete inventories can be defined in OT.

    b. *Broad empirical claim 2.* Inventories in natural languages frequently are harmonically complete but not definable in OT.

The problem can be cast somewhat more formally in terms of an important property introduced in Prince and Smolensky 1993/2004, Chap. 9.

(71) The challenge of strong harmonic completeness (SHARC)

    a. A typology has the **strong harmonic completeness (SHARC) property** if and only if every inventory in the typology is harmonically complete and every harmonically complete inventory is in the typology.

b. *Central problem.* Broadly, actual typologies seem to have the SHARC property, but the typologies generated by OT do not.

c. Major case: **BOWOW inventories**, which "ban only the worst of the worst." The following type of **BOWOW diagram** will be used often in the remainder of the chapter:

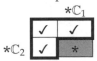

The white cells denote legal elements (here marked '✓') while the gray cell denotes an element excluded from the inventory ('*'). The gray cell corresponds to an element that incurs both of the marks $*\mathbb{C}_1$ and $*\mathbb{C}_2$. The two white cells directly above and left of the gray cell correspond to elements that incur only one of the marks ($*\mathbb{C}_1$ and $*\mathbb{C}_2$, respectively). The elements represented by the top left cell incur neither of these two marks. The only illegal form is the one violating both constraints: violators of $\mathbb{C}_1$ are "the worst," but among those, structures that also violate $\mathbb{C}_2$ are "the worst of the worst."

(72) Example BOWOW inventory: English obstruents (small subset)

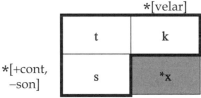

a. An obstruent can be marked for place (here, velar): ✓ *k*.

b. An obstruent can be marked for continuancy: ✓ *s*.

c. But an obstruent cannot be marked for *both* place and continuancy: **x*.

Local constraint conjunction is the solution proposed to meet this challenge; it was introduced in Chapter 12 (43), and the definition is restated here.

(73) Local conjunction of constraints

a. *Informal theoretical claim 3.* With a simple augmentation to the theory, local conjunction, the typologies generated by OT have the SHARC property.

b. Given a domain type $\mathcal{D}$ and two constraints A and B that can be evaluated over a $\mathcal{D}$-domain, the **local conjunction** of A and B relative to $\mathcal{D}$, denoted $A \&_{\mathcal{D}} B$, is violated in a particular $\mathcal{D}$-domain if and only if A and B are *both* violated in that *single* domain. (When not explicitly identified, $\mathcal{D} \equiv$ segment.)

Stating and proving these theoretical claims formally is not as simple as one

Box 1

might expect; the formalities are relegated to the Appendix (see also Box 2). The results derived in the Appendix can be summarized as follows (simplifying slightly):

(74) Constraint conjunction and strong harmonic completeness

    a. *Definition.* A **basic inventory** consists of

        i. A universe $\mathcal{U}$ of potential outputs that can be described by a set of properties, or binary 'features', $\varphi_1, \varphi_2, \dots, \varphi_n$, such that every combination of $\pm$ values for these features describes a potential output; $\mathcal{U}$ is also the set of possible inputs

        ii. A set of markedness constraints $\mathcal{M} \equiv \{ *[\varphi_1 = +], *[\varphi_2 = -], \dots, *[\varphi_n = -] \}$

        iii. A set of faithfulness constraints $\mathcal{F} \equiv \{ \text{ID}[\varphi_1], \text{ID}[\varphi_2], \dots, \text{ID}[\varphi_n] \}$

        iv. A ranking G of $Con \equiv \mathcal{M} \cup \mathcal{F}$

        The set of all outputs derived from all inputs $\mathcal{U}$ is a basic inventory I_G.

    b. *Definition.* The collection of all I_G arising from all rankings G is a **basic typology**.

    c. *Theorem.* A basic inventory is harmonically complete. A basic typology is *not* strongly harmonically complete.

    d. *Theorem.* If Con is augmented with all conjunctions of markedness constraints, the resulting factorial typology *is* strongly harmonically complete.

Box 2. Why does proving such simple results get so complex?

Desired result

If there is some language in which an element X is ungrammatical, then X violates a markedness constraint.

Desired argument

To be ungrammatical, any output O containing X must be suboptimal. What could make every such O lose? It can't be a faithfulness constraint concerning X, since those favor output X whenever X is in the input. It can't be a faithfulness constraint concerning some input element Y, since this would fail for any input not containing Y. So it must be a markedness constraint M; M must be violated by every output containing X, so M is $*X$.

    Trivial and obvious, right?

Complexities

(1) What if X is not present in *any* output? Then it would be ungrammatical in every language, even if no markedness constraint penalized it. Stupid, of course; but a formal theorem must protect itself from all counterexamples, no matter how inane. So henceforth let us assume that

    A_1. X is present in some output of *Gen*.

    Of course, it must also be that X is *absent* from some output in *Gen(I)* for every I, since otherwise X would necessarily appear in the optimal output for I

and thus it could not be ungrammatical.

(2)   Suppose *Con* contains a set of constraints $\mathbb{C}_k$: 'If the input contains Y_k, the output must not contain X'. Suppose too that every input to *Gen* must contain some Y_k. If these constraints are top ranked, no output containing X can be optimal. But there is no markedness constraint penalizing X: the constraints $\mathbb{C}_k$ do penalize X in the context of an input containing Y_k, but this is not a markedness constraint because it inspects the input as well as the output. Neither is $\mathbb{C}_k$ a faithfulness constraint, since it is not demanding one-to-one correspondence between input and output. So we assume that

A_2.   Every constraint in *Con* is either a markedness constraint or a faithfulness constraint.

(3)   Suppose every output containing X that is generated by *Gen* also contains some Y_k in a set $\mathcal{Y}$ not containing X (e.g., in the Basic CV Syllable Theory, X = onset and Y = syllable). Suppose *Con* contains $*Y_k$, for all $Y_k \in \mathcal{Y}$, but *Con* contains no constraint that even mentions X. If the $*Y_k$ constraints are undominated, no output containing X can be optimal, but X is not marked if this means 'penalized by a constraint'. So henceforth let us assume that

A_3.   For every set of structures $\mathcal{Y}$ not including X, if there is a candidate in *Gen*(I) that contains both X and an element of $\mathcal{Y}$, then there is another candidate in *Gen*(I) that contains X but no element of $\mathcal{Y}$.

Now these assumptions are getting very difficult to satisfy. Suppose $\mathcal{Y}$ is the set of *all* structures except X. A_3 can only be satisfied if there is an output containing X and nothing else! For many structures X, there is no such output. But even putting aside this seemingly serious problem, there are still more complications to deal with.

(4)   Suppose no *input* contains X (perhaps X = a syllable, in a theory banning underlying prosodic structure). Suppose, however, there is a faithfulness constraint F_D (like DEP) that prohibits an X in an output that is not in correspondence with an input X. Then if F_D is top ranked, X is ungrammatical—but because of a faithfulness constraint, not a markedness constraint. So let us assume that

A_4.   If *Con* contains a DEP-type faithfulness constraint F_D—violated by an output X with no input correspondent—then necessarily there are inputs that contain X, and a MAX-type faithfulness constraint F_M requiring an output X that corresponds to any input X.

Now F_D cannot block all output Xs, and indeed F_M compels them for X-containing inputs.

(5)   (This is essentially (3) using *Con* rather than *Gen* to tie X to other structure.) Suppose that *Con* contains $*Y$ and a single constraint that mentions X, namely, $\mathbb{C}$: 'If X is present, then Y must be present' (e.g., $X = \sigma$ and Y = Nucleus). Now if $*Y$ and $\mathbb{C}$ are top ranked, no output containing X can be optimal: X is ungrammatical. Does X violate a markedness constraint? There is no con-

Box 2

straint "*X"; but it might be said that $\mathbb{C}$ asserts that X is marked in specific contexts, namely, those lacking Y. A definition of 'marked' or 'violates a markedness constraint' must be attuned to this possibility. Perhaps,

> "*Definition*." Suppose M is a markedness constraint that is violated by a structure containing X, but not violated (or less violated) by the structure when X is removed. Then X is "M-marked."

But this definition is not rigorously well defined, since "the structure when X is removed" is undefined: for many X there will be no sensible definition.

The bottom line is that despite the apparent obviousness and triviality of the sought-after result here, it is not even clear that there is any useful formalization of the intended argument that actually works. And the topic of this chapter is considerably more complex than that of this box.

4 VOWEL HARMONY

In this section, a markedness-driven theory of vowel harmony is constructed using the techniques developed in the previous two sections: local conjunction and headed feature domains.

4.1 Lango

This section addresses in detail the vowel harmony system of Lango, a Nilotic language spoken in Uganda. In this language, as in many of its relatives, the advanced tongue root feature ATR spreads, subject to complex conditions that can be understood in terms of the relative markedness of [±ATR] when this feature co-occurs with other features. The proposed analysis builds directly upon the insights of the previous analyses of this system by Woock and Noonan (1979), Poser (1982), and Archangeli and Pulleyblank (1994). (Data come from Okello 1975; Woock and Noonan 1979; and Noonan 1992.) Archangeli and Pulleyblank (1994) clearly identify the role of markedness in shaping the system, and formalize the role of markedness by imposing a schema structure on autosegmental spreading rules, a schema that restricts the possible rules to those that are "phonetically grounded" in markedness. The goal of the present analysis is to show how the independently motivated formalisms of ranked markedness constraints and feature domains already restrict vowel harmony systems in this way, with no need to impose additional superstructure. The restricted descriptive capability follows inevitably from the basic apparatus of grammar under OT. The relevant inventory will be seen to be consistent with markedness principles, in the formal sense of being harmonically complete, as previewed in (68). The highly complex Lango inventory is one that derives from multiple local conjunctions of the basic markedness constraints.

4.1.1 Data

Lango's ATR harmony system will be studied by examining its inventory of ATR domains $\mathcal{D}$[ATR]. Vowel harmony renders ungrammatical many candidate ATR domains—disharmonic domains.

The first datum in (75) illustrates a case of [+ATR] harmony. As in nearly all relevant cases, the input contains a disharmonic pair of vowels; in this case, the first is [−ATR] and the second [+ATR]. The output, however, is harmonic: a single [+ATR] domain spanning both vowels. The head of this domain is the vowel underlyingly bearing the surface ATR value, [+ATR]; as usual, this is denoted by the location of the head marker '°'. The competing output ATR domains are shown in (75a): the faithful, disharmonic output, consisting of a sequence of two domains [−ATR][+ATR], and the harmonic output, consisting of a single [−ATR] domain. The head of the latter is, again, the vowel underlyingly specified for the surface feature. For single-vowel domains, as in the disharmonic output, each vowel is necessarily the head of its own domain, but this is not explicitly marked.

(75)   Lango ATR harmony: 'your_{SG/PL} stew'

     a.   dɛ̀k + C í   →   * dɛ̀k. k í   ☞ dɛ̀k. k í   * dɛ̀k. k í

     ATR: −   +   [−] [+]   [+ +°]   [−° −]

     b.   dɛ̀k + wú   → ☞ dɛ̀k.wú   * dɛ̀k.wú   * dɛ̀k.wʊ́

The input for the second datum (75b) has the same ATR structure, but the output does not. Now the optimal candidate is the faithful, disharmonic one.[20] The critical difference, as noted by Archangeli and Pulleyblank (1994), is the degree of markedness of the feature [+ATR] in two cases. Where [+ATR] harmony is optimal, the underlying [+ATR] feature co-occurs with the feature [+front] in the input vowel /i/; where [+ATR] harmony is suboptimal, [+ATR] co-occurs with the feature [−front] in /u/. As Archangeli and Pulleyblank discuss, [−front] and [+ATR] make antagonistic demands on the tongue, the articulatory basis for the markedness constraints (76a); likewise for [−ATR, +front]. Similar antagonism between [+ATR] and [−high] motivates the constraints (76b).[21]

(76)   Markedness of [±ATR] features

     a.   *[+ATR, −fr]   *[−ATR, +fr]

     b.   *[+ATR, −hi]   *[−ATR, +hi]

     c.   *V_{+A}C.   No [+ATR] vowels in closed syllables.

Thus, the [+ATR]-harmony candidate in (75b) has a more marked head (*u*: [+ATR, −fr]) than does its counterpart in (75a) (*i*: [+ATR, +fr]): this is what makes it suboptimal in (75b) although it was optimal in (75a). In autosegmental terminology, "a [−front]

***

[20] According to Noonan (1992, 33) this lack of harmony is characteristic of only "some speakers."

[21] I have used [±front] to denote the feature values conventionally written [∓back]. This is purely for mnemonic ease: as evident in (76), with [±fr], the unmarked feature combinations are those in which the sign of [±ATR] is the same as that of [±fr] and [±hi].

Box 2

vowel is a worse source for [+ATR] spread than its [+front] counterpart because the feature [+ATR] is marked in co-occurrence with [−front] but unmarked with [+front]."

The change of a single feature between (75a) and (75b) suffices to change the outcome from [+ATR] harmony to no harmony. In fact, the Lango ATR harmony system is sensitive in this way to *six* binary dimensions of the input: there are $2^6 = 64$ distinct environments that must be analyzed. This is graphically displayed in (77), which represents the 2 examples in (75) and 62 other analogous examples.[22] (For examples of actual Lango forms, see (108), page 95.) This display of the ATR domain inventory will be used many times in this analysis. It encapsulates a large quantity of information that we must now unpack.

Each cell in table (77) indicates the output for an input containing one [+ATR] and one [−ATR] vowel: these are the inputs where real (nonvacuous) harmony can potentially manifest itself. In the left half of the table, the [+ATR] vowel precedes the [−ATR] vowel, as indicated in the label '/V_{+A} (C)C $V_{−A}$/'. In the right half of the table, the [+ATR] vowel follows the [−ATR] vowel. In autosegmental terms, this difference determines whether [+ATR] and [−ATR] spread would be progressive or regressive. This is the first of the six dimensions represented in (77); these dimensions are listed in (78).

(77)   Lango ATR harmony data

					V_{+A} (Potential: +ATR source; −ATR target)							
					/V_{+A} (C).C $V_{−A}$/				/$V_{−A}$ (C).C V_{+A}/			
					+hi		−hi		+hi		−hi	
					+fr	−fr	+fr	−fr	+fr	−fr	+fr	−fr
					i _	u _	e _	o/ə _	_ i	_ u	_ e	_ o/ə
$V_{−A}$ (Potential: −ATR source; +ATR target)	C	+fr	+hi	ι	[i° i]	[u° i]	[e° i]	[o° i]	[i i°]	[i u°]	ι e	ι o
			−hi	ε	[i° e]	[u° e]	[e° e]	[o° e]	[e i°]	[e u°]	ε e	ε o
		−fr	+hi	ʊ	[i° u]	[u° u]	[e° u]	[o° u]	[u i°]	[u u°]	[ʊ° ε]	[ʊ° ɔ]
			−hi	ɔ/a	[i° o]	[u° o]	[e° o]	[o° o]	[o i°]	[o u°]	[ɔ° ε]	[ɔ° ɔ]
	C.C	+fr	+hi	ι	[i° i]	[u° i]	e ι	o ι	[i i°]	[i u°]	ι e	ι o
			−hi	ε	[i° e]	[u° e]	e ε	o ε	[e i°]	ε u	ε e	ε o
		−fr	+hi	ʊ	[i° u]	[u° u]	e ʊ	o ʊ	[u i°]	[u u°]	[ʊ° ε]	[ʊ° ɔ]
			−hi	ɔ/a	[i° o]	[u° o]	e ɔ	o ɔ	[o i°]	ɔ u	[ɔ° ε]	[ɔ° ɔ]

Key: | /$V_+V_−$/ | [+° +] | + − | [− −°] | /$V_−V_+$/ | [+ +°] | − + | [−° −] |
| | +ATR→ | | ←−ATR | | ←+ATR | | −ATR→ |

---

[22] The table is constructed from the rules of Archangeli and Pulleyblank 1994.

(78)   Dimensions of variation conditioning ATR harmony

    a.   [+ATR] vowel precedes/follows [−ATR] vowel:

          $/V_{+A}$ (C).C $V_{−A}/$ versus $/V_{−A}$ (C).C $V_{+A}/$.

    b.   [+ATR] vowel is [+hi]/[−hi].

    c.   [+ATR] vowel is [+fr]/[−fr].

    d.   [−ATR] vowel is [+hi]/[−hi].

    e.   [−ATR] vowel is [+fr]/[−fr].

    f.   Initial syllable is open/closed: intervening C versus C.C (with '.' = syllable boundary).

Within the left half of the table are columns for the different [+ATR] vowels of Lango, grouped by their features [±hi], [±fr]. These vowels are {i, u, e, o, ə}. In the Lango ATR harmony system, the two vowels /o/ and /ə/ pattern identically: they differ phonologically only in the feature [±rd] to which the ATR system is not sensitive. (From an articulatory point of view, this is perhaps not surprising, since the articulator implementing the feature [±rd], the lips, is independent of the tongue, which implements [±ATR], [±hi], and [±fr].) The table shows the cases with /o/; the corresponding data with /ə/ in its place are identical, with [−rd] replacing [+rd].

The top half of the table pertains to cases in which the input has a single consonant intervening between its [+ATR] and [−ATR] vowels. In the lower half, two consonants (possibly a geminate consonant) intervene. This is relevant to ATR harmony via the markedness constraint (76c), which states that in closed syllables, [+ATR] vowels are marked.[23] Within each half, sorted by the features [±fr] and [±hi], the rows distinguish among the [−ATR] vowels of Lango: {ɪ, ɛ, ʊ, ɔ, a}. The pair ɔ/a is the [−ATR] counterpart of the pair o/ə and again the entries in table (77) show only the [+rd] case, ɔ.[24]

Thus, the two examples of (75) are located in the table as follows. The first, /dèk+Cí/ → [dèk.kí], is the cell containing the ATR domain [e i°]; it is in the row labeled 'ɛ' in the lower half of the table labeled 'C.C', and the column labeled '_i' in the right half of the table, labeled '/$V_{−A}$(C).CV_{+A}/'. The second example (75b), /dèk+wú/ → [dèk.wú], is the cell labeled 'ɛ u' in the row C.C/ɛ, column /$V_{−A}$ (C).C V_{+A}/_u. 'ɛ u' abbreviates the ATR domain structure [$_{−A}$ ɛ°][$_{+A}$ u°].

The shading scheme of table (77) indicates the winner of harmonic competition. In the white cells, [+ATR] harmony wins; in the black cells, [−ATR] harmony; in the gray cells, neither: the faithful, disharmonic output is optimal. This is shown in the key at the bottom of the table. The left and right halves of the table have separate

---

[23] Thanks to John McCarthy and Rolf Noyer, who independently suggested that this was the relevant constraint. An alternative is a constraint declaring that a vowel feature domain spanning two consonants is more marked than one spanning a single consonant. The former but not the latter offers an explanation of why in Lango it is the [+ATR], not the [−ATR], harmony domains that are sensitive to the open/closed syllable distinction.

[24] For those to whom International Phonetic Association symbols are not completely transparent, it may be helpful to note that with the choice of displaying the [+rd] vowels o/ɔ, the [+ATR] vowels are all and only those denoted by letters of the Roman alphabet.

Box 2

keys because they differ in the linear order of the [+ATR] and [−ATR] vowels.

The inventory of input-output mappings of ATR domains in Lango includes all those shown in table (77). As noted before, replacing /o/ with /ə/ or /ɔ/ with /a/ yields additional valid input-output pairs. All other ATR domain input-output mappings of an underlyingly disharmonic pair of vowels are banned from the inventory of Lango. Most importantly, for every white or black cell the faithful mapping /x y/ → [x] [y] is banned from the inventory.

The shading scheme used in table (77) can be related to that used in the earlier diagram (71c) as follows. Consider the structure of a single [+ATR] domain spanning the word. The inputs for which this is grammatical are indicated in table (77) with white cells. These constitute the inventory of harmonic [+ATR] domains. All nonwhite cells are banned from this inventory. This corresponds quite directly to the conventions of the simple BOWOW diagram (71c). Now consider the structure of a single [−ATR] domain spanning the word. The inputs for which this is grammatical are indicated in (77) by black shading. All nonblack cells are excluded from this inventory.

The task at hand is to use simple, universal markedness constraints to explain the exact shapes of these inventories.

The remarkably complex structure of the Lango ATR domain inventory can be explored by examining in some detail table (77), reproduced below in (79).[25] Consider the gray cell in (79) labeled 'ɛ u'; it represents example (75b) and is identified with a heavy solid border; the labels for its column and row are also marked with a matching border. This cell corresponds to the input $I_0 \equiv$ /ɛCCu/, and its gray shading specifies that the optimal output is faithful, that is, disharmonic: neither [+ATR] harmony (white) nor [−ATR] harmony (black) is optimal. This outcome—disharmony—is extremely sensitive to properties of the input. If we change the feature [−fr] of the [+ATR] vowel in this input, we follow the horizontal white arrow and move left one cell to the location marked with a heavy dashed border. The cell is labeled '[e i°]' and this move has changed the cell color from gray to white: the optimal output is no longer faithfully disharmonic; it is now a single [+ATR] harmony domain. This is example (75a).

Table (79) shows the effects of changing each of the values of the six dimensions corresponding to the gray cell 'ɛ u', with input I_0 = /ɛCCu/. The horizontal white arrow, we have just seen, indicates that changing the [−fr] feature of the [+ATR] vowel /u/ in this input I_0 changes the optimal output from disharmony to [+ATR] harmony. The vertical white arrow shows that changing the [−ATR] vowel from [−hi] /ɛ/ to [+hi] /ɪ/ also changes the optimal output in the same way. The vertical gray arrow shows that changing I_0 to /ɛCu/, with one rather than two intervening Cs, also changes the optimum—as does reversing the input sequence to /uCCɛ/, as shown by the horizontal heavy solid gray arrow.

---

[25] Lango forms exemplifying those cells of (79) discussed in the text can all be found in the tableaux (108).

Changing the [+hi] of /u/ does not change the outcome, however; as the horizontal dashed arrow shows, the input /ɛCCo/ surfaces disharmonically, like I_0. Similarly, the dashed vertical gray line shows that disharmony remains optimal when we change the [+fr] of /ɛ/, yielding /ɔCCu/. But when we make *both* changes, from I_0 = /ɛCCu/ to /ɔCCo/, the outcome is different: here [−ATR] harmony wins, as indicated by the black cell [ɔ° ɔ].

(79)   Sensitivity of harmonic outcome to input features

Lango — ATR domain inventory				**V**+A (*Potential: +ATR source; −ATR target*)							
				/V+A (C).C V−A/				/V−A (C).C V+A/			
				+hi		−hi		+hi		−hi	
				+fr	−fr	+fr	−fr	+fr	−fr	+fr	−fr
				i	u	e	o	i	u	e	o
V−A (*Potential: −ATR source; +ATR target*) — **C**	+fr	+hi	ɪ	[i° i]	[u° i]	[e° i]	[o° i]	[i i°]	[i u°]	ɪ e	ɪ o
		−hi	ɛ	[i° e]	[u° e]	[e° e]	[o° e]	[e i°]	[e u°]	ɛ e	ɛ o
	−fr	+hi	ʊ	[i° u]	[u° u]	[e° u]	[o° u]	[u i°]	[u u°]	[ʊ ɛ]	[ʊ° ɔ]
		−hi	ɔ	[i° o]	[u° o]	[e° o]	[o° o]	[o i°]	[o u°]	[ɔ° ɛ]	[ɔ° ɔ]
C.C	+fr	+hi	ɪ	[i° i]	[u° i]	e ɪ	o ɪ	[i i°]	[i u°]	ɪ e	ɪ o
		−hi	ɛ	[i° e]	[u° e]	e ɛ	o ɛ	[e i°]	ɛ u	ɛ e	ɛ o
	−fr	+hi	ʊ	[i° u]	[u° u]	e ʊ	o ʊ	[u i°]	[u u°]	[ʊ ɛ]	[ʊ° ɔ]
		−hi	ɔ	[i° o]	[u° o]	e ɔ	o ɔ	[o i°]	ɔ u	[ɔ° ɛ]	[ɔ° ɔ]

Key: /V+V−/ [+° +] +ATR→ + − [− −°] ←−ATR ‖ /V−V+/ [+ +°] ←+ATR − + [−° −] −ATR→

4.1.2 The challenge

To explain the ATR harmony system of Lango within a theory of universal grammar, we face a major challenge.

(80)   Needed is a grammatical framework
   a.   able to handle the nightmarish descriptive complexity of (79), while
   b.   staying strictly within the confines of restrictive, rigidly universal principles.

We need a grammatical formalism with expressive power sufficient to handle the complexity of this harmony system, but restrictive enough to prevent generation of harmony systems inconsistent with universal markedness principles.

Box 2

4.1.3 Rule-based account (Archangeli and Pulleyblank)

How does rule-based phonology fare against the challenge of (80)? Within an autosegmental perspective, Archangeli and Pulleyblank (1994) account for these Lango facts by positing six spreading rules: two progressive [+ATR] rules, three regressive [+ATR] rules, and one progressive [−ATR] rule. With the notation being employed here, these rules can be expressed as in (81). Note the high degree of complexity internal to the conditions of these rules, necessitated by the complex sensitivity of harmony to multiple structural dimensions.

(81)   Spreading rules

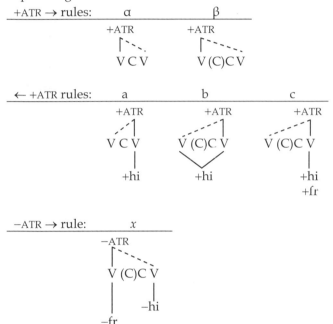

How these six rules account for the data is shown in (82). In each cell appears the label of the rules that apply to the corresponding input. For every white cell, (at least) one of the [+ATR] spreading rules applies; for every black cell, the [−ATR] rule applies. For the gray cells, neither rule applies.

Thus, Autosegmental Phonology meets the first half of the challenge of (80): it provides the descriptive power demanded by these data. The problem is the second half. Autosegmental Phonology per se is equally disposed to a rule system just like (81) except that each occurrence of [+hi] is replaced by [−hi]. Such a harmony system runs counter to markedness theory; for example, rule b becomes a rule preferring to create [+ATR] domains with a [−hi] rather than a [+hi] target. And indeed such systems have no place in Archangeli and Pulleyblank's typological survey, which documents the consistency between harmony systems and markedness theory. Archangeli and Pulleyblank deal with this by imposing a superstructure on autosegmental rules that prevents formulation of markedness-violating harmony systems.

(82)   Derivation of inventory by spreading rules

Lango				$\mathbf{V}_{+A}$ *(Potential: +ATR source; −ATR target)*							
Rule-based account				/$\mathbf{V}_{+A}$ (C).C $\mathbf{V}_{-A}$/				/$\mathbf{V}_{-A}$ (C).C $\mathbf{V}_{+A}$/			
				+hi		−hi		+hi		−hi	
				+fr	−fr	+fr	−fr	+fr	−fr	+fr	−fr
				i _	u _	e _	o/ə _	_ i	_ u	_ e	_ o/ə
$\mathbf{V}_{-A}$ *(Potential: −ATR source; +ATR target)*	C	+fr	+hi ɩ	α β	α β	α	α	a b c	a b		
			−hi ɛ	α β	α β	α	α	a c	a		
		−fr	+hi ʊ	α β	α β	α	α	a b c	a b	*x*	*x*
			−hi ɔ/a	α β	α β	α	α	a c	a	*x*	*x*
	C.C	+fr	+hi ɩ	β	β			b c	b		
			−hi ɛ	β	β			c			
		−fr	+hi ʊ	β	β			b c	b	*x*	*x*
			−hi ɔ/a	β	β			c		*x*	*x*

Key: | /V₊V₋/ | [+° +] +ATR→ | + − | [− −°] ← −ATR | /V₋V₊/ | [+ +°] ←+ATR | − + | [−° −] −ATR→ |

4.1.4 ATR domain inventory governed by markedness

Can the shape of the Lango ATR domain inventory be formally explained directly by markedness principles? To begin, the inventory map (77) is repeated in (83) with the markedness of [±ATR] values indicated. The labels of rows and columns for [+hi] are white cells, indicating that the unmarked ATR value is [+ATR] for [+hi]; the labels of rows and columns for [−hi] are black cells, indicating that the unmarked value is [−ATR]. Similarly, [+fr] labels are white, [−fr] labels black. The label 'C.C' for the lower half of the table is black because the initial closed syllable disfavors [+ATR], in accordance with (76c). Finally, the label for the right half of the table, '/V₋ₐ (C).C **V**₊ₐ/' is black because for such an input, [−ATR] harmony is 'progressive' (left-headed), while [+ATR] harmony is 'regressive' (right-headed). Progressive or left-headed domains are evidently preferred in Lango, as we will see; this preference is encoded in the ranking HD-L[ATR] ≫ HD-R[ATR]. I will take this to be a language-particular ranking, lacking arguments for its universality.

Markedness considerations, then, favor [+ATR] (white) for cells in rows and columns with white labels, and favor [−ATR] (black) for cells with black labels. And in-

Box 2

deed this is visible in (83). The lower-right corner, outlined with a solid gray border, is black, and the corresponding column and row labels are predominantly black. The same is true for the upper-left corner, outlined with a dashed gray border, with white replacing black. The gray cells fall where row and column labels mix black and white in roughly equal proportions.

This extremely vague style of "explanation" seems quite hopeless as the basis of a formal account. And so markedness-based explanation can often appear. But as formalized in OT, we will now see that just this approach to explanation can provide an account that is formally explicit, demonstrably correct, and explanatorily powerful, showing precisely how the complexity of these data emerges from interactions of simple, universal markedness principles.

(83)   ATR domain inventory and markedness

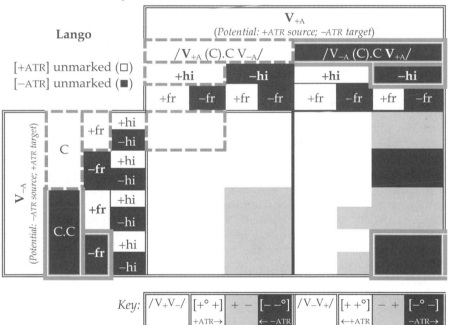

4.1.5 Encapsulated ranking

The overall organization of the ranking in the proposed OT account of Lango ATR harmony is shown in (84).

(84)   Encapsulated ranking
    a.   UNDOM ≫ M($\mathcal{D}$[ATR]) ≫ AGREE[ATR] ≫ F[ATR] ≫ M[ATR]
    b.   UNDOM ≡ {MAX, DEP, F[fr], F[hi], F[ATR] & *HD[ATR]}

    c.   M($\mathcal{D}$[ATR]): $\mathcal{D}$[ATR]-markedness constraints (to be determined)

    d.   AGREE[ATR] ≡ *HD[ATR]

    e.   F[ATR] ≡ IDENT[ATR]

    f.   M[ATR] ≡ {*[−ATR, +fr], *V$_{+A}$C., ...} (to be determined)

Undominated MAX and DEP ensure that neither deletion nor epenthesis is optimal. Undominated faithfulness constraints F[fr] and F[hi] ensure that it is also suboptimal to change [fr] or [hi] values to meet markedness constraints; F[φ] ≡ IDENT[φ]. Only ATR features can be changed for this purpose: F[ATR] is dominated by AGREE[ATR], the harmony-inducing markedness constraint, which is just *HD[ATR] (59). Thus, ATR values will be changed to achieve harmony, except when the resulting ATR domain would violate one of the markedness constraints in M($\mathcal{D}$[ATR]): these dominate AGREE[ATR]. It is exactly these constraints we must uncover in the analysis to follow.

    While it is crucial that F[ATR] be sufficiently low ranked (below AGREE[ATR]), we can now see that it is also crucial that F[ATR] & *HD[ATR] be sufficiently high ranked (above M($\mathcal{D}$[ATR])). This conjunction has as domain the segment; it is just the enhancement of F[ATR] at the head of ATR domains (59d). This constraint is needed for harmonic *inputs*, as we will now see.

4.1.6 Harmonic inputs

Consider inputs with two vowels that agree in ATR: harmonic inputs. These simply surface faithfully in Lango; they are not among the central data of interest, which concern disharmonic inputs (77).

    Yet harmonic inputs would pose a problem for the analysis if F[ATR] & *HD[ATR] were not highly ranked. For harmonic inputs may contain vowels that are marked with respect to ATR; we do not want the ATR markedness constraints to prevent these marked vowels from surfacing faithfully. For example, the schematic disharmonic input /CɛCe/ surfaces faithfully, without harmony, according to (77). On the present account, this must be because the harmonic alternative [₋ Cɛ°.Cɛ] violates some markedness constraint M in M($\mathcal{D}$[ATR])—say, something like *[−ATR, +fr]. But now consider the corresponding harmonic input /CɛCɛ/. The output [₋ Cɛ°.Cɛ] is now faithful, but M must still be violated: markedness constraints see only the output, and only the input here is different. Thus, the faithful candidate will be less harmonic than a candidate like [₊ Ce°.Ce] that satisfies M (and AGREE[ATR]) and merely violates low-ranked F[ATR].

    This problem is simply resolved by undominated F[ATR] & *HD[ATR]. This constraint ensures that unfaithfulness to ATR can only be optimal in *nonhead position*: an unfaithful head violates both F[ATR] and *HD[ATR].

    Now consider the harmonic input /CɛCɛ/. The faithful output does violate M, but the alternatives are still worse. Changing the ATR value of one vowel V (e.g. [₋Cɛ°].[₊Ce°]) creates a new ATR domain headed by V: this is an unfaithful head. Changing the ATR values of both vowels ([₊ Ce°.Ce]) fares no better, as one of the

Box 2

vowels must be the domain head and it will necessarily be unfaithful.

That F[φ] & *HD[φ] is high ranked is not surprising: this constraint insists that the head of a [+φ] domain be underlyingly [+φ], analogous to the autosegmental account, where the source of [+φ] spread must be underlyingly [+φ].

Thus, the overall ranking (84) ensures that ATR values in the output will be faithful to those in the input, except when an altered ATR value on a single vowel V allows V to agree in ATR with the other vowel, and the resulting two-vowel ATR domain does not violate a markedness constraint in the set M($\mathcal{D}$[ATR]). We now proceed to identify that set.

4.1.7 [−ATR] domains: Admitting only the best of the best

Let us begin by considering the fairly restricted set of environments where [−ATR] harmony obtains: the black cells in (83), where a single (left-headed) [−ATR] domain is output. This inventory of [−ATR] domains is in fact a case of 'only the best of the best of the best'. This is illustrated in table (85).

(85)   [−ATR] domains: Only the best$_Z$ of the best$_Y$ of the best$_X$

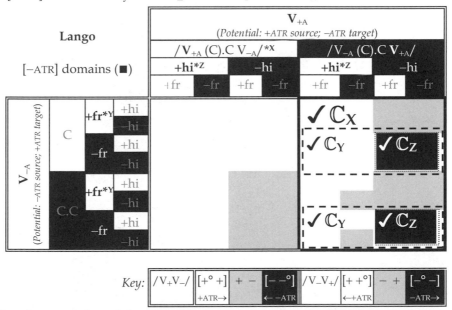

First, harmonic [−ATR] domains (black cells) occur only in the right half of the table, beneath the black label '/V$_{−A}$ (C).C V$_{+A}$/'. As discussed above, these environments are the 'best' for a [−ATR] harmonic domain because such a domain can be left-headed (the underlying [−ATR] vowel being the leftmost one). These 'best' environments are indicated in (85) by a heavy solid black border around the right half of the table, labeled '✓ $\mathbb{C}_X$'. $\mathbb{C}_X$ is the constraint favoring left-headed [−ATR] domains: it is simply HD-L[−ATR], the first of the [−ATR] constraints listed in (87) below. The cells in which a harmonic [−ATR] domain violates $\mathbb{C}_X$ are shown in (86). The label of the half of the table violating $\mathbb{C}_X$ is marked with a superscript X, as it is in (85).

(86) $\mathbb{C}_X$ violations by [−ATR] harmonic domains

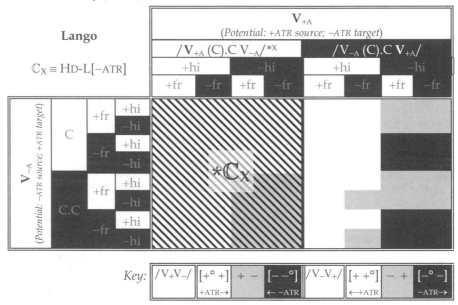

(87)   [−ATR] constraints

    a. $\mathbb{C}_X$ ≡ HD-L[−ATR]

             A [−ATR] domain must be left-headed.

             "No regressive [−ATR] spread."

    b. $\mathbb{C}_Y$ ≡ *[−ATR, +fr] & *HD[ATR] & $_{\mathcal{D}[A]}$ F[ATR]

             No [+fr] head of an unfaithful [−ATR] domain.

             "No [−ATR] spread from a [+fr] vowel."

    c. $\mathbb{C}_Z$ ≡ *[−ATR, +hi]

Of the 'best' environments for [−ATR] harmony—those satisfying $\mathbb{C}_X$—the 'best of the best' are those in which the underlying [−ATR] vowel—the head of the [−ATR] harmony domain—is [−fr]; these feature values form an unmarked combination (76a), satisfying another markedness constraint $\mathbb{C}_Y$. These environments are indicated in (85) with a heavy dashed border, labeled '✓ $\mathbb{C}_Y$'. Table (89) shows the cells where the [−ATR] harmony candidate violates $\mathbb{C}_Y$. $\mathbb{C}_Y$ asserts the markedness of harmonic [−ATR] domains in which the head vowel is [+fr], that is, violates *[−ATR, +fr] (76a). This constraint targets the head of the domain only: it is the conjunction of the feature

Box 2

co-occurrence constraint *[−ATR, +fr] with the constraint *HD[−ATR], violated by the head of a [−ATR] domain.

(88)   *[−ATR, +fr] & *HD[−ATR]

This is simply a case of markedness enhancement at a head, introduced in a general context in (59d); it instantiates Head Markedness Propagation (66): marked heads make marked domains.

(89) $\mathbb{C}_Y$ violations by [−ATR] harmonic domains

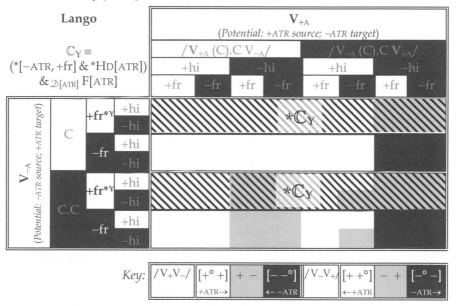

Now for a disharmonic input with a [−ATR, +fr] vowel, not only the [−ATR] harmony candidate, but also the faithful candidate, has a [−ATR, +fr] head: the [−ATR] domain spans two vowels in the harmonic candidate, and only one vowel in the disharmonic candidate, but the same segment is the [−ATR] domain head in each case. In order for $\mathbb{C}_Y$ to render the [−ATR] harmony candidate more marked than the faithful candidate in the region shown in (89), it suffices to ensure that $\mathbb{C}_Y$ is violated only when a [−ATR] domain with a marked [+fr] head contains a vowel unfaithful to ATR — a vowel that has harmonized. This is achieved by conjoining our existing constraint (88) with F[ATR], where the domain of conjunction is the feature domain $\mathcal{D}$[ATR]. This yields the final result (90), previously given in (87b).

(90) $\mathbb{C}_Y \equiv$ (*[−ATR, +fr] & *HD[−ATR]) & $_{\mathcal{D}[ATR]}$ F[ATR]

$\mathbb{C}_Y$ asserts that a [−ATR, +fr] vowel is a poor head of a domain resulting from the spread of [−ATR] to an underlyingly [+ATR] vowel.

Finally, of the 'best of the best' environments for [−ATR] — where both $\mathbb{C}_X$ and $\mathbb{C}_Y$

are satisfied—the 'best of the best of the best' are those in which the underlying [+ATR] vowel is [–hi]; changing this vowel to [ATR] via [–ATR] harmony results in the unmarked combination [–ATR, –hi] (76b). These environments satisfy a third constraint $\mathbb{C}_Z$, and are labeled '✓$\mathbb{C}_Z$' in (85); they are exactly the black cells, the environments in which [–ATR] harmony is optimal. $\mathbb{C}_Z$ can take either of two forms. If we define it as in (91), then it is violated by a [–ATR, +hi] segment that is unfaithful to ATR: an underlyingly [+ATR, +hi] segment that is the *target* of [–ATR] spread. The region in which a [–ATR] harmony domain violates constraint (91) is shown in table (93).

(91) $\mathbb{C}_Z \equiv {}^*[-\text{ATR}, +\text{hi}] \,\&\, F[\text{ATR}]$

It is in fact possible to give $\mathbb{C}_Z$ the simpler definition in (92).

(92) $\mathbb{C}_Z \equiv {}^*[-\text{ATR}, +\text{hi}]$

Now, in addition to the region shown in (93), a [–ATR] harmony domain will violate $\mathbb{C}_Z$ when the underlyingly [–ATR] vowel (the *source* of spreading) is [+hi]. But note that these additional violations also now appear on the faithful (disharmonic) candidate; if the would-be source of [–ATR] harmony is [+hi], *[–ATR, +hi] is violated at this segment whether or not it induces harmony on an adjacent vowel. Thus, the simpler definition of $\mathbb{C}_Z$ in (92) yields the same optimal outputs as (91). On the simpler definition, the region labeled '*$\mathbb{C}_Z$' in (93) is still the relevant one: it is the region in which the [–ATR] harmony candidate is more marked with respect to $\mathbb{C}_Z$ than is the disharmonic candidate.

(93) $\mathbb{C}_Z$ violations by [–ATR] harmonic domains

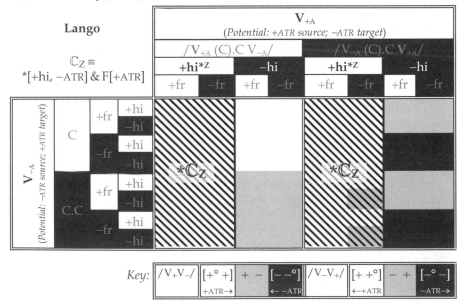

Box 2

Definition (92) completes our derivation of the three [−ATR] domain markedness constraints previewed in (87). These constraints are the [−ATR] subset of the markedness constraints M($\mathcal{D}$[ATR]), part of the encapsulated ranking given in (84). Thus, the ranking that yields the [−ATR] domain inventory—admitting only the best (✓ $\mathbb{C}_Z$) of the best (✓ $\mathbb{C}_Y$) of the best (✓ $\mathbb{C}_X$)—is that given in (94).

(94) {$\mathbb{C}_X$, $\mathbb{C}_Y$, $\mathbb{C}_Z$} ≫ AGREE[ATR] ≫ F[ATR]

AGREE[ATR] is the harmony-driving constraint that is best satisfied by a harmonic word. (Recall that AGREE[ATR] is just another name for *HD[ATR].) In the inputs we are considering, one vowel is [+ATR] and the other [−ATR], so satisfying AGREE[ATR] requires violating faithfulness to ATR, F[ATR]. The ranking AGREE[ATR] ≫ F[ATR] in (94) entails that underlying ATR values will be altered to achieve agreement in the output: a harmonic candidate is optimal unless some higher-ranked constraint is violated by the resulting ATR domain. And the constraints $\mathbb{C}_X$, $\mathbb{C}_Y$, and $\mathbb{C}_Z$ are just such constraints: in order for a harmonic [−ATR] domain to be optimal, this domain must satisfy all three of these [−ATR] domain markedness constraints. That is, [−ATR] harmony occurs only in the intersection of the three constraint-satisfying regions shown in (86), (89), and (93)—only when the resulting [−ATR] domain is the best of the best of the best, as illustrated in (85).

What about the competing outputs consisting of harmonic [+ATR] domains? The constraints governing such domains constitute the remaining constraints in this Lango analysis. They must render [+ATR] harmony suboptimal in the nonwhite cells of the data table.

4.1.8 [+ATR] domains: Banning only the worst of the worst

The set of environments in which [+ATR] harmony is optimal—the white cells of (77)—is considerably more complex than the set we just looked at, where [−ATR] harmony is optimal—the black cells. The analysis proceeds by taking the six dimensions (78) plotted in (77) and examining them a few at a time. This makes it possible to see within the [+ATR] domain inventory several BOWOW subinventories that ban only the worst of the worst.

To begin, consider the left half of the data table, which in table (95) has been carved into four subregions. On the horizontal axis, only the [±hi] dimension of the [+ATR] vowel is considered; on the vertical axis, only the 'C versus C.C' dimension. The result is shown in compact form in (96). The [+ATR] domain inventory consists of the white region. Excluded is the gray region, where the [+ATR] harmonic output loses to the faithful, disharmonic output. This picture is obviously a classic case of the BOWOW pattern, first introduced in (71c). Such an inventory is the result of a high-ranking conjunction $\mathbb{C}$ & $\mathbb{C}'$, where $\mathbb{C}$ and $\mathbb{C}'$ are the horizontal and vertical markedness dimensions of the diagram.

(95) $\mathbb{C}_1 \equiv (*[+\text{ATR},-\text{hi}] \ \& \ *V_{+A}C. \ \& \ *H_D[+\text{ATR}]) \ \&_{\mathcal{D}[\text{ATR}]} F[\text{ATR}]$

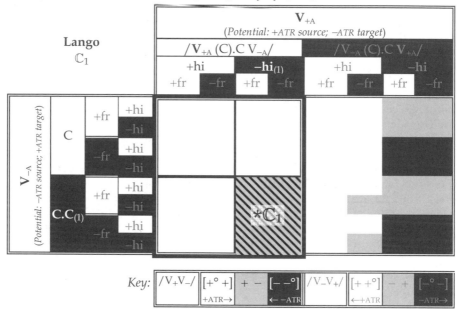

(96)   BOWOW diagram for $\mathbb{C}_1$

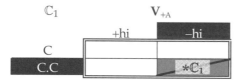

In the present case, on the horizontal axis, $\mathbb{C}$ is simply *[+ATR, −hi] (76b). On the vertical axis, $\mathbb{C}'$ is just $*V_{+A}C.$ (76c), which prohibits [+ATR] vowels in closed syllables. The conjunction of these constraints is (97).

(97) $*[+\text{ATR}, -\text{hi}] \ \& \ *V_{+A}C.$

It remains to consider the dimensions specific to the environments of the left half of (95), to which the diagram (96) is restricted. There, the head of the [+ATR] harmony candidate is on the left, in the syllable relevant to the open/closed vertical dimension. Thus, to single out the hatched gray region of (95), the conjunction (97) must be violated at the domain head; we have enhancement of (97) at the head, achieved, as in $\mathbb{C}_Y$, by the further conjunction with *H_D: (98).

(98) $*[+\text{ATR}, -\text{hi}] \ \& \ *V_{+A}C. \ \& \ *H_D[+\text{ATR}]$

Finally, all the data in table (95) involve disharmonic inputs, for which the [+ATR] harmony candidate requires unfaithfulness to ATR at the underlyingly [−ATR] vowel.

Box 2

As in (91), this demands conjunction of F[ATR], with domain $\mathcal{D}$[ATR]. This yields (99), the first of the [+ATR] domain constraints in (100a).

(99) $\mathbb{C}_1 \equiv$ (*[+ATR, −hi] & *V$_{+A}$C. & *Hd[+ATR]) & $_{\mathcal{D}[ATR]}$ F[ATR]

This final conjunction with F[ATR] is needed because without it, $\mathbb{C}_1$ would be violated not just in the [+ATR] harmonic candidate, but also in the faithful candidate, in the case of an underlying [+ATR, −hi] initial vowel in a closed syllable: in both candidates, this marked vowel heads a [+ATR] domain. Thus, in such a case, the conjunction with F[ATR] — which limits $\mathbb{C}_1$ violations to cases of actual 'spread' of [+ATR] — is necessary in order for $\mathbb{C}_1$ to achieve its function of rendering the faithful candidate optimal in the hatched gray region of (95).

(100)   [+ATR] conjunctive constraint interactions

a. $\mathbb{C}_1 \equiv$ (*[+ATR,−hi] & *Hd[+ATR] & *V$_{+A}$C.) & $_{\mathcal{D}[ATR]}$ F[ATR]
An unfaithful [+ATR] domain cannot be headed by a [−hi] vowel in a closed syllable.
"No [+ATR] spread from a [−hi] source in a closed syllable."

b. $\mathbb{C}_2 \equiv$ *[+ATR, −hi] & Hd-L[+ATR]
A [+ATR] domain cannot have a [−hi] head that is not leftmost.
"No regressive [+ATR] spread from a [−hi] source."

c. $\mathbb{C}_3 \equiv$ (*[+ATR, −fr] & Hd-L[ATR]) & $_{\mathcal{D}[ATR]}$ (*[+ATR, −hi] & *V$_{+A}$C. & F[ATR])
A [+ATR] domain with a [−fr] head that is not leftmost must be faithful at a [−hi] vowel in a closed syllable.
"No regressive [+ATR] spread from a [−fr] source onto a [−hi] vowel in a closed syllable."

It is important to recall that the verbal descriptions of the constraints in (100) are merely that: they translate into English; they do not define the constraints. The definition of each constraint is automatically determined by the general definition of constraint conjunction (73) and the basic definitions of the elementary constraints being conjoined (feature domains: (59)–(60); ATR feature: (76)).

The second [+ATR] domain constraint, (100b), can be derived with the help of table (101). Here the data are divided into four classes, drawn in more compact form in (102). Now the two dimensions are [±hi] for the [+ATR] vowel, and directionality: whether the head of the [+ATR] harmony candidate is on the left or right (or, whether [+ATR] spread is progressive or regressive).

(101) Region of violation of $\mathbb{C}_2$ by [+ATR] harmony candidates

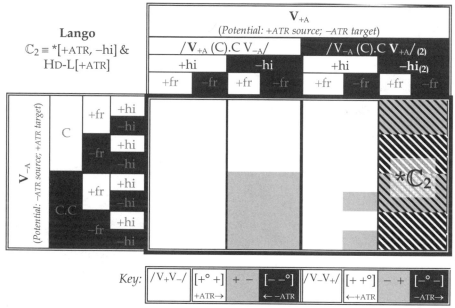

(102) BOWOW diagram for $\mathbb{C}_2$

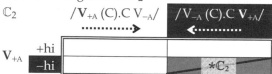

The horizontal constraint here is simply HD-L[+ATR], demanding left-headedness. The vertical constraint is *[+ATR, –hi] (76b). The resulting conjunction is (103).

(103) $\mathbb{C}_2 \equiv$ *[+ATR, –hi] & HD-L[+ATR]

The only structure violating HD-L[+ATR] is a [+ATR] domain spanning two vowels that are underlyingly [–ATR] followed by [+ATR]: /– +/ → [+ +°]. This HD-L[+ATR] violation does not occur in the faithful, disharmonic candidate, so the final conjunction '& $_{\mathcal{D}[ATR]}$ F[ATR]' needed for $\mathbb{C}_1$ is not needed here. Furthermore, the locus of a HD-L[+ATR] violation is the (right-aligned) head. Thus, violations of the conjunction (103) are already limited to [+ATR, –hi] vowels that are heads; therefore, the conjunction '& *HD[+ATR]' needed in $\mathbb{C}_1$ is also not needed here. The simple conjunction (103) suffices: we have derived (100b).

For the final constraint, consider the four cells surrounded with a heavy border in (104), where one of the cells is labeled '*$\mathbb{C}_3$'. These cells are isolated in (105).

Box 2

(104) $\mathbb{C}_3$

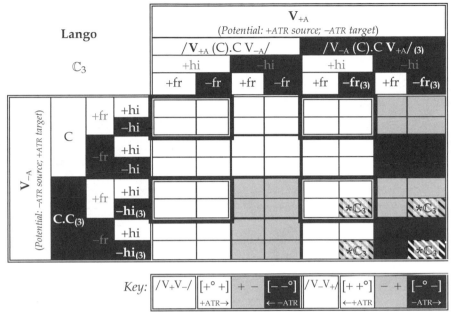

(105) BOWOW diagram for $\mathbb{C}_3$

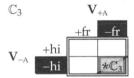

Again we see the BOWOW pattern, with horizontal constraint *[+ATR, −fr] (76a) and vertical constraint *[+ATR, −hi] (76a). The conjunction of these two constraints, sufficiently high ranked, can render the [+ATR] harmony candidate suboptimal in the gray cell of (105). But as is, this conjunction would erroneously have this same effect on cells in (104) that are white: the conjunction is violated by the [+ATR] harmony candidate in every cell located both in a row labeled [−hi] and in a column labeled [−fr], as well as every cell located both in a column labeled [−hi] and in a row labeled [−fr]. As shown in (105), the violations of $\mathbb{C}_3$ must be limited to those in which the *head* /V$_{+A}$/ is [−fr] and the nonhead /V$_{−A}$/ is [−hi], and must further be restricted to those falling in the lower right quadrant of (104), the four cells labeled '*$\mathbb{C}_3$'. This requires that the conjunction defining $\mathbb{C}_3$ include the constraint HD-L[ATR], which is violated in the right half of the table, and the constraint *V$_{+A}$C., which is violated in the lower half. And to ensure that it is the head vowel that violates *[+ATR, −fr], we can conjoin it with HD-L[ATR], with the segment as domain. To ensure that it is the nonhead (unfaithful) vowel that violates *[+ATR, −hi] , we conjoin it with F[ATR]. The result is (106), that is, (100c).

(106)　$\mathbb{C}_3 \equiv$ (*[+ATR, −fr] & HD-L[ATR]) &$_{\mathcal{D}[ATR]}$ (*[+ATR, −hi] & *V$_{+A}$C. & F[ATR])

4.1.9　The Optimality Theory account

Putting all the ATR domain constraints together, we get (107).

(107)　OT derivation of inventory

Lango OT account				/V+A (C).C V−A/ *X				/V−A (C).C V+A/ (2,3)			
				+hi*Z		−hi(1)		+hi*Z		−hi(2)	
V−A (Potential: −ATR source; +ATR target)				+fr	−fr	+fr	−fr	+fr	−fr(3)	+fr	−fr(3)
C	+fr*Y	+hi		X Y Z	X Y Z	X Y	X Y	Y Z	Y Z	Y(2)	Y(2)
		−hi		X Y Z	X Y Z	X Y	X Y	Y Z	Y Z	Y(2)	Y(2)
	−fr	+hi		X Z	X Z	X	X	Z	Z	(2)	(2)
		−hi		X Z	X Z	X	X	Z	Z	(2)	(2)
C.C(1,3)	+fr*Y	+hi		X Y Z	X Y Z	X Y(1)	X Y(1)	Y Z	Y Z	Y(2)	Y(2)
		−hi(3)		X Y Z	X Y Z	X Y(1)	X Y(1)	Y Z	Y Z(3)	Y(2)	Y(23)
	−fr	+hi		X Z	X Z	X(1)	X(1)	Z	Z	(2)	(2)
		−hi(3)		X Z	X Z	X(1)	X(1)	Z	Z(3)	(2)	(23)

Key: | /V+V−/ | [+° +] (+ATR→) | + − | [− −°] (← −ATR) | /V−V+/ | [+ +°] (←+ATR) | − + | [−° −] (−ATR→) |

Cells marked with 'X', 'Y', or 'Z' are inputs for which the [−ATR] harmony output candidate violates the indicated constraint(s), $\mathbb{C}_X$, $\mathbb{C}_Y$, or $\mathbb{C}_Z$: see diagrams (86), (89), and (93). Similarly, cells marked with '1', '2', or '3' are inputs for which the [+ATR] harmony candidate violates $\mathbb{C}_1$, $\mathbb{C}_2$, or $\mathbb{C}_3$, following (95), (101), and (104). The faithful, disharmonic candidate violates none of these constraints,[26] but violates AGREE[ATR]. Since AGREE[ATR] ≫ F[ATR] (84), the faithful candidate loses to a harmonic candidate, provided the harmony domain does not violate one of the ATR domain constraints. Thus, if a cell bears none of the marks X, Y, or Z, the [−ATR] harmony candidate is optimal (black); if a cell bears none of 1, 2, or 3, then the [+ATR] harmony candidate is optimal (white). Otherwise—in cells with both one of X, Y, Z and one of 1, 2, or 3—the disharmonic candidate wins (gray). In principle, there could be an environment

---

[26] For this purpose, I consider $\mathbb{C}_Z$ to be defined as in (91). As explained above, the simpler alternative definition (92) yields the same outcome, but generates a more complicated version of (107).

Box 2

with no marks whatever, in which case neither [+ATR] harmony nor [−ATR] harmony is blocked, and the determination of which type of harmony is optimal would arise from a further ranking (of the two harmony-driving constraints, *HD[+ATR] and *HD[−ATR]). As it happens, however, this does not arise, since the complexity of the data requires a set of [−ATR] and [+ATR] domain constraints which are rich enough that no cell escapes violating at least one of them.

Conventional OT tableaux for a number of forms are given in (108).[27] As indicated in the key in the upper left corner of (108), [±ATR] values are shown above vowels, [±hi] values directly below vowels, and [±fr] values further below. In harmonic candidates, the location of the sign of ATR marks the head of the domain, the extension of which is marked with '…'. Marks incurred by optimal forms are indicated '⊛'.

(108) Tableaux of selected Lango forms

$\pm$ATR V $\perp$hi $\pm$fr		+ATR			−ATR				
		$\mathbb{C}_1$	$\mathbb{C}_2$	$\mathbb{C}_3$	$\mathbb{C}_X$	$\mathbb{C}_Y$	$\mathbb{C}_Z$	AGREE[ATR]	F[ATR]
− + pɪ+wu + + + − 'for you' ☞ …+ piwu									⊛
− + pɪwu								*!	
− … pɪwʊ					*!	*			*
− ꟾ lɛ+wu − + + − 'your axe' ☞ …+ lewu									⊛
− + lɛwu								*!	
− … lɛwʊ					*!	*			*
− + jɔ+wu − + − − 'your people' ☞ …+ jowu									⊛
− + jɔwu								*!	
− … jɔwʊ						*!			*

---

[27] The harmony-inducing constraint AGREE[ATR] ≡ *HD[ATR] marks a disharmonic, faithful candidate relative to its [+ATR] harmonic and [−ATR] harmonic competitors. The disharmonic candidate violates *HD[ATR] twice, the harmonic candidates only once. In the tableaux, rather than two marks versus one, this preference is indicated with one mark versus zero, in effect precanceling the one *HD[ATR] mark shared by all candidates. There is no harm in this abbreviation, since *HD[ATR] is completely satisfied only when no vowels at all appear in the output, which is declared nonoptimal by undominated MAX (84).

±ATR V ±hi ±fr		+ATR			−ATR			AGREE[ATR]	F[ATR]
		$\mathbb{C}_1$	$\mathbb{C}_2$	$\mathbb{C}_3$	$\mathbb{C}_X$	$\mathbb{C}_Y$	$\mathbb{C}_Z$	AGREE[ATR]	F[ATR]
− + ɲiŋ+wu + + + − 'your name'	☞ ......+ ɲiŋwu								⊛
	− + ɲɪŋwu							*!	
	−......... ɲɪŋwʊ					*!	*		*
− + dɛk+wu − + + − 'your stew'	......+ dekwu			*!					*
	☞ − + dɛkwu							⊛	
	−......... dɛkwʊ					*!	*		*
− + lʊt+wu + + − − 'your stick'	☞ ......+ lutwu								⊛
	− + lʊtwu							*!	
	−......... lʊtwʊ						*!		*
− + lɪm+Co + + + − 'to visit'	.........+ limmo	*!							*
	☞ − + lɪmmo							⊛	
	−......... lɪmmɔ					*!			*
− + lwɔk+Co − − − − 'to wash'	......+ lwokko	*!	*						*
	− + lwɔkko							*!	
	☞ − ...... lwɔkkɔ								⊛
− + lʊb+Co + − − − 'to follow'	......+ lubbo	*!							*
	− + lʊbbo							*!	
	☞ − ...... lʊbbɔ								⊛

Box 2

±ATR V ±hi ±fr			+ATR			−ATR				
			C_1	C_2	C_3	C_X	C_Y	C_Z	AGREE[ATR]	F[ATR]
+ − cull+ɛrɛ + −	☞	+········· cullere								⊛
− + 'penis 3SG ALIEN'		+ − cullɛrɛ							*!	
		·········− cullɛrɛ				*!	*	*		*
+ − ciŋ+a + −		··· − cıŋa				*!	*			
+ − 'hand 1SG INAL'		+ − ciŋa							*!	
	☞	+ ··· ciŋə								⊛
+ − pig+na + −		········− pɪgga				*!	*			*
+ − 'juice 1SG ALIEN'		+ − pigga							*!	
	☞	+······ pɪggə								⊛
+ − gwen+na		······ − gwɛnna				*!				*
+ − 'chicken 1SG ALIEN'	☞	+ − gwenna							⊛	
		+······ gwennə	*!							*

4.1.10 WOW diagrams

To make contact with the way inventories are represented in the Appendix, I close the discussion of Lango ATR harmony with two diagrams, each depicting a cross-section of the ATR domain inventory across four of the six dimensions of the full data space. These **WOW diagrams** reveal the harmonic completeness of the inventory; they are merely multidimensional analogues of the basic BOWOW diagram (71b).

The inventory is of the /input/ → [output] mappings of [+ATR] domains in Lango. In the first diagram, (109), the inputs are specified in the top headers as either /**V**$_{+A, +H, ±F}$ (C).CV$_{−A, +F, ±H}$/ (left subcube) or /V$_{−A, +F, ±H}$(C).**CV**$_{+A, +H, ±F}$/ (right subcube), with the remaining distinctions specified by the labels for the three dimensions internal to the subcubes: C versus CC, [+hi] versus [−hi], [+fr] versus [−fr] (the marked pole of each opposition, in a [+ATR] domain, is marked '*'). Thus, for example, the cell labeled '[eC.Cu°]' denotes the mapping /εCCu/ → [eC.Cu°]. Each cell denotes a mapping from a disharmonic input to an output with [+ATR] harmony. The white cells are the legal mappings; the gray cell is barred from the inventory. That is, for this input, /εCCu/, the output with [+ATR] harmony is not grammatical; the grammatical mapping is actually faithful, with a disharmonic output. The *illegal* [+ATR] harmony output labels the gray cell in the diagram; this is the structure ruled out of the inventory. The actual grammatical output for this input, [ε°]C.C[u°], is shown pointing to the cell.

(109) Subinventory of harmonic [+ATR] domains: head {i u}, nonhead {i e}

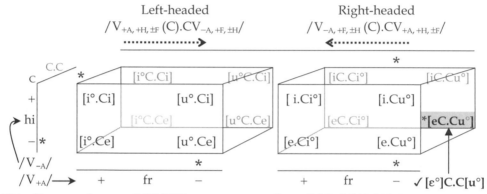

This diagram shows a BOWOW pattern—actually, a BOWOWOWOW pattern since the only banned element is worst on *four* dimensions. The harmonic completeness of this subinventory is exhibited by the fact that from any white cell, a move toward decreased markedness on any dimension leads to another white cell.

(110) Subinventory of harmonic [+ATR] domains: head {u o}, nonhead {i e}

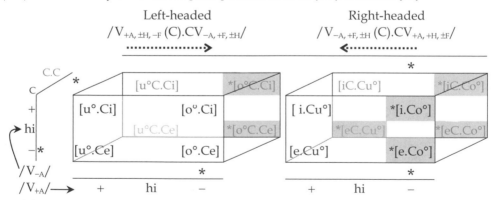

   The picture in (109) changes to (110) if in the underlying [+ATR] vowel we consider [±hi, −fr] instead of [+hi, ±fr]. Now considerably more [+ATR] domains are

Box 2

barred from the inventory. But the harmonic completeness of this subinventory is exhibited graphically just as before. (The harmonic completeness of this part of the inventory was displayed in another form in (68d).)

4.2 Typology of vowel harmony

In Chapter 12 (2a) and (72a), OT was described as having the property of **inherent typology**: every language-particular analysis is necessarily also a theory of universal typology. The representations and constraints proposed in the Lango analysis do have typological consequences. Close to home, the same constraints with different conjunctive interactions are at work in many languages related to Lango (Archangeli and Pulleyblank 1994); the harmony systems are different, and different autosegmental rules are required to describe them—but the universal constraints generating them in OT are the same as for Lango. Somewhat further afield, other harmony systems involving different features are predicted by the conjunctive interactions of the same types of markedness constraints as those at work in Lango. This is the topic of the present subsection. In the next subsection, still wider-ranging typological extrapolations of the Lango analysis are explored.

In the Lango analysis, the focus was on the conjunctive interactions among markedness constraints: M & M conjunctions. But faithfulness constraints figured crucially in these interactions too. Now the analysis will focus on M & F—markedness and faithfulness—conjunctions. The markedness constraints posited will sometimes stand in for conjunctions of more basic markedness constraints, but since it is the M & F rather than the M & M interactions that are of principal interest now, the reduction of markedness constraints to interactions of elementary constraints will be mostly overlooked.

For harmony, two general ranking schemas can be discerned.

(111) Markedness-driven harmony systems

    a. 'Harmonize except when highly marked domains result'.

        $\mathbb{C}_{blocking}[\varphi] \gg_{iii} \text{AGREE}[\varphi] \gg_{ii} F[\varphi] \gg_i M[\varphi]$

        where $\text{AGREE}[\varphi] \equiv *\text{HD}[\varphi]$; $F[\varphi] = \text{IDENT}[\varphi]$; $M[\varphi] = (\text{e.g.}) *[+\varphi, -\psi]$

      i. $F[\varphi] \gg M[\varphi]$ admits $M[\varphi]$-marked segments into the inventory.

      ii. $\text{AGREE}[\varphi] \gg F[\varphi]$ forces φ harmony in the general case.

      iii. $\mathbb{C}_{blocking}[\varphi] \gg \text{AGREE}[\varphi]$ blocks φ harmony if the result is $\mathbb{C}_{blocking}$-marked.

    b. 'Harmonize only when highly unmarked domains result'.

        $\mathbb{C}_{inducing}[\varphi] \gg_{iii} F[\varphi] \gg_{ii,i} \{\text{AGREE}[\varphi], M[\varphi]\}$

      i. $F[\varphi] \gg M[\varphi]$ admits $M[\varphi]$-marked segments into the inventory.

      ii. $F[\varphi] \gg \text{AGREE}[\varphi]$ blocks φ harmony in the general case.

      iii. $\mathbb{C}_{inducing}[\varphi] \gg F[\varphi]$ forces φ harmony if disharmony is $\mathbb{C}_{inducing}$-marked.

As the analysis of Sections 4.2.1–4.2.4 will show, the markedness of feature domains

referred to in (111a–b) can be controlled by the markedness of the domain head—
'source-conditioned' harmony (64)—or the markedness of the domain nonhead—
'target-conditioned' harmony (63)—or the markedness of a domain in relation to a
parallel domain—'sharing-conditioned' or 'parasitic' harmony (65).

4.2.1   Target-conditioned harmony I: Contrastive case (Lango)

Target-conditioned harmony can be generally characterized as follows:

(112)   Target-markedness-conditioned harmony

Harmony spreads feature φ *except* when doing so would create an especially
marked segment (or, *only* when doing so would create an especially *unmarked*
segment).

Examples of this type of harmony condition can be found in the Lango ATR harmony
system analyzed in Section 4.1. In the fragment of the Lango system shown in (113),
the now-familiar BOWOW inventory pattern can be observed—the kind of inventory
shown in Section 3 to require local constraint conjunction.

Consider the nonhead (left) position of a [+ATR] domain, and the markedness
constraint M = *[+ATR, –hi] (76a). If it is faithful, an M-marked segment (*e*) is legal:
/e u/ → [e u°] (lower left cell; gray shading shows site of M violation). If it is not M-
marked (*i*), an unfaithful segment is legal: /ɪ u/ → [i* u] (upper right cell; the '*' locates the site of unfaithful ATR, where an underlying [–ATR] *ɪ* has surfaced as [+ATR]
i). But a segment that is *both* marked *and* unfaithful (⍟) is illegal: /ɛ u/ ↛ [e* u]
(lower right cell; the oval marks the *F and *M incurred by a single segment). Examples of the disharmonic inputs (two rightmost cells) are given in (113). Subscripts
show [±ATR] values.

(113)   BOWOW diagram: Target-conditioned [+ATR] harmony in Lango

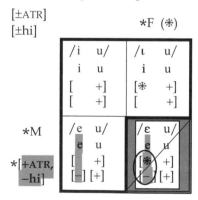

Box 2

(114) Target-conditioned [+ATR] harmony in Lango

    a. /ɲì₋ₐŋ+wú₊ₐ/ → ɲì₊ₐŋwú₊ₐ *ɲì₋ₐŋwú₊ₐ 'your_PL name'

    b. /dè₋ₐk+wú₊ₐ/ → dè₋ₐkwú₊ₐ *dè₊ₐkwú₊ₐ 'your_PL stew'

The basic conjunction at work here is M & F ≡ *[+ATR, –hi] & F[ATR]. The full conjunction involves further constraints, since the pattern shown in (113) is restricted to cases where the initial syllable is closed and the final syllable has a [+ATR, –fr] vowel (*u, o*). The full constraint was derived in Section 4.1.8: it is $\mathbb{C}_3$ of (100c). It plays the role of $\mathbb{C}_{blocking}$ in the general schema (111a); the entire schema is instantiated in the ranking shown in (84).

(115) Regressive ATR harmony conditioned by target markedness

	M & F	AGREE ≡ *HD[ATR]	F[ATR]	M ≡ *[+ATR,–hi]
/gwèn/ 'chickens'				
a. *faithful* ☞ gw[₊è]n		*		⦿ *
b. *unfaithful* gw[₋ɛ̀]n		*	*!	
/ɲìŋ+wú/ 'your_PL name'				
c. *faithful* ɲ[₋ì°]ŋw[₊ú°]		*!*		
d. *harmonic* ☞ ɲ[₊ìŋwú°]		*	⦿ *	
/dèk+wú/ 'your_PL stew'				
e. *faithful* ☞ d[₋ è°]kw[₊ú°]		*ɛ *u		
f. *harmonic* d[₊èkwú°]	*e!	*u	*e	*e

Tableaux (115) show how the conjunction conditions harmony. Subscripts show the vowels at which constraints are violated. Individual violations of M and F in optimal candidates are marked with a dotted circle; the two violations triggering the conjunction M & F are indicated with a solid oval. Other candidates are ruled out by other constraints; the full analysis of this highly complex harmony system is given in Section 4.1.

(116) Summary: Target-conditioned harmony I (contrastive)

    a. $\mathbb{C}_{blocking}$ ≡ M[φ] & F[φ] blocks φ harmony when it would produce an M[φ]-marked segment

    b. M[φ] & F[φ] permits an M[φ]-marked segment if it is underlying.

    c. This is correct when φ is contrastive, but not in the following case, where φ is noncontrastive.

4.2.2 Target-conditioned harmony II: Noncontrastive case (Kirghiz)

The conjunction schema M & F, where F = IDENT[φ] for some feature φ, gives rise to target-conditioned harmony in languages like Lango where ATR is contrastive when not subject to harmony (e.g., stem vowels will harmonize in ATR with suffix vowels under certain conditions, but are contrastive in ATR in other conditions, such as unsuffixed forms). Thus, in Lango, ATR is contrastive in the environment $V_{\pm A, -H, +F}$CCu: both /eCCu/ and /ɛCCu/ surface faithfully. Regressive [+ATR] harmony does not apply in /ɛCCu/ because the resulting initial vowel *e* would be too marked. But it is not too marked to surface in that position if it is there underlyingly. The markedness constraint violated by *e*, M, is lower ranked than F[ATR], but the conjunction M & F is higher ranked than F[ATR], blocking unfaithfulness—harmony—that would create *e*.

Suppose, however, that φ is not contrastive in an environment where harmony might occur—where its value is fixed by the environment when harmony does not apply. Benua and Smolensky (2001) analyzed such a case: progressive rounding harmony in the Turkic language Kirghiz (Hebert and Poppe 1963; Korn 1969; Johnson 1980; Steriade 1981; Kaun 1995). A suffix vowel must agree in backness with the stem, and must agree in roundness with the stem except when this would produce *o*, in which case *o*'s [−rd] counterpart, *a*, must appear (except under height agreement, to be discussed in Section 4.2.4.2). Thus, in Kirghiz we find the past definite *tut-tu* 'hold' and the past participle *kör-gön* 'see', but the past participle *tut-kan* (**tut-kon*).

In every case, the only contrastive feature of the suffix vowel is [±hi]: the surface values of [±bk] and [±rd] are fixed by the stem. By Richness of the Base, we are not entitled to assume any particular underlying values for the noncontrastive features. Underlying surface *tut-kan* might be /tut-kon/, in which case the faithful candidate must be suboptimal. But unlike in the contrastive case (Lango), here M & F[rd] will not work: the faithful output for /tut-kon/ of course satisfies F[rd], hence M & F[rd]. Here M ≡ M₀ is the relevant markedness constraint, violated by *o* but satisfied by *a*, *ö*, and *u*.[28]

But the theory of headed feature domains developed in Section 2 provides a second faithfulness constraint, F°[rd], which requires an underlying [+rd] vowel to have an output correspondent that *heads* a [+rd] domain (and similarly for [−rd]). The conjunction M & F°[rd] achieves the necessary results when it is ranked above F[ATR] (and M and F°[ATR] are ranked sufficiently low). With left-headed [rd] domains, M & F°[rd] targets noninitial vowels. The initial stem vowel heads a [rd] domain, satisfying F°[rd] and hence M & F°[rd], so the conjunction tolerates *o* in stem-initial position. In any other output position within a [rd] domain, however, *o* violates the conjunction, and is banned, even if the segment is underlying /o/: see tableaux (117) (*bol* 'become').

---

[28] The exact formulation of M₀ is not relevant here, and while it is not clear just how to best define M₀, the relative markedness of *o* in Turkic is evident. That Turkic [rd] harmony favors targets that are high or front is clear from the typological surveys of Korn 1969 and Kaun 1995, 27, 60-64.

Box 2

This analysis predicts the impossibility of *CuCo* morphemes, and indeed Kirghiz lacks stems and disyllabic affixes with *CuCo* melody; unharmonized *CuCa* is found, however.

A BOWOW diagram for the conjunction M&F°[rd] is shown in (118). At a [rd] head, an M-marked segment (*o*) is legal: /o u/ → [o° u] violates M at *o* (gray shading) and violates F°[rd] at *u* (dotted circle), but these are different segments and the local conjunction is satisfied. At a [rd] nonhead, an M-unmarked segment (*ö*) is legal: /u ö/ → [u° ö] violates F°[rd] at *ö* but this segment satisfies M (which penalizes only *o*). But a single segment that is *both* marked *and* a nonhead is illegal: */u o/ → [u° o] violates both M and F°[rd] in the same segment *o*, violating the high-ranked conjunction that blocks [rd] harmony (the grammatical output for /u o/ is [u°][a°]). The result is summarized in (119).

(117) Kirghiz harmony in noncontrastive [rd]

			M & F°[rd]	Hᴅ-L[rd]	*Hᴅ[rd]	F°[rd]	F[rd]	M
/bol + dɨ/								
a.	*faithful*	bo°ldɨ°			*o *ɨ!			*o
b.	[−*rd*] *harmony*	baldɨ°		*ɨ	*ɨ	*a	*a	
c.	[+*rd*] *harmony* ☞	bo°ldu			*o	*u	*u	*o
/tut + ɢon/								
d.	*antiharmonic* ☞	tu°tka°n			*u *a	*a	*a	
e.	*harmonic*	tu°tkon	*o!		*u	*o		*o

(118) BOWOW diagram: Kirghiz [rd] domains

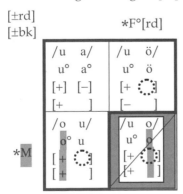

(119) Summary: Target-conditioned harmony II (noncontrastive)

    a. $\mathbb{C}_{blocking}$ ≡ M[φ] & F°[φ] permits an M[φ]-marked segment only at a φ head. Suppose HD-L[φ] undominated; then:

    b. M[φ] & F°[φ] blocks φ agreement when that entails a noninitial M[φ]-marked segment X ...

          ... whether X is underlying or created by spread;

          this is essential for target-conditioned harmony when φ is noncontrastive, by Richness of the Base.

    'Noninitial' means 'not the leftmost segment of a contiguous string of [±φ]-bearing segments'.

4.2.3 Source-conditioned harmony (Lango)

Target-conditioned harmony systems are obviously to be expected within OT, where the harmonic output competes with a nonharmonic output and markedness of the target segment can make the decision. Less obvious is source-conditioned harmony.

(120) Source-markedness-conditioned harmony

    Harmony spreads feature φ except when the source is especially marked (or, only when the source is especially unmarked).

In the competition between the harmonic and nonharmonic outputs, the target segments differ in their φ values, but the sources are identical. The markedness of the source contributes equally to the Harmony of both candidates, and cancels; how can it matter?

On the theory developed here, the explanation is to be sought not in the markedness of *segments* but in the markedness of *feature domains*. In the harmonic candidate, source and target are in the same φ domain; in the disharmonic candidate, they are not. The harmonic domain has a degree of markedness determined by the markedness of the segments it spans, relative to their structural roles within the domain: say that the source is the domain head, and the target is a nonhead. In the case of interest, the target is unfaithful: its underlying φ value is altered on the surface to agree with that of the source. Thus, the competition determining whether harmony occurs is between the harmonic candidate in which the source heads a domain that includes the φ-unfaithful target, and the faithful candidate in which the source and target are in different φ domains.

Source-markedness-conditioned harmony arises from a well-formedness constraint $\mathbb{C}_{blocking}$ evaluating φ domains in which the constraint violations of the source and the target interact conjunctively. More specifically, it is the markedness of the head, M°[φ], and the faithfulness of the target, F[φ] ≡ IDENT[φ], that conjoin. Schematically:

(121) $\mathbb{C}_{blocking}$ = M°[φ] & $_{\mathcal{D}[φ]}$ F[φ]

Box 2

The domain of conjunction is obviously the φ domain, since the constraint evaluates φ domains: its ranking governs the inventory of such domains in a language.

The markedness of a domain's head M°[φ] is evaluated by the conjunction M°[φ] ≡ M[φ] & *HD[φ]: M[φ] assesses the markedness of the head segment qua segment, *HD[φ] is violated at the domain head, and the conjunction evaluates the markedness of the segment qua domain head; the conjunction domain is clearly the segment. Thus, (121) becomes (122).

(122) Constraint inducing source-markedness-conditioned harmony

$$\mathbb{C}_{\text{blocking}} \equiv (M[\varphi]\ \&\ {}^*HD[\varphi])\ \&_{\mathcal{D}[\psi]}\ F[\varphi]$$

(123) BOWOW diagram: Lango harmonic [−ATR] domains

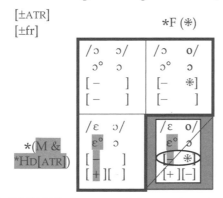

A BOWOW diagram of this conjunctive interaction (122) is shown in (123). The domain constraint (122) is in fact exactly $\mathbb{C}_Y$ (90) in the Lardil analysis with φ ≡ [−ATR]. Progressive [−ATR] harmony does not occur when the source violates the markedness constraint *[−ATR, +fr] ≡ M: it does not occur with source ε, but does with ɔ. '❋' indicates an unfaithful segment, while shading identifies a marked head, violating M[φ] & *HD[φ]. Examples and tableaux are provided in (124) and (125). As (123) shows, if its $\mathcal{D}$[ATR] is faithful, an M-marked head [ε°] is legal: /ε ɔ/ → [ε° ɔ] (gray in lower left cell; (124a.i)). If its head is M-unmarked [ɔ°], an unfaithful $\mathcal{D}$[ATR] is legal: /ɔ o/ → [ɔ° ɔ] (❋ in upper right cell; (124b.ii)). But a $\mathcal{D}$[ATR] that is *both* headed by a marked segment *and* unfaithful is illegal: /ε o/ ↛ [ε° ɔ] (oval in lower right cell; (124b.i)).

(124) Lango data

    a. Alternation of -o/ɔ (object marker, transitive verb, nominal object)

        In environment εC—, o/ɔ may be determined by underlying lexical ATR value; in ɔC—, only ɔ may appear. (Examples from Woock and Noonan 1979.)

    i.   àpyɛ́tɔ̀ kàl   'I sieved the millet'
    ii. àwɛ́kò àtín   'I left the child'
    iii. àlwɔ́kɔ̀ àtín   'I washed the child'
    iv. *⋯ɔCo

  b.   Alternation of -Co (infinitive marker)
       In environment εC—, only Co appears; in ɔC—, only Cɔ.
       i.   nɛnno   'to see'
       ii. lwɔkkɔ   'to wash'

(125) Progressive [−ATR] harmony conditioned by source markedness

	(M & *Hᴅ) & $\mathcal{D}_{[ATR]}$ F	Aɢʀᴇᴇ[ATR] ≡ *Hᴅ[ATR]	F	M
/lwɔk + Co/ *unmarked source*				
a. *faithful* lw[−ɔ°]kk[₊o°]		*ɔ *o!		
b. *harmonic* ☞ lw[₊ɔ° kk…ɔ.]		*ɔ	*ɔ	
/nɛn + Co/ *marked source*				
c. *faithful* ☞ n[−ɛ°]nn[₊o°]		*ɛ *o		*ɛ
d. *harmonic* n[₊ɛ° nn…ɔ.]	*𝒟!	(*ɛ)	(*ɔ)	(*ɛ)

4.2.4 Sharing-conditioned ('parasitic') harmony

In previous sections, we have considered implications of constraints M[φ] & F[φ] where M[φ] is a feature co-occurrence constraint determining the markedness of [±φ] in different featural contexts. A new structure introduced in the headed feature domain theory, the head itself, introduces a new markedness constraint, *Hᴅ[φ]—the instance of the *Sᴛʀᴜᴄᴛᴜʀᴇ family pertaining to the new structure. And feature domain heads add a new type of faithfulness constraint, F°[φ], which asserts that beyond expressing the underlying [±φ] feature in virtue of lying in a matching [±φ] domain, a segment must express the feature in the way distinguished by the head—it must 'project a [±φ] head'.

    Applying the same constraint schema above—conjoined markedness and faithfulness—to the new markedness and new faithfulness constraints yields a surprising result. (126) successively paraphrases the meaning of this M & F.

(126) M & F = *Hᴅ[φ] & F°[ψ]
    For example: *Hᴅ[ATR] & F°[hi]
    a.   A *Hᴅ[ATR] violator must be an F°[hi] satisfier.

Box 2

b. The head of an ATR domain must be a faithful head of a [hi] domain.
c. A [±ATR] initiator must be a [±hi] initiator.
d. If *X* doesn't initiate [±hi], *X* can't initiate [±ATR].
e. If *X* shares [±hi], *X* must share [±ATR].
f. **Parasitic harmony**. ATR harmony is dependent on [hi] agreement.

Yet another formulation: since *HD[φ] = AGREE[φ], the conjunction *HD[ATR] & F°[hi] "turns on" AGREE[ATR] when F°[hi] is violated—that is, when [hi] is shared.

It has been *segmental* markedness that regulates harmony in the previous discussions, but here it is *feature domain* markedness. In fact, it is the markedness of the *relations between domains* that is critical—specifically, the relative positions of their *heads*.

Section 4.2.4 briefly summarizes part of an analysis of parasitic harmony due to Benua and Smolensky (2001).

4.2.4.1 Javanese ATR harmony

The harmony system we now consider is the height-stratified ATR harmony in Eastern Javanese (Schlindwein 1988; Archangeli and Pulleyblank 1994): vowels harmonize in [±ATR] if they agree in height. The relevant conjunction is exactly the one spelled out in (126). The vowel inventory is that of Lango (77): a symmetrical 10-vowel inventory, with [+ATR] and [−ATR] at each place. The basic distribution of [ATR] is determined by vowel height and syllable structure—two factors also operating in Lango ATR harmony. High and mid vowels are [+ATR], except in closed syllables, where they are [−ATR]; low vowels are [−ATR], except in word-final open syllables, where they are [+ATR]. Thus, dominating F[ATR] are the constraints relating [±ATR] and [±hi] (76b); dominating these are constraints relating [±ATR] and syllable structure, including $*V_{+A}C$. (76c). And dominating these is the harmony-inducing conjunction *HD[ATR] & F°[hi] (126). The tableaux in (127) illustrate.

In the first input, the vowels do not agree in height, and the optimal output has ATR values determined by the height- and syllable-structure-dependent phonotactic constraints. In the second input, the vowels share height and harmony is optimal. (The sign of this harmonic [±ATR] domain is determined by the phonotactics. Dotted circles identify F°[hi] violations; gray shading, *HD violations; and solid ovals, violations of the conjunction.) Note that the optimal candidate (127b′) violates both constraints in the conjunction, but at different vowels, so it does not violate the *local* conjunction. Candidate (127d′) shows that the heads of the ATR and [hi] domains coincide in the optimal candidate; whether the heads are left- or right-aligned is not phonologically significant in Javanese, since it is not directionality but phonotactics that determines the [±ATR] value.

(127) ATR harmony stratified by [hi]: Eastern Javanese

[±ATR] [±hi]		*HD[ATR] & F°[hi]	*V_{+A}C.	*[−ATR, +hi]	AGREE[ATR] ≡ *HD[ATR]	F°[hi]
/V_{±A, +H} j V_{±A, −H} n/						
a. *phonotactic* ☞	i jɛn [+][−] [+][−]				**	
b. *harmonic* [−ATR]	ɪ jɛn [−] [+][−]			*!	*	
c. *harmonic* [+ATR]	i jen [+] [+][−]		*!		*	
/t V_{±A, +H} l V_{±A, +H} s/						
a'. *phonotactic*	tu lɪs [ ][ ] [ ]	*ɪ!		*ɪ	*u (*ɪ)	(*ɪ)
b'. *harmonic* ☞ [−ATR]	tʊ lɪs [ ] [+]			**	(*ʊ)	(*ɪ)
c'. *harmonic* [+ATR]	tu lis [+] [ ]		*!		*u	*i
d'. *harmonic* [−ATR] (*variant*)	tʊ lɪs [ ] [ ]	*ɪ!		*ɪ	(*ɪ)	(*ɪ)

A diagram of the BOWOW pattern corresponding to the harmony-inducing conjunction is given in (128).

(128) BOWOW diagram: Javanese ATR harmony parasitic on [hi]

[±ATR] [±hi]

*F°[hi]

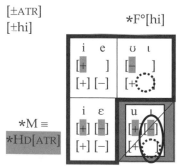

*M ≡ *HD[ATR]

Box 2

The marks defining the cells in (128) concern the second vowel. If it is a [hi] head, satisfying F°[hi], an ATR head is legal, despite its violation of *HD[ATR] (gray shading): [i][ɛ] is a grammatical configuration of [+ATR] and [hi] domains. If the second vowel is not an ATR head, thereby satisfying *HD[ATR], a [hi] nonhead is legal, notwithstanding its violation of F°[hi] (dotted circle): [ʊ ɪ] too is legal. But a segment that is *both* an ATR head *and* a [hi] nonhead violates the conjunction *HD[ATR] & F°[hi] (oval) and renders the structure *[u][ɪ] illegal.

4.2.4.2 Kirghiz [round] harmony, continued

The methods developed here can be used to complete the description of Benua and Smolensky's (2001) account of Kirghiz [rd] harmony. The complication remaining after the analysis summarized in Section 4.2.2 involves a sharing-conditioned exception. Recall from Section 4.2.2 that Kirghiz progressive [+rd] harmony is generally blocked when it would create the M_0-marked vowel [+rd, –hi, +bk] *o* (/tut + gV$_{-H}$n/ → *tutkan*, **tutkon* 'held'). Exceptionally, however, marked *o* is created by harmony when source and target share height: /bol + gV$_{-H}$n/ → *bolgon* 'became'. Tableaux (129) show the effect of the sharing-conditioned-harmony-inducing constraint F°[hi] & *HD[rd] dominating the target-conditioned-harmony-blocking constraint M_0 & F°[rd]. Since [rd] is not contrastive in Kirghiz, the suffix /-gV$_{-H}$n/ must produce the correct output whether the underlying vowel is *a* or *o*; both inputs are shown in (129), with parenthesized marks resulting when the underlying vowel is *o*. (The candidates evaluated all have left-headed [rd] and [hi] domains, satisfying the corresponding undominated HD-L constraints.)

(129) Blocking$_{\text{sharing harmony}}$ blocking$_{\text{target harmony}}$ in Kirghiz [rd] harmony

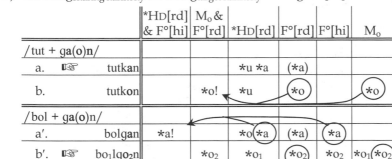

	*HD[rd] & F°[hi]	M_0 & F°[rd]	*HD[rd]	F°[rd]	F°[hi]	M_0
/tut + ga(o)n/						
a. ☞ tutkan			*u *a	(*a)		
b. tutkon		*o!	*u	(*o)		*o
/bol + ga(o)n/						
a'. bolgan	*a!		*o(*a)	(*a)	*a	
b'. ☞ bo₁lgo₂n		*o₂	*o₁	(*o₂)	*o₂	*o₁(*o₂)

In (129a'), the higher-ranked conjunction blocks the blocking normally resulting from the lower-ranked conjunction (129b).

4.2.4.3 Summary

Target-conditioned harmony systems are governed by the markedness of an individual *segment*, the target; such systems are immediately predicted by the markedness-driven competition in OT. Source-conditioned systems are more subtle, but these too are predicted by OT competition given the notion of *feature domain*, a structure whose markedness depends on the markedness of its constituents: crucially, the segmental markedness of its head—the harmony 'source'. Segmental markedness effects are evident in these systems—but not in sharing-conditioned systems, which would seem to be completely unrelated to the others. Yet the existence of *heads* of feature domains entails markedness constraints integral to OT—economy of structure, or *STRUCTURE constraints—and we have seen that this new type of markedness is what unifies parasitic harmony systems with the others.

(130) Summary: Sharing-conditioned ('parasitic') harmony

    a. Sharing-conditioned harmony occurs only when compelled by the conjunction *HD[φ] & F°[ψ].

    b. If ψ is shared, then φ domains must be minimized. That is, a head of a φ domain must be a faithful head of a ψ domain.

4.3 Summary

Four kinds of conjunctions of the form M & F have been seen to give rise to harmony systems of different types.

(131) Harmony systems from conjunction of markedness and faithfulness constraints

    a. M[φ] & F[φ]: target-conditioned harmony, φ contrastive

    b. M[φ] & F°[φ]: target-conditioned harmony, φ noncontrastive

    c. *HD[φ] & F°[ψ]: φ harmony parasitic on ψ agreement

    d. (M[φ] & *HD[φ]) &$_{\mathcal{D}[\varphi]}$ F[φ]: source-conditioned harmony

5 TYPOLOGY OF CONJUNCTIVE FEATURE-DOMAIN INTERACTIONS

We have just seen that headed feature domains, evaluated by basic constraints interacting via ranking and conjunction, generate vowel harmony systems shaped by the markedness of the harmony target, the harmony source, and the relationships between domain heads for different features. Systematic exploration of the full typology of systems arising from the possible conjunctive interactions of basic headed-feature-domain constraints is an enormous task, and the analyses of the previous section constitute only the beginning of this project. This section attempts a first, speculative look at the wider typology generated by conjunctive interaction of feature domain constraints. The modest objective is simply to begin to characterize the *types of patterns* predicted by this typology. Particular phonological phenomena will be used to instantiate these patterns, but that is merely for the sake of rendering the abstract patterns concrete; no empirical claims whatever are intended. Should it ultimately prove possible to develop these fragmentary phonological illustrations into empirically adequate theories, the typology explored here would provide an interesting formal integration of a diverse range of seemingly unrelated phonological phenomena.

Box 2

Table (132) depicts a typological space in which basic constraints of headed feature domains interact conjunctively: a given cell concerns the conjunction of the constraints labeling its row and column. All but one are conjunctions of two constraints; a single three-way conjunction, *[φ, φ'] & *HD[φ'] & $_{\mathcal{D}[φ']}$ F[φ'], appears in the lower left corner (❶), to include the analysis of source-conditioned harmony from Section 4.2.3. (See also Itô and Mester 2002 regarding the implications some of these conjunctions have for the analysis of phonological opacity phenomena, and Łubowicz 2002 for markedness/faithfulness conjunction accounts of "derived environment" effects.)

(132) Typology: Binary conjunctions of basic headed-feature-domain constraints

&		MARKEDNESS — *[φ, φ'']	MARKEDNESS — *HD[φ]	FAITHFULNESS — F[φ]	FAITHFULNESS — F°[φ]
MARKEDNESS	*[φ, φ']	No φ'-marked where φ''-marked: [BOWOW] ❷	φ-marked segment only created by spreading ③	φ-marked segment not created by spreading (φ contrastive): target-conditioned harmony ❸	φ-marked segment not created by spreading (φ noncontrastive): target-conditioned harmony ❹ ⑦
	↑ → Source-	*HD[φ']	φ head must receive φ' by spreading: nasal place assimilation ②	No φ' head where φ unfaithful: epenthetic weakness ⑤	No φ head at φ' nonhead: φ' harmony parasitic on φ agreement (underlying or derived) ❺
FAITHFULNESS	condi-tioned	harmony → ❶	F[φ']	No φ' unfaithful where φ unfaithful: chain shift ①	If share φ, must be faithful to φ': geminate inalterability ⑥
				F°[φ']	If share φ, must be a φ' head: OCP ④

There are 10 binary conjunctions in this table; 4 of them have already been considered, and are shaded gray. These include the basic conjunction of two featural markedness constraints yielding the central BOWOW pattern, *[φ, φ'] & *[φ, φ''] (❷; Section 3); the conjunction of featural markedness and faithfulness, yielding target-conditioned harmony for a feature that is contrastive (*[φ, φ'] & F[φ], ❸; Section 4.2.1) or noncontrastive (*[φ, φ'] & F°[φ], ❹; Section 4.2.2); and the conjunction of head markedness with head faithfulness, HD[φ] & F°[ψ], resulting in parasitic harmony (❺; Section 4.2.4). We will return in Section 5.7 for a glimpse of another type of behavior from the conjunction $*[\varphi, \varphi'] \& F°[\varphi]$.

To address the remaining six cells in the most space-efficient fashion, in each of the following subsections I briefly sketch one example that illustrates one of the predicted conjunctive interactions. The circled numbers (white disks) in table (132) indicate the relevant subsection (e.g., the conjunction type $*HD[\varphi'] \& F[\varphi]$, labeled ⑤, is considered in Section 5.5). I repeat that these illustrations are not proposed as serious phonological analyses. In particular, the constraints posited are designed purely for convenience in illustrating the range of patterns of conjunctive constraint *interaction*.

5.1 $F[\varphi] \& F[\varphi']$: Chain shifts

The conjunction $F[\varphi] \& F[\varphi']$ was proposed by Kirchner (1995, 1996) to explain synchronic chain shifts (vowel raising). Tableaux (133) illustrate with a chain shift in child English reported by Smith (1973, 149): *sick* comes out [θɪk] but *thick* is pronounced [fɪk]. Such chain shifts exemplify a class of opacity phenomena known in rule-based theory as **counterfeeding**: one shift along the chain fails to feed the next one. In OT terms, these cases manifest **overfaithfulness**: by refusing to move more than one step in the chain, each element remains more faithful than it would be if it moved to fully minimize markedness. It makes intuitive sense that such overfaithfulness is the conjunctive effect of multiple faithfulness constraints.

(133) Chain shift: Child English

		F[strident] & F[place]	M_s	M_θ	M_f	F[strident]	F[place]
/θɪk/ →							
a.	[sɪk]		*!			*	
b.	[θɪk]			*!			
c. ☞	[fɪk]				⊛		⊛
/sɪk/ →							
a'.	[sɪk]		*!				
b'. ☞	[θɪk]			⊛		⊛	
c'.	[fɪk]	*!			*	*	*

5.2 $*HD[\varphi] \& *HD[\varphi']$: Nasal place assimilation

To satisfy the constraint $*HD[\varphi] \& *HD[\varphi']$, a φ head X must not be also a φ' head. That is, X must share φ' with another segment that can serve as the domain head; in processual terms, X must receive its φ' value by spreading. In languages such as Lardil (Prince and Smolensky 1993/2004, Chap. 7), a noncoronal coda nasal must share place with a following consonant; onset nasals are unrestricted. Consider first

Box 2

the noncoronal case. The conjunction *HD[+nas(al)] & *HD[place] & NOCODA is violated by a coda segment that heads a [+nas] domain and also a place domain. The legal NC clusters will have the place head at C and the [nas] head at N. Rather than presenting multiple tableaux, in (134) I show how various configurations fare with respect to the conjunction; violations (solid ovals) occur just in the cases that violate the assimilation requirement. Assume HD-L[nas] is undominated; only left-headed [nas] domains can be optimal.

(134) Nasal assimilation: $\mathbb{C} \equiv$ *HD[+nas] & *HD[place] & NOCODA

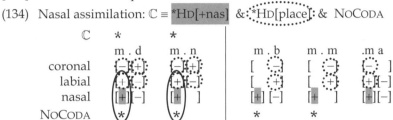

Now a grammar like Lardil's requiring that a coda nasal assimilate to a following segment if there is one, and neutralize to the least marked place [cor], *n*, otherwise, can be constructed as follows. Express the universal place markedness hierarchy as [*HD$_{[lab]}$ ≫ *HD$_{[cor]}$] = $\mathcal{H}_{Pl}$, and conjoin this hierarchy with *I ID[+nas] & NOCODA, preserving the universal ranking; this generates two place-specific versions of $\mathbb{C}$ (134), ranked [$\mathbb{C}_{[lab]}$ ≫ $\mathbb{C}_{[cor]}$] ≡ $\mathbb{C}_{Pl}$. Then rank F[place] as $\mathbb{C}_{Pl}$ ≫ F_{Pl} ≫ $\mathcal{H}_{Pl}$, and rank other faithfulness constraints so as to block any unfaithfulness except to the nasal's place. Then /onba/ → *omba*, *onba* (*$\mathbb{C}_{[cor]}$), while /om/ → *on* (*$\mathbb{C}_{[cor]}$), *om* (*$\mathbb{C}_{[lab]}$).

5.3 *HD[φ] & *[φ, φ′]: Vowel nasalization

To satisfy the conjunction *HD[φ] & *[φ, φ′], a featurally marked segment *X* violating *[φ, φ′] must not head a φ domain: *X* must be a nonhead of a shared φ domain. *X* "can only be derived by spreading"; it cannot surface as result of faithfulness to an input *X*. Consider a language in which vowels are nasalized if and only if they precede a nasal consonant, as in English (Hammond 1999, 8ff.). The idea of the analysis is that, relative to consonants, vowels are marked as heads of [nas] domains—both [+nas] and [−nas]. The role of the constraint *[φ, φ′] is played by the markedness hierarchy *V$_{+N}$ ≡ *Ṽ ≡ *[+nas, +voc(oid), +syll(abic)] ≫ *[−nas, +voc, +syll] ≡ *V$_{−N}$; *HD[φ] is *HD[nas]. The conjunction of interest is between *HD[nas] and the hierarchy; this yields *HD[nas] & *V$_{+N}$ ≫ *HD[nas] & *V$_{−N}$. Actually, it suffices for present purposes to encapsulate this simply as *HD[nas] & *V$_{±N}$; the distinction in ranking of the two conjunctions is not critical.

Assume HD-R[nas] is undominated. For the relevant faithfulness constraint, F[nas] ≡ IDENT[nas], distinguish between consonant and vowel: F_C[nas] and F_V[nas]. Then the tableaux (135) illustrate a ranking that gives the correct distribution.

The difference between the pattern here and the one in Section 5.2 is that here, the segments eliminated by neutralization (Ṽ) are marked in a context free sense; in place assimilation, the segment eliminated is not the one with most marked place in the context-free sense: it is not neutralization to *n* but neutralization to the following consonant's place, no matter how marked. In the latter case, the conjunction *HD[+nas] & *HD[Pl] says, 'If X is a source of nasality, X can't be a source of place'; in the present case, *HD[nas] & *V$_{\pm N}$ says, 'If X is a source of nasality, X can't be a vowel'. Crucially, it doesn't say, 'If X is nasal, X can't be a vowel': that's what the basic markedness constraint *Ṽ says. X *can* be both nasal and a vowel, as long as it is not the *source* of nasality; this is what the conjunction prohibits.

(135)   Vowel nasalization: *HD[nas] & *V$_{\pm N}$ ≡ {*HD[nas] & *V$_{-N}$ ≫ *HD[nas] & *V$_{+N}$}

	*HD[nas] & *V$_{\pm N}$	F$_C$[nas]	*Ṽ	F$_V$[nas]	*HD[nas]	*V$_{-N}$
/nã/ →						
nã°	*ã		(*ã)		(*ã)	
☞ n°a°	*a			*a	*n(*a)	(*a)
/tãk/ →						
t°ã°k°	*ã!		(*ã)		*t(*ã)*k	
t°ãŋ°		*ŋ!	*ã		*t *ŋ	*a
☞ tak°				*a	*k	
/tan/ →						
ta°n°	*a!				(*a)*n	(*a)
☞ t°ãn°			*ã	*ã	*t *n	
nãn°		*n!	*ã	*ã	*n	
tat°		*t!			*t	*a
/tãn/ →						
☞ t°ãn°			*ã		*t *n	
ta°n°	*a!			*a	(*a)*n	(*a)

5.4 F°[φ] & F°[φ′]: Obligatory Contour Principle effects

A segment violating F°[φ] is necessarily similar to an adjacent segment in at least one respect: they have the same value of [±φ]. To violate the conjunction F°[φ] & F°[φ′], a segment must be similar to its neighbors in at least the features φ and φ′. Consider the example in (136), which shows seven pairs of consonants adjacent on the consonantal tier; it is assumed that HD-L[φ] and HD-L[φ′] are undominated. The pairs that violate the conjunction F°[place] & F°[cont(inuant)] & F°[son(orant)] ≡ ℂ, the first four pairs, are exactly those that violate the following generalization: if adjacent consonants agree in place, they can't agree in manner. This generalization was stated for the consonants of an Arabic root by McCarthy (1994), who attributed this type of ef-

Box 2

fect to the Obligatory Contour Principle (OCP; Leben 1973; Goldsmith 1976; McCarthy 1979). Just like the OCP, $\mathbb{C}$ penalizes tier-adjacent consonants that are identical in some respects.

This example is intended to help unpack the meaning of constraints of type $F°[\phi]$ & $F°[\phi']$; to become a serious proposal for explaining the Arabic facts, the analysis would need to overcome a number of obstacles. For example, the constraint may be violated if a segment shares some of the targeted features with a left neighbor, and the others with a right neighbor, but not all of them with either neighbor; similarly, if some (but not all) of the domains in (136) are made right-headed, pairs that share all features do not violate the constraint. (Note, however, that both problems are eliminated if the relevant domains are required to be all left- or all right-headed.) Analysis of the OCP as local conjunction (without feature domains) has been proposed by Itô and Mester (1996, 1998); Alderete (1997); Suzuki (1998); and Fukazawa (1999).

(136)   OCP: Arabic root consonants. $\mathbb{C} \equiv F°[Pl]$ & $F°[cont]$ & $F°[son]$; 'c/d' = [coronal/dorsal] place

5.5 F[φ] & *Hᴅ[φ']: Epenthetic weakness

In the conjunction $F[\phi]$ & *Hᴅ$[\phi']$, let the faithfulness constraint be Dᴇᴘ, rather than Iᴅᴇɴᴛ: $F[\phi] \equiv$ Dᴇᴘ. Then the conjunction is violated by an epenthetic segment (violating Dᴇᴘ) that is the head of a φ' domain. That is, to satisfy this constraint, an epenthetic segment must share φ' with an adjacent segment. For example, in Lardil, subminimal (monosyllabic) words are augmented with a final syllable, by inserting either a final vowel, or an entire final CV. In the latter case, the place of the epenthetic C must be shared with that of the preceding consonant. This can be seen as simply the result of conjunctive interaction of Dᴇᴘ[C] and *Hᴅ[place]. In fact, many sorts of 'epenthetic weakness', where epenthetic segments do not 'license' properties found in other segments, can in this way be understood simply as conjunctive interaction between a faithfulness constraint of the Dᴇᴘ family and a markedness constraint of the *Hᴅ family (137). To take just one more example, Dᴇᴘ[V] & *Hᴅ[Foot] is violated if an epenthetic vowel is the head of a foot, that is, stressed; this is Hᴇᴀᴅ-Dᴇᴘ of Alderete 1995, 1999. This proves to be a profitable way of understanding the tendency for epenthetic vowels to be 'invisible' to stress.

(137)   Dᴇᴘ[φ] & *Hᴅ[φ']: Epenthetic weakness

An epenthetic φ segment must receive its φ' value from a neighbor.

More generally, any constraint of the form DEP[φ] & M requires that an epenthetic φ segment not be an M-marked segment.

5.6 F°[φ] & F[φ']: Geminate inalterability

To satisfy the conjunction F°[φ] & F[φ'], a segment that shares φ must be faithful in φ'; sharing φ strengthens faithfulness to φ'. It may be possible to illustrate this type of conjunctive interaction with geminate inalterability. Two segments constituting a geminate share features, and in some cases this might conceivably be the origin of the greater faithfulness exhibited by geminates, resisting "processes" that corresponding nongeminates undergo.

In the Semitic language Tigrinya, postvocalic velar consonants spirantize—except geminates (Kenstowicz 1982; Schein and Steriade 1986). Assuming undominated HD-L[vel(ar)], tableaux (138) show how conjunctive interaction of F[cont] and F°[vel] can enable geminates to resist the spirantization demanded by a constraint we can gloss as SPIR. Violations of F°[vel] are marked with ✳; gray shading marks violations of F[cont].

(138) F°[vel] & F[cont]: Geminate inalterability in Tigrinya

[±vel] [±cont]	F°[vel] & F[cont]	SPIR	F[cont]	F°[vel] ✳
/ak/ ☞ a x [+] [+]			⊛	
a k [+] [−]		*!		
/akk/				
a x k (✳ +] [+][−]	*!		*	*
a x x (✳ +] [+]	*!		*	*
☞ a k k (✳+] [✳ −]		⊛		⊛

(Note that this analysis proceeds identically if spirantization is treated as spreading of [+cont] from the vowel to the following consonant. What matters is only that the consonant is unfaithful to [cont]; whether it heads its [+cont] domain is irrelevant. For

Box 2

this reason, it also makes no difference whether the [+cont] domain of the geminate velar fricative *xx* is left- or right-headed.)

5.7 *[φ, φ'] & F°[φ]: Lexically conditioned phonological markedness

I would like to close this section by pointing out an interesting type of application for the conjunction type *[φ, φ'] & F°[φ], different from noncontrastive target-conditioned harmony, to which it was applied in Section 4.2.2. The idea is to consider the possibility that φ is a nonphonological feature. Specifically, suppose [±φ] ≡ [±Yam(ato)], a feature indicating whether a morpheme is part of the native Yamato stratum of the Japanese lexicon; in this stratum, Lyman's Law asserts that a morpheme may contain at most one voiced obstruent (Itô and Mester 1986). This constraint relates to markedness because the class of segments in which [+voi(ce)] is marked is exactly the class of obstruents—so Lyman's Law permits only one segment with a *marked* [+voi] specification: there is no restriction on voicing in sonorants. In other words, the constraint *[+voi, −son] may be violated at most once in a Yamato morpheme.[29] This constraint is interesting from the perspective of the Underspecification Theory of markedness, the topic of Section 1: if unmarked [+voi] specifications are absent from underlying representations, then the constraint becomes simply that only one [+voi] specification is possible underlyingly. The challenge then becomes to introduce the unmarked [+voi] features during the derivation in a way that allows them to function properly. (For discussion of this problem and an OT analysis, see Itô, Mester, and Padgett 1995.)

Lyman's Law can be understood in present terms as the result of the conjunctive interaction of *[+voi, −son] with F°[Yam] (139).

(139)   Lyman's Law: *[+voi, −son] & F°[+Yam] ≫ F[voi] ≫ *[+voi, −son]

Suppose that the Yamato feature value for a morpheme is specified underlyingly for all segments of the morpheme, with value [+Yam] for morphemes in the Yamato lexical stratum and [−Yam] for the others. Suppose correspondingly that in the output, a [±Yam] domain spans the entire morpheme (perhaps the result of high-ranked *HD[Yam]). There is thus exactly one [±Yam] head per morpheme; this segment satisfies F°[Yam] while all others violate it. At every position except the head, a voiced obstruent triggers a violation of the conjunction in (139), which, given the ranking, forces unfaithfulness to [voi] if necessary to ensure that any obstruent is unvoiced. At the segment heading a [+Yam] domain, the constraint F°[+Yam] is satisfied, so the conjunction is too, allowing an underlying voiced obstruent to surface faithfully. Note that the conjunction does not *require* that the [+Yam] head be voiced: it simply *permits* it, by exempting the head from the elevated prohibition on marked [+voi, −son] segments that holds in nonhead positions. If there is a segment that is underly-

---

[29] For a different use of local conjunction to analyze Lyman's Law, see Itô and Mester 1996, 1998; Suzuki 1998.

ingly [+voi, −son], it is optimal to locate the head on such a segment: this allows F[voi] to be satisfied once among all underlyingly [+voi, −son] segments, while locating the head elsewhere allows no such segment to satisfy F[voi]. And finally, in a [−Yam] word, F°[+Yam] is vacuously satisfied; hence, so is the conjunction, and the ranking F[voi] ≫ *[+voi, −son] means that there is no limitation on the distribution of voiced obstruents.

6 SONORITY AND THE OBLIGATORY CONTOUR PRINCIPLE

In previous sections, we have seen how local conjunction provides a general means of characterizing harmonically complete inventories in terms of the interaction of basic markedness constraints. This type of analysis begins with markedness constraints of the familiar OT sort; the conjunctions are then built from these constraints. Another style of analysis begins with a familiar markedness constraint and *deconstructs* it, revealing it to be a conjunction of more elementary constraints. Such analyses show the power of conjunction to reduce the elementary constraints in *Con*, enabling a deeper explanation—in some sense—than is possible with the unanalyzed original constraints. The cost of reduction of course is that what was previously simple and atomic—and stipulated—becomes complex and internally structured when analysis shifts to a deeper level.

This section illustrates the reductive use of local conjunction in the context of the sonority structure of syllables, building on Clements 1990, McCarthy and Prince 1993, Prince 1983, Itô and Mester 1994, and Prince and Smolensky 1993/2004, Chap. 8 (excerpted in Box 13:1). Sonority is a multivalued phonological scale; the structural dimensions we have considered so far have been characterized by binary features. If dimensions are scales with more than two levels, local conjunction can still be used to generate harmonically complete inventories, but it needs to be used in a slightly new way: conjoining a constraint *with itself*. As in Clements 1990 and Prince and Smolensky 1993/2004, the empirical component of the analysis consists of broad empirical generalizations rather than detailed language-particular facts.

6.1 Local self-conjunction and power hierarchies

Suppose relative markedness of a scalar dimension is formalized as follows. Posit the constraint $\mathbb{C}$, which I will call the **generating constraint** for the markedness scale. At the unmarked pole of the dimension, $\mathbb{C}$ issues one mark; at the next level of the scale, it issues one more mark, and so on. For example, consider the margin Harmony scale of Prince and Smolensky 1993/2004, Chap. 8, which evaluates the markedness of segments in the syllable margin (onset, let's say) according to an eight-level sonority scale, lower-sonority segments being less marked.

(140) Margin Harmony scale

Ons/a ≺ Ons/y ≺ Ons/l ≺ Ons/n ≺ Ons/z ≺ Ons/s ≺ Ons/d ≺ Ons/t

Box 2

The markedness scale generating constraint $\mathbb{C}$ assesses one mark to t in the onset, as it has least sonority; it assesses d one more mark, as it occupies the next level up in sonority; it assesses s one more mark than d; z one more mark than s; and so on.[30]

Suppose that, like the markedness scale (140) determined by $\mathbb{C}$, there is a corresponding faithfulness scale determined by F, such that F issues one mark when an underlying segment α surfaces as a segment β, where α and β differ in sonority by one level; F issues two marks when β's sonority differs from α's by two levels, and so on. Then a ranking employing only $\mathbb{C}$ and F can generate an inventory of onset segments that includes only t, and an inventory that includes all segments: the former when $\mathbb{C} \gg F$, the latter when $F \gg \mathbb{C}$.

But there are other harmonically complete inventories: those admitting into the onset all segments with a sonority value equal to or lower than some cutoff. These inventories were generated in Prince and Smolensky 1993/2004 (see Box 13:1) by using, instead of a single constraint $\mathbb{C}$, a *hierarchy* of constraints — the margin hierarchy, here specialized to the only marginal position under discussion, the onset (141).

(141) Onset hierarchy

$$*\text{Ons}/a \gg *\text{Ons}/y \gg \cdots \gg *\text{Ons}/s \gg *\text{Ons}/d \gg *\text{Ons}/t$$

Now different sonority levels correspond not to differing numbers of marks at a single rank in the constraint hierarchy — that of $\mathbb{C}$ — but to single marks at differing ranks. Now, many rankings are possible: if F is ranked between the margin hierarchy constraint for sonority level $n+1$ and that for sonority level n, the inventory of onset segments generated consists of those with sonority value less than or equal to n.

The margin hierarchy is generated in Prince and Smolensky 1993/2004 by an important general operation, **Harmonic** (or **Prominence**) **Alignment** (Box 13:1). Another perspective on the margin hierarchy is made possible with local conjunction: a construction based on the single markedness-scale-generating constraint $\mathbb{C}$. This construction is developed in Box 3 below. The result is (142).

(142) Local self-conjunction and power hierarchies

    a.   Let $\mathbb{C}$ be a binary constraint[31] defined over a domain $\mathcal{D}$. The **local self-conjunction** of $\mathbb{C}$ with respect to $\mathcal{D}$, $\mathbb{C} \,\&_{\mathcal{D}}\, \mathbb{C} \equiv \mathbb{C}^2$, is violated once for each domain of type $\mathcal{D}$ in which there are exactly two distinct violations of $\mathbb{C}$.

    b.   Generally, $\mathbb{C}^k$, the kth **power** of $\mathbb{C}$, is violated once for each domain of type $\mathcal{D}$ in which there are exactly k distinct violations of $\mathbb{C}$.

---

[30]An alternative version of $\mathbb{C}$, which I will actually employ in Sections 6.2–6.4, assesses no mark to the least marked element, Ons/t, and then successively one *more* to each consecutive level of the scale. For most purposes, the two definitions are equivalent, but the definition in the text is advantageous when the $\mathbb{C}$-markedness scale is conjoined with another markedness constraint M: then an M violation coincident with even the least marked element of the $\mathbb{C}$ scale registers a violation of the conjunction. For an example on a two-point scale, see $*\text{V}_{+\text{N}} \gg *\text{V}_{-\text{N}}$ in Section 5.3. See also Footnotes 12:28–29.

[31] That is, there is some configuration X such that $\mathbb{C}$ assesses a structure S one violation mark $*\mathbb{C}$ for each distinct instance of X in S. A nonbinary constraint assesses several types of violation marks, arrayed along a scale from least to most Harmony. The vast majority of constraints proposed in the OT literature are binary in this sense.

c. The constraints $\{\mathbb{C}^k\}$ are universally ranked in the following **power hierarchy** over $\mathbb{C}$:

$$\cdots \gg \mathbb{C}^3 \gg \mathbb{C}^2 \gg \mathbb{C}.$$

d. If $\mathbb{C}$ is the generating constraint for a markedness scale, the power hierarchy over $\mathbb{C}$ is a **universal markedness hierarchy**.

So suppose $\mathbb{C}$ is the generating constraint for the onset sonority markedness scale. Then, with $\mathcal{D}$ = onset, the power hierarchy over $\mathbb{C}$ is exactly the hierarchy (141) posited in Prince and Smolensky 1993/2004:[32] in an onset, a segment α of sonority level k generates a violation of $\mathbb{C}^k$, the kth-ranked constraint in the hierarchy. (That is, Ons/α $\equiv \mathbb{C}^{\mathrm{son}(\alpha)}$, where son($\alpha$) is the sonority level of segment α, with the sonority levels represented by $t, d, \ldots, a$ assigned values $1, 2, \ldots, 8$.)

So far, $\mathbb{C}$ is a constraint stipulated to assess Ons/α more marks as the sonority of α increases. The goal now is to recognize $\mathbb{C}$ as an independently motivated constraint, such that the number of marks it assesses follows from more basic considerations rather than stipulation. To do this, we need to derive sonority itself from more basic properties.

The proposed analysis draws heavily on the classic paper Clements 1990. Following Clements, I will henceforth work with the five-level sonority scale in (143), derived from distinctive features as in (144). I will use Φ to denote the set of four features given in (144).

(143) Sonority scale

O(bstruent) > N(asal) > L(iquid) > G(lide) > V(owel)

(144) Sonority determined by distinctive features

[syll]	−	−	−	−	+
[voc]	−	−	−	+	+
[approx(imant)]	−	−	+	+	+
[son]	−	+	+	+	+
	O	N	L	G	V

As the sonority scale is mounted, one by one the features [son] … [syll] of Φ go from − to +; the number of features with value + equals the sonority level, from 0 to 4. I will let **V** be the set of positive feature values, which characterize vowels: {[+son], …, [+syll]}. Analogously, **C** will denote the set of negative values, {[−son], …, [−syll]}. I will consider **V** and **C** to be **feature classes** in the sense of Padgett 1995, 2001, 2002b: constraints can refer directly to these classes.

The constraints relevant here derive directly from those of the Alignment Theory of Syllable Structure developed by McCarthy and Prince (1993) and Itô and Mester (1994).

---

[32] This analysis of Prince and Smolensky 1993/2004 treats only the case of onsets consisting of at most one segment.

Box 2

(145)　Alignment Theory of Syllable Structure

　　a.　ONSET ~ ALIGN-L(σ, C)

　　b.　NoCoda, CodaCond ~ ALIGN-L(C, σ)

ALIGN-L(σ, C) requires every syllable to begin with a consonant, hence is a version of ONSET (145a), the constraint requiring every syllable to have an onset (see Chapter 13). ALIGN-L(C, σ) requires every consonant to appear at the beginning of a syllable, a version of NoCoda. If 'C' denotes 'C-place', ALIGN-L(C, σ) requires that C-place be specified only syllable-initially—in other words, that coda consonants have no C-place specification (domain head) of their own, a kind of 'Coda Condition' in the sense of Steriade 1982 and Itô 1986 (see also Section 1.4.4).

　　The constraints used below, which are listed in (146), are adapted from (145) and the feature domain faithfulness constraints in (60).

(146)　Constraints

　　a.　ONS ≡ ALIGN-L(σ, **C**): For each [$-\varphi$] ∈ **C**, ALIGN-L(σ, [$-\varphi$]).

　　b.　COD ≡ CODACOND ≡ ALIGN-L(**C**, σ): For each [$-\varphi$] ∈ **C**, ALIGN-L([$-\varphi$], σ).

　　c.　F: For each φ ∈ Φ, corresponding segments of the input and output have the same values of φ.

　　d.　F°: For each φ ∈ Φ, an input segment that is [$+\varphi$] (or [$-\varphi$]) corresponds to an output segment that heads a [$+\varphi$] (or [$-\varphi$]) domain.

ONS (a distinct constraint from ONSET) requires that every syllable begin with [$-\varphi$], for each consonantal feature value [$-\varphi$] ∈ **C**. For a given syllable, for each feature φ that does not have the value [$-\varphi$] required of a φ in **C**, ONS assesses one violation.

(147)　Initial segment of a syllable　　　　　Marks assigned by ONS

O	
N	*
L	**
G	***
V	****

This is spelled out with feature domains for O, N, and L in (148). Here and henceforth, we are only considering syllables in isolation, or more specifically, assuming that feature domains do not span syllables, so we can analyze syllables independently. (Interesting consequences follow from this analysis if feature domains span syllables, but this would take us too far afield.)[33]

---

[33] When domains span syllables, the interpretation of the ONS power hierarchy in (150b) needs to be revised; ONS^k is satisfied when the sonority *drop* at a syllable boundary is $4-k$ levels, for each level of drop entails a fresh [$-\varphi$] domain at the syllable onset. (The case treated in the text is equivalent to assuming that the syllable under examination is preceded by a V.) The location of a relevant faithfulness constraint—say, DEP—in the ONS hierarchy then determines a minimal sonority *drop* at a syllable boundary. If this is set at 1 via the ranking ONS⁴ ≫ DEP ≫ ONS³, then syllable contact is required to have a positive sonority drop; otherwise, a V will be epenthesized. This is the Syllable Contact Law

The typological markedness generalizations concerning the role of sonority in the onset inventory that will be examined here are summarized in (149). A markedness relation $x \prec y$ (x is less harmonic, or more marked, than y) entails an implicational universal $x \Rightarrow y$: if an inventory contains x, then it contains y (Section 1.5.1). This entailment follows from a universal ranking amounting to $*x \gg_{UG} *y$. Recall that in OT, this means that for any grammar G admitted by UG, if G maps some input I_x to an output containing x, then there is an input I_y that G maps to an output containing y. Richness of the Base asserts that the pool of potential inputs from which I_x and I_y are drawn is rich and universal. For inventory theory, the input-output mapping of the grammar is not itself relevant: it does not matter *which* output a given input is mapped to. All that matters is the set of structures z appearing in all the grammar's outputs when it is fed all the potential inputs. So below, what matters for a grammar is that no input gets parsed into syllables of type, say, LV; this means an underlying form /LV/ must get mapped to something else, say, .NV. The conclusion is *not* that there are lexical forms /LV/ in this language and the grammar nasalizes the liquid! What it means is exactly this: the syllable inventory of the language includes no .LV. syllables. (See the extended discussion of Richness of the Base and lexicon optimization in Sections 12:1.6–1.7.)

(148)

Output structures	ONS ≡ ALIGN-L(σ, **C**)
O V syll $\begin{bmatrix}-\end{bmatrix}\begin{bmatrix}+\end{bmatrix}$ voc $\begin{bmatrix}-\end{bmatrix}\begin{bmatrix}+\end{bmatrix}$ approx $\begin{bmatrix}-\end{bmatrix}\begin{bmatrix}+\end{bmatrix}$ son $\begin{bmatrix}-\end{bmatrix}\begin{bmatrix}+\end{bmatrix}$	
N V syll $\begin{bmatrix}-\end{bmatrix}\begin{bmatrix}+\end{bmatrix}$ voc $\begin{bmatrix}-\end{bmatrix}\begin{bmatrix}+\end{bmatrix}$ approx $\begin{bmatrix}-\end{bmatrix}\begin{bmatrix}+\end{bmatrix}$ son $\begin{bmatrix}+\quad\end{bmatrix}$	*
L V syll $\begin{bmatrix}-\end{bmatrix}\begin{bmatrix}+\end{bmatrix}$ voc $\begin{bmatrix}-\end{bmatrix}\begin{bmatrix}+\end{bmatrix}$ approx $\begin{bmatrix}+\quad\end{bmatrix}$ son $\begin{bmatrix}+\quad\end{bmatrix}$	* *

(149) Onset markedness

 a. Less sonorous onsets are less marked: for example, LV $\prec$ NV (Vennemann 1988, 13; Clements 1990, (17); Prince and Smolensky 1993/2004, Chap. 8).

 b. **Sonority Sequencing Principle**. In unmarked complex onsets, sonority does not fall; for example, LOV $\prec$ OLV (Hooper 1972; Clements 1990, (2)).

(Vennemann 1988, 40; Clements 1990, (28)). Thus, for /CVC$_1$C$_2$V/, the output is .CVC$_1$.C$_2$V. if son(C$_1$) > son(C$_2$), but otherwise .CV.C$_1$v.C$_2$V., with epenthetic 'v'.

Box 2

    c.   **Minimum sonority distance**. In unmarked syllables, consecutive segments from onset to peak are separated by a sonority distance of at least d (Steriade 1982; Clements 1990, 317).

    d.   In complex onsets with monotonically rising sonority, less-marked onsets have a steady sonority rise: ONV $\prec$ OLV (Clements 1990, (18)).

Box 3. Deriving power hierarchies from self-conjunction

The construction begins with a refinement of the definition of local conjunction (73b) and proceeds to draw the implications for conjoining a constraint with itself.

(1)   Local self-conjunction

    a.   *Definition.* The local conjunction of constraints A and B in domain $\mathcal{D}$, $A \mathbin{\&}_{\mathcal{D}} B$, is the constraint violated when there are *distinct* violations of A and B in a single domain of type $\mathcal{D}$. One violation is incurred for every distinct pairing of a violation of A and a distinct violation of B.

    b.   Suppose $A \equiv \mathbb{C}$ and $B \equiv \mathbb{C}$ refer to the same constraint. It follows that $A \mathbin{\&}_{\mathcal{D}} B = \mathbb{C} \mathbin{\&}_{\mathcal{D}} \mathbb{C} \equiv \mathbb{C}^{(2)}$ is violated when, in a single domain of type $\mathcal{D}$, there is a violation of $A \equiv \mathbb{C}$ distinct from a violation of $B \equiv \mathbb{C}$; that is, when a violation of $A \equiv \mathbb{C}$ is ignored, there remains a violation of $B \equiv \mathbb{C}$. For each domain of type $\mathcal{D}$, $\mathbb{C}^{(2)}$ assesses one violation for every pair of distinct violations of $\mathbb{C}$ in that domain.

    c.   Let $A \equiv \mathbb{C}$ and $B \equiv \mathbb{C}^{(2)}$. It follows that $A \mathbin{\&}_{\mathcal{D}} B = \mathbb{C} \mathbin{\&}_{\mathcal{D}} \mathbb{C}^{(2)} \equiv \mathbb{C}^{(3)}$ is violated when, in a single domain of type $\mathcal{D}$, there is a violation of $A \equiv \mathbb{C}$ distinct from a violation of $B \equiv \mathbb{C}^{(2)}$; that is, when a violation of $A \equiv \mathbb{C}$ is ignored, there remains a violation of $B \equiv \mathbb{C}^{(2)}$. For each domain of type $\mathcal{D}$, $\mathbb{C}^{(3)}$ assesses one violation for every pair of a violation of $\mathbb{C}$ and a distinct set of violations of $\mathbb{C}^{(2)}$ (a pair of distinct $\mathbb{C}$ violations).

Clearly, this recursive process can be continued to generate further $\mathbb{C}^{(k)}$.

    To illustrate with the onset sonority example: consider s in an onset, Ons/s. Since s is in the third sonority level, Ons/s incurs three distinct violations of the ONSET-generating constraint $\mathbb{C}$: $\{*_1, *_2, *_3\}$. (Coincidentally,) it incurs three violations of $\mathbb{C}^{(2)}$ as well, since there are three distinct pairings of a violation of $\mathbb{C}$ with a distinct violation of $\mathbb{C}$: $\{(*_1, *_2), (*_1, *_3), (*_2, *_3)\}$. Ons/$s$ is (coincidentally) also assessed three violations of $\mathbb{C}^{(3)}$, one for each of the pairs $\{((*_1, *_2), *_3), ((*_1, *_3), *_2), ((*_2, *_3), *_1)\}$. Ons/$s$ incurs no violations of $\mathbb{C}^{(4)}$, as no marks remain once the three needed for $\mathbb{C}^{(3)}$ are exhausted. And Ons/s therefore incurs no marks from $\mathbb{C}^{(5)}$, and hence none from $\mathbb{C}^{(6)}$, and so on.

    The number of violations of $\mathbb{C}^{(k)}$ generated by $n \geq k$ violations of $\mathbb{C}$ grows quickly with n and k. The following proposition is thus helpful:

(2)   *Proposition.* Let $\mathcal{H}$ be a constraint hierarchy employing constraints $\mathbb{C}$, $\mathbb{C}^{(2)}$, … and let $\mathcal{H}'$ be the hierarchy obtained by replacing $\mathbb{C}^{(k)}$ by $\mathbb{C}_k$, defined as fol-

---

lows: to a structure that incurs n distinct marks from $\mathbb{C}$, $\mathbb{C}_k$ assesses no marks if $n < k$, and $n - k + 1$ marks otherwise. ($\mathbb{C}_k$ assesses one mark if $n = k$, and one additional mark for each remaining $\mathbb{C}$ mark.)

Then $\mathcal{H}'$ determines the same input-output mapping as $\mathcal{H}$.

Proof. Let $n(c)$ be the number of violations of $\mathbb{C}$ incurred by candidate c. Consider any input I and the optimization over $\mathcal{H}$ to select the correct output. The initial candidate set $Gen(I)$ is filtered by each constraint, successively down the hierarchy; at each point, only the most harmonic candidates are passed through. Consider the step at which $\mathbb{C}^{(k)}$ filters the candidates, passing through only those candidates with the fewest violations. If any candidates c remain with $n(c) < k$, these satisfy the constraint, and they are the ones that pass. The same result obtains if $\mathbb{C}_k$ is used in place of $\mathbb{C}^{(k)}$, since the same candidates satisfy the two constraints. On the other hand, if there are no remaining candidates c with $n(c) < k$, then $\mathbb{C}^{(k)}$ passes those candidates with the fewest violations. Because the number of $\mathbb{C}^{(k)}$ violations grows monotonically (and quickly) with $n(c) - k$, the candidates with minimal violation are those with the smallest $n(c)$ value. But these are the same as the candidates with the fewest violations of $\mathbb{C}_k$, so again substituting $\mathbb{C}_k$ for $\mathbb{C}^{(k)}$ does not affect optimization. Thus, $\mathcal{H}'$ yields the same output as $\mathcal{H}$. (This result is an immediate corollary of the formal results of Prince 1997; the proofs of this box are simple applications of the methods developed in that work.)☐

(3)   *Proposition.* Let $\mathcal{H}$ be a constraint hierarchy employing the constraints $\mathbb{C}$, $\mathbb{C}_2$, $\mathbb{C}_3$, ... defined in (2). Suppose for some k, $\mathbb{C}_{k+1}$ is ranked below $\mathbb{C}_k$. Then reranking $\mathbb{C}_{k+1}$ directly above $\mathbb{C}_k$ in $\mathcal{H}$ produces a hierarchy $\mathcal{H}'$ that defines the same mapping as $\mathcal{H}$.

Proof. For a given input, consider the filtering of candidates at $\mathbb{C}_k$ in $\mathcal{H}$. Following the same reasoning as in the previous proof, the candidates c that pass $\mathbb{C}_k$ either all have $n(c) < k$ (i.e., fewer than k violations of $\mathbb{C}$) or all have the same (minimal) value of $n(c) - k$. The same is true therefore of the subset of these candidates that are received by lower-ranked $\mathbb{C}_{k+1}$. In the former case, each c has $n(c) < k + 1$, so they all pass and $\mathbb{C}_{k+1}$ has no effect. In the latter case, all candidates c have the same value of $n(c) - (k + 1)$, hence all the same number of violations of $\mathbb{C}_{k+1}$, hence again $\mathbb{C}_{k+1}$ is inactive. Thus, the optima of $\mathcal{H}$ are the same as those of $\mathcal{H}_0$, the hierarchy created by simply removing $\mathbb{C}_{k+1}$ from $\mathcal{H}$. We now see that in turn, $\mathcal{H}_0$ has the same optima as $\mathcal{H}'$, giving the result.

Now consider an optimization in $\mathcal{H}_0$ at the point of filtering candidates at constraint $\mathbb{C}_k$; let C be the set of candidates entering the filter, and C' be those that pass it. The same set C arrives at $\mathbb{C}_{k+1}$ in $\mathcal{H}'$; we must show that the same set C' passes $\mathbb{C}_{k+1}$ followed immediately by $\mathbb{C}_k$—in other words, that inserting $\mathbb{C}_{k+1}$ directly above $\mathbb{C}_k$ has no effect on what survives $\mathbb{C}_k$.

There are two cases to consider. In the first case, some c in C have $n(c) <$

Box 3

k; these then are the candidates C' that satisfy (hence pass) $\mathbb{C}_k$ in $\mathcal{H}_0$. All these candidates also satisfy (hence pass) $\mathbb{C}_{k+1}$ in $\mathcal{H}'$, and then pass through $\mathbb{C}_k$. Any c' in C with $n(c') = k$ will also satisfy (hence pass) $\mathbb{C}_{k+1}$, but these will be filtered out immediately by $\mathbb{C}_k$, leaving the same ultimate survivors C'. In the second case, no c in C has $n(c) < k$. The minimal violators then of $\mathbb{C}_k$ are those c in C with least $n(c) - k$, that is, with lowest $n(c)$. These constitute C' in this case. Now in $\mathcal{H}'$, these same candidates C' with lowest $n(c)$ also have lowest $n(c) - [k + 1]$, hence minimally violate $\mathbb{C}_{k+1}$; these then are the survivors of $\mathbb{C}_{k+1}$, which are fed to $\mathbb{C}_k$, which assigns them all the same number of marks, $n(c) - k$, hence simply passes them all. So C' is the set of candidates that are passed on by $\mathbb{C}_k$ both in $\mathcal{H}$ and in $\mathcal{H}_0$. $\square$

(4) *Proposition.* Let $\mathcal{H}$ be a constraint hierarchy employing the $\mathbb{C}$, $\mathbb{C}_2$, $\mathbb{C}_3$, … defined in (2). Then there is another hierarchy $\mathcal{H}'$ with the same optima as $\mathcal{H}$, where in $\mathcal{H}'$ the relative ranking of these constraints is

$$\cdots \gg \mathbb{C}_3 \gg \mathbb{C}_2 \gg \mathbb{C}.$$

Proof. Consider $\mathbb{C}_2$. If in $\mathcal{H}$ it is ranked below $\mathbb{C}$, by (3) we can rerank it just above $\mathbb{C}$, yielding a hierarchy $\mathcal{H}_2$ with the same optima as $\mathcal{H}$. If $\mathbb{C}_2$ is already ranked above $\mathbb{C}$ in $\mathcal{H}$, simply let $\mathcal{H}_2 \equiv \mathcal{H}$. Now consider $\mathbb{C}_3$; if in $\mathcal{H}_2$ it is ranked below $\mathbb{C}_2$, rerank it just above $\mathbb{C}_2$, yielding $\mathcal{H}_3$, with the same optima as $\mathcal{H}_2$, hence as $\mathcal{H}$. If $\mathbb{C}_3 \gg \mathbb{C}_2$ in $\mathcal{H}_2$, simply define $\mathcal{H}_3 \equiv \mathcal{H}_2$. Continuing in this fashion, we can ultimately construct the desired $\mathcal{H}'$. $\square$

(5) *Proposition.* Let $\mathcal{H}$ be a constraint hierarchy employing $\mathbb{C}$, $\mathbb{C}_2$, $\mathbb{C}_3$, … that satisfies the ranking requirement of (4). Let $\mathbb{C}^k$ be defined as the constraint that is violated once for each domain of type $\mathcal{D}$ in which $\mathbb{C}_k$ is violated and $\mathbb{C}_{k+1}$ is unviolated. Define $\mathcal{H}'$ as the hierarchy constructed from $\mathcal{H}$ by replacing each $\mathbb{C}_k$ with $\mathbb{C}^k$. Then $\mathcal{H}'$ has the same optima as $\mathcal{H}$.

$\mathbb{C}^k$ is the same constraint as defined in the text: it is violated once for each domain of type $\mathcal{D}$ in which $\mathbb{C}$ is violated exactly k times.

Proof. Let C be the candidate set received by $\mathbb{C}_k$ during an optimization over $\mathcal{H}$, hence also the candidate set received by $\mathbb{C}^k$ during the corresponding optimization over $\mathcal{H}'$. The goal is to show that the same candidates are passed on in both cases. Now since $\mathbb{C}_{k+1} \gg \mathbb{C}_k$ in $\mathcal{H}$, the candidate set has already been filtered by $\mathbb{C}_{k+1}$. Thus, either (i) all c in C satisfy $\mathbb{C}_{k+1}$ or (ii) all violate it, equally. In case (i), $n(c) < k + 1$ for all c in C. In subcase (a), $n(c) = k$ for all c in C. Then all c violate $\mathbb{C}_k$ equally; hence, all pass in $\mathcal{H}$. Also, all violate $\mathbb{C}^k$ equally (once); hence, all pass in $\mathcal{H}'$. In subcase (b), $n(c) < k$ for some c in C. Then those c satisfy $\mathbb{C}_k$, hence pass it. They also satisfy $\mathbb{C}^k$, hence pass it in $\mathcal{H}'$. If in addition $n(c) = k$ for some c in C, they violate $\mathbb{C}_k$ and are filtered out in $\mathcal{H}$; just the same is true for $\mathbb{C}^k$ in $\mathcal{H}'$. In case (ii), all c in C violate $\mathbb{C}_{k+1}$ equally, so $n(c)$ is the same for all of them, and because they violate $\mathbb{C}_{k+1}$, $n(c) > k$. Since $n(c)$ is the same for all c in C, they all equally violate $\mathbb{C}_k$; hence, all pass it in $\mathfrak{H}$. Since $n(c) > k$ for all c in C, they all satisfy $\mathbb{C}^k$; hence, all pass it in $\mathfrak{H}'$. In every case, the same candidates survive in $\mathfrak{H}$ and $\mathfrak{H}'$.

The bottom line is that, given the ranking of the $\{\mathbb{C}_k\}$, when a given $\mathbb{C}_k$ is active in winnowing the candidate set, it receives a set C of candidates c in which $n(c) = k$ for some c, and $n(c) < k$ for others: only the latter survive. But in just this situation, $\mathbb{C}^k$ achieves the same result. In all other situations, either all c in C have $n(c) < k$, in which case they all satisfy both $\mathbb{C}_k$ and $\mathbb{C}^k$, or all c in C have the same $n(c) \geq k$, in which case they all pass in $\mathfrak{H}$ because they all equally violate $\mathbb{C}_k$, and all pass in $\mathfrak{H}'$ because they all satisfy $\mathbb{C}^k$. $\square$

The net result of these propositions is that when local conjunction freely operates on a constraint $\mathbb{C}$, recursively generating self-conjunctions $\mathbb{C}^{(k)}$, any hierarchy including these constraints is equivalent to a hierarchy employing the more simply defined constraints $\mathbb{C}^k$ of the text (142b), satisfying the universally fixed ranking (142c).

6.2 First result: Onset hierarchy derived

It is evident from (147) that for our five-point sonority scale (143), $\text{O{\small NS}}$ is the generating constraint '$\mathbb{C}$' introduced at the beginning of Section 6.1.

(150) $\text{O{\small NS}}$ hierarchy: The power hierarchy over $\text{O{\small NS}}$

    a. $\text{O{\small NS}}^4 \gg \text{O{\small NS}}^3 \gg \text{O{\small NS}}^2 \gg \text{O{\small NS}}$

    b. $*.V \gg *.G \gg *.L \gg *.N$

Suppose segment α is syllable initial. Then, as illustrated in (148), it incurs k violations of $\text{O{\small NS}}$, where k is the sonority level of α. Thus, it violates $\text{O{\small NS}}^k$. (For an obstruent, O, $k = 0$; this violates no constraint of the onset hierarchy.) Thus, (150a) is equivalent to (150b), where $*.X$ is violated by syllable-initial segments of sonority level X (and as always '.' denotes a syllable boundary). The hierarchy (150b) is a version of the onset hierarchy (141) in which 'Ons' is treated not as a structural constituent, but as syllable-initial position.[34]

The first implicational universal, exemplified in (149a) as LV $\prec$ NV, asserts that if an onset inventory includes some sonority level (e.g., L), then it also includes lower sonority levels (e.g., N), which form less-marked onsets. This follows from the $\text{O{\small NS}}$ power hierarchy (150a). The three tableaux in (151) show a ranking in which L (leftmost tableau), but not G (middle tableau), is a legal sonority level for a syllable-initial segment (marks of optimal candidates are denoted '$\circledast$'). An input /LV/ surfaces faithfully, but /GV/ does not: /GV/ $\rightarrow$ [LV]. This is because the critical faithfulness constraint F (146c) is ranked between $\text{O{\small NS}}^3 \equiv *.G$ and $\text{O{\small NS}}^2 \equiv *.L$. For /GV/, changing

---

[34] The syllable-initial formulation clearly relates directly to the Syllable Contact Law (Vennemann 1988), which forbids a rise in sonority across a syllable boundary. The empirical basis for this law includes systems in which a sequence VCC'V is syllabified V.CC'V if C has lower sonority than C', but VC.C'V otherwise. Equivalently, the syllable boundary is located so as to minimize the sonority of the syllable-initial consonant, just what is favored by the onset hierarchy (150).

Box 3

a **V** feature [+voc] to a **C** feature [–voc] incurs a violation of F, but reduces an ONS^3 violation to an ONS^2 violation; this change is optimal because of the ranking $\text{ONS}^3 \gg F \gg \text{ONS}^2$. For an input /LV/, however, changing a **V** feature [+approx] to a **C** feature [–approx] incurs an F violation while only reducing an ONS^2 violation to an ONS^1 violation, a suboptimal change given that $F \gg \text{ONS}^2 \gg \text{ONS}^1$. This reasoning shows clearly that a ranking admitting L into the onset inventory must rank F higher than $\text{ONS}^2 \equiv {*}.L$, so that /LV/ surfaces faithfully; it follows from the universal relation $\text{ONS}^2 \gg \text{ONS}^1$ that F outranks $\text{ONS}^1 \equiv {*}.N$, so /NV/ must surface faithfully—hence, N is also in the onset inventory (right tableau in (151)). This argument clearly generalizes, deriving the implicational universal (149a).

(151) Onset inventory {L, N, O}; $\mathbb{C} \equiv \text{ONS} \equiv \text{ALIGN-L}(\sigma, \mathbf{C})$

Output	Input	$\mathbb{C}^3\equiv$ *.G	F	$\mathbb{C}^2\equiv$ *.L	$\mathbb{C}^1\equiv$ *.N	Input	$\mathbb{C}^3\equiv$ *.G	F	$\mathbb{C}^2\equiv$ *.L	$\mathbb{C}^1\equiv$ *.N	Input	$\mathbb{C}^3\equiv$ *.G	F	$\mathbb{C}^2\equiv$ *.L	$\mathbb{C}^1\equiv$ *.N
syll	− +					− +					− +				
voc	+ +					− +					− +				
approx	+ +					+ +					− +				
son	+ +					+ +					− +				
	/GV/					/LV/					/NV/				
.G V. [−][+] [+ [+ [+			}*!				*	}*!				}*!	*	*	
.L V. [−][+] [−][+] [+ [+		☞	⊛ }⊛				☞	}⊛						*! }*	*
.N V. [−][+] [−][+] [−][+] [+				* *!	*				*!	*		☞			⊛
.O V. [−][+] [−][+] [−][+] [−][+]				* *! *					*! *					*!	

The import of the *locality* of conjunction here can be seen simply by comparing /LVLV/ and /GV/. In the inventory produced by the ranking in (151), /GV/ does not surface faithfully because the output .GV. violates ONS^3: at the left edge of the single output syllable, three features are in **V** rather than **C**; that is, three features violate ONS. In contrast, /LVLV/ does surface faithfully as .LV.LV., even though ONS is violated more times in this output (four) than in the illegal output .GV. for /GV/. This is because the four violations of ONS are not all co-local. To determine the marks assessed to .LV.LV. by the ONS ≡ ALIGN-L(σ, **C**) ('Every σ ...') hierarchy, each output syllable is examined independently, and the resulting marks are combined: two violations of ONS^2, not one violation of ONS^4, are assessed. Because F strictly dominates ONS^2 in this ranking, it is suboptimal to violate F to avoid .LV., no matter how many times ONS^2 ≡ *.L is violated, that is, no matter how many .LV. syllables may appear in the output.

6.3 Second result: Sonority Sequencing Principle

According to the second universal generalization (149b), syllables in which sonority *decreases* between the left syllable edge and the syllable peak are marked: they are excluded from the syllable inventories of many languages, and in no language are they required. So, for example, on the markedness dimension under consideration, the syllable .OLV. is unmarked, while .LOV. is marked and hence can be excluded from syllable inventories. (Of course, .OLV. can be excluded because of its markedness on dimensions other than onset sonority rise — for example, onset complexity.)

This result is a consequence of the constraint COD introduced in (146b); it exploits the notion of feature domain in an interesting way. Tableaux (152) show how COD penalizes sonority declines. The critical point is that a sonority decline corresponds to *initiation of a **C** domain after the syllable onset*. That is, the left edge of a **C** domain is not aligned with the left edge of the syllable, exactly the configuration marked by COD ≡ ALIGN-L(**C**, σ). When COD dominates the faithfulness constraint F, it eliminates from the inventory syllables with onset sonority decline.

Tableaux (152) treat two inputs. The left half of the table concerns the declining-sonority input /LOV/. In the faithful output, two **C** domains, [−son] and [−approx], begin at the second segment O. Because O's sonority is lower than that of the first segment L, it has more **C** domains than the first segment; that is, some [+φ] feature values for L must change to [−φ] for O, initiating a new [−φ] domain away from the left syllable edge. This means COD is violated (twice, in this case, once for each of [−son] and [−approx]; the number of COD violations is the number of levels of sonority decline). The optimal output .OOV. eliminates the COD violations,[35] incurring only lower-ranked F violations (one for each feature involved in the decline). Thus, .LOV. is barred from the syllable inventory by this ranking.

The right half of (152) shows that for the increasing-sonority input /OLV/, in the faithful candidate all **C** domains are initiated at the left syllable edge, satisfying COD. Thus, .OLV. is admitted into the inventory.

The version of the Sonority Sequencing Principle derived here is one that identifies as marked onsets xyV for which son(x) > son(y). The markedness of sonority plateaus, where son(x) = son(y), will now be shown to be marked on other grounds.

---

[35] .LLV. incurs the same COD and F violations as .OOV. but ONS favors .OOV.

Box 3

(152) Markedness of onset sonority decline: Sonority Sequencing Principle

Output	Input	COD ≡ ALIGN-L(**C**, σ)	F	Input	COD ≡ ALIGN-L(**C**, σ)	F
syll	– – +			– – +		
voc	– – +			– – +		
approx	+ – +			– + +		
son	+ – +			– + +		
	/L O V/			/O L V/		
.L O V. [–][+] [–][+] [+][–][+] [+][–][+]		*! *				*!* * *
. O O V. [–][+] [–][+] [–][+] [–][+]	☞		⊛			*! *
.O L V. [–][+] [–][+] [–][+] [–][+]			*!* * *	☞		

6.4 Third result: Minimal sonority distance

In addition to deriving the markedness of declining-sonority onsets, we have the means to derive the markedness of equal-sonority sequences or, more generally, of onsets with small sonority distances between consecutive segments — generalization (149c) (Steriade 1982; Clements 1990). The relevant generating constraint is F° (146d), which requires each underlying feature to head an output domain. The power hierarchy over F° evaluates sonority distances.

The tableaux in (153) show two inputs, /GV/ and /LV/, with sonority distances of 1 and 3 separating consecutive segments, respectively. As shown in (153), a sonority distance of 1 in .GL. incurs a violation of $[F°]^3$. A sonority distance of 1 means one of four features changes; hence, three are shared between the adjacent segments, meaning that for three features, one segment does not have a domain head. (The nonheads in these domains are circled in (153). These domains are assumed to be left-headed; right-headed domains would produce the same results.) With F ranked between $[F°]^3$ and $[F°]^2$, it is optimal to be unfaithful to one feature, yielding output .LV.; this increases the sonority distance by 1, reducing the $[F°]^3$ violation to an $[F°]^2$ mark. The second input in (153), /LV/, has sonority distance 2 and surfaces faithfully. Thus, with this ranking, an onset C in .CV. must be separated from V by at least 2 sonority levels.

(153)   Minimal sonority distance

Output	Input	‖[F°]³	F	[F°]²	[F°]¹	Input	‖[F°]³	F	[F°]²	[F°]¹
syll	− +					− +				
voc	+ +					− +				
approx	+ +					+ +				
son	+ +					+ +				
	/G V/					/L V/				
.G V. [−][+] [+○] [+○] [+○]		*!					*!	*		
. L V. ☞ [−][+] [−][+] [+○] [+○]	☞		⊛	⊛		☞			⊛	
. N V. [−][+] [−][+] [−][+] [+○]			* *!		*				*!	*

The same analysis applies to a complex onset, like that of CCV. For the same ranking as (153), the tableaux in (154) show two inputs, /ONV/ and /OLV/, the former having sonority distances 1,3 separating its segments, and the latter sonority distances 2,2. Again we see that this ranking yields a syllable inventory in which consecutive segments (through V) must be separated by at least 2 sonority levels: .OLV. is in the inventory, but .ONV. is not. This shows how in the unmarked syllable, sonority rises steadily to the peak, maximizing sonority distance between adjacent segments: the fourth generalization (149d).

The explanation provided here for minimal sonority distance conditions is, in an intuitive sense, based in the OCP. The nonheads of feature domains that violate F° arise when adjacent segments are identical with respect to these features: adjacent identicals are marked, where 'identical' is assessed, of course, through sharing of Φ features. (See also the OCP effect induced by F° conjunction in Section 5.4.)

Box 3

(154) Sonority dispersion

Output	Input	[F°]³	F	[F°]²	[F°]¹	Input	[F°]³	F	[F°]²	[F°]¹
syll	− − +					− − +				
voc	− − +					− − +				
approx	− − +					− + +				
son	− + +					− + +				
	/O N V/					/O L V/				
.O N V. [−◯][+] [−◯][+] [−◯][+] [−][+◯]			*!		*		*!	*		
.O L V. [−◯][+] [−◯][+] [−][+◯] [−][+◯]	☞		*	*		☞			*	*
.O G V. [−◯][+] [−][+◯] [−][+◯] [−][+◯]			*!	*	*		*!		*	*

6.5 Summary

This section has shown that several central properties of the optimal sonority profile of syllable onsets (149) can be derived by bringing together a number of independently motivated concepts: headed feature domains (including F°), power hierarchies formed by local conjunction, sonority defined via stricture features, classes of such features, and the characterization of the unmarked position of consonantal material in syllables via alignment constraints. (155) provides a summary, connecting several levels of description, from the most low-level, mechanical definitions of the key constraints, up to their universal markedness implications.

(155) Summary ($\varphi \in \Phi \equiv \{[son], [approx], [voc], [syll]\}$)

> ALIGN-L(σ, C)
>
> > The left edge of a syllable must coincide with the left edge of a $[-\varphi]$ domain.
> > $\equiv$ ONS: Syllables begin with consonantal material.
> > ONS hierarchy $\equiv$ power hierarchy over ONS: A syllable-initial segment has low sonority.
> > Implicational universals such as .LV. $\Rightarrow$. NV.

ALIGN-L(C, σ)

>The left edge of a [−φ] domain must coincide with the left edge of a syllable.
>
>≡ COD: Consonantal material is syllable initial.
>
>Syllable-initial sequences do not decrease in sonority: Sonority Sequencing.
>
>Implicational universals such as .LOV. ⇒ .OLV.

F°

>An underlying [±φ] feature corresponds to the head of an output [±φ] domain.
>
>Power hierarchy over F°: Syllable-initial sequences increase sonority maximally.
>
>Minimum sonority-distance conditions
>
>OCP[φ]: No similar adjacent φ values
>
>Dispersion: Sonority rises steadily to the syllable peak.
>
>Implicational universals such as .ONV. ⇒ .OLV.

6.6 Numerology

Clements (1990) derived the above results from a complexity hierarchy based on a numerical evaluation of onsets of a given length. Complexity predicts implicational universals as follows: if an inventory contains a structure x of complexity c, then it will also contain any structure y of complexity less than c. This of course is exactly a numerical formulation of harmonic completeness.

The complexity of an onset $C_1 \cdots C_n$ of length n is the rank, among all onsets of length n, of its numerical **dispersion** value D, defined in (156): the sum, over all pairs of segments x, y in $C_1 C_2 \ldots C_n V$, of the inverse of the square of the sonority distance between x and y. D actually evaluates the **demisyllable** $C_1 C_2 \ldots C_n V$, not just the onset $C_1 \ldots C_n$; thus, V is one of the segments examined in computing D.

(156)   Clements's dispersion function D

$$D(C_1 \cdots C_n V) \equiv \sum_{\substack{x \neq y \, \in \\ \{C_1, \cdots, C_n, V\}}} \frac{1}{(\text{son}[x] - \text{son}[y])^2}$$

The lower the dispersion value D, the less marked the onset: small D means large differences of sonority. Computing all possible values of D for a given n allows these onsets to be ordered from smallest to largest: the position in this order is the complexity of an onset.

Can this numerical computation be rationalized in some way via the preceding analysis of onset markedness? Why does the dispersion function have the particular, and peculiar, inverse-sum-of-squares form? Are there general constraints on what form such a function should take?

On this general question, Clements says of the formula defining D:

Box 3

(157) "It can be noted in passing that other ways of defining the value of D are possible in principle. For example, it might be more appropriate to restate [(156)] over the sum of sonority distances for *adjacent* pairs of segments only. As it happens, this version of [(156)] gives only slightly different values of D, since the value of d^2 [*sic*] is always small for nonadjacent pairs, and proves to yield no differences in actual demisyllable rankings. Other possible versions, involving some simple summation of the distance between members instead of the inverse of the square, prove not to yield the desired complexity rankings." (1990, 304, emphasis original; rather than '$d^{2'}$', it is actually $1/d^2$ that is intended, where d is a sonority distance)

Given the equivalence of the definition (156) for D and the simpler definition in which only adjacent pairs of segments x, y contribute, I will assume the simpler form henceforth.

The basic idea of the following analysis is to use a numerical implementation of OT — specifically, of the syllable theory elements proposed above — to connect numerical evaluation with the general principles that have been derived from the OT analysis in this section.

As discussed at some length in Chapters 6 and 20, an OT ranking can be implemented as a **harmonic grammar**. Each violation of constraint $\mathbb{C}_k$ contributes an **H-penalty** $-h_k$ to the numerical Harmony H of a candidate; these contributions are simply summed to get the total Harmony. The penalty h_k from a violation of $\mathbb{C}_k$ is greater than the penalty h_j if in the OT ranking, $\mathbb{C}_k \gg \mathbb{C}_j$. But much more is required of the penalties: the penalty h_k must actually be greater than the sum of the penalties incurred by all possible violations of constraints ranked lower than $\mathbb{C}_k$; this is the numerical counterpart of strict domination. In general, this requires exponentially increasing penalties; we will see this arise in the present case shortly.

The OT grammar of interest is the power hierarchy over F°, shown in tableaux (153)–(154). Henceforth, let '$\mathbb{C}$' denote F°.

What conditions must the penalty h_k satisfy in order to realize the power hierarchy $\cdots \gg \mathbb{C}^k \gg \mathbb{C}^{k-1} \gg \cdots \gg \mathbb{C}^3 \gg \mathbb{C}^2 \gg \mathbb{C}^1$? For the moment, we will restrict attention to onsets with two consonants, CCV. The analysis is compactly expressed in (160). What we need to ensure is that one violation of $\mathbb{C}^k$ is more costly than the maximum cost achievable by violating only the lower-ranked constraints $\mathbb{C}^{k-1}$, ..., $\mathbb{C}^2$, $\mathbb{C}^1$. A violation of $\mathbb{C}^k$ by an onset means a sonority distance of $4 - k$ between some pair of adjacent segments in that onset. So the strict domination requirement

(158) H-penalty(Best onset violating $\mathbb{C}^k$)

> H-penalty(Worst onset satisfying all of $\mathbb{C}^k$, $\mathbb{C}^{k+1}$, $\mathbb{C}^{k+2}$, ...)

is equivalent to

(159) H-penalty(Best onset with minimum sonority distance d)

> H-penalty(Worst onset with all sonority distances > d),

where $d \equiv 4 - k$.

The table in (160) computes such requirements for each value of d. The subscripts in onsets such as 'G$_3$O$_4$V' simply make explicit the sonority distance between adjacent segments. Note that 'best' and 'worst' hold *only with respect to sonority distance*. The 'best' onsets are terrible, in fact, but (except for OOV) that must be handled by other constraints; in the analysis above, for example, these 'best' onsets are penalized by COD because they are not rising in sonority. Since the Harmony penalty increases with decreasing sonority distance, the 'best' CCV onset with minimal sonority distance d will have one sonority change of size d, and the other sonority change as large as possible (4). And the worst CCV onset with all sonority distances $> d$ will have both its sonority changes as close as possible to $(d+1)$.

(160)   Dispersion analysis of CCV

		$\mathbb{C}^4$	$\mathbb{C}^3$	$\mathbb{C}^2$	$\mathbb{C}^1$	
a.	$\mathbb{C}^k$					
b.	Sonority distance d	0	1	2	3	4
c.	Best CCV onset with minimal sonority distance d	O$_0$O$_4$V	N$_1$O$_4$V	L$_2$O$_4$V	G$_3$O$_4$V	—
d.	Worst CCV onset with all sonority distances $> d$	L$_1$G$_1$V	O$_2$L$_2$V	G$_3$O$_4$V	—	—
e.	$\mathbb{C}^k \gg \mathbb{C}^{k-1}$ condition	$h_0 + h_4$ $> 2h_1$	$h_1 + h_4$ $> 2h_2$	$h_2 + h_4$ $> h_3 + h_4$		
f.	Does D meet condition?	$\infty + 1/16$ $> 2(1)$ ✓	$1 + 1/16$ $> 2(\frac14)$ ✓	$h_2 = 1/4 >$ $1/9 = h_3$ ✓		
g.	$D: h_d \equiv 1/d^2$	$1/0 = \infty$	1	1/4	1/9	1/16
h.	Condition if $h_4 = 0$	$h_0 > 2h_1$	$h_1 > 2h_2$	$h_2 > h_3$		

In the table (160), the power hierarchy over $\mathbb{C}$ is given in row (a), and the corresponding values of the sonority distances are given in row (b). In the column for sonority distance d, row (c) gives the best onset with minimal sonority distance equal to d, and row (d) gives the worst onset with all sonority distances greater than d. The strict domination requirement (159) is that the H-penalty of the former must exceed that of the latter; this is spelled out in row (e), where the H-penalty of a sonority distance d is h_d. Using the values of h_d given by D, shown in row (g), row (f) checks whether the strict domination condition is met. In each case, it is: this explains why the numbers assigned by D yield the correct relative markedness results.

The final row (h) of (160) shows what the domination conditions become if h_4 is set to zero. In fact, a sonority distance of 4 incurs no violation of the $\mathbb{C}$ hierarchy, so assigning zero penalty is what the OT analysis suggests. With $h_4 \equiv 0$, the domination conditions become quite transparent, and the canonical exponential growth condition is clearly seen in the conditions $h_d > 2h_{d+1}$. (That the requirement for $d = 2$ is less stringent—$h_2 > h_3$—arises from the idiosyncrasy that no CCV onset can have two sonority distances of 3.)

Box 3

(161) Dispersion analysis of CCCV

		$\mathbb{C}^4$	$\mathbb{C}^3$	$\mathbb{C}^2$	$\mathbb{C}^1$	
a.	$\mathbb{C}^k$					
b.	Sonority distance d	0	1	2	3	4
c.	Best CCCV onset with minimal sonority distance d	$G_0G_3O_4V$	$L_1G_3O_4V$	$N_2G_3O_4V$	$O_3G_3O_4V$	–
d.	Worst CCCV onset with all sonority distances > d	$N_1L_1G_1V$	$L_2O_2L_2V$	$O_3G_3O_4V$	–	–
e.	$\mathbb{C}^k \gg \mathbb{C}^{k-1}$ condition	$h_0+h_3+h_4 > 3h_1$	$h_1+h_3+h_4 > 3h_2$	$h_2+h_3+h_4 > 2h_3+h_4$		
f.	Does D meet condition?	$\infty+1/9+1/16 > 3(1)$ ✓	$1+1/9+1/16 > 3(\tfrac{1}{4})$ ✓	$h_2=1/4 > 1/9=h_3$ ✓		
g.	$D: h_d \equiv 1/d^2$	∞	1	1/4	1/9	1/16
h.	Condition if $h_4 = 0$	$h_0 + h_3 > 3h_1$	$h_1 + h_3 > 3h_2$	$h_2 > h_3$		

Clements is careful to insist that only onsets of the same length are to be compared using D.[36] This is the reason that all onsets considered in (160) have the same number of consonants: 2. The same analysis can be repeated for other onset lengths. For onsets CV, the computation is trivial, and the conclusion is just the obvious one: the H-penalties must increase as the sonority distance decreases. Clearly, D meets this criterion. So the cases of CV and CCV are now accounted for. These are the only two cases that have been examined in the preceding OT analysis. But analyses of CCCV (161) and CCCCV (162) yield the same results: the numbers generated by the formula for D meet the strict domination conditions.

There are infinitely many sets of H-penalties other than those given by D (156) that also meet the strict domination conditions in (160)–(162); there is presumably nothing special about the particular formula defining D other than that it happens to meet these requirements. At this point, I do not see any deeper connection between the OT analysis and the 'inverse-square law' given by the formula for D; Clements also explicitly states (in the passage (157) quoted above) that he has no reason to believe this particular formula has special significance.

---

[36] If onsets of different lengths *are* compared, the formula for D does not yield the same results as strict domination. There are of course other sets of H-penalties that *would* produce results equivalent to the OT analysis; if it should turn out that comparison of different-length onsets in the OT analysis is empirically relevant, then these alternative H-penalties could replace D in a numerical analysis of the sort proposed by Clements. An example of a set of penalties that would suffice for onsets of no more than four consonants — the longest considered by Clements — is given by $h_k \equiv 5^{k-1}$; then one violation of $\mathbb{C}^{k+1}$ is more costly than four violations of all $\mathbb{C}^j$ with $j \leq k$, and no more than four violations are possible with such onsets:

$$\Sigma_{j=1,\ldots,k}\, 4h_j = \Sigma_{j=1,\ldots,k}\, 4[5]^{j-1} = 4(1-5^k)/(1-5) = 5^k-1 = h_{k+1}-1 < h_{k+1}.$$

(Here the identity $\Sigma_{j=0,\ldots,n}\, r^j = (1-r^{n+1})/(1-r)$ has been employed.) This illustrates the exponential growth characteristic of strict domination; see Chapter 20.

(162) Dispersion analysis of CCCCV

		$\mathbb{C}^4$	$\mathbb{C}^3$	$\mathbb{C}^2$	$\mathbb{C}^1$	
a.	$\mathbb{C}^k$					
b.	Sonority distance d	0	1	2	3	4
c.	Best CCCCV onset with minimal sonority distance d	$O_0O_3G_3O_4V$	$N_1O_3G_3O_4V$	$L_2O_3G_3O_4V$	$G_3O_3G_3O_4V$	–
d.	Worst CCCCV onset with all sonority distances $> d$	$O_1N_1L_1G_1V$	$O_2L_2O_2L_2V$	$G_3O_3G_3O_4V$	–	–
e.	$\mathbb{C}^k \gg \mathbb{C}^{k-1}$ condition	$h_0 +2h_3 + h_4 > 4h_1$	$h_1 +2h_3 + h_4 > 4h_2$	$h_2 + 2h_3 + h_4 > 3h_3 +h_4$		
f.	Does D meet condition?	$\infty+2/9+1/16 > 4(1)$ ✓	$1+2/9+1/16 > 4(¼)$ ✓	$h_2 = 1/4 > 1/9 = h_3$ ✓		
g.	$D: h_d \equiv 1/d^2$	∞	1	1/4	1/9	1/16
h.	Condition if $h_4 = 0$	$h_0 + 2h_3 > 4h_1$	$h_1 + 2h_3 > 3h_2$	$h_2 > h_3$		

7 CONJUNCTION, RESTRICTIVENESS, AND EXPLANATION IN OPTIMALITY THEORY

Given the enormous variety and complexity of phonological patterns—for example, Lango ATR harmony (Section 4.1)—what could possibly be universal? The answer proposed by generative grammar has two parts: representations and principles. The representational assumption is relatively uncontroversial (within generative linguistics, if not within cognitive science as a whole).

(163) **Representational Universality**

The space of possible linguistic representations is universal.

Both OT and rule-based grammatical frameworks, by and large, adopt this assumption. At issue is the form of universal principles. Rule-based grammars assume the following:

(164) **Processual Universality**

Primitive operations of algorithms constructing linguistic representations are universal; they are *recombined* to create language-particular grammars.

A prime example is Autosegmental Phonology, which assumes the universality of autosegmental representations, and the universality of processes of linking, delinking, and spreading that manipulate associations among constituents. These operations are applied to specific types of constituents (e.g., features or autosegments) in a language-particular fashion, and combined into language-particular rules. It is not

Box 3

the rules themselves that are universal, but the elements of which they are constructed. A combinatorial explosion of language-particular combinations accommodates the great diversity of phonological grammars, yet universality is present nonetheless, residing at the subrule level of elementary processes.

OT of course adopts a different form of principle universality.

(165) **OT Markedness Universality**

The well-formedness polarity of dimensions of linguistic representations is universal; the *interaction* of markedness (and faithfulness) along these dimensions—especially, the adjudication of their conflicts—is language particular.

What type of 'interactions' are there among markedness dimensions? In OT, the markedness of dimensions d, d' are formalized via constraints $\mathbb{C}$, $\mathbb{C}'$. (For example, d = [±nas], $\mathbb{C}$ = *[+nas]; d' = '[±coda]', $\mathbb{C}'$ = NoCoda.) The fundamental mode of interaction is formalized in OT by constraint ranking: d and d' interact either as $\mathbb{C} \gg \mathbb{C}'$ or as $\mathbb{C}' \gg \mathbb{C}$.

In this chapter, we have explored the further possibility of *conjunctive interaction* of d and d'. This has been implemented in constraint ranking by means of additional constraints: conjunctions of basic constraints, $\mathbb{C} \& \mathbb{C}'$. Several points concerning conjunctive interaction deserve mention.

First, note that local conjunction provides OT a language-particular combinatorial structure. Under Processual Universality (164), it is elementary universal *processes* that recombine; in local conjunction, it is elementary well-formedness *constraints* that recombine.

Second, this chapter has provided evidence that conjunctive interaction is empirically observed, and that constraint conjunction allows the generalizations inherent in these interactions to be captured in the grammar. The descriptive complexity of Lango ATR harmony demands that complex rules be created in a rule-based analysis, or that complex conjunctive constraints be created in an OT analysis. The crucial point of comparison is that, in an important sense, the OT analysis is more restrictive: the rule-based analysis cannot capture a fundamental generalization that is inherent in the OT analysis. The argument goes as follows.

The combinatorial possibilities of processual Autosegmental Phonology allow the Lango grammar to create a rule such as (81a), repeated here:

(166)

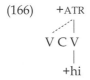

But the combinatorial options make this rule no more or less acceptable for a grammar than the following rule (with [+hi] replaced by [−hi]):

(167)   +ATR

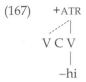

           V C V
              |
            –hi

Crucially, however, as Archangeli and Pulleyblank (1994) have shown, this sort of rule is in fact just what we *don't* find in ATR harmony systems — because [–hi] is a *marked* bearer of [+ATR] and it is *unmarked* vowels that best serve as sources of spreading.

For rule-based grammars, markedness can provide informal commentary *about* the grammar (perhaps commenting that (166) is a "good" rule, while (167) is not). In Grounded Phonology (Archangeli and Pulleyblank 1994), this is formalized as a descriptive superstructure *over* grammar, declaring certain rules to be dispreferred. In rule-based grammars, markedness is not an integral part of the grammar; additional stipulations must be made to rule out markedness-violating rules.

But in OT, markedness *is* the grammar, and UG simply does not provide the material for building grammars exhibiting the effects of unnatural rules like (167) — grammars producing harmonically incomplete inventories. The conjunctive interaction corresponding to the unnatural rule (167) — "*[+ATR, +hi] & HD-L[+ATR] ≫ F[ATR]" (cf. $\mathbb{C}_2$, (100b)) — simply cannot be created, because that conjunction would require a constraint "*[+ATR,+hi]", and no such constraint exists in *Con*: among [+ATR] vowels, the universal polarity of markedness *favors* [+hi]. The absence of *[+ATR, +hi] from *Con* is the formal statement, present in every OT grammar, that the co-occurrence of [+ATR] and [+hi] is unmarked.[37]

The overarching generalization here is that harmony systems respect markedness; that is, inventories of vowel feature domains are harmonically complete. The OT analysis via conjunctive interaction captures this generalization directly: it is solely through the interaction of elementary markedness constraints (like *[+ATR,–hi]) that inventories of harmonic feature domains are fashioned. This conclusion can be maintained, however, only if the constraint interactions possible in OT include conjunctive interactions.

The third point is that conjunctive interaction is from a formal point of view entirely natural in OT; indeed, in an important sense, its *absence* would be *unnatural*. By

---

[37] This discussion assumes the simpler formalization of markedness in which $\alpha \prec \beta$ is expressed as '∃ *$\alpha \in Con$ but ∄ *$\beta \in Con$', rather than the alternative '*$\alpha \gg_{UG}$ *β'. (See Footnotes 12:28–29.) In the latter formalization, the argument proceeds as follows: since conjunction respects universal markedness hierarchies (Chapter 12 (44)), *HD-L[ATR] & *[+ATR,–hi] ≫ *HD-L[ATR] & *[+ATR,+hi], so the needed ranking in the text *HD-L[ATR] & *[+ATR,+hi] ≫ F[ATR] entails *HD-L[ATR] & *[+ATR,–hi] ≫ F[ATR] as well. Thus, any ranking that attempts to "block regressive spread of [+ATR] from a [+hi] vowel" — to achieve the intent of the unnatural rule (167), that spread is *restricted to* [–hi] vowels — will inevitably also "block regressive spread of [+ATR] from a [–hi] vowel"; that is, all regressive spread is blocked. This gives the equivalent of the rule (167) with no height specification, and hence no markedness breach.

Box 3

this I mean simply that without conjunction, basic OT typologies are not strongly harmonically complete, but with conjunction, they are. Harmonic completeness is the central organizing principle by which OT formalizes the broad generalization that "typologies of inventories are consistent with markedness." Thus, the necessity and sufficiency of conjunctive interaction for SHARC typologies constitutes a strong basis for claiming that, formally speaking, OT with conjunction is more natural than OT without it.

The fourth point is that, as implemented through constraint conjunction, conjunctive interaction preserves the strict domination structure of OT; the need for conjunction is not evidence for (indeed, not even consistent with) the claim that it is weighted numerical interaction, not strict domination, that provides the evaluative calculus for linguistic well-formedness. This point is demonstrated and illustrated in Section 20:1.1.3.

The final point is that while conjunctive interactions do not appear to be rare, it does seem that constraint interaction is overwhelmingly nonconjunctive. From the numerical perspective of Section 20:1.1.3, conjunctive interaction corresponds to *nonlinear* interaction, and nonconjunctive to linear. It is perhaps not inappropriate then to regard conjunctive interaction as a kind of *higher-order* effect, with the first-order baseline provided by nonconjunctive interaction. Grammars may constitute yet another of the multitude of natural systems for which linear theories provide an excellent first-order description, with higher-order, nonlinear effects profitably viewed as deviations from the norm.

The admission of conjunctive interaction into OT raises many obvious questions: Which constraints can interact conjunctively? What determines the domain of conjunctive interaction? How are conjunctive interactions learned? At this point, it is premature to seriously address these important, but empirically and theoretically enormous, questions. They must be left for ongoing and future research.

I will close by briefly considering two less obvious questions. The first is, are *self*-conjunctions necessary or desirable? The serious problem posed by self-conjunctions is their ability to count. Generally speaking, in a power hierarchy of self-conjoined constraints $\cdots \mathbb{C}^3 \gg \mathbb{C}^2 \gg \mathbb{C}^1$, if a conflicting constraint $\mathbb{C}'$ interrupts the hierarchy between $\mathbb{C}^n$ and $\mathbb{C}^{n-1}$, then the grammar distinguishes between n and $n-1$ violations of $\mathbb{C}$, producing different types of output in the two cases. Such counting is not generally regarded as possible within human grammars, as discussed in Section 20:1.2.1.1. Thus, it may be that the kind of counting required for the definition of self-conjunctions is not within the computational power of the human language faculty.

It is worth noting that the cases of self-conjunction employed in this chapter (Section 6) are special as regards counting. There are four sonority-determining segmental features and instances of general constraints for each of the four. Combining these features into a set $\mathbf{C}$ and defining a single constraint $\mathbb{C}_{\mathbf{C}}$ in terms of $\mathbf{C}$ makes violations of $\mathbb{C}$ for different features into multiple violations of the same constraint. But if the features are kept separate in distinct constraints $\mathbb{C}_1, \ldots, \mathbb{C}_4$, then instead of multiple violations of a single constraint we have a single violation of each of several constraints — which can be handled without *self*-conjunction.

While this move succeeds in avoiding self-conjunction, in general it misses the generalization that numbers capture: instead of a single constraint $\mathbb{C}^2$, we have multiple constraints $\mathbb{C}_1 \& \mathbb{C}_2$, $\mathbb{C}_1 \& \mathbb{C}_3$, ... one for each pair of features. These must all be ranked together in order to do the work of $\mathbb{C}^2$. Why are these all ranked together? Because they each register *two* violations! That all pairs $\mathbb{C}_i \& \mathbb{C}_j$ are ranked alike is a generalization requiring the number 2 for its statement — precisely what is captured in the self-conjunction $\mathbb{C}^2$.

It is unclear whether such problems arise in the case of the ONS power hierarchy, because the features within a single segment are not independent (144). Since a [−son] segment must also be a [−approx] segment, a segment that violates ALIGN-L(σ, [−approx]) must also violate ALIGN-L(σ, [−son]). Thus, the conjunction ALIGN-L(σ, [−approx]) & ALIGN-L(σ, [−son]) is violated just when ALIGN-L(σ, [−approx]) is violated. It is just conjunctions of this type, ALIGN-L(σ, [−f_1]) & ALIGN-L(σ, [−f_2]), that make up ONS^2; they can be reduced from a conjunction to a single ALIGN constraint. So self-conjunction may be convenient for constructing the ONS hierarchy, but it is not necessary (as already suggested in (150)).

However, self-conjunction does seem integral to the F° power hierarchy used to derive the sonority distance generalization; there, constraint violations within different features of a segment are independent (153)–(154). But then it is hardly surprising that counting is an issue in an account of a generalization that relies crucially on numerical differences (between sonority levels). If it is true that grammars can't count, then this would seem to be a generalization that cannot be explained — or even stated — by grammatical theory. Given the limited empirical evidence for the generalization,[38] the theory without self-conjunction may in fact prove to be empirically as well as theoretically more sound.

Finally, consider the question, which constraints heretofore seen as atomic should now be decomposed as conjunctions of more basic constraints, as has been done here for ONSET? For example, should *[+ATR, −hi] be regarded as the conjunction *[+ATR] & *[−hi]? While I have no knockdown argument, I would say no. I view conjoined constraints as merely the implementation within strict domination hierarchies of a general nonlinear effect whereby two independently marked configurations are especially marked when they fall within a single local domain — superadditive interaction.

But *[+ATR, −hi] expresses the markedness of the *combination* [+ATR, −hi] — that is, [−hi] is marked here *only because* it is combined with [+ATR]. From this perspective, it exemplifies the same general structure not of NOCODA & *[lab] but rather of *ONS/a.

---

[38] Concerning the inadequacy of sonority distance for characterizing inventories of onset clusters, see, for example, Rice 1992 and Morelli 2002.

Box 3

[lab] is not a marked place *because* it is in coda—it is always a marked place, but its markedness is especially pronounced in a context that itself is independently marked, the coda. This is the canonical conjunctive interaction. But *Ons/*a* asserts that *a* is marked *as an onset*; it is only the *combination* Ons and *a* that is marked. This is not the conjunctive interaction of the general markedness of onsets and the general markedness of *a*—which general markedness most likely does not even exist. The internal combinatorial structure of *Ons/*a* is not that of conjunction; rather, it is that of Harmonic Alignment (Chapter 12 (42)).

Analogously, the internal structure of *[+ATR, −hi] might profitably be analyzed as the result of the (articulatorily motivated) alignment of two phonetic scales, as in (168).

(168)   Feature co-occurrence constraints as Harmonic Alignment

    a.   Scales
        i.   ATR   [+ATR] > [−ATR]
        ii. [hi]   [+hi] > [−hi]

    b.   Harmonic alignments[39]
        i.   [+ATR, +hi] ≻ [+ATR, −hi]
        ii.   [−ATR, −hi] ≻ [−ATR, +hi]
        iii. [+ATR, +hi] ≻ [−ATR, +hi]
        iv. [−ATR, −hi] ≻ [+ATR, −hi]

    c.   Constraint hierarchies
        i.   *[+ATR, −hi] ≫ *[+ATR, +hi]
        ii.   *[−ATR, +hi] ≫ *[−ATR, −hi]
        iii. *[−ATR, +hi] ≫ *[+ATR, +hi]
        iv. *[+ATR, −hi] ≫ *[−ATR, −hi]
        or alternatively, more simply,[40]
        v.   *[+ATR, −hi], *[−ATR, +hi] ∈ *Con*
        vi. *[+ATR, +hi], *[−ATR, −hi] ∉ *Con*

8 SUMMARY

Does OT provide a satisfactory formal theory of markedness? In outline, the argument developed in this chapter has gone as follows:

(169)   Synopsis

    a.   OT formalization of markedness ⇒ invisibility of the unmarked, with no need to stipulate underspecified representations

---

[39] The definition of Harmonic Alignment is asymmetric. One scale must be binary; but if both are binary, then either can serve in either alignment role. In (168b–c), one alignment yields (i)–(ii) and the other yields (iii)–(iv).
[40] See also Footnotes 12:28–29.

  b. Strong harmonic completeness ⇔ Local constraint conjunction
  c. Local conjunction + Headed feature domains ⇒
    i. Markedness-governed vowel harmony systems
    ii. Syllable structure constraints
    iii. A wide range of markedness-governed inventories

Bringing the primary part of this chapter to a close, the following points summarize each of the subarguments and central concepts referred to in the synopsis (169): the formal character of markedness in OT (170); conjunctive constraint interaction and harmonic completeness (171); and the notion of headed feature domain upon which the empirical analyses of the chapter rest (172). The Appendix, an extended formal analysis of basic inventories, follows.

(170) Markedness
  a. Along an individual dimension d of structural variation, there is typically a marked pole. Let the two poles of d be denoted by $[\pm\varphi]$, where $[+\varphi]$ is the marked pole.
  b. Structures falling at the marked end of the dimension d will violate a markedness constraint that we can write '$*[+\varphi]$'. Structures falling at the unmarked pole of d violate a constraint $*[-\varphi]$ that is universally lower ranked than $*[+\varphi]$ (or nonexistent).
  c. These simple principles entail that in OT, less-marked material is necessarily less phonologically active than more-marked material. Nearly all the effects of coronal underspecification, for example, follow inevitably, without stipulating underspecified representations. Unmarked material is "invisible" to the grammar, although present in representations, because the grammar sees only 'marks' (constraint violations).
  d. Whatever the mechanics of markedness combination, the result must be inventories of linguistic forms that 'respect markedness' in the following sense. If x is in a language's inventory of structures of some type, and x is modified along a single dimension d to a less-marked φ value, then the newer structure must be in the inventory as well: 'If a more-marked structure is legal, then a less-marked structure must be also'. Contrapositively, 'If a less-marked structure is illegal, then a more-marked structure must be also'. Here comparison is along a single structural dimension d.
  e. An inventory that 'respects markedness' in this sense is dubbed 'harmonically complete' in OT.
  f. A crosslinguistic typology has the SHARC (strong harmonic completeness) property if it declares an inventory possible if and only if it is harmonically complete.
  g. This is relatively straightforward if only a single dimension d is involved. But linguistic structures vary along many dimensions; a critical problem for markedness theory is combination of multiple markedness dimensions.

Box 3

(171) Local constraint conjunction

    a. OT combines markedness dimensions by regulating, through ranking, the interaction of the corresponding markedness constraints.

    b. Generally speaking, the inventories OT generates are harmonically complete.

    c. Generally speaking, however, OT does not generate all harmonically complete inventories, so OT typologies lack the SHARC property.

    d. An important class of examples is the BOWOW inventory, which bans only the worst of the worst. These are harmonically complete but not generable by basic OT.

    e. Suppose that in addition to interacting via simple ranking, two markedness constraints A and B can also interact more strongly: the disharmony generated by violating both A and B is amplified when the two violations occur within a common domain $\mathcal{D}$. This can be implemented within strict domination via the operation of local conjunction, which yields a constraint $A \,\&_{\mathcal{D}}\, B$ that is only violated when A and B are both violated within a common domain $\mathcal{D}$.

    f. Adding conjunctive constraint interaction to ranking preserves the result that the inventories generated are harmonically complete.

    g. Adding conjunctive interaction in fact yields typologies that are strongly harmonically complete.

(172) Headed feature domains

    a. To incorporate the insights of Autosegmental Phonology in nonderivational OT, a new formalism is needed to capture autosegmental "processes" representationally.

    b. In an output, a contiguous span of segments bearing a common feature value [±φ] forms a [±φ] domain.

    c. Such a feature domain has a left and right edge; these can be used

        i. to formulate a harmony or spreading imperative, requiring alignment of, say, the right edge of a feature domain and the right edge of a word;

        ii. to define syllable-structure constraints by requiring that left edges of consonantal feature domains align with left edges of a syllable;

        iii. to show how basic syllable structure constraints, like ONSET, and sonority conditions emerge from a still more basic level, through the interactions of the domains of multiple features.

    d. A feature domain is a constituent with a Harmony of its own.

        i. The Harmony of a domain reflects the Harmony of the elements within it; markedness violations within a single domain, even if they are incurred by different segments, can interact conjunctively in determining the Harmony of the domain.

    ii. A vowel harmony system can be analyzed as a (harmonically complete) inventory of permitted vowel feature domain configurations.

e. A feature domain has a head segment.

    i. The notion 'head' is a descendent of the concept "source of spreading" in a rule-based account.

    ii. Thus, left-headed domains descend from "progressive harmony" processes; right-headed ones, from "regressive harmony."

    iii. There are several levels of faithful expression of an underlying feature value [±φ]: it can surface unfaithfully as [∓φ]; it can appear in the output as a *member* of a [±φ] domain; or, most faithful of all, it can surface as the *head* of a [±φ] domain.

f. Headed feature domains interacting by local conjunction explain complex markedness effects in vowel harmony systems and predict a typology that unifies a wide range of disparate phonological patterns.[41]

[41] For valuable comments and suggestions on the work presented here, I am grateful to many audience members. Section 1—excluding (36)–(48)—was presented in October 1993 at the Rutgers Optimality Workshop (ROW–1) and in 1994 at a University of California, Santa Cruz linguistics colloquium. Section 2 originated in work presented at ROW–1 and at linguistics colloquia at the University of Arizona and UCLA in 1995. Sections 4.1 and 7 were presented at the 1997 Hopkins Optimality Theory Workshop/University of Maryland Mayfest (HOT-97). Section 4.2 summarizes joint work with Laura Benua presented at linguistics colloquia in 2001 at the State University of New York at Stony Brook and the University of Massachusetts at Amherst. Section 5 and the Appendix were presented at the 2001 Phonology Forum, Chiba University, Japan. Section 6 was presented in 1995 linguistics colloquia at the University of Arizona and UCLA. Various bits of the work discussed in this chapter were presented in 2002 at the annual meeting of the Linguistic Society of America, a linguistic colloquium at Rutgers University, and a session of the Korean Phonological Society in Seoul, and in 2003 at the MIT Workshop on Markedness and the Lexicon. While fading memory doubtless obscures many valuable conversations, among the members of these audiences who I would like to thank particularly are Laura Benua, Ellen Broselow, Paul de Lacy, Matt Goldrick, Bruce Hayes, Junko Itô, Linda Lombardi, John McCarthy, Armin Mester, Elliott Moreton, Geoffrey Pullum, Donca Steriade, Bruce Tesar, Colin Wilson, Cheryl Zoll, and especially Alan Prince. The reader is referred to McCarthy 2004 for arguments that *HD is the right spreading-inducing constraint; that work appeared after this book went into production.

Box 3

APPENDIX. STRONG HARMONIC COMPLETENESS AND LOCAL CONJUNCTION: FORMAL ANALYSIS OF BASIC INVENTORIES

(173) Assume given a set of (underlying) inputs $\mathcal{U}$ and a set of (surface) outputs S; the set of input-output pairs is $\mathcal{U} \times S$. The notation will be /u/ or u $\in \mathcal{U}$, [s] or $s \in S$, and π or /u/ $\to$ [s] or u $\to s \in \mathcal{U} \times S$.

(174) Basic definitions and assumptions

    a. A **constraint** $\mathbb{C}$ is a function assigning to each input-output pair $\pi = u \to s$ a **Harmony value** on some scale.

        i. To denote that $\mathbb{C}(\pi_1)$ is lower on the Harmony scale than $\mathbb{C}(\pi_2)$, we write '$\mathbb{C}(\pi_1) \prec \mathbb{C}(\pi_2)$' or '$\pi_1 \prec_{\mathbb{C}} \pi_2$'. '$\pi_1 \succ_{\mathbb{C}} \pi_2$' means '$\pi_2 \prec_{\mathbb{C}} \pi_1$'; '$\pi_1 \sim_{\mathbb{C}} \pi_2$' means '$\mathbb{C}$ assigns π_1 and π_2 equal Harmony': $\mathbb{C}(\pi_1) = \mathbb{C}(\pi_2)$. '$\pi_1 \succcurlyeq_{\mathbb{C}} \pi_2$' means '$\pi_1 \succ_{\mathbb{C}} \pi_2$ or $\pi_1 \sim_{\mathbb{C}} \pi_2$'; and so on.

        ii. $\mathbb{C}(\pi)$, the Harmony of π with respect to $\mathbb{C}$, is also called the '**set** (or **sequence**) **of marks** assigned to π by $\mathbb{C}$'. The marks assigned by distinct constraints are distinct.

    b. $Con = \mathcal{M} \cup \mathcal{F}$, where $\mathcal{M}$ is the set of **markedness** constraints and $\mathcal{F}$ is a disjoint set of **faithfulness** constraints.

        i. When $\mathbb{C}$ is a markedness constraint, $\mathbb{C}(u \to s)$ depends only on s, and we write it '$\mathbb{C}(s)$'.

        ii. When $s \prec_{\mathbb{C}} s'$, $\mathbb{C}$ a markedness constraint, we say that s is **more marked** than s' with respect to $\mathbb{C}$.

    c. The **Harmony** of an input-output pair π, denoted '$H(\pi)$', is the set of marks assigned it by all the constraints $\mathbb{C} \in Con$. The **M-Harmony** of a structure π, denoted 'MARK(π)', is the set of marks assigned it by all the constraints in $\mathcal{M}$; the **F-Harmony**, denoted 'FAITH(π)', the corresponding set for $\mathcal{F}$.

    d. '$H(\pi_1) \prec_{\mathcal{G}} H(\pi_2)$' (or '$\pi_1 \prec_{\mathcal{G}} \pi_2$') means that the Harmony of π_1 is lower than that of π_2 with respect to a (total) ranking $\mathcal{G}$ of the constraints in Con; this means that π_1 has lower Harmony than π_2 with respect to the constraint that is highest ranked in $\mathcal{G}$ among those constraints that assign different Harmony values to π_1 and π_2. That is, if $\mathcal{G} = [\mathbb{C}_1 \gg \mathbb{C}_2 \gg \cdots \gg \mathbb{C}_n]$, then $\pi_1 \prec_{\mathcal{G}} \pi_2$ if and only if

        $\exists k \in \{1, \ldots, n\}$ such that $\pi_1 \prec_{\mathbb{C}_k} \pi_2$ and $\forall j < k$, $\pi_1 \nprec_{\mathbb{C}_j} \pi_2$.

        $H(\pi_1) \sim_{\mathcal{G}} H(\pi_2)$ (or $\pi_1 \sim_{\mathcal{G}} \pi_2$) means that $\forall \mathbb{C} \in Con$, $\pi_1 \sim_{\mathbb{C}} \pi_2$.

    e. An input-output pair u $\to s$ is **optimal** with respect to $\mathcal{G}$ — written '$\mathcal{G}$: u $\to s$' — if and only if there is no s' such that u $\to s \prec_{\mathcal{G}}$ u $\to s'$.

    f. The (output) **language** specified by $\mathcal{G}$ is $\mathcal{L}_{\mathcal{G}} \equiv \{s \mid \exists u$ such that $\mathcal{G}$: u $\to s\}$.

    g. It will be convenient to abbreviate '$s \in \mathcal{L}$' by '✓s' and '$s \notin \mathcal{L}$' by '*s'.

(175) Structure u (unmarked) is **universally less marked** than structure m (marked), written '$u \gtrsim m$', if and only if $\exists M_0 \in \mathcal{M}$ such that $M_0(u) \succ M_0(m)$ and $\forall M \in \mathcal{M}$, $M(u) \succcurlyeq M(m)$. '$x \backsim y$' means $\forall M \in \mathcal{M}$, $M(x) \sim M(y)$. '$x \gtrsim y$' means $x \succ y$ or $x \backsim y$.

Figure 1. Φ-space

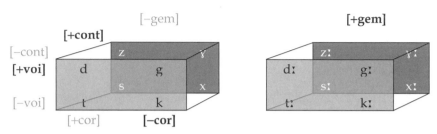

(176) A language $\mathcal{L}$ is **harmonically complete** if and only if $m \in \mathcal{L}$ and $u \succeq m$ imply $u \in \mathcal{L}$. (Equivalently, if and only if $u \notin \mathcal{L}$ and $u \succeq m$ imply $m \notin \mathcal{L}$. That is, in a harmonically complete language, if $u \succeq m$, then ✓$m \Rightarrow$ ✓u – an **implicational universal** – and $*u \Rightarrow *m$.)

(177) A **basic inventory** is defined by the following elements:

a. A set S of **output** ('surface') **linguistic structures**. The set of input structures $\mathcal{U}$ is also S. To emphasize the role of a structure as input or output, '/s/' or 's' denotes a structure considered as an input, and '[s]' or 's' denotes the same structure considered as an output.

   For example, segments: /n/→t, /t/→t; vowel tiers: /u e/→[u o]

b. A set of functions $\Phi = \{\varphi_1, \varphi_2, ..., \varphi_n\}$ called **features**; Φ assigns to each $s \in S$ a list of **feature values** $[\varphi_1(s), \varphi_2(s), ..., \varphi_n(s)]$.

   i. S is represented in **Φ-space** by assigning to s the coordinates that are its feature values (see Figure 1: segments, with $n = 4$):
   $$s_\Phi \equiv [\varphi_1(s), \varphi_2(s), ..., \varphi_n(s)].$$

   ii. S is **featurally decomposable**: for every sequence $[f_1, f_2, ..., f_n]$, where f_i is a possible value of feature φ_i, there is a structure s with this feature list (i.e., $\exists s \in S$ such that $s_\Phi = [f_1, f_2, ..., f_n]$).

c. A set of **markedness constraints** $\mathcal{M} = \{M_1, M_2, ..., M_n\}$.

   i. Each $M \in \mathcal{M}$ assigns to each $s \in S$ a markedness value $M(s)$ that is determined by the feature values s_Φ of s.

   ii. The markedness values of each constraint M form a binary scale: for the two values m_+ and m_-, one – say, m_+ – indicates less markedness (greater Harmony), and we write '$m_+ \succ m_-$'.

   iii. S is represented in **M-space** by assigning to s the coordinates that are its markedness values: $s_M \equiv [M_1(s), M_2(s), ..., M_N(s)]$ (see Figure 2).

   iv. $\mathcal{M}$ is **featurally decomposable**: if $s_\Phi = [f_1, f_2, ..., f_n]$, then
   $$M(s) = M_1[f_1] \cup M_2[f_2] \cup \cdots \cup M_n[f_n].$$
   That is, M_i assesses the markedness of the corresponding feature φ_i. Let the least marked ('best') value of φ_i be denoted 'b_i', and the most-marked ('worst') value, 'w_i': $M_i(b_i) = m_+ \succ m_- = M_i(w_i)$.

Figure 1   *Box 3*

Figure 2. M-space

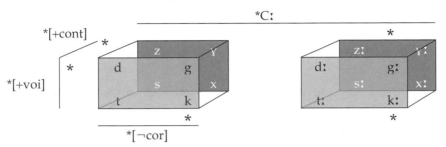

d. A set of **faithfulness constraints** $\mathcal{F} = \{F_1, F_2, ..., F_n\}$

   i. Given any input-output pair $u \rightarrow s$, each $F \in \mathcal{F}$ assigns a Harmony value determined by the features u_Φ of u and the features s_Φ of s.

   ii. The Harmony values of each faithfulness constraint F form a scale.

   iii. When input = output, $F(s \rightarrow s) = \varnothing$, the highest Harmony value.

   iv. $\mathcal{F}$ is **featurally decomposable**; if $u_\Phi = [f_1, f_2, ..., f_n]$ and $s_\Phi = [f_1', f_2', ..., f_n']$, then
$$F(s) = F_1[f_1 \rightarrow f_1'] \cup F_2[f_2 \rightarrow f_2'] \cup \cdots \cup F_n[f_n \rightarrow f_n'].$$

   v. Thus each F_i evaluates faithfuless with respect to feature φ_i. For all i, $F_i[f_i \rightarrow f_i'] = \varnothing$ whenever $f_i = f_i'$, and $F_i[f_i \rightarrow f_i'] \prec \varnothing$ whenever $f_i \neq f_i'$ (any featural change lowers the F-Harmony).

e. For a ranking $\mathcal{G}$ of the constraints in *Con*, the **inventory** is defined by
$$I_\mathcal{G} \equiv \{s \in S \mid \mathcal{G} : s \rightarrow s\}.$$
   $I_\mathcal{G}$ is the set of inputs that are mapped to themselves by the grammar: the set of s such that there is no s' such that $s \rightarrow s'$ has higher Harmony than $s \rightarrow s$.[42]

f. An inventory arising from an OT system satisfying all the above properties is a **basic inventory**.

g. The set of inventories defined by all rankings $\mathcal{G}$ of *Con* define the (**factorial**) **typology** of *Con*, denoted $\mathcal{T}_{Con}$. When *Con* has all the above properties, $\mathcal{T}_{Con}$ is a **basic typology**.

(178) *Theorem.* Suppose $I_\mathcal{G}$ is a basic inventory and $s_\Phi = [f_1, f_2, ..., f_n]$. Let *J* be the set of all *j* such that the markedness of f_j with respect to M_j is not the lowest possible—that is, for each $j \in J$, there is another value f_j' of φ_j such that $M_j(f_j') \succ M_j(f_j)$. Then $s \in I_\mathcal{G}$ if and only if $[\forall j \in J, F_j \gg M_j \text{ in } \mathcal{G}]$.

---

[42] In general, in OT the inventory is the set of all possible outputs, that is, the set of all s such that for *some* u, $u \rightarrow s$: it is not necessary that $u = s$ (174f). The case where u cannot be s amounts to a chain shift: $u \rightarrow s$ but $s \rightarrow s' \neq s$. In the simplified setting of a basic inventory, however, the definition in the text is correct because whenever there exists a u such that $u \rightarrow s$, then necessarily also $s \rightarrow s$. This follows from the logic of the proof of Theorem (178).

Proof. '*Only if*' part: Suppose $s \in I_{\mathcal{G}}$ where s is as defined in the theorem; then we must show that $[\forall j \in J, F_j \gg M_j \text{ in } \mathcal{G}]$. Let j be any element of J. Let s' be the structure in S with the same feature values as s, except that f_j is replaced by f_j'; such an s' exists by (177b.ii). Since $s \in I$, $s \to s$ is optimal (177e); hence

$$H(s \to s) \succcurlyeq H(s \to s') \qquad\qquad \text{def. of optimality (174e)}$$
$$\Rightarrow M(s) \cup F(s \to s) \succcurlyeq M(s') \cup F(s \to s') \qquad Con = \mathcal{M} \cup \mathcal{F} \text{ (174b)}$$
$$\Rightarrow M(s) \cup \varnothing \succcurlyeq M(s') \cup F(s \to s') \qquad F(x \to x) = \varnothing \text{ (177d.ii)}$$
$$\Rightarrow M_1(f_1) \cup \cdots \cup M_j(f_j) \cup \cdots \cup M_n(f_n) \qquad \mathcal{M} \text{ decomposable (177c.iii)}$$
$$\succcurlyeq M_1(f_1) \cup M_2(f_2) \cup \cdots \cup M_j(f_j') \cup \cdots \cup M_n(f_n) \cup F(s \to s')$$
$$\Rightarrow M_j(f_j) \succcurlyeq M_j(f_j') \cup F(s \to s') \qquad \text{mark cancellation}$$
$$\Rightarrow M_j(f_j) \succcurlyeq \qquad\qquad \mathcal{F} \text{ decomposable (177d.iii)}$$
$$M_j(f_j') \cup F_1(f_1 \to f_1) \cup F_2(f_2 \to f_2) \cup \cdots \cup F_j(f_j \to f_j') \cup \cdots \cup F_n(f_n \to f_n)$$
$$\Rightarrow M_j(f_j) \succcurlyeq M_j(f_j') \cup F_j(f_j \to f_j') . \qquad F_k(f_k \to f_k) = \varnothing \text{ (177d.iii)}$$

By hypothesis, $M_j(f_j) \prec M_j(f_j')$. Now $M_j(f_j) \succcurlyeq M_j(f_j') \cup F_j(f_j \to f_j')$ can only result from $F_j \gg M_j$—it is the higher ranked of F_j and M_j that makes the decision, and M_j favors f_j', not f_j; the higher-ranked constraint must therefore be F_j: $F_j \gg M_j$, Q.E.D. Since $F_j(f_j \to f_j') \neq \varnothing$ (177d.iii), with $F_j \gg M_j$, F_j does indeed make the decision in favor of f_j, ensuring that $M_j(f_j) \succ M_j(f_j') \cup F_j(f_j \to f_j')$.

'*If*' part: Suppose s is as defined in the theorem and $F_j \gg M_j$ for all j in J; then we must show that $s \in I_G$, that is, that $\mathcal{G}{:}s \to s$. Consider any $s' \in S$, with $s'_\Phi = [f_1', f_2', \ldots, f_n']$.

$$H(s \to s') = M(s') \cup F(s \to s') \qquad Con = \mathcal{M} \cup \mathcal{F} \text{ (174b)}$$
$$= [M_1(f_1') \cup M_2(f_2') \cup \cdots \cup M_n(f_n')] \cup \qquad \mathcal{M} \text{ decomposable (177c.iii)}$$
$$[F_1(f_1 \to f_1') \cup \cdots \cup F_n(f_n \to f_n')] \qquad \mathcal{F} \text{ decomposable (177d.iii)}$$
$$= [M_1(f_1') \cup F_1(f_1 \to f_1')] \cup \qquad \cup \text{ commutative, associative}$$
$$\cdots \cup [M_n(f_n') \cup F_n(f_n \to f_n')].$$
$$H(s \to s) = M(s) \cup F(s \to s) \qquad Con = \mathcal{M} \cup \mathcal{F} \text{ (174b)}$$
$$= M(s) \cup \varnothing \qquad F(x \to x) = \varnothing \text{ (177d.ii)}$$
$$= M_1(f_1) \cup M_2(f_2) \cup \cdots \cup M_n(f_n). \qquad \mathcal{M} \text{ decomposable (177c.iii)}$$

s will only fail to be optimal if $\exists s' \in S$ such that $H(s \to s') \succ H(s \to s)$ (174e). Now in order for $H(s \to s') \succ H(s \to s)$, the highest-ranked uncanceled mark between them must be one of the marks of $H(s \to s)$, that is, one of the marks $M_k(f_k)$. This uncanceled mark $M_k(f_k)$ must outrank all the uncanceled marks of $H(s \to s')$, so in particular it must outrank all the uncanceled marks in $[M_k(f_k') \cup F_k(f_k \to f_k')]$. Now no F marks in $[M_k(f_k') \cup F_k(f_k \to f_k')]$ can be canceled because $H(s \to s)$ has no F marks; and the mark $M_k(f_k')$ can't be canceled because it would have to be canceled by $M_k(f_k)$ and by assumption this is an uncanceled mark. Thus, $M_k(f_k)$ would have to outrank all the marks in $M_k(f_k') \cup F_k(f_k \to f_k')$. Thus, we are ensured that no such s' will exist—ensured that s is optimal—if $\forall k$,

(i) $M_k(f_k') \cup F_k(f_k \to f_k') \preccurlyeq M_k(f_k).$

If for some k, $f_k' = f_k$, then (i) is trivially satisfied because both sides reduce to the same mark $M_k(f_k)$. If for some k, f_k' is more marked than f_k, then (i) is satisfied because then $M_k(f_k') \cup F_k(f_k \to f_k') \prec M_k(f_k') \prec M_k(f_k)$. The interesting cases are those k for which f_k' is less marked than f_k—such a k must lie in the set J defined in the theorem. In such a case, because $M_k(f_k') \succ M_k(f_k)$, (i) will fail if M_k is the decisive constraint, and (i) will hold if F_k is decisive, since $\varnothing \neq F_k(f_k \to f_k') \prec \varnothing$. By hypothesis, $F_k \gg M_k$ for all k in J, so (i) cannot fail. Thus, $s \to s$ is optimal and $s \in I_G$.

Figure 2   *Box 3*

(179) *Corollary.* Suppose I_G is a basic inventory, and $s_\Phi = [f_1, f_2, \ldots, f_n]$. Let J be the set of all j such that the markedness of f_j with respect to M_j is not the lowest possible — that is, for each $j \in J$, there is another value f_j' of φ_j such that $M_j(f_j') \succ M_j(f_j)$. Then $s \notin I_G$ if and only if $[\exists j \in J$ such that $M_j \gg F_j$ in $G]$.

> *Proof.* The contrapositive of the preceding theorem: $p \Leftrightarrow q$ is equivalent to $\neg p \Leftrightarrow \neg q$;
>
> $\neg[\ \forall j \in J, F_j \gg M_j\ ] \equiv \exists j \in J, \neg[F_j \gg M_j]$
>
> by de Morgan's Law. Since G is a total ranking,
>
> $\neg[F_j \gg M_j] \equiv [M_j \gg F_j]$.

(180) *Theorem.* A basic inventory I_G is harmonically complete.

> *Proof.* We show that if $s \notin I_G$ and $s' \precsim s$, then $s' \notin I_G$ (176). Let $s_\Phi = [f_1, f_2, \ldots, f_n]$ be an element not in the inventory. By Corollary (179), there is some k such that f_k is not the least marked value of φ_k and $M_k \gg F_k$ in G. Now let $s' = [f_1', f_2', \ldots, f_n']$ be an element universally more marked than s: $s' \precsim s$. By definition (175), this means that f_i' is at least as marked as f_i for all i; so in particular, f_k' is at least as marked as f_k. Thus, since f_k is not the least marked value of φ_k, f_k' is also not the least marked value. For this k, we already know $M_k \gg F_k$. Thus, by Corollary (179), $s' \notin I_G$.

(181) The **harmonic upper bound set (HUB)** of x is

$$\text{HUB}(x) \equiv \{y \mid y \succsim x\} = \{y \mid \forall i, M_i(y) \succsim M_i(x)\}.$$

In M-space, $M_i(y)$ is the ith coordinate of y, so $\text{HUB}(x)$ is the m-dimensional rectangle with one corner at the origin and the other at x, where m is the number of $\varphi_i(x)$ that are not the least marked value. For the other coordinates i — those for which $\varphi_i(x) = b_i$ — $\text{HUB}(x)$ is of zero length along the dimension M_i. (Recall that 'b_i' and 'w_i' denote the most and least harmonic values of feature φ_i, respectively (177c.i).)

In Figure 3, and subsequent such WOW diagrams, the white cells identify the segments of an inventory; the black cells contain segments, marked with '*', excluded from the inventory. The inventories shown in these figures are largely hypothetical, designed to illustrate the theoretical results being derived. Figure 4, however, shows a four-dimesional slice of an actual segment inventory, the consonants of Thai (Hudak 1987, 760).[43]

---

[43] The aspirated fricatives occupying the [+cont, +asp] subspace are highly marked, but they do merit membership in this space as they are attested, for example, in Burmese (Ladefoged and Maddieson 1996, 179). The other two dimensions are [±voi], [cor/ ¬cor].

Figure 3. Two harmonically complete (hypothetical) inventories each of which is a single HUB

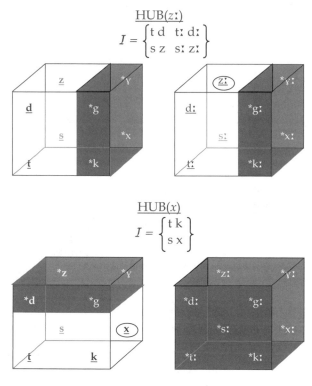

HUB(zː)

$$I = \left\{ \begin{matrix} \text{t d} & \text{tː dː} \\ \text{s z} & \text{sː zː} \end{matrix} \right\}$$

HUB(x)

$$I = \left\{ \begin{matrix} \text{t k} \\ \text{s x} \end{matrix} \right\}$$

(182) *Lemma.* $z \in$ HUB(x) if and only if $\forall i[\varphi_i(x) = b_i \Rightarrow \varphi_i(z) = b_i]$.

> *Proof.* By definition (181), $z \in$ HUB(x) $\Leftrightarrow \forall i[M_i(z) \succcurlyeq M_i(x)]$. Consider any i. If $\varphi_i(x) = b_i$, then $M_i(z) \succcurlyeq M_i(x) = M_i(b_i) \Leftrightarrow \varphi_i(z) = b_i$ since b_i is the least marked ('best') value of φ_i. Since our constraints are binary valued, if $\varphi_i(x) \neq b_i$, then $\varphi_i(x) = w_i$, the 'worst' value of M_i, so for any z at all, it must be that $M_i(z) \succcurlyeq M_i(x) = M_i(w_i)$. Thus, $\forall i[M_i(z) \succcurlyeq M_i(x)]$ is equivalent to the condition in the lemma, $\forall i[\varphi_i(x) = b_i \Rightarrow \varphi_i(z) = b_i]$.

(183) *Theorem.* A basic inventory $I_{\mathcal{G}}$ is a single HUB.

> *Proof.* Let J be the set of j for which $F_j \gg M_j$ in $\mathcal{G}$. By Theorem (178), $s \in I_{\mathcal{G}}$ if and only if for each $k \notin J$, $\varphi_k(s)$ is the least marked feature value b_k. Thus, $I_{\mathcal{G}}$ is the set of s such that $\varphi_i(s)$ is any feature value when $j \in J$, and the least marked value b_i when $j \notin J$. By Lemma (182), this is HUB(x), where $\varphi_i(x)$ is the most marked feature value when $i \in J$, and the least marked feature value when $i \notin J$. That is, $s \in I_{\mathcal{G}}$ if and only if $s \succsim x$.

Figure 3   *Box 3*

Figure 4. Thai consonant inventory: Four-dimensional subspace

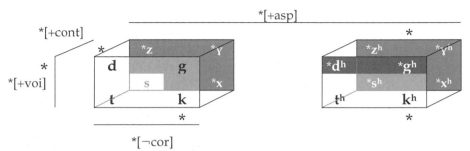

(184) *Lemma.* Let H_1 and H_2 be two HUBs such that neither $H_1 \subset H_2$ nor $H_2 \subset H_1$. Then $H_1 \cup H_2$ is not a HUB.

> *Proof.* Let $H_1 = HUB(x)$ and $H_2 = HUB(y)$. Now there must be an i such that $\varphi_i(x) = b_i$ and $\varphi_i(y) \neq b_i$. For if no such i existed, it would be the case that $\forall i\ [\varphi_i(x) = b_i \Rightarrow \varphi_i(y) = b_i]$, which by Lemma (182) would mean that $y \in HUB(x)$, which in turn would mean that $H_2 = HUB(y) \subset HUB(x) = H_1$, contrary to the hypothesis of the lemma. By symmetrical reasoning, there must be a j such that $\varphi_j(y) = b_j$ and $\varphi_j(x) \neq b_j$. Now consider the z such that $\varphi_i(z) = \varphi_i(y) \neq b_i$, $\varphi_j(z) = \varphi_j(x) \neq b_j$, and $\varphi_k(z) = b_k$ for $k \neq i, j$. Now, $z \notin H_1 \cup H_2$: $\varphi_i(x) = b_i$ but $\varphi_i(z) \neq b_i$ so by Lemma (182), $z \notin HUB(x) = H_1$; by symmetrical reasoning concerning j, $z \notin HUB(y) = H_2$. But z must be in any HUB containing both x and y. For if v is such that $x, y \in HUB(v)$, then by Lemma (182) it must be the case that $\varphi_i(v) = w_i$ (since $\varphi_i(y) = w_i$) and $\psi_j(v) = w_j$ (since $\varphi_j(x) = w_j$); from this it follows, again by Lemma (182), that $z \in HUB(v)$. Since any HUB containing x and y must contain z, but $z \notin H_1 \cup H_2$, it cannot be that $H_1 \cup H_2$ (which contains both $x \in H_1$ and $y \in H_2$) is a HUB.

(185) *Theorem.* Any harmonically complete inventory I is the union of HUBs and any union of HUBs is a harmonically complete inventory.

> *Proof.* For the first part, we show that $X \equiv \cup\{HUB(s) \mid s \in I\}$ is in fact just I. Clearly, since $s \in HUB(s)$, if $s \in I$, then $s \in X$, so $I \subset X$. If $s' \in X$, then $s' \in HUB(s)$, that is, $s' \gtrsim s$, for some $s \in I$, by the definition of X; and since I is harmonically complete, this entails $s' \in I$. Thus, $X \subset I$, and we have proved that $X = I$, so I is a union of HUBs. For the second part, define $I \equiv \cup\{HUB(s) \mid s \in Y\}$ for any Y. Now if $s' \in I$, then $s' \in HUB(s)$ for some $s \in Y$; that is, $s' \gtrsim s$. If $s'' \gtrsim s'$, then $s'' \gtrsim s' \gtrsim s$, so $s'' \in HUB(s)$; hence, $s'' \in I$. Thus, I is harmonically complete.

Figure 5 shows the segments of a hypothetical harmonically complete inventory. This inventory is shown to be the union of six HUBs; each HUB is shown in a separate diagram, with the segments of the HUB underlined and outlined with a double border. This same inventory is enumerated and analyzed in Figure 6.

Figure 5. Viewing an inventory as a union of HUBs

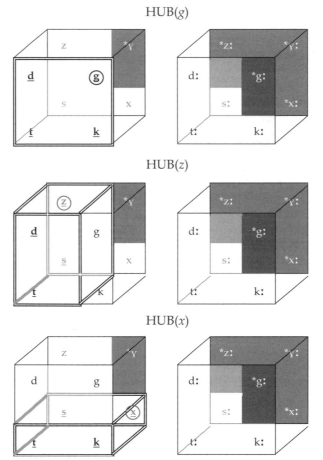

(186)   *Corollary.* Basic typologies exist that are not strongly harmonically complete.

Proof. Consider a simple Φ-space of two dimensions, with $\varphi_i(s) \in \{+, -\}$ for $i = 1, 2$, and $b_i = -$ (i.e., '$-$' is the unmarked value of both φ_1 and φ_2). Now let H_1 be HUB(x), where $x_\Phi \equiv [-, +]$. HUB(x) = $\{z \mid z_\Phi \in \{[-,+], [-,-]\}\}$; that is, $z \in$ HUB(x) if and only if $\varphi_1(z) = -$. Similarly, let H_2 be HUB(y), where $y_\Phi \equiv [+, -]$. Thus, HUB(y) = $\{z \mid z_\Phi \in \{[+,-], [-,-]\}\}$; that is, $z \in$ HUB(y) if and only if $\varphi_2(z) = -$. Note that $x \notin$ HUB(y) and $y \notin$ HUB(x), so neither $H_1 \subset H_2$ nor $H_2 \subset H_1$. Now define the inventory $I \equiv H_1 \cup H_2$. By Lemma (184), I is not a HUB, which by Theorem (183) means I is not a basic inventory, that is, not part of a basic typology. Yet by Theorem (185), I is harmonically complete. Thus, the basic typology determined by $\{M_1, M_2\}$ over this two-dimensional Φ-space is not strongly harmonically complete.

Figure 5 (cont.). Viewing an inventory as a union of HUBs

HUB(*d*ː)

HUB(*k*ː)

HUB(*s*ː)

(187) Given a basic inventory, the corresponding **basic conjunctive typology** is the set of inventories each of which is determined by a ranking of the faithfulness constraints, the markedness constraints, and a set of **markedness conjunctions** $M_{i[1]}$ & $M_{i[2]}$ & $\cdots$ & $M_{i[k]}$, where each of $M_{i[1]}, \cdots, M_{i[k]}$ is a distinct markedness constraint. A structure s violates the conjunction $M_{i[1]}$ & $M_{i[2]}$ & $\cdots$ & $M_{i[k]}$ if and only if it violates *each* of the conjoined markedness constraints $M_{i[1]}, \cdots, M_{i[k]}$. Every combination of markedness conjunctions contributes to the typology.

(188) *Theorem.* A basic conjunctive typology is strongly harmonically complete.

Proof. Let I be any harmonically complete inventory. Let $X \equiv \{s \mid s \notin I\}$ be the excluded outputs. For any s_0, let $\mathbb{C}(s_0) \equiv M_{i[1]}$ & $M_{i[2]}$ & $\cdots$ & $M_{i[k]}$, where $\{M_{i[1]}, \cdots, M_{i[k]}\} \equiv \{M_j \mid$

$\varphi_j(s_0) \neq b_j\}$. Let $\mathcal{G}$ be a constraint ranking consistent with the following stratified hierarchy: $C \gg \mathcal{F} \gg M$, where $\mathcal{F} \equiv \{F_i\}$ as always, $C \equiv \{\mathbb{C}(s) \mid s \in X\}$, and M contains all remaining markedness constraints: $M \equiv \{M_j \mid M_j \notin C\}$. It will be shown that the inventory specified by the ranking $\mathcal{G}$, $I_\mathcal{G}$, is the desired inventory I. More specifically, if $s \in I$, then $[s] \rightarrow s$ is optimal under $\mathcal{G}$, and if $s \notin I$, then $[s] \rightarrow s \prec_\mathcal{G} [s] \rightarrow u$, so $[s] \rightarrow s$ is not optimal under $\mathcal{G}$, where u is the least marked element: $\forall i, \varphi_i[u] = b_i$.

First, suppose $s \notin I$. Then $s \in X$, so $\mathbb{C}(s) \in C$, so $\mathbb{C}(s) \gg \mathcal{F}$ in $\mathcal{G}$. Now $s \rightarrow s$ violates $\mathbb{C}(s)$ because $\mathbb{C}(s)$ is the conjunction of all the M_i that are violated by s. $s \rightarrow u$ violates faithfulness constraints in $\mathcal{F}$, but, since u is the completely unmarked output, no markedness constraints, hence no conjunctions. Since $\mathbb{C} \gg \mathcal{F}$ in $\mathcal{G}$, $s \rightarrow s \prec_G s \rightarrow u$, and hence $s \notin I_G$ as desired.

Now suppose $s \in I$. It cannot be that s violates any of the conjunctions in C. For if s were to violate $\mathbb{C}(s_0)$ for some $s_0 \in X$, then s would violate M_i for each i such that $\varphi_i(s_0) \neq b_i$; that is, for each such i, $\varphi_i(s) \neq b_i$ as well, which would mean that $s \preceq s_0$. But I is harmonically complete, and $s_0 \notin I$, so it would then follow that $s \notin I$, a contradiction. Now since s violates no conjunction in C, $s \rightarrow s$ must be optimal with respect to $\mathcal{G}$, for any unfaithful mapping would violate at least one faithfulness constraint in $\mathcal{F}$, and all constraints in $\mathcal{F}$ outrank all the unconjoined markedness constraints in M that s may happen to violate. Hence, $s \in I_\mathcal{G}$, as desired.

The same harmonically complete inventory shown in Figure 5 is shown in Figure 6 as an inventory in the basic conjunctive typology, generated by four conjunctive constraints. The region excluded from the inventory by each conjuction is shown with a double or heavy border.

(189) Note: Extending to markedness scales with more than two values requires power hierarchies over $M[\varphi]$.

(190) Note: In defining an inventory of structures of a given type $\mathcal{T}$, we only evaluate *individual* structures of type $\mathcal{T}$, so the violations of a conjunctive constraint must coexist within a single structure of type $\mathcal{T}$—they must be *co-local* to a *domain* defined by the structural type $\mathcal{T}$ (e.g., segment; syllable). When larger structures are built up by combining multiple elements of this type (e.g., strings of segments or syllables), the inventory of elements of type $\mathcal{T}$ will be preserved only if we define a violation of a conjunctive constraint as resulting from simultaneous violations of all of the individual conjoined constraints *within a single element or domain of type $\mathcal{T}$*. For this reason, these conjunctive constraints are termed **local** *conjunctions*—'local' relative the domain type $\mathcal{T}$.

The results of this Appendix are likely to generalize to less restricted OT systems, such as those defined by the following conditions.

(191) Generalizations

a. MARKEDNESS is **featurally monotonic**: if x and y differ only in features $\varphi_1 \ldots \varphi_n$ and on each such φ_k, x has a less-marked value than y, then $x \prec y$.

b. FAITHFULNESS is **symmetric** and **translation invariant**: $[-\varphi_k] \rightarrow [+\varphi_k]$ violates the same faithfulness constraint as $[+\varphi_k] \rightarrow [-\varphi_k]$, irrespective of the other feature values.

Figure 5   *Box 3*

Figure 6. A harmonically complete inventory derived conjunctively

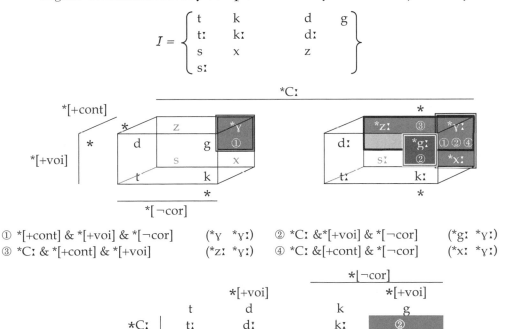

① *[+cont] & *[+voi] & *[¬cor]   (*ɣ *ɣː)   ② *Cː &*[+voi] & *[¬cor]   (*gː *ɣː)
③ *Cː & *[+cont] & *[+voi]   (*zː *ɣː)   ④ *Cː &[+cont] & *[¬cor]   (*xː *ɣː)

(192) *Con* is **homogeneous**: suppose x and x' have the same values for features $\varphi_1 \ldots \varphi_n$, and that y differs from x only in these features, that y' differs from x' only in these features, and that y' has the same values as y for these features:

$$x_\Phi = [\alpha_1\varphi_1, \ldots, \alpha_n\varphi_n, \gamma_{n+1}\varphi_{n+1}, \ldots, \gamma_N\varphi_N],$$
$$x'_\Phi = [\alpha_1\varphi_1, \ldots, \alpha_n\varphi_n, \gamma'_{n+1}\varphi_{n+1}, \ldots, \gamma'_N\varphi_N],$$
$$y_\Phi = [\beta_1\varphi_1, \ldots, \beta_n\varphi_n, \gamma_{n+1}\varphi_{n+1}, \ldots, \gamma_N\varphi_N],$$
$$y'_\Phi = [\beta_1\varphi_1, \ldots, \beta_n\varphi_n, \gamma'_{n+1}\varphi_{n+1}, \ldots, \gamma'_N\varphi_N].$$

Then, regardless of ranking,

$$F[x \to x'] \cup M[x'] \succ M[x] \Leftrightarrow F[y \to y'] \cup M[y'] \succ M[y].$$

Let $\Delta M[x \to x']$ be the MARKEDNESS marks of x, after cancellation of marks shared with x'. Then the above condition can be rewritten

$$F[x \to x'] \succ \Delta M[x \to x'] \,\&\, M[x'] \succ M[x] \Leftrightarrow$$
$$F[y \to y'] \succ \Delta M[y \to y'] \,\&\, M[y'] \succ M[y].$$

Note that under the assumptions for a basic inventory, the homogeneity of *Con* follows from the stronger invariances

$$F[x \to x'] = F[y \to y'] = F_{n+1}[\gamma_{n+1} \to \gamma'_{n+1}] \cup \cdots \cup F_N[\gamma_N \to \gamma'_N]$$

and

$$Z \cup M[x'] \prec M[x] \Leftrightarrow Z \cup M[y'] \prec M[y].$$

The latter holds because

$$Z \cup M[x'] \prec M[x]$$
$$\Leftrightarrow Z \cup M_1[\alpha_1] \cup \cdots \cup M_n[\alpha_n] \cup M_{n+1}[\gamma'_{n+1}] \cup \cdots \cup M_N[\gamma'_N]$$
$$\prec M_1[\alpha_1] \cup \cdots \cup M_n[\alpha_n] \cup M_{n+1}[\gamma_{n+1}] \cup \cdots \cup M_N[\gamma_N]$$
$$\Leftrightarrow Z \cup M_{n+1}[\gamma'_{n+1}] \cup \cdots \cup M_N[\gamma'_N] \prec M_{n+1}[\gamma_{n+1}] \cup \cdots \cup M_N[\gamma_N],$$

and by analogous logic this last condition is equivalent to

$$Z \cup M[y'] \prec M[y]$$

(for $y \to y'$ the marks $M_i[\beta_i]$, $i = 1, \ldots, n$ cancel just as do the marks $M_i[\alpha_i]$ for $x \to x'$). In other words,

$$\Delta M[x \to x'] = M_{n+1}[\gamma_{n+1}] \cup \cdots \cup M_N[\gamma_N] = \Delta M[y \to y'].$$

Departing from homogeneity through feature co-occurrence constraints such as $*[-\varphi, +\varphi']$ makes it possible to generate 'diagonal' inventories, such as $(\alpha\varphi, \alpha'\varphi') \in I \Leftrightarrow \alpha = \alpha' \in \pm$, for example, by a ranking that generates the mapping $[\pm\varphi, \alpha\varphi'] \to [\alpha\varphi, \alpha\varphi']$:

$$\{F[\varphi'], *[-\varphi, +\varphi']\} \gg \{F[\varphi], *[+\varphi], *[+\varphi']\}.$$

Figure 6   *Box 3*

References

ROA = Rutgers Optimality Archive, http://roa.rutgers.edu

Alderete, J. 1995. Faithfulness to prosodic heads. Ms., University of Massachusetts at Amherst. ROA 94.

Alderete, J. 1997. Dissimilation as local conjunction. In *Proceedings of the North East Linguistic Society 27.* ROA 175.

Alderete, J. 1999. Faithfulness to prosodic heads. In *The derivational residue in phonological Optimality Theory,* eds. B. Hermans and M. van Oostendorp. Benjamins. ROA 453.

Archangeli, D. 1984. Underspecification in Yawelmani phonology and morphology. Ph.D. diss., MIT.

Archangeli, D. 1988. Aspects of underspecification theory. *Phonology* 5, 183–207.

Archangeli, D., and D. Pulleyblank. 1994. *Grounded Phonology.* MIT Press.

Baković, E. 2000. Harmony, dominance, and control. Ph.D. diss., Rutgers University.

Battistella, E. L. 1990. *Markedness: The evaluative superstructure of language.* State University of New York Press.

Battistella, E. L. 1996. *The logic of markedness.* Oxford University Press.

Beckman, J. 1997. Positional faithfulness, positional neutralization, and Shona vowel harmony. *Phonology* 14, 1–46.

Benua, L., and P. Smolensky. 2001. Preconditions on vowel harmony. Talk presented at the Linguistics Department Colloquium, State University of New York at Stony Brook.

Boersma, P. 1998. *Functional phonology: Formalizing the interactions between articulatory and perceptual drives.* Holland Academic Graphics.

Cassimjee, F. 1998. *Isixhosa tonology: An optimal domains theory analysis.* Lincom Europa.

Cassimjee, F., and C. W. Kisseberth. 1998. Optimal domains theory and Bantu tonology: A case study from Isixhosa and Shingazidja. In *Theoretical aspects of Bantu tone,* eds. L. Hyman and C. W. Kisseberth. CSLI Publications. ROA 176.

Clements, G. N. 1976. Vowel harmony in nonlinear generative phonology: An autosegmental model. Distributed by Indiana University Linguistics Club.

Clements, G. N. 1977. Neutral vowels in Hungarian vowel harmony: An autosegmental interpretation. In *Proceedings of the North East Linguistic Society 7.*

Clements, G. N. 1990. The role of the sonority cycle in core syllabification. In *Papers in laboratory phonology I: Between the grammar and the physics of speech,* eds. J. Kingston and M. Beckman. Cambridge University Press.

Clements, G. N., and E. Sezer. 1982. Vowel and consonant disharmony in Turkish. In *The structure of phonological representations, vol. II,* eds. H. van der Hulst and N. Smith. Foris.

Cole, J. S., and C. W. Kisseberth. 1994. Optimal domains theory. Technical report, University of Illinois.

de Lacy, P. 2002. The formal expression of markedness. Ph.D. diss., University of Massachusetts. ROA 542.

Firth, J. R. 1948. Sounds and prosodies. *Transactions of the Philological Society,* 127–52.

Fukazawa, H. 1999. Theoretical implications of OCP effects on features in Optimality Theory. Ph.D. diss., University of Maryland. ROA 307.

Gafos, A. 1996. *The articulatory basis of locality in phonology.* Garland.

Goldsmith, J. A. 1976. Autosegmental phonology. Ph.D. diss., MIT.

Goldsmith, J. A. 1990. *Autosegmental and metrical phonology.* Blackwell.

Greenberg, J. 1978. *Universals of human language.* Vol. 2, *Phonology.* Stanford University Press.

Grignon, A.-M. 1984. Phonologie lexicale tri-dimensionnelle du japonais. Ph.D. diss., Université de Montréal.

Hale, K. 1973. Deep-surface canonical disparities in relation to analysis and change: An Australian example. *Current Trends in Linguistics* 11, 401–58.

Hammond, M. 1999. *The phonology of English: A prosodic optimality-theoretic approach.* Oxford University Press.

Hebert, R. J., and N. Poppe. 1963. *Kirghiz manual.* Indiana University Publications.

Hooper, J. B. 1972. The syllable in linguistic theory. *Language* 48, 525–40.

Hudak, T. J. 1987. Thai. In *The world's major languages*, ed. B. Comrie. Oxford University Press.

Itô, J. 1986. Syllable theory in prosodic phonology. Ph.D. diss., University of Masschusetts at Amherst.

Itô, J., and R. A. Mester. 1986. The phonology of voicing in Japanese: The theoretical consequences of morphological accessibility. *Linguistic Inquiry* 17, 49–73.

Itô, J., and R. A. Mester. 1994. Reflections on CODACOND and alignment. In *Phonology at Santa Cruz [PASC] 3*, eds. J. Merchant, J. Padgett, and R. L. Walker. Linguistics Research Center, University of California at Santa Cruz. ROA 141.

Itô, J., and R. A. Mester. 1996. Rendaku 1: Constraint conjunction and the OCP. Talk presented at the Kobe Phonology Forum. ROA 144.

Itô, J., and R. A. Mester. 1998. Markedness and word structure: OCP effects in Japanese. Ms., University of California at Santa Cruz. ROA 255.

Itô, J., and R. A. Mester. 2002. On the sources of opacity in OT: Coda processes in German. In *The optimal syllable*, eds. C. Féry and R. van de Vijver. Cambridge University Press. ROA 347.

Itô, J., R. A. Mester, and J. Padgett. 1995. Licensing and redundancy: Underspecification in Optimality Theory. *Linguistic Inquiry* 26, 571–614.

Iwasaki, S. 2002. *Japanese.* Benjamins.

Johnson, C. D. 1980. Regular disharmony in Kirghiz. In *Issues in vowel harmony: Proceedings of the City University of New York Linguistics Conference on Vowel Harmony, 14th May 1977*, ed. R. M. Vago. Benjamins.

Kaun, A. 1995. The typology of rounding harmony: An optimality theoretic approach. Ph.D. diss., UCLA. ROA 227.

Kenstowicz, M. 1982. Gemination and spirantization in Tigrinya. *Studies in the Linguistic Sciences* 12, 103–22.

Kiparsky, P. 1973. How abstract is phonology? In *Three dimensions of linguistic theory*, ed. O. Fujimura. TEC.

Kiparsky, P. 1981. Vowel harmony. Ms., MIT.

Kiparsky, P. 1982. Lexical phonology and morphology. In *Linguistics in the morning calm*, ed. I. S. Yang. Hanshin.

Kiparsky, P. 1985. Some consequences of Lexical Phonology. *Phonology* 2, 84–108.

Kiparsky, P. 1994. Remarks on markedness. Talk presented at the Tri-Lateral Phonology Weekend-2.

Kirchner, R. 1993. Turkish vowel harmony: An optimality-theoretic analysis. Ms., UCLA. ROA 4.

Kirchner, R. 1995. Going the distance: Synchronic chain shifts in OT. Ms., UCLA. ROA 66.

Kirchner, R. 1996. Synchronic chain shifts in Optimality Theory. *Linguistic Inquiry* 27, 341–50. ROA 66.

Korn, D. 1969. Types of labial harmony in the Turkic languages. *Anthropological Linguistics* 11, 98–106.

Ladefoged, P., and I. Maddieson. 1996. *The sounds of the world's languages.* Blackwell.

Leben, W. 1973. Suprasegmental phonology. Ph.D. diss., MIT.

Lewis, G. L. 1967. *Turkish grammar.* Oxford University Press.

Lombardi, L. 2002. Coronal epenthesis and markedness. *Phonology* 19, 219–51. ROA 579.

Łubowicz, A. 2002. Derived environment effects in Optimality Theory. *Lingua* 112, 243–80. ROA 239.

McCarthy, J. J. 1979. Formal problems in Semitic phonology and morphology. Ph.D. diss., MIT.

McCarthy, J. J. 1994. The phonetics and phonology of Semitic pharyngeals. In *Papers in laboratory phonology III: Phonological structure and phonetic form,* ed. P. Keating. Cambridge University Press.

McCarthy, J. J. 2004. Headed spans and autosegmental spreading. Ms., University of Massachusetts at Amherst. ROA 685.

McCarthy, J. J., and A. Prince. 1993. Prosodic Morphology I: Constraint interaction and satisfaction. Technical report RuCCS-TR-3, Rutgers Center for Cognitive Science, Rutgers University, and University of Massachusetts at Amherst. ROA 482, 2001.

McCarthy, J. J., and A. Prince. 1995. Faithfulness and reduplicative identity. In *University of Massachusetts occasional papers in linguistics 18: Papers in Optimality Theory,* eds. J. Beckman, L. Walsh Dickey, and S. Urbanczyk. Graduate Linguistic Student Association, University of Massachusetts at Amherst. ROA 60.

McCarthy, J. J., and A. Taub. 1992. Review of Carole Paradis and Jean-François Prunet, The special status of coronals. *Phonology* 9, 363–72.

Mester, R. A., and J. Itô. 1989. Feature predictability and underspecification: Palatal prosody in Japanese mimetics. *Language* 65, 258–93.

Mohanan, K. P. 1989. On the bases of underspecification. Ms., Stanford University.

Mohanan, K. P. 1991. On the bases of radical underspecification. *Natural Language and Linguistic Theory* 9, 285–325.

Morelli, F. 2002. The relative harmony of /s+stop/ onsets: Obstruent clusters and the Sonority Sequencing Principle. In *The optimal syllable,* eds. C. Féry and R. van de Vijver. Cambridge University Press.

Morris, R. E. 2002. Coda obstruents and local constraint conjunction in north-central peninsular Spanish. In *Current issues in linguistic theory: Selected papers from the 29th Linguistic Symposium on Romance Languages,* eds. D. Cresti, T. Satterfield, and C. Tortora. Benjamins. ROA 383, 2000.

Noonan, M. 1992. *A grammar of Lango.* Mouton.

Okello, J. 1975. Some phonological and morphological processes in Lango. Ph.D. diss., Indiana University.

Olli, J. B. 1958. *Fundamentals of Finnish grammar.* Northland Press.

Padgett, J. 1995. Feature classes. In *University of Massachusetts occasional papers in linguistics 18: Papers in Optimality Theory,* eds. J. Beckman, L. Walsh Dickey, and S. Urbanczyk. Graduate Linguistic Student Association, University of Massachusetts at Amherst.

Padgett, J. 2001. The *unabridged* feature classes in phonology. Ms., University of California at Santa Cruz.

Padgett, J. 2002a. Constraint conjunction versus grounded constraint subhierarchies in Optimality Theory. Ms., University of California at Santa Cruz. ROA 530.

Padgett, J. 2002b. Feature classes in phonology. *Language* 78, 81–110.

Palmer, F. R. 1970. *Prosodic analysis.* Oxford University Press.

Paradis, C., and J.-F. Prunet, eds. 1991. *The special status of coronals: Internal and external evidence.* Academic Press.

Poser, W. 1982. Phonological representation and action-at-a-distance. In *The structure of phonological representations,* eds. H. van der Hulst and N. Smith. Foris.

Prince, A. 1983. Relating to the grid. *Linguistic Inquiry* 14, 19–100.

Prince, A. 1984. Phonology with tiers. In *Language sound structure,* eds. M. Aronoff and R. Oehrle. MIT Press.

Prince, A. 1997. Topics in Optimality Theory. LSA Linguistic Institute course, Cornell University.

Prince, A., and P. Smolensky. 1993/2004. *Optimality Theory: Constraint interaction in generative grammar.* Technical report, Rutgers University and University of Colorado at Boulder, 1993. ROA 537, 2002. Revised version published by Blackwell, 2004.

Pulleyblank, D. 1983. *Tone in lexical phonology.* Reidel.

Rice, K. D. 1992. On deriving sonority: A structural account of sonority relationships. *Phonology* 9, 61–99.

Schachter, P. 1987. Tagalog. In *The world's major languages,* ed. B. Comrie. Oxford University Press.

Schein, B., and D. Steriade. 1986. On geminates. *Linguistic Inquiry* 17, 691–744.

Schlindwein, D. 1988. The phonological geometry of morpheme concatenation. Ph.D. diss., UCLA.

Smith, J. 2002. Phonological augmentation in prominent positions. Ph.D. diss., University of Massachusetts at Amherst.

Smith, N. V. 1973. *The acquisition of phonology: A case study.* Cambridge University Press.

Smolensky, P. 1993. Harmony, markedness, and phonological activity. Handout of talk presented at the Rutgers Optimality Workshop–1. ROA 87.

Smolensky, P. 1997. Constraint interaction in generative grammar II: Local conjunction (or, Random rules in Universal Grammar). Talk presented at the Hopkins Optimality Theory Conference.

Steriade, D. 1981. Parameters of metrical harmony rules. Ms., MIT.

Steriade, D. 1982. Greek prosodies and the nature of syllabification. Ph.D. diss., MIT.

Steriade, D. 1995. Underspecification and markedness. In *Handbook of phonological theory,* ed. J. A. Goldsmith. Blackwell.

Suzuki, K. 1998. A typological investigation of dissimilation. Ph.D. diss., University of Arizona. ROA 281.

Trubetzkoy, N. 1939/1969. *Principles of phonology* (translation of *Grundzüge der Phonologie*). University of California Press.

Vago, R. M. 1973. Abstract vowel harmony systems in Uralic and Altaic languages. *Language* 49, 579–605.

Vago, R. M., ed. 1980. *Issues in vowel harmony.* Benjamins.

Välimaa-Blum, R. 1986. Finnish vowel harmony as a prescriptive and descriptive rule: An autosegmental account. In *Proceedings of the Eastern States Conference on Linguistics 3.*

Vennemann, T. 1988. *Preference laws for syllable structure and the explanation of sound change.* Mouton de Gruyter.

Walker, R. L. 1998. Nasalization, neutral segments, and opacity effects. Ph.D. diss., University of California at Santa Cruz. ROA 405.

Williams, E. 1976. Underlying tone in Margi and Igbo. *Linguistic Inquiry* 7, 463–84.

Woock, E., and M. Noonan. 1979. Vowel harmony in Lango. In *Proceedings of the Chicago Linguistic Society 15.*

Yip, M. 1991. Coronals, clusters, and the Coda Condition. In *The special status of coronals: Internal and external evidence,* eds. C. Paradis and J.-F. Prunet. Academic Press.

Zoll, C. 1998. Positional asymmetries and licensing. Ms., MIT. ROA 282.

15

Optimality in Syntax I: Case and Grammatical Voice Typology

Géraldine Legendre, William Raymond,
and Paul Smolensky

The majority of the empirical tests of Optimality Theory concern phonology. Does the OT framework shed light on problems in syntax and semantics? For determining the range of language phenomena for which the symbolic level of the Integrated Connectionist/Symbolic Cognitive Architecture (ICS) may provide insight, this is clearly an important question about the theory/data bridge ② of Figure 6 in the ICS map of Chapter 2.

In this chapter, we argue that with violable constraints, even extremely simple, intuitive constraints on the mapping between semantic (thematic) and syntactic (case) roles can produce nontrivial and empirically sensible linguistic typologies. The chapter reprints, with minor elaborations, very early work, the first published application of OT outside phonology (Legendre, Raymond, and Smolensky 1993). The basic ideas have since been greatly extended and refined (e.g., Aissen 1999, 2003; Sells 2001).

Contents

1 INTRODUCTION

In this chapter, we explore the consequences of the hypothesis that universal grammar (UG) contains formal counterparts of extremely simple constraints like these: agents surface as subjects; low-prominence arguments do not surface as subjects or objects; low-'animacy' arguments surface as objects. Using Optimality Theory (OT; Prince and Smolensky 1991, 1993/2004) to formally manage the necessary violations of such constraints as they come into conflict, we show that such simple universal principles governing the mapping of semantic roles to surface morphosyntactic roles can provide formal explanation of empirical crosslinguistic typologies of case and grammatical voice systems. (See Box 1 for background.)

OT provides a general means for constructing particular grammars from universal constraints, and of generating theoretical typologies of possible languages from the same constraints (Chapter 12).[1] In Section 2, we present the universal constraints that constitute our proposed theory of case and voice. In this chapter, we take a grammatical voice to be a particular mapping of thematic roles to surface abstract cases. In Section 3, we show how the theory entails three possible intransitive case-marking systems: nominative/accusative, ergative/absolutive, and active/stative. In Section 4, we illustrate how the theory treats one example language from each of these three systems, including voice distinctions and intransitive case. In Section 5, we state a set of implicational universals entailed by the theory and use these universals to derive analytic typologies of case/voice systems with substantial empirical validity. In Section 6, we briefly sketch some extensions.

Box 1. Case, thematic roles, and grammatical voice

Case and thematic roles

We have previously identified the **grammatical functions** of the two **arguments** of the verb *play* in the sentence *boys play games*: *boys* is the **subject** and *games* the **direct object** (Box 12:1). If we replace the two NPs with their pronominal counterparts, we see a striking difference between them: *they play them*. *They* and *them* are 3rd person plural pronouns that differ in **morphological case**. *They* bears **nominative** case, the case associated with the subject grammatical function, while *them* bears **accusative** case, associated with the direct object grammatical function. Substituting full noun phrases for pronouns, we may assert that in *boys play games*, *boys* also bears nominative case and *games* accusative case. In many languages, this distinction is marked morphologically by different affixes (e.g., suffixes): *der Junge* ('the boy', NOM) versus *den Jungen* ('the boy', ACC) in German, for example. In English, however, morphological case marking

---

[1] In this chapter, we assume that all rankings of the universal constraints are possible. In other applications, restrictions on possible rankings are also part of UG (Prince and Smolensky 1993/2004, Sec. 8.1.2; McCarthy and Prince 1993).

has been lost, except for a few pronouns such as *they* (NOM) and *them* (ACC). Instead, case in English is encoded by strict word order: *NOM Verb ACC*. The concept of case is therefore a fairly abstract one; it subsumes both morphological case and case distinctions encoded by word order. (Abstract case is often simply called 'Case' with uppercase C.) The **nominative/accusative** case system is not the only one found in languages of the world; two others will be described below.

Grammatical functions (or syntactic roles) are crucially related to **semantic** or **thematic** (or **θ-)roles** (Fillmore 1968; Gruber 1976). As linguistically represented in natural language, events have a schematic structure. In our example, *boys* denotes the **agent**: a participant that is the primal causer of the event (typically volitionally). The agent role is common to many different types of events. The **patient** is an event participant that is acted upon: *games* in our example. (The term 'theme' can, for our purposes, be equated with 'patient'.) Other thematic roles such as **experiencer, instrument**, and **location** are self-explanatory. The point is that although events differ enormously from one another, their cognitive representations have in common a few general roles filled by event participants. And this means that a few syntactic roles shared by sentences can identify the few semantic roles shared by event participants.

Each verb V has a **thematic** (or **θ-)grid** that identifies which thematic roles are involved in the cognitive representation of the type of event V denotes. This is an important part of V's **lexical entry** — V's contribution to the mental dictionary. The thematic grid for *hear* has an experiencer and a **stimulus**. The thematic grid for *play* consists of an agent and a patient.

The lexical entry for each verb includes its **argument structure**, which identifies the grammatical functions that are obligatory for the verb, those that are optionally present, and the canonical (default; unmarked) relation between these syntactic roles and thematic roles. For example, the argument structure of *sheathe* specifies that a subject and a direct object are obligatory and that they canonically correspond to agent and patient, respectively. The argument structure of *put* requires a subject agent, a patient direct object, and a goal indirect object: *Josh sheathed his foil* versus *Josh put his foil in its sheath*. A verb requiring a subject and a direct object is **transitive**; a verb requiring only a subject is **intransitive**; and a verb requiring a subject, direct object, and indirect object is **ditransitive**. (Indirect objects bear **dative** case.) In *boys play games*, *play* is transitive. *Play* can also be used as an intransitive verb, as in *boys play*. One common analysis of this dual argument structure is to say that there are two versions of *play* in the English lexicon.

The transitive/intransitive distinction is crucially relevant to the **ergative/absolutive** case system. This system is best introduced by comparing two versions of English with alternative case systems: (real) English versus (hypothetical) 'Erglish'. In English, the subject and the object bear nominative case and accusative case, respectively, regardless of whether the verb is transitive or intransitive. The form of the subject pronoun is the same in both: *they* (NOM) in transitive *they love them* and intransitive *they die*. The subject canonically precedes the verb regardless of its transitivity status.

Box 1

In an ergative/absolutive case system, transitivity status matters. In Erglish, we would say *they love them* as in real English for the transitive verb *love*. But for intransitive *die*, we would say *them die*. In an ergative/absolutive case system, the subject of an intransitive verb and the object of a transitive verb share the same case, labeled **absolutive (ABS)**. The subject of a transitive verb bears its own unique case, labeled **ergative (ERG)**. Typically, these cases are expressed morphologically. Therefore, transitive clauses are easily identified in ergative languages like Erglish.

The third and last pure case system to be introduced is the **active/stative** system (we do not discuss mixed systems here). Let's invent 'Actish' as a prototypical active/stative language. As in real English and Erglish, in Actish we would say *they love them* for the transitive verb *love*. But with an intransitive verb, we would have two choices: *they run* (**active, ACT**) and *them die* (**stative, STA**). The choice is typically grounded in semantic roles. Roughly, when a verb takes an agent-like argument, the argument appears with active case; when a verb takes a patient-like argument, the argument appears with Stative case. The hallmark of an active/stative language is a case split among intransitive verbs (see Legendre and Rood 1992 for illustration).

Grammatical voice

In *boys play games,* the subject refers to the agent, while the direct object denotes the patient. This is the canonical **active voice**: a grammatical voice is a correspondence relation between syntactic and semantic roles. That canonical relation changes if the patient is given higher discourse **prominence** than the agent. The subject position is the canonical locus of high prominence: to promote the prominence of the patient, it is placed in subject position. In the **passive voice** (e.g., *games are played by boys),* the subject denotes the patient; there is no direct object, and the agent may be denoted by the object of the preposition *by* or simply left out (the ultimate prominence demotion). This demotion of the agent makes the passive voice a favorite of politicians and lawyers. The passive voice in English is marked by distinct morphology: *auxiliary-be + V-past-participle*, as in *are played*.

Since the meaning of a sentence has been defined here to include the cognitive properties that distinguish the topic (what the sentence is about), the meanings of *boys play games* and *games are played by boys* are different; the topic in the active voice (subject) *boys* differs from the topic of the passive, *games*. In both sentences, however, the semantic roles have the same values. This can be written 'play(boys, games)' where by convention the first-listed argument is the agent or experiencer. This is the **predicate-argument structure** for the sentence — the major component of its meaning.

In the **antipassive voice**, the patient is not a direct object; it is demoted to an even less-prominent syntactic role, as the agent is in the passive voice. The antipassive voice is typical of ergative languages. In Erglish, it would result in something like *boys play-AP (with games),* where 'AP' stands for an antipassive inflection on the verb to signal the change of voice (parallel to the distinct morphology of the English passive). Arguably, the intransitive version of English *play* could in fact be the antipassive counterpart (with zero morphology) to transitive *play*. In *boys play with a football,* the verb *play* is intransitive: *a football* is not a direct object, and is optional. This is arguably the antipassive form of *boys play football*; this version of *play* has an agent but no patient. Indeed, this analysis is adopted in the present chapter.

The multiplicity of terminology inherited from traditional descriptions of these languages makes it difficult to compare them and provide a unified analysis. What we need is a notion of abstract case that subsumes all three systems. In this chapter, we therefore introduce two concepts: **abstract case C₁** which subsumes all possible cases associated with transitive subjects, and **abstract case C₂**, which subsumes those associated with transitive direct objects. Thus, C_1 encapsulates nominative, ergative, and active cases, while C_2 encapsulates accusative, absolutive, and stative cases. These are the **core** cases. All noncore cases (goal, instrumental, etc.) can be subsumed under the term **oblique case**, denoted **C₄**.

A final grammatical voice transparently called **reversal** (but **inverse** in the traditional voice literature) is discussed in the chapter. In such a voice (e.g., as found in Navajo), the agent and the patient exchange their respective cases: the agent surfaces with abstract case C_2 and the patient with abstract case C_1.

2 A MINIMAL THEORY OF ABSTRACT CASE

2.1 Inputs

Here, an input to be assigned a structural description by a grammar is simply a clause or a predicate-argument complex. Each argument in the input is labeled with its thematic role; here, we treat only agent and patient.[2] In addition, each argument is labeled with an abstract 'prominence' level, high or low. The voice alternations we treat are driven by prominence demotions in the input: the abstract 'passive' we consider arises from an input consisting of a low-prominence agent and a high-prominence patient. We denote this input '**aP**', using '{a,p}' to denote low- and '{A,P}' high-prominence agents and patients, respectively. Our abstract 'antipassive' arises from the input **Ap**, with prominence-demoted patient. Simple transitives (active voice) derive from the input **AP**. Our two intransitive inputs are **A** and **P**, depending on whether the argument is a thematic agent or patient. (The predicate itself is not made explicit in the input.)

2.2 Outputs

The output a grammar assigns to an input consists in the input arguments themselves, together with a value for each argument of what we will call an **abstract case**

---

[2] A natural extension would decompose the cover terms 'agent' and 'patient' into features, and the universal constraints would evaluate feature configurations rather than thematic roles per se. This would facilitate extension to a fuller spectrum of thematic roles — case marking of experiencers being of particular interest.

Box 1

(see Box 1). We take such cases to be realized by overt morphological case on the NPs in some languages, by word order in others, and by verbal cross-referencing in still others (Box 11:1). We do not explicitly treat verbal morphology or auxiliaries that may be associated with certain voices.

For our initial work restricted to two thematic roles, we assume only three possible abstract cases: C_1, C_2, and C_4. As shown in Section 2.4, the theory entails that, in all languages, C_1 and C_2 are the abstract cases respectively assigned to the arguments A and P for the simple transitive input **AP**; therefore, in any given language, we take C_1 and C_2 to be realized through whatever surface means are used to identify the agent and the patient in a simple transitive sentence. In the simple account here, C_4 subsumes all lower cases, including dative or oblique overt case on NPs, as well as failure of an argument to appear on the surface at all.

We notate outputs by simply subscripting each thematic argument with the number of the case it is assigned; for example, the simple transitive input **AP** is universally assigned the output A_1P_2 (as we show in Section 2.4). We assume that the candidate set of possible outputs made available by UG excludes every structure in which two different arguments are assigned the same **core case** C_1 or C_2; thus, for example, A_1P_1 and a_2P_2 are not possible outputs.[3]

In all languages, intransitive arguments are taken to bear case C_1 or C_2 when they are realized on the surface like the agents or the patients, respectively, in simple transitive sentences. This will permit all languages to be treated using a common set of universal constraints governing the assignment of abstract case.

The traditional names associated with C_1/C_2 vary depending on the intransitive case assignment strategy of the language. Their relation to traditional terminology is spelled out in (1), which also summarizes previous notation.

(1) Notation
    a. Inputs: X/x = high/low prominence; A = agent; P = patient
        AP active input
        aP passive input (agent demoted in prominence)
        Ap antipassive input (patient demoted in prominence)
    b. Abstract cases C_1/C_2 correspond to
        'Nominative/accusative' (NOM/ACC): traditionally used when intransitive arguments are all marked like transitive agents—in our terms, when intransitive arguments are assigned C_1, regardless of whether they are thematic agents or patients

        'Ergative/absolutive' (ERG/ABS): traditionally used when intransitive arguments are all marked like transitive patients — in our terms, all assigned C_2

        'Active/stative' (ACT/STA): traditionally used when intransitive

---

[3] Empirically, this principle is occasionally violated; one case in Lakhóta was given a multistratal OT analysis in Legendre and Rood 1992.

agents are assigned C_1 but intransitive patients are assigned C_2

c.   Outputs

For input $\alpha\pi$, with α = a or A and π = p or P, outputs are $\alpha_j\pi_k$ where j, k = 1, 2, or 4, and not $j = k = 1$ or $j = k = 2$.

Our first result is a derivation of the typology of case-marking systems for intransitive clauses: we show that nominative/accusative, ergative/absolutive, and active/stative systems arise from different domination rankings of a single universal set of constraints. But first we must present these constraints.

2.3 The universal constraints

We propose the following set of constraints:[4]

(2)   Universal constraints governing abstract case

a. $A{\rightarrow}C_1$ Agents receive abstract case C_1.

b. $P{\rightarrow}C_2$ Patients receive abstract case C_2.

c. $A{\nrightarrow}C_2$ Agents do not receive abstract case C_2.

d. $P{\nrightarrow}C_1$ Patients do not receive abstract case C_1.

e. $\alpha{\nrightarrow}C_4$ Core arguments (agents and patients) do not receive abstract case C_4.

f. $\alpha{\rightarrow}C_2$ Some argument receives abstract case C_2.

g. $X{\rightarrow}C_1$ High-prominence arguments receive abstract case C_1.

h. $x{\nrightarrow}C_{1,2}$ Low-prominence arguments do not receive core case (are not assigned C_1 or C_2).

Note: '$A{\rightarrow}C_1$' applies to all agents, prominent (**A**) or not (**a**). Similarly for all 'A' and 'P' appearing in constraint names.

Most of these constraints arise from the natural assumption that the mappings between thematic roles and cases that are manifest in simple transitives satisfy the universal mapping constraints: agents receive C_1 and not C_2 or C_4 (2a,c,e); patients receive C_2 and not C_1 or C_4 (2b,d,e). Some argument is case-marked C_2 (2f) (and another is marked C_1; a constraint to that effect is redundant with (2g), since in all inputs considered here, at least one argument is of high prominence). The constraints sensitive to abstract prominence (2g,h) reflect the fact that prominence demotion as manifest in passive and antipassive voices is expressed through loss of core case by core arguments (2h), and, in the case of passive, the opportunity for a high-prominence patient to be promoted to C_1 (2g). These constraints formally capture aspects of the functional correlation between subjecthood and discourse prominence (e.g., Givón 1984, 1989). The formal mechanism is **Prominence Alignment** (Chapter 12(42); see Prince

---

[4] It is possible that this constraint set could be modified without affecting the results established below. However, as we will show, fully exploring the consequences of each alternative constraint set is a lengthy matter, and we have not extensively investigated alternatives. Some of the more obvious simplifications of the account, however, are not empirically adequate.

Box 1

and Smolensky 1993/2004, Chap. 5). This operation ($\otimes$) generates constraints favoring configurations in which a feature with high prominence on one scale is paired with a feature with high prominence on the aligned scale, and similarly for low prominence paired with low prominence.

(3)   Universal case constraints express prominence alignments

    a.   Core roles: case $[C_1 > C_2] \otimes \theta$-role $[A > P]$: (2a–d)

    b.   Core versus noncore roles: case $[C_{1,2} > C_4] \otimes \theta$-role $[A, P > $ oblique$]$: (2e)

    c.   Discourse $[X > x] \otimes$ case $[C_1 > C_2]$ and $[X > x] \otimes [C_{1,2} > C_4]$: (2g–h)

It is important to note that these proposed constraints and the input-output representations they presume are neutral with respect to many syntactic assumptions. Our cases might be primitive elements in a syntactic theory (analogous to the MAPs of Gerdts 1993, and references therein). On the other hand, while it is not made explicit in the minimalist notation we employ, constituent structure of considerable complexity is consistent with the theory we explore here. Our abstract cases could be taken to encode structural properties, the constraints (2) forming a module of a theory containing other structure-related constraints; the constraints (2) would then presumably serve to license the structural elements or movement required in the optimal structure (e.g., as suggested for another syntactic domain in Grimshaw 1993).

2.4 Active voice

The means used in a given language to mark the abstract cases C_1 and C_2 are determined by how that language marks the agents and patients in simple transitive sentences. This follows, we asserted, from the fact that our theory of abstract case entails that the input for such sentences, **AP** (high-prominence agent, high-prominence patient), is *always* assigned the output A_1P_2 (i.e., A receives C_1, P receives C_2), regardless of the way the language ranks the universal constraints (2) in its language-particular domination hierarchy. We now demonstrate this.

The first step is to determine the set of possible outputs for the input **AP**: the candidate set provided by UG. Following (1c), this is $\{A_1P_2, A_1P_4, A_2P_1, A_2P_4, A_4P_1, A_4P_2, A_4P_4\}$. (As stated in Section 2.2, assigning both A and P the same core case — A_1P_1 or A_2P_2 — is assumed to be prohibited by UG.) Now, since there are two high-prominence arguments and at most one can receive C_1, every candidate must violate constraint (2g) $X \rightarrow C_1$ at least once — only A_1P_1 satisfies this constraint fully, and UG (*Gen*) does not provide this structure as a candidate output. The output A_1P_2 satisfies all the other constraints, however. All other candidate outputs violate additional constraints; for example, A_4P_2 also violates $A \rightarrow C_1$ and $a \nrightarrow C_4$. Thus, no matter how a grammar ranks the universal constraints (2), A_1P_2 is the most harmonic candidate: it incurs only the mark $*X \rightarrow C_1$, whereas all the alternatives incur this same mark and others as well. Therefore, the theory entails that, in all languages, the structural description assigned to **AP** is A_1P_2.

3 DEDUCING THE TYPOLOGY OF INTRANSITIVE CASE SYSTEMS

Consider the two possible (high-prominence) intransitive inputs: **A**, corresponding to an intransitive predicate taking a thematic agent as argument, and **P**, for a patient-taking predicate. The possible outputs for **A** are just $\{A_1, A_2, A_4\}$; for **P**, $\{P_1, P_2, P_4\}$. The constraints in (2) that bear on these alternatives are given in (4).

(4)   Intransitive case-marking typology

Constraint	Input: P	Input: A
$P \rightarrow C_2$	$\Rightarrow$ choose C_2	
$P \nrightarrow C_1$	$\Rightarrow$ choose C_2	
$\alpha \rightarrow C_2$	$\Rightarrow$ choose C_2	$\Rightarrow$ choose C_2
$X \rightarrow C_1$	$\Rightarrow$ choose C_1	$\Rightarrow$ choose C_1
$A \rightarrow C_1$		$\Rightarrow$ choose C_1
$A \nrightarrow C_2$		$\Rightarrow$ choose C_1
RESULT:	*choose C_2 unless* $X \rightarrow C_1$ *dominates* $P \rightarrow C_2$, $P \nrightarrow C_1$, *and* $\alpha \rightarrow C_2$	*choose C_1 unless* $\alpha \rightarrow C_2$ *dominates* $X \rightarrow C_1$, $A \rightarrow C_1$, *and* $A \nrightarrow C_2$

		A_1	A_2
	P_2	Act/Stat	Erg/Abs
	P_1	Nom/Acc	IMPOSSIBLE

Consider first the input **P**, and two of the possible outputs, P_1 and P_2. As the table shows, three of the constraints will be satisfied if and only if P is assigned C_2, that is, if and only if the output is P_2. The fourth constraint is satisfied only if the output is P_1. Which output is more harmonic? In OT, we do *not* answer this by majority vote; rather, we consult the language's domination hierarchy. If the fourth constraint $X \rightarrow C_1$ dominates the other three, it wins, and P_1 is the more harmonic; otherwise, it is P_2. According to OT, the typology of crosslinguistic variation is generated by all possible rankings of universal constraints, so the theory predicts that P will receive case C_1 in some languages (those that rank $X \rightarrow C_1$ highest) and case C_2 in others. These two possibilities are indicated in the bottom two lines of the table (shaded).

We have ignored the remaining candidate, P_4. Regardless of how the constraints are ranked, this structure can never be more harmonic than P_2: the only mark incurred by P_2 is $*X \rightarrow C_1$, and P_4 incurs this mark *as well as* the marks $*P \rightarrow C_2$, $*\alpha \rightarrow C_2$,

Box 1

and $*\alpha\!\to\!C_4$. (P_4 is **harmonically bounded** by P_2; see Section 12:1.6.) Thus, P_1 and P_2 are the only two possible optimal structures.

The case of agentive intransitives is analogous: it is treated in the rightmost column of table (4). Again, there are two possibly optimal candidates, A_1 and A_2; the latter will be optimal only in languages that rank $\alpha\!\to\!C_2$ higher than the other three relevant constraints, all of which are violated by A_2.

Assuming the universal constraints (2), factorial typology (Section 12:1.6) thus predicts the typology of intransitive case-marking systems given in the shaded lower-right portion of (4). Depending on its ranking of the universal constraints, a given language will fall into one of the three possible cells: the fourth cell, a language systematically assigning intransitive agents C_2 and patients C_1, is predicted to be impossible because it would require that $X\!\to\!C_1 \gg \alpha\!\to\!C_2$ (for P_1) and, in the same domination hierarchy, that $\alpha\!\to\!C_2 \gg X\!\to\!C_1$ (for A_2). The three predicted systems correspond to the traditional active/stative (A_1, P_2), ergative/absolutive (A_2, P_2), and nominative/accusative (A_1, P_1) systems.

4 TREATMENT OF EXAMPLE LANGUAGES

How a language's grammar ranks the universal constraints (2) determines the cases assigned to all the possible inputs considered here, not just the intransitive inputs considered in Section 3. We now illustrate the patterns of case assignment across several different inputs, for three different domination hierarchies corresponding to the three typological language families in (4). The Appendix provides a summary by language of the actual case/voice systems we refer to here; relevant references are marked in the reference list.

4.1 A nominative/accusative example

An OT constraint tableau for a typological family that includes English is shown in (5). Across the top of the tableau is a ranking of the universal constraints (2), with the most dominant to the left. (Certain modifications of the ranking would not affect the results.) Comparing the domination hierarchy against the shaded intransitive typology of (4), we see that the conditions are met for a nominative/accusative system: $X\!\to\!C_1$ *does* dominate all three constraints $P\!\to\!C_2$, $P\!\nrightarrow\!C_1$, and $\alpha\!\to\!C_2$, so **P** will be assigned C_1; on the other hand, $\alpha\!\to\!C_2$ does *not* dominate $X\!\to\!C_1$, so **A** will also be assigned C_1. Both high-prominence intransitive arguments **A** and **P** must be assigned C_1 in order to satisfy the most dominant constraint, $X\!\to\!C_1$. The most dominant mark incurred by P_2, $*X\!\to\!C_1$, is a higher-ranked violation than that of P_1, $*\alpha\!\to\!C_2$, so P_1 is more harmonic than P_2; P_1 is the optimal candidate, and therefore the output. (The candidate P_4 is not shown in (5) because, as previously explained, it is harmonically bounded by — universally less harmonic than — P_2.) Similarly, for input **A**, the optimal candidate is A_1. This domination hierarchy gives rise to a nominative/accusative intransitive system.

(5)   Constraint tableau for English-type languages

Input	Output	$X\to C_1$	$x\not\to C_{1,2}$	$\alpha\to C_2$	$A\not\to C_2$	$A\to C_1$	$P\not\to C_1$	$P\to C_2$	$\alpha\not\to C_4$
A	☞ A_1			$\circledast$					
	A_2	*!			*	*			
P	☞ P_1			$\circledast$			$\circledast$	$\circledast$	
	P_2	*!							
aP	a_1P_2	*!	*						
	a_2P_1		*!		*	*	*	*	
	☞ a_4P_1			$\circledast$		$\circledast$	$\circledast$	$\circledast$	$\circledast$
	a_4P_2	*!				*			*
Ap	A_1p_2		*!						
	☞ A_1p_4			$\circledast$				$\circledast$	$\circledast$
	A_2p_4	*!			*	*		*	*

The remainder of tableau (5) concerns the passive input **aP** and the antipassive input **Ap**. The candidate outputs shown are all those that are not harmonically bounded (universally less harmonic than some competitor, Section 12:1.6; see Section 3). For **aP**, the optimal candidate is a_4P_1: the highest-ranking mark incurred by this structure, $*\alpha\to C_2$, is a less serious violation than the highest-ranking mark of each of its competitors. Since the output of **aP** is a_4P_1, in this language, passive is realized with an agent demoted to C_4 (in English, either a *by* phrase or absent) and a patient promoted to C_1 (NOM). This configuration, the traditional passive, we dub 'Passive₁', the subscript labeling the case of the high-prominence argument (P). The antipassive input **Ap** produces output A_1p_4 — 'Antipassive₁' — in which the patient is demoted to C_4 (in English, typically realized through absence on the surface; e.g., *John ate*).

The domination hierarchy shown in (5), therefore, yields a language with nominative/accusative intransitive case marking, and Passive₁ and Antipassive₁ voices. English is of course just one representative of this large typological class.

4.2 An ergative/absolutive example

If the constraint $X\to C_1$ topping the preceding hierarchy (boxed column in (5)) is ranked a bit lower and all other relative rankings remain unchanged, the typological class changes from one including English to one exemplified by Inuit. As shown in (6), the intransitive case-marking system is now ergative/absolutive: intransitive A and P both receive case C_2 (ABS). The optimal parse of **aP** is now a_4P_2 — 'Passive₂': the agent demotes to C_4 (in Inuit, either an OBL or surface-absent NP) while the patient receives C_2 (ABS), like intransitive arguments. The output for **Ap** is now A_2p_4 —

Box 1

'Antipassive₂': the patient demotes to C_4 (OBL or surface-absent in Inuit) and the agent receives C_2 (ABS). This is the traditional antipassive structure.

(6)   Constraint tableau for Inuit-type languages

Input	Output	$x \nrightarrow C_{1,2}$	$a \rightarrow C_2$	$X \rightarrow C_1$	$A \nrightarrow C_2$	$A \rightarrow C_1$	$P \nrightarrow C_1$	$P \rightarrow C_2$	$a \nrightarrow C_4$
A	A_1		*!						
	☞ A_2			⊛	⊛	⊛			
P	P_1		*!				*	*	
	☞ P_2			⊛					
aP	a_1P_2	*!		*					
	a_2P_1	*!			*	*	*	*	
	a_4P_1		*!			*	*	*	*
	☞ a_4P_2			⊛		⊛			⊛
Ap	A_1p_2	*!							
	A_1p_4		*!					*	*
	☞ A_2p_4			⊛	⊛	⊛		⊛	⊛

4.3 An active/stative example

If we modify the English-type ranking (5) by moving the pair of constraints $A \rightarrow C_1$, $P \nrightarrow C_1$ (dashed columns in (5)) to the top of the hierarchy, we move to a typological class including Lakhóta. Tableau (7) shows that the intransitive case-marking system is now active/stative, with A_1 and P_2 optimal. The output for **aP** is now a_1P_2, the same case assignment as in active voice. That is, whether the agent is of high (**AP**) or low prominence (**aP**) makes no difference: the optimal parse assigns C_1 to the agent in either case. This is a language *without* a passive voice: the top-ranked constraint $A \rightarrow C_1$ ensures that agents receive C_1, regardless of their level of prominence. There is, however, an antipassive voice: input **Ap** produces output A_1p_4 — Antipassive₁ (C_4 = surface absence in Lakhóta).

5 GENERAL ANALYSIS

In Section 4, we showed 3 possible case/voice systems that may arise through appropriate ranking of the universal constraints (2). What are all the possible such case/voice systems? There are 8! = 40,320 rankings in all, so careful analysis is required. In the end, we will show that only 13 distinct case/voice systems are predicted possible.

(7)   Constraint tableau for Lakhóta-type languages

Input	Output	$A{\to}C_1$	$P{\not\to}C_1$	$X{\to}C_1$	$x{\not\to}C_{1,2}$	$\alpha{\to}C_2$	$A{\not\to}C_2$	$P{\to}C_2$	$\alpha{\not\to}C_4$
A	☞ A_1					⊛			
	A_2	*!		*			*		
P	P_1		*!			*		*	
	☞ P_2			⊛					
aP	☞ a_1P_2			⊛	⊛				
	a_2P_1	*!	*		*		*	*	
	a_4P_1	*!	*			*	*	*	*
	a_4P_2	*!		*					*
Ap	A_1p_2				*!				
	☞ A_1p_4					⊛		⊛	⊛
	A_2p_4	*!		*			*	*	*

5.1   A typology of passives

The possible structures that can in fact surface as outputs from the low-prominence-agent input **aP** are these: a_4P_1 = Passive$_1$; a_4P_2 = Passive$_2$; a_2P_1 = Reversal; and a_1P_2 = No Passive. Only these four can be optimal for some constraint ranking — these are the possibly optimal structures. Examination of all other possible outputs (a_2P_4, a_4P_4, etc.) reveals that each such output L is harmonically bounded—universally less harmonic than some other, possibly optimal, alternative W: L incurs all the marks incurred by W, and some others as well, so $W \succ L$, universally (Section 12:1.6; Prince and Smolensky 1993/2004, Sec. 9.1.1).

Of the four possibly optimal outputs for **aP**, two are surface intransitive: in a_4P_1 and a_4P_2, only P bears a core case (C_1 or C_2). In a_2P_1, agent and patient reverse the cases they receive relative to active voice; this Reversal form of passive is exhibited in, for example, Navajo (Jelinek 1990). When a_1P_2 is optimal, the language lacks a passive, as discussed above for the Lakhóta class.[5]

While there are four possibly optimal outputs for **aP**, only one is optimal for a given language (determined by its domination hierarchy). In the simple form presented here, the present theory provides only one possible input for generating passive structures, and since each input generates only one output, multiple passive constructions in a single language cannot be treated. An extension to a richer input representation capable of distinguishing different inputs would allow for multiple pas-

---

[5] 'No Passive' here means no *personal* passive. Impersonal passives, briefly considered in Section 6.1, derive not from the personal passive input **aP** but rather from aP: the agent is *absent* from the input.

Box 1

sives within a single language.

For subsequent analysis, it is important to identify the exact conditions on a domination hierarchy that will ensure that a given passive structure is optimal. Here is one such **constraint domination condition**; others can be deduced for Passive$_2$, Reversal, and No Passive.

(8)   A language has Passive$_1$ if and only if its constraint ranking obeys these conditions:

   a.   either $X{\rightarrow}C_1$ or $x{\nrightarrow}C_{1,2}$ dominates each of $a{\nrightarrow}C_4$ and $A{\rightarrow}C_1$; and

   b.   either $A{\nrightarrow}C_2$ or $x{\nrightarrow}C_{1,2}$ dominates each of $a{\rightarrow}C_2$ and $a{\nrightarrow}C_4$; and

   c. $X{\rightarrow}C_1$ dominates each of $a{\rightarrow}C_2$, $P{\rightarrow}C_2$, and $P{\nrightarrow}C_1$.

It may be verified that the 'English' hierarchy (5) but not the 'Inuit' (6) or 'Lakhóta' (7) hierarchy, satisfies (8); Passive$_1$ occurs only in the English case.

5.2 A typology of antipassives

For the input **Ap,** there are only three possibly optimal structural descriptions: A_2p_4 = Antipassive$_2$; A_1p_4 = Antipassive$_1$; and A_1p_2 = No Antipassive. The same reasoning used with passives will show that the remaining parses of **Ap** are suboptimal regardless of the constraint ranking. And again, for each of the three possibly optimal parses of **Ap**, it is possible to derive a constraint domination condition, analogous to (8), under which that type of antipassive will be present in a language.

5.3 Implicational universals of case and grammatical voice systems

By examining the various constraint domination conditions analogous to (8), it is possible to determine which combinations of passive and antipassive voices and intransitive case systems can simultaneously obtain in a single language (i.e., derive from a single constraint ranking). (9) gives the results ('$\Rightarrow$' = 'implies'; '$\neg$' = 'not').

(9)   *Theorem.* Implicational universals

   1.   Reversal $\Rightarrow \neg$Antipassive$_{1,2}$
   2.   Passive$_2 \Rightarrow \neg$Accusative
   3.   Antipassive$_1 \Rightarrow \neg$Ergative
   4.   Antipassive$_2 \Rightarrow$ Passive$_2$
   5.   Antipassive$_2 \Rightarrow$ Ergative
   6.   Passive$_1 \Rightarrow \neg$Active
   7.   Passive$_1 \Rightarrow \neg$Ergative
   8.   Reversal $\Rightarrow \neg$Active

This set of implications is nonredundant (each one rules out a combined voice/case system not ruled out by the rest) and complete (every voice/case system not ruled out by these implications can be realized through a ranking of the constraints (2)).

5.4 Compound typologies

These implicational universals determine the typology shown in (10). Each gray cell represents an impossible combination, ruled out by the universal(s) labeled by the indicated number(s). We locate in the typology of (10) a number of languages from a survey of voice systems. The predictions of this extremely simple theory are borne out fairly well empirically: although one of the Dyirbal and one of the Mam passives fall into predicted-impossible (gray) cells, and examples have not yet been found for two systems predicted possible (empty white cells), the great majority of languages examined fall in the predicted-possible (white) cells and nearly all cells are occupied.

(10)   The combined case/voice typology

Accusative	Antipassive$_1$	Antipassive$_2$	No Antipassive
Passive$_1$	Arabic, English, Saramaccan	4 5	Bambara, Finnish
Passive$_2$	2 Dyirbal(1st/2nd)	2 5	2
Reversal	1	1 4 5	Navajo
No Passive	Ewe, Mojave	4 5	Ute

Ergative	Antipassive$_1$	Antipassive$_2$	No Antipassive
Passive$_1$	3 7	4 7 Mam	7
Passive$_2$	3	Dyirbal(3rd), Mam, Chamorro, Inuit	Burushaski
Reversal	1 3	1 4	
No Passive	3	4	Enga

Active	Antipassive$_1$	Antipassive$_2$	No Antipassive
Passive$_1$	6	4 5 6	6
Passive$_2$	Lezgian	5	
Reversal	1 8	1 4 5 8	8
No Passive	Lakhóta	4 5	Choctaw

Box 1

6 EXTENSIONS

A number of fairly straightforward extensions of the theory, such as to other thematic and case roles, are clearly needed. We mention two less obvious extensions here.

6.1 Impersonal constructions

A dummy can be treated as a case-receiving element in the output that is not present in the input—analogous to epenthesis in phonology. Certain kinds of impersonal passives (Footnote 11:13) can then be analyzed, as, for example, $\mathbf{a}P \to a_1P_2$ = Impersonal Passive$_{1,2}$, where '$\mathbf{a}$' denotes a missing agent in the input, and 'a_1' a dummy assigned C_1.[6] As in the OT treatment of epenthesis, this would violate a constraint FILL, which says that surface structural positions must be filled by underlying material (Prince and Smolensky 1993/2004). Impersonal constructions would appear only in languages where FILL is sufficiently low ranked.

6.2 Split ergativity and the ergative/accusative asymmetry

As indicated in (4), the constraint $a \to C_2$ is necessary for the existence of ergative languages, but not accusative ones. In fact, compared with accusative languages, *pure* ergative languages are relatively rare; they are most often split, typically with nominals high on an **animacy** hierarchy exhibiting an accusative pattern and lower-animacy nominals exhibiting the ergative pattern. This suggests that a more accurate version of the constraint $a \to C_2$ might be (11).

(11) $[-\mathbf{An}] \to \mathbf{C_2}$: Some low-animacy argument should receive abstract case C_2.

The ergativity we have seen resulting from $a \to C_2$ (when sufficiently highly ranked) would then appear only with low-animacy arguments, explaining why in ergative systems, but not accusative ones, splitting seems to be the unmarked case. Similar treatment may be possible for aspect- or tense-based splits.

---

[6] This dummy may be silent. In the Appendix, this has been indicated in the last column by [a]—in null-subject languages offering independent evidence for a silent dummy.

APPENDIX. LANGUAGES OF THE TYPOLOGY

The passive, antipassive, and impersonal passive constructions of the languages shown in the typology (10) are described in the following table. Language sources are identified in the references.

Language			Passive (V-morph)		Antipassive		Impersonal: aP
Arabic	N	Acc	1 (*ʔin-*)		1 (-0)		
(Palestinian) Semitic			A:0	P:NOM	A:NOM	P:0	
Bambara	N	Acc	1 (-*ra*)		—		
Mande			A:0,OBL	P:ACC			
Burushaski	N[7]	Erg	2 (-0/ *d-*)		—		
S. Asian isolate			A:0/0,OBL	P:ABS			
Chamorro	N	Erg	2 (-*ma*; -*in*)		2 (-*man*; -*fan*)		
Austronesian			A:OBL	P:ABS	A:ABS	P:0,OBL	
Choctaw	V	Act	—		—		
Muskogean							
Dyirbal	N	Erg*	2 (-0)		2 (-*ŋay*)		
Pama-		(3rd)	A:0	P:ABS	A:ABS	P:0,OBL	
Nyungan		Acc*	2 (-0)		1 (-*ŋay*)		
		(1st,2nd)	A:0	P:ACC	A:NOM	P:0,OBL	
Enga	N	Erg*	—		—		
Papuan							
English	N	Acc	1 (periphrastic *be*)		1 (-0)		
Germanic			A:0,OBL	P:NOM	A:NOM	P:0	
Inuit	NV	Erg	2 (-*(g)au-*)		2 (-0; -*i-*)		
(Greenlandic) Eskimo			A:0,OBL	P:ABS	A:ABS	P:0,OBL	
Ewe	N	Acc	—		1 (-0)		
Kwa/Niger-Congo					A:NOM	P:0	
Finnish	N	Acc	1 (-*(t)AAn*)		—		12 (-*(t)AAn*)
Finno-Ugric			A:0,OBL	P:NOM			a:NOM P:ACC
							(pronoun only)
Lakhóta	V	Act*	—		1 (*wa-*)		12 (-0)
Siouan					A:ACT	P:0	a:ACT P:STA
Lezgian	N	Act[8]	2 (-0)		1 (-0)		
NE Caucasian			A:0	P:STA	A:ACT	P:0	

[7] We treat the noun-marking system of Burushaski; there is also a verbal cross-referencing system, which is not completely aligned with the noun-marking system.
[8] Lezgian is described as ergative/absolutive by Mel'cuk (1988); his discussion, however, clearly shows what in our terms is an active/stative system.

Box 1

Language	Passive (V-morph)	Antipassive	Impersonal: aP

Mam V Erg
Mayan
	2 (-*eet*; -*j*; -*ʔn*)
	   A:0,OBL P:ABS
	2 (-*njtz*)
	   A:0,OBL P:ABS
	   (A:3rd, underived V)
	1 (-*njtz*)
	   A:0 P:ERG
	   (general truths)
		2 (-*n*)
		   A:ABS P:0,OBL	

Mojave V Acc
Yuman
	—	1 (-0)
		   A:NOM P:0
			12 (-*č*)
			   a:NOM P:ACC

Navajo N Acc Athapaskan	Reversal (*bi*-) A:ACC P:NOM	—	

Saramaccan N Acc
Creole
	1 (-0)
	   A:0 P:ACC
		1 (-0)
		   A:NOM P:0	

Ute N Acc Uto-Aztecan	—	—	12 (-*ta*-) a:NOM P:ACC

Notes: 'N'= abstract case realized by morphology on noun and/or word order, 'V'= verbal cross-referencing; '1' and '2' under Passive or Antipassive headings denote Passive₁,₂ or Antipassive₁,₂; 'Erg' = ergative/absolutive, 'Acc' = nominative/accusative, 'Act' = active/stative; 'Erg*', 'Acc*', 'Act*' = split system; OBL includes DAT; '0' = surface absence; [a] = silent dummy

References

ROA = Rutgers Optimality Archive, http://roa.rutgers.edu

Aissen, J. 1999. Markedness and subject choice in Optimality Theory. *Natural Language and Linguistic Theory* 17, 673–711.

Aissen, J. 2003. Differential object marking: Iconicity vs. economy. *Natural Language and Linguistic Theory* 21, 435–83.

Comrie, B. 1975. The antiergative: Finland's answer to Basque. In *Proceedings of the Chicago Linguistic Society 11.* (Finnish)

Comrie, B. 1989. *Language universals and linguistic typology.* University of Chicago Press.

Cooreman, A. 1988. The antipassive in Chamorro: Variations on the theme of transitivity. In *Passive and voice*, ed. M. Shibatani. Benjamins. (Chamorro)

Dixon, R. M. W. 1972. *The Dyirbal language of North Queensland.* Cambridge University Press. (Dyirbal)

England, N. C. 1983. *A grammar of Mam, a Mayan language.* University of Texas Press. (Mam)

Fillmore, C. J. 1968. The case for case. In *Universals in linguistic theory*, eds. E. Bach and R. T. Harms. Holt, Rinehart and Winston.

Gerdts, D. 1993. Mapping transitive voice in Halkomelem. In *Proceedings of the Berkeley Linguistics Society 19.*

Givón, T. 1984. *Syntax: A functional-typological introduction.* Vol. 1. Benjamins.

Givón, T. 1989. *Mind, code, and context: Essays in pragmatics.* Erlbaum.

Glock, N. 1972. Clause and sentence in Saramaccan. *Journal of African Languages* 11, Part 1, 45–61. (Saramaccan)

Grimshaw, J. 1993. Minimal projection, heads, and optimality. Technical report RuCCS-TR-4, Rutgers Center for Cognitive Science, Rutgers University. ROA 68.

Gruber, J. S. 1976. *Lexical structure in syntax and semantics.* North Holland.

Jelinek, E. 1990. Grammatical relations and coindexing in inverse systems. In *Grammatical relations: A cross-theoretical perspective*, eds. K. Kziwirek, P. Famlee, and E. Jejias-Bicardi. CSLI Publications. (Navajo)

Keenan, E. L. 1985. Passive in the world's languages. In *Language typology and syntactic description.* Vol. 1, *Clause structure*, ed. T. Shopen. Cambridge University Press. (Arabic)

Koopman, H. 1992. On the absence of case chains in Bambara. *Natural Language and Linguistic Theory* 10, 555–94. (Bambara)

Legendre, G., W. Raymond, and P. Smolensky. 1993. An optimality-theoretic typology of case and grammatical voice systems. In *Proceedings of the Berkeley Linguistics Society 19.* ROA 3.

Legendre, G., and D. S. Rood. 1992. On the interaction of grammar components in Lakhóta: Evidence from split intransitivity. In *Proceedings of the Berkeley Linguistics Society 18.*

McCarthy, J. J., and A. Prince. 1993. Prosodic Morphology I: Constraint interaction and satisfaction. Technical report RuCCS-TR-3, Rutgers Center for Cognitive Science, Rutgers University, and University of Massachusetts at Amherst. ROA 482, 2001.

Mel'cuk, I. A. 1988. *Dependency syntax: Theory and practice.* SUNY Press. (Lezgian)

Morin, Y.-C., and E. Tiffow. 1988. Passive in Burushaski. In *Passive and voice*, ed. M. Shibatani. Benjamins. (Burushaski)

Munro, P. 1976. *Mojave syntax.* Garland. (Mojave)

Munro, P., and L. Gordon. 1982. Syntactic relations in Western Muskogean: A typological perspective. *Language* 58, 81–115. (Choctaw)

Prince, A., and P. Smolensky. 1991. Notes on connectionism and Harmony Theory in linguistics. Technical report CU-CS-533-91, Computer Science Department, University of Colorado at Boulder.

Prince, A., and P. Smolensky. 1993/2004. *Optimality Theory: Constraint interaction in generative grammar*. Technical report, Rutgers University and University of Colorado at Boulder, 1993. ROA 537, 2002. Revised version published by Blackwell, 2004.

Rood, D. S., and A. R. Taylor. 1997. Sketch of the Lakhóta language. In *Handbook of North American Indians*. Vol. 17. Smithsonian Institution. (Lakhóta)

Sadock, J. M. 1980. Noun incorporation in Greenlandic: A case of syntactic word formation. *Language* 56, 300–19. (Inuit)

Sells, P. 2001. Form and function in the typology of grammatical voice systems. In *Optimality-theoretic syntax*, eds. G. Legendre, S. Vikner, and J. Grimshaw. MIT Press.

Van Valin, R. D., Jr. 1980. On the distribution of passive and antipassive constructions in Universal Grammar. *Lingua* 50, 303–27. (Enga, Lakhóta)

Westermann, D. 1930. *A study of the Ewe language*. Oxford University Press. (Ewe)

Witherspoon, G. 1980. Language in culture and culture in language. *International Journal of American Linguistics* 46, 1–13. (Navajo)

Woodbury, A. C. 1977. Greenlandic Eskimo, ergativity, and Relational Grammar. In *Syntax and semantics*. Vol. 8, *Grammatical relations*, eds. P. Cole and J. M. Sadock. Academic Press. (Inuit)

16

Optimality in Syntax II:
Wh-Questions

Géraldine Legendre, Colin Wilson, Paul Smolensky,

Kristin Homer, and William Raymond

Can complex syntactic phenomena be explained via the interaction of simple, universal, violable constraints? The rich phenomena surrounding information questions (*wh*-questions) have been at the center of much of the theoretical development of modern generative syntax; they are therefore critical to the empirical assessment of Optimality Theory (Figure 2:6 ②). Question formation has often been analyzed derivationally, through the movement of *wh*-phrases; the constraints on possible movements have been a central object of study.

An important syntactic principle at work in these phenomena is economy of movement: movement is not gratuitous, but must be driven to satisfy some constraint. And when movement does occur, it is often required to be local, that is, "as short as possible." The comparison inherent in principles that disfavor longer relative to shorter movement (or none at all) suggests that OT might provide a natural computational platform for such an economy principle. Here we argue that this is indeed the case, showing how OT can be used to explain cross-linguistic question formation systems and to derive a central 'Relativized Minimality' effect as an emergent property arising from simple principles that refer to neither minimality nor relativization. We also argue for the importance of faithfulness in syntax, as part of a general analysis of the nature of syntactic competition.

Sections 1–3 are slightly revised versions of sections of Legendre et al. 1995. Sections 4–6 are extracted from Legendre, Smolensky, and Wilson 1998.

Contents

1 ISSUES

T he study of *wh*-question formation has historically provided the empirical basis for major concepts in syntactic theory. Illustrations from Government-Binding Theory (GB; Chomsky 1981) include the Empty Category Principle (ECP), the existence of Logical Form (LF) as a separate level of representation — motivated in part by the abstract *wh*-movement-at-LF analysis of *wh*-in-situ languages like Chinese (Huang 1982) — and the central issue of which principles apply at which levels of representation. (For example, using data from Chinese, Huang (1982) argues that the ECP applies at both S-Structure and LF while Subjacency and his Condition on Extraction Domain (CED) apply only at S-Structure.)

Crosslinguistic investigations have revealed that these ideas are actually hard to formalize in a simple and unified fashion, and a brief survey reveals problems. (i) Standard GB offers no unified treatment of *wh*-fronting: languages that observe movement constraints are analyzed as involving movement; languages that do not observe movement constraints are analyzed as not involving movement (e.g., Palauan *wh*-fronting involves base generation; Georgopoulos 1985, 1991). (ii) No unified treatment of *wh*-in-situ is offered either: languages like Chinese and Japanese that observe (at least some) movement constraints have been analyzed as involving overt movement of a null operator coindexed with an in-situ *wh*-variable at S-Structure (Aoun and Li 1993; Cole and Hermon 1994); Malay and Ancash Quechua, which do not observe movement constraints, are analyzed as involving, not movement, but interpretation in situ (Cole and Hermon 1994). (iii) *Wh*-in-situ languages offer contradictory evidence about the level at which Subjacency applies: S-Structure in Chinese (Huang 1982) and Japanese (Lasnik and Saito 1992), LF in Hindi (Srivastav 1991). (iv) Languages with several *wh*-strategies show different degrees of constraint for each strategy: in Ancash Quechua, overt movement is more constrained than LF movement (Cole and Hermon 1994), while the reverse is true of Iraqi Arabic (Wahba 1991). While parameterization offers ways of resolving the contradictions in (iii) and (iv), such parameterization raises serious challenges for a theory of parameters that seeks to limit parameters to the lexicon or to functional categories. (v) Last but not least, we observe a proliferation of principles bearing the same name, the ECP. Some are clearly distinct in content — Chomsky (1986) seeks to reduce the ECP to antecedent government, Cinque (1990) to head government — while others are formally distinct — conjunctive (Aoun et al. 1987; Rizzi 1990) or disjunctive (Chomsky 1981, 1986; Lasnik and Saito 1992; Manzini 1992).

In this chapter, we propose to start addressing the issues outlined above by testing the hypothesis that different patterns of extractability across languages result from different rankings of universal constraints realizing a few simple principles. The scope of this chapter does not permit us to address all these issues; we can only set up the basic framework and explore a few of its consequences. In particular, we limit ourselves here to languages that observe movement constraints, whether they make use of *wh*-fronting (English, Bulgarian) or *wh*-in-situ (Chinese). The framework we develop is a version of GB that incorporates the two fundamental constructs of OT, **soft** constraints and **ranking** of soft constraints. In content, some of our constraints are reminiscent of similar constraints in the GB literature; they are, however, formally quite different because of their intrinsic violability and because of the way they interact: they can be violated in well-formed structures, and the force of a given constraint is greater in some languages than in others.[1]

Economy plays a well-known role in *wh*-question formation, ranging from the ultimate economical strategy — in-situ *wh* — to successive-cyclic movement (which some languages register morphologically, e.g., Irish, Chamorro). Instantiating the minimalist intuition that shorter movements are better than longer ones (Chomsky 1993), OT allows a precise formalization of economy in the MINLINK constraints defined below.

The chapter proceeds as follows. In Section 2, we discuss three *wh*-strategies and illustrate the basics of the OT analysis by showing how the distinct *wh*-strategies of English, Chinese, and Bulgarian arise from different rankings of three constraints. In Section 3, we turn to the technical focus of the chapter, an OT treatment of what traditionally falls under the ECP and Subjacency. For reasons of space, we limit our illustration to *wh*-islands and extraction out of the complement of *think*-type verbs. In Section 4, we consider the formal structure of the proposed MINLINK constraint. In Section 5, we discuss how Relativized Minimality effects arise in this theory from constraints formulated without either relativization or minimality. There, we also address two fundamental conceptual issues facing any optimization-based theory of syntax: the nature of the input to the grammar and the status of faithfulness in syntax. In Section 6, we review the main arguments of the chapter.

Box 1. Information questions: Semantic and syntactic structure

Note.   More background in syntax is needed to understand the technical details of this chapter than any other in the book. The chapter is included here for both empirical and theoretical reasons. It addresses crosslinguistic empirical questions surrounding *wh*-questions—called **extraction phenomena** for reasons to be explained in this box. These questions have been at the core of (generative) syntax since Ross's classic dissertation on extraction phenomena (Ross 1967, 1986), and they eventually took center stage in syntactic research of the 1980s (e.g., **Government-Binding Theory** (**GB**); Chomsky 1981). The literature on extraction phenomena of that era is vast. More recent research programs, including the **Minimalist Program** (Chomsky 1995), have sought to eliminate

---

[1] Our account is comparatively simple, by at least two measures of simplicity. (i) The constraints we posit are simple: for example, the ECP is reduced to head government; barriers are defined in terms of L-marking. (ii) Our account does not invoke antecedent government, minimality barriers (rigid or relativized), a distinction between inherent barrierhood and barrierhood by inheritance, gamma-marking, adjunction to VP in order to void the barrierhood of VP, and so on. The violability of constraints apparently renders these mechanisms unnecessary.

Box 1

many of the relevant constructs of the GB era and replace them with fewer, more fundamental principles, including an economy-of-movement principle referred to as **Shortest Move** (Chomsky 1993) or the **Minimal Link Condition** (Chomsky 1995). An OT conception of the Minimal Link Condition is the topic of this chapter.

The most general theoretical issues addressed in this chapter concern the nature of competition in OT syntax. One particularly important topic is the phenomenon of language-particular **ineffability**: the fact that in language $\mathcal{L}$ there is a grammatical expression for a given meaning but in language $\mathcal{L}'$ there is none. This poses a challenge to OT because the theory defines a grammatical output for every optimization. In this chapter (excerpted from papers written around 1994), we propose a solution on which much current discussion in OT syntax circles is based.

As explained at the end of Box 12:1, according to the X′ Theory of phrase structure, a clause can belong to one of several grammatical categories. The simplest clause is VP, with a lexical head V: a verb. More complex is IP, with a functional head I (sometimes written 'Infl'), which is the locus of inflectional features such as tense and number. The complement of the I head is a VP. CP is a still more complex clause, with a functional head C (sometimes written 'Comp'), the complement of which is an IP. When the clause is an argument of a verb, C is often a complementizer, like *that* in *she believed that boys play games*; here, the clause *that boys play games* is an argument of *believe*. Such a clause is a type of **subordinate clause**, as opposed to a **matrix clause** (or **root clause**), which is a simple, complete, stand-alone sentence.

C can function in other ways too. Intuitively, the functional features in C identify the **illocutionary force** of the clause: for example, a simple **declarative**, a command (**imperative**), or a question (**interrogative**). A question is a clause in which C bears the feature [+wh].

The semantics of a question involves a **question operator** we'll call $\mathbf{Q}$. Intuitively, an operator takes one proposition as input—for example, *play(boys, games)*—and produces a related proposition as output—here, *not(play(boys, games))*, the result of the **negation** operator. The input to this operator is the meaning of *boys play games*, while the output is the meaning of *it is not the case that boys play games*, or more simply, *boys do not play games*. In a semantic structure, the **scope** of an operator is the proposition serving as input to that operator. Negation has different scope in *she said that boys do not play games* and in *she did not say that boys play games*. In the first case—**narrow scope**—*not* operates on *play(boys, games)*, whereas in the second case—**wide scope**—it operates on *said(she, play(boys, games))*; what is negated is *playing* in the former but *saying* in the latter.

A more complex type of operator is involved in information questions. In the question *what has Felix eaten?*, one of the arguments of the *eat* proposition is missing—that's why the question is being asked. So while the answer might express *eaten(Felix, Mickey)*, the question has a blank where *Mickey* would go: *eaten(Felix, x)*. x is unknown, and the information question requests its value. The question operator Q takes *eaten(Felix, x)* and produces *Qx.eaten(Felix, x)*, expressed by *for what x is it the case that Felix has eaten x?* An operator like Q that **binds** a **variable** like x is a **quantifier**.

Like all operators, quantifiers have scope. *What does Hillary think Bill plays?* is, as a whole, an information question in which *what* has scope over everything else. *Hillary wonders what Bill plays* is not a question but a declarative assertion about Hillary: *what* has scope only over *Bill plays*, and *what Bill plays* is an **indirect question** that is an argument of *wonder*.

Thus, semantically, an information question results from taking a proposition p containing a variable x and giving it as input to the Q-operator, which is a quantifier that binds x; the scope of Q is p.

Syntactically, an information question is formed from an IP containing a variable x. This IP is the complement of a C head containing the feature [+wh]; the specifier of CP is the operator Q binding x. The syntactic realization of the quantifier-variable binding relationship is a chain connecting Q_i in SpecCP with x_i, a constituent within IP. This chain is often regarded as the description of movement from the location of x_i to the specifier of the CP defining the scope of Q_i. This view is useful in part because the material "passed over" during this movement matters for determining whether the result is grammatical. Such movement is called **extraction**: in *what has Felix eaten?*, *what* is said to have been 'extracted from' the clause *Felix has eaten what*. The syntactic structure is shown in tree form in (1a) and in the more compact bracketed form in (1b). In the tree, the **wh-movement** of *what$_m$* is indicated with a dashed arrow; the dotted arrows show other types of movement discussed in Box 12:1.

In English, the *wh*-phrase is pronounced at the location of Q, at the front of the sentence.[2] In other languages, including Chinese and Japanese, the *wh*-phrase is pronounced **in situ**, that is, in the position of the variable x: the counterpart of *Felix has eaten what* is itself the grammatical form in these languages. However, even in in-situ languages, the chain from x_i (where the *wh*-phrase is pronounced) to Q_i (where nothing is pronounced) can still be relevant to grammaticality. This chain is often interpreted as **covert movement**. Whether *wh*-phrases are fronted or in situ, the meaning of the question is the same.

According to this view, in both English and Chinese a *wh*-phrase moves from the position of x_i to the position of Q_i, but in English this movement occurs *before* determining pronunciation, whereas in Chinese it occurs *after*. In all languages, at the level of **D(eep)-Structure**, *wh* is in its base position, and at the level of **Logical Form** (**LF**), it is in the extracted position of Q. In between lies **S(urface)-Structure**, which determines pronunciation. In English, *wh*-movement occurs before the level of S-Structure, while in Chinese, it occurs after S-Structure. In the Chinese case, *wh*-movement occurs in the part of the derivation that creates LF from S-Structure; this is therefore sometimes called **LF movement** (or 'movement at LF').

---

[2] **Echo** questions like *Felix ate WHAT?*, with heavy sentential stress on the *wh*-phrase, are not requests for new information: they presuppose that the answer is already known. As their interpretation requires special discourse contexts, we do not consider them here. See also Footnote 14.

Box 1

(1)   A simple *wh*-question

a.   Tree form

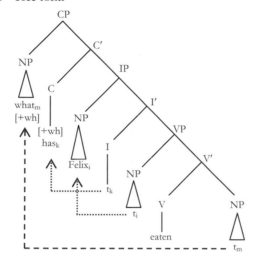

b.   Bracketed form

[CP what$_m$ has$_k$ [IP Felix$_i$ t$_k$ [VP t$_i$ eaten t$_m$]]]

The movement of the *wh*-phrase can be thought of as the result of a requirement that there be **specifier-head agreement** with respect to the question feature [+wh]. To be a question is to have [+wh] in C. To be a *wh*-phrase is to carry the feature [+wh]. If the *wh*-phrase moves to SpecCP, a configuration is created in which there is agreement between the specifier and the head of CP: both bear [+wh]. This is parallel to subject-verb agreement in number: after movement, the subject is in SpecIP and verb is in the head of IP; for correct agreement, both specifier and head must bear [+plural] (*boys play*) or [−plural] (*a boy plays*).

There are important constraints on *wh*-movement; these are the topic of Box 3.

In the perspective adopted in this chapter, there is no literal *wh*-movement in the derivational sense; "movement" is just a locution referring to *wh*-chains. In the standard case, either the *Q* at the head of the chain or the *t* at the foot is silent; the other hosts the overt *wh*-phrase. But it can happen that *both Q* and *t* are overt. In this case, the *wh*-phrase appears in *Q* and a pronoun appears in *t*: this is a **resumptive pronoun.**

Box 2. Multiple *wh*-questions

Questions involving multiple *wh*-phrases pose a syntactic challenge, which languages meet in different ways. The question *what did Dick know when?* would be structured

Dick when knew what? in Chinese and *when what knew Dick?* in Bulgarian. In Chinese, both *wh*-phrases remain in situ; in Bulgarian, both phrases are fronted; in English, one phrase remains in situ while the other is fronted. We assume that these questions ask for *pairs* of answers: *Dick knew <u>about the break-in</u> <u>months ago</u> and <u>about the cover-up</u> <u>the whole time</u>*. The meaning of the question can be taken to be 'for which x and y did Dick know x at time y' or *Qxy. know(Dick, x; y)*. Here the question operator binds two variables: this is the syntactic challenge.

Syntactically, SpecCP must house the structure that binds two variables. With only a single *wh*, this structure is an operator Q_i heading a chain with the variable t_i at its foot. Their coindexation encodes the binding. A *wh*-phrase will be pronounced at either the location of Q or the location of t. To bind two variables, one possibility is to have two chains, $Q_j Q_n$ *Dick know* $t_j t_n$; the two Qs form the structure in SpecCP binding the two variables. This structure is **adjunction to SpecCP**, sometimes notated with '+'; see (1).

(1)   Multiple *wh*: Adjunction candidate

$[_{CP} [_{NP} what_j + when_n] [_{IP} Dick_i knew_l [_{VP} [_{VP} t_i t_l t_j] t_n]]]$

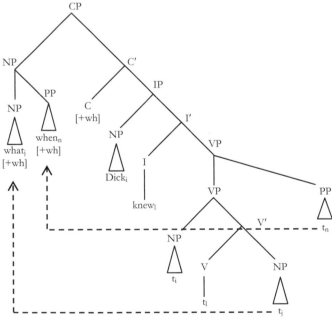

Another means of binding two variables is to put a single Q in SpecCP but to co-index it with both variables: $Q_{j[n]}$. For one index, j, the pair $Q_j \ldots t_j$, as before, are the head and foot of a chain: the result of movement, if you like. For the other index, n, there is no chain, no movement. The use of $Q_{j[n]}$ to bind both t_j and t_n is called **absorption**: 'The operator Q_n has been absorbed by the operator Q_j'.

Box 2

The relationship between the doubly indexed operator and the second variable t_n—marked by the common index n—is rather like the coindexing in *John$_i$ thinks Jane likes him$_i$*: for the purposes of interpretation, the coindexation asserts that the interpretation of *him$_i$* is dependent on—equal to—the interpretation of *John$_i$*. But there is no movement here, no chain linking *John$_i$* and *him$_i$*. There is an interpretive dependency but no syntactic dependency: *John$_i$* and *him$_i$* do not have to come or go as a unit the way $Q_k \dots t_k$ do. The coindexing of $Q_{j[n]}$ and the second variable t_n is also a marking of the interpretive (rather than syntactic) dependency between the operator and the variable: the interpretation of t_n is dependent on $Q_{j[n]}$ because this operator marks the scope of the operator-variable binding. The contrast between (2) and (3) shows the dependence of the interpretation of t_n on its coindexed operator. In (2) (and (1)), the scopes of t_n and t_j encompass the same clause; the single specifier of this CP hosts the Q-operator(s) binding these two variables. In (3), the two variables have different scopes; one Q lies in SpecCP of the matrix clause, the other in SpecCP of the embedded clause.

(2) Multiple *wh*: Absorption candidate
[CP what$_{j[n]}$ did$_l$ [IP Dick$_i$ t$_l$ [VP [VP t$_i$ know t$_j$] when$_n$]]]

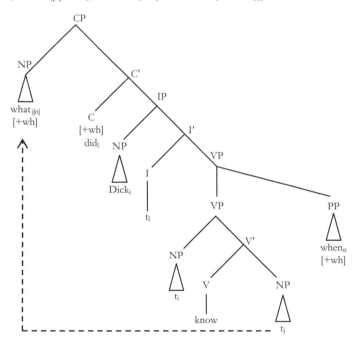

(3)   Multiple *wh*: Different scopes

*[$_{CP}$ what$_j$ did$_l$ [$_{IP}$ Josh$_i$ t$_l$ [$_{VP}$ t$_i$ ask [$_{CP}$ who$_p$ [$_{IP}$ t$_p$ had [$_{VP}$ t$_p$ bought t$_j$]]]]]]

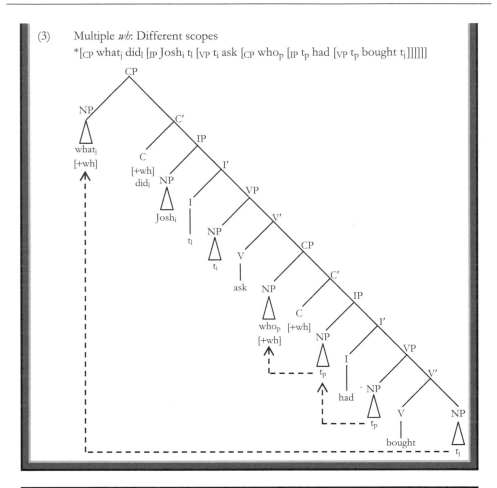

Box 3. Constraints on *wh*-questions

Wh-movement is a transformation whereby a *wh*-phrase moves to the specifier of CP. The output of this transformation is subject to a number of well-formedness constraints (or 'filters') that figure in the OT analysis of this chapter. Much technical terminology in the OT analysis is transparently borrowed or adapted from GB Theory (Chomsky 1981), including the central concept of government.

Ross (1967) identified certain syntactic contexts as **islands**: constituents out of which a *wh*-phrase cannot move. Among them are the **complex NP island** and the **wh-island**. Compare (1a) and (1b).

Box 3

(1) Complex NP island for extraction

    a. [$_{CP}$ What$_j$ did [$_{IP}$ Josh claim [$_{CP}$ e$_j$ that [$_{IP}$ he read t$_j$ in the newspaper]]]]?

    b. *[$_{CP}$ What$_j$ did [$_{IP}$ Josh make [$_{NP}$ the claim [$_{CP}$ e$_j$ that [$_{IP}$ he read t$_j$ in the newspaper]]]]]?

The difference in grammaticality is attributed to an 'island' effect. In (1b), the *wh*-phrase *what$_j$* has been extracted from (moved out of) a complex NP island—*the claim that he read t$_j$ in the newspaper*—so the result is ungrammatical.

Such contrasts led to characterizing certain kinds of nodes as **bounding nodes** (or boundaries to movement). In cases like (1b), the bounding node is NP: this is what must be crossed in *wh*-movement out of a complex NP. Bounding nodes matter because of the Subjacency Condition (Chomsky 1973).

(2) Subjacency Condition

    Wh-movement may not cross more than one bounding node.

Another key contrast is shown in (3): extraction out of a *that*-complement is grammatical, while extraction out of a *wh*-island—the complement of a verb like *wonder*—is not.

(3) *Wh*-island for extraction

    a. [$_{CP}$ What$_j$ do [$_{IP}$ you think [$_{CP}$ e$_j$ that [$_{IP}$ Josh opened t$_j$]]]]?

    b. *[$_{CP}$ What$_j$ do [$_{IP}$ you wonder [$_{CP}$ who opened$_n$ [$_{IP}$ t$_n$ t$_j$]]]]?

The *wh*-island extraction (3b) will violate Subjacency if, like NP above, IP is a bounding node. But the contrast between (3a) and (3b) rests on a subtle difference: in (3a), the embedded CP has *that* in C but nothing in SpecCP. Thus, the *wh*-movement can proceed in two steps: first, *what$_j$* moves from its original direct object position up to the specifier of the embedded CP; then it moves from there to the specifier of the outer CP. This leaves a silent trace at the intermediate "hopping" point; we have marked this *e$_j$* to distinguish this intermediate position in the *j* chain from the base position containing *t$_j$*. This kind of movement—**successive-cyclic movement**—is registered morphologically in some languages (including Irish, Chamorro, and others): as the *wh*-phrase "hops through" an intermediate SpecCP, its passage is marked on the complementizer ('that') heading SpecCP. The point is that via successive-cyclic movement, each step of movement—or each link of the total chain—crosses only one IP bounding node: this satisfies Subjacency.

Why, then, is (3b) ungrammatical? It is because the "escape hatch" in (3a) enabling successive-cyclic movement—an intermediate empty SpecCP—is not available in (3b). The embedded CP is now an indirect question, with a *wh*-phrase *who* in its specifier position. The extracted *wh*-phrase *what$_j$* cannot "hop through" the intermediate specifier: it must move directly to its final position, the specifier of the outer CP. Instead of two short links, the *j* chain is now a single long link. This link crosses *two* IP bounding nodes, violating Subjacency.

Returning to (1b), we observe that *what* raises first to the intermediate SpecCP, crossing only one bounding node (IP); but in a second step, it crosses NP and IP, violating Subjacency. As a result, (1b) is ungrammatical.

An intuitive gloss of this explanation for the contrast in (3) between *that*-complements and *wh*-complements is this. *Wh*-extraction moves through specifier positions, and this is the same position occupied by a *wh*-phrase at the front of a *wh*-complement; thus, the latter *wh* interferes with the former *wh*. This interference arises directly from the fact that the two elements in question are of the same type—*wh*-phrases—and therefore compete for the same structural position—SpecCP. In contrast, *that* is a complementizer, occupying the CP-head position C; this does not interfere with *wh*-movement, which targets SpecCP.

A similar intuition is captured directly in the OT analysis proposed in this chapter, but with a twist. A structure for extracting a *wh*-phrase from a *wh*-complement has two SpecCP positions available for *wh*-phrases, one marking narrow scope, the other, wide scope. These literally compete, making it more difficult to achieve wide scope *wh*-extraction. This competition does not arise in a structure for extracting a *wh*-phrase from a *that*-complement, which has only one SpecCP available for a *wh*-phrase: the wide scope position. In the OT account, the intermediate SpecCP is available for a *wh*-phrase extracted from a *wh*-complement, but not from a *that*-complement. The reverse holds in the GB analysis, where the intermediate SpecCP is available for a *that*- but not a *wh*-complement. See Section 3.2.1.

Perhaps the most important of the structural relations in syntax is **c-command** ('c' for 'constituent'; Reinhart 1976). Informally, a node c-commands its sister (the node that shares the same mother) and all the daughters, granddaughters, and so on, of its sisters. For example, V c-commands its complement under V′ and all the subconstituents of that complement.

The formal definition is given in (4). (4a) gives a traditional tree-oriented definition, while (4b) gives an equivalent phrase-oriented definition, using the following terminology: A **strictly contains** B if and only if A contains B and A ≠ B.

(4)   C-command

    a.   Node A c-commands node B if and only if every branching node dominating A also dominates B, and neither A nor B dominates the other.

    b.   Phrase A c-commands phrase B if and only if A *does not* strictly contain B, but any phrase strictly containing A *does* strictly contain B.

Government is simply a local version of c-command. It is the structural relation that holds between a head (V, P, I, C, etc.) and an element that is governed (its sister). Unlike c-command, head government does not reach down to terminal nodes.

Government pervaded analyses of many syntactic phenomena in the 1980s including case (see Box 15:1) and *wh*-movement. For example, subjects typically differ from objects with respect to extraction. Specifically, it is possible to extract the subject from (5a) but not (5b). In contrast, extraction of the object in (5c) is possible whether or not there is an overt complementizer *that* (the irrelevance of *that* is indicated by enclosing it in parentheses).

Box 3

(5)   *That*-trace effect

    a.   [$_{CP}$ Who$_i$ did [$_{IP}$ you think   [$_{IP}$ t$_i$ came]]]?

    b.   *[$_{CP}$ Who$_i$ did [$_{IP}$ you think [$_{CP}$ that [$_{IP}$ t$_i$ came]]]]?

    c.   [$_{CP}$ What$_j$ did [$_{IP}$ you think [$_{CP}$ (that) [$_{IP}$ Josh found t$_j$]]]]?

The subject-object asymmetry in (5a–c) is commonly referred to as the ***that*-trace (*that-t*) effect**. Chomsky (1981) proposed that (5b) is ungrammatical because it violates (6).

(6)   Empty Category Principle (ECP)

    An empty category must be **properly governed**. Lexical categories (V, P, etc.) are proper governors; functional categories (I, C) are not.

It is as though the overt presence of lexical categories robustly indicates the arguments required, so the presence of empty elements is implied by the absence of overt arguments; but the ephemeral functional categories do not provide such information.

    Given the definition of proper governor, an object trace is always properly governed because it is governed by a lexical category (V). A subject trace typically is not. Specifically, (5b) is ungrammatical because the trace of the extracted subject fails to be properly governed when the complementizer *that* (a functional category) is realized. In its absence, the subject trace t_i is properly governed via an extension of the concept of proper government to include **antecedent government**: the subject trace has a c-commanding antecedent, the fronted *wh*-phrase *who$_i$* in SpecCP with which it is co-indexed. The (extended) ECP is satisfied. Returning to the ungrammatical (5b), one could posit that the subject trace is neither head-governed (as just stated) nor antecedent-governed (which is defined so that the complementizer in C blocks the government relation between the subject trace and its c-commanding antecedent).

    A principle close (and eventually reduced) to the ECP was introduced in Huang 1982 to explain the ungrammaticality of extracting a *wh*-phrase *what$_j$* out of an adjunct like *after eating t$_j$* in **after eating t$_j$* in *what$_j$ did Josh drink milk after eating t$_j$?* (Adjuncts are assumed not to be properly governed by the verb *drink*.)

(7)   Condition on Extraction Domain (CED; Huang 1982)

    No constituent may be extracted from a domain that is not properly governed.

The concept of **barrier** was introduced in Chomsky 1986 in an attempt to unify Bounding Theory and the ECP. Simply stated, structures that are complements of lexical categories (**L-marked** phrases) are not barriers, whereas structures that are not complements of lexical categories are. In reality, Chomsky's Barrier Theory is very complex, well beyond what the reader needs in order to understand our proposed constraint MINLINK. One addition to the definition of barrier that is relevant, however, is the **Minimality Condition** that Chomsky (1986) introduces to (i) formalize the intuition that government is a unique relationship (if an element is governed by one element, it cannot be by another), and (ii) formalize within Barrier Theory the idea that the complementizer is a 'barrier' to antecedent government of the subject trace. Given the Minimality Condition, the complementizer *that* in C is a more minimal governor of the subject than the *wh*-element in SpecCP. The node immediately dominating the nearest governor can become a barrier to government.

Barrier Theory (including the Minimality Condition) was eventually reformulated in terms of Relativized Minimality in Rizzi 1990.

(8)   Relativized Minimality

An element minimally governs its trace if there is no other 'typical potential governor' that is closer to the trace.

Under Rizzi's proposal, what counts as a governor is relativized to what is being governed. Thus, a typical potential governor for the trace of a head X is another head X; a typical potential governor for an element in an 'A-chain' (e.g., passivization) is another antecedent governor in an 'A-position' (e.g., SpecIP), and a typical potential governor for an element in an 'A-bar chain' (e.g., a *wh*-chain) is an antecedent governor in another 'A-bar position' (e.g., SpecCP).

Finally, the ECP was abandoned and Bounding Theory was reduced to (9).

(9)   Minimal Link Condition (Chomsky 1995)

Movement must target the closest potential position.

2 AN OPTIMALITY THEORY ANALYSIS OF *WH*-STRATEGIES

Chinese, Bulgarian, and English exemplify the three distinct *wh*-strategies we focus on in this chapter: Chinese leaves *wh*-phrases in situ; Bulgarian obligatorily fronts all available *wh*-phrases, despite having relatively free word order elsewhere; English obligatorily fronts one *wh*-phrase, and only one. Relevant facts are illustrated in (1).

(1)   a.   Lisi *zenmeyang* chuli   zhe-jian shi?

Lisi how   handle this   matter

'How did Lisi handle this matter?'

(what is the means or manner *x* such that Lisi handled this matter by *x*)

(Tsai 1994)

b.   *Koj   kakvo na kogo*   e   da   t t?*

who what to whom has given

'Who gave what to whom?'

(Rudin 1988)

c.   *Who* gave *what to whom*?

Our unified approach starts with a representation of scope in terms of **chains**, not movement. Following May (1985) and others, we retain the basic idea of modeling the representation of *wh*-interpretation on quantifier-variable binding, but we modify the standard representation in the following way. A *wh*-chain contains an operator as its head (in highest specifier position of a clause) and a variable as its foot; the latter marks the D-Structure position of a questioned element, the former the scope of its

Box 3

interpretation.[3] The *wh*-fronting strategy places the overt *wh*-operator at the head of the chain, with an empty trace *t* at the foot of the chain; the *wh*-in-situ strategy places an empty operator Q at the head of the chain and the overt *wh*-phrase at its foot. What matters is (i) the relationship between Q and the variable it binds, namely, the chain (Q, x); (ii) that only one of Q or x can be overt "for free" (if both are overt, a resumptive pronoun results, violating a FILL constraint, as discussed in Section 3.2.3); and (iii) that any empty variables (and intermediate traces) obey constraints on traces. (Following Aoun and Li (1993), we assume that overt question markers such as optional *ne* in Chinese are generated in C position in the presence of a Q-operator via the mechanism of specifier-head agreement.)

In OT, a grammar specifies a function that maps inputs to outputs. Inputs consist of raw materials from which the candidate outputs are built: skeletal structures containing predicate-argument structure and scope information. These materials are those employed to express the basic meaning (including discourse properties) and provide the basic building blocks (NP, V, P, C, etc.) and single clausal brackets. For every input, *Gen* generates the set of candidate outputs, or 'parses', with scope relations (roughly a combination of S-Structure, D-Structure, and LF). *Gen* generates all relevant brackets in accordance with standard X' Theory. *Gen* marks as overt Q or x (or both, in which case a resumptive pronoun realizes x). Each candidate output for an input contains that input ('containment'). *Gen* also generates unfaithful candidates that fail to parse some element of the input (e.g., the [wh] feature or the scope of Q, as discussed below). *Gen* is also responsible for placing Q in the highest specifier position of a clause.[4] In OT, the optimal form is grammatical: roughly, it is the form that least violates the lowest-ranked constraints, relative to its competitors. The set of candidates entering the competition is universal.

Consider the candidate set for questioning, say, a direct object out of a simple clause. The universal input is schematically shown in (2), and a subset of the corresponding universal candidate set to be evaluated by the constraints is shown in (3).

(2) Universal input for questioning a direct object out of a simple clause

$[Q_j [...t_j...]]$

(3) Universal candidate set for (2)

    a. $[Q_j [...wh_j...]]$ faithful parse

    b. $[wh_j [...t_j...]]$ faithful parse

    c. $\langle Q_j \rangle [...NP/\langle wh_j \rangle...]$ unfaithful parse

(3a) represents *wh*-in-situ, the winning strategy in Chinese; (3b) represents fronting of

---

[3] This proposal goes back to Baker (1970) and has been revived in recent work by a number of linguists. Our proposal is close to that of Aoun and Li (1993) in several respects, with a crucial difference: they posit overt movement of a null Q-operator in Chinese at S-Structure. Our system has a single level of optimization that subsumes D-Structure, S-Structure, and LF, and it involves no movement.

[4] In principle, *Gen* also generates all word orders, candidates being evaluated against word order constraints that are ranked along with other constraints. In lieu of an OT theory of word order, here we artificially limit candidate sets to candidates observing the surface word order of the language.

a *wh*-phrase to a scope position, the winning strategy in English and Bulgarian. In candidate output (3c), the [wh] feature is not parsed: it is unfaithful to the semantics of the input. We admit unfaithful parses in our candidate set because in some instances, there is no grammatical way of expressing some input. The structure corresponding to a failure to parse [wh] in (3c) is not a question; rather, it is a statement with a [–wh] NP in lieu of a [+wh] NP. A language for which candidate (3c) is optimal is a language in which direct objects cannot be directly extracted out of simple clauses, as is the case in Bahasa Indonesia (Saddy 1991), Kwakwala (Anderson 1984), Malagasy (Keenan 1976), Tagalog (Guilfoyle, Hung, and Travis 1992), and other languages. (See Section 3.2.1, and general discussion of ineffability and faithfulness in Section 5.)

We now turn to constraints and rankings. Chinese, as shown in (1a), obviously has a relatively strong constraint against "overt movement" of *wh*-phrases, which we state with maximal generality: *t or 'No traces'. (This is Grimshaw's (1997) constraint STAY; compare Chomsky's (1993) proposals regarding economy of derivation.) We suppose that Bulgarian (1b) shows the effects of a constraint that has the opposite effect, namely, forcing *wh*-phrases to front: *Q or 'No empty *Q*-operators'. English seems to have both constraints at work simultaneously: a constraint against leaving *wh*-phrases in situ that prevails for one element and one element only, and a constraint against fronting that prevails for all remaining *wh*-phrases (1c). According to OT, of course, conflicts between *t and *Q are resolved by ranking; the three languages obey the same constraints, but the constraints are ranked differently. In Chinese, *t ranks higher than *Q. The situation is reversed in Bulgarian, where *Q ranks higher than *t.[5] That only one *wh*-phrase moves in English results from a third constraint that ranks higher than *t in Bulgarian but lowest in English. Drawing on a standard feature of the analysis of English multiple *wh*-questions with the same scope (Higginbotham and May 1981), we propose that this constraint is one against absorption of *Q*s, *ABSORB. In English, *ABSORB ranks low, with the result that English allows one operator to mark the scope of two variables. In Bulgarian, *ABSORB ranks relatively high; in effect, Bulgarian does not allow two *Q*s to be combined.

The constraints are summarized in (4), and the language-particular rankings are given in the standard OT tableau format in (6a–c), using the notation in (5).

(4)   Constraints

*t	No traces.
*Q	No empty *Q*-operators.
*ABSORB	No absorption of *Q*-operators.

---

[5] The effect of *Q is very close to Grimshaw's (1997) OPSPEC 'Operators must be in specifier position'. Our representations are quite different, however: *Q is violated by a *Q*—an empty operator—that heads a *wh*-chain in our structures; such an element (and chain) is simply not present in Grimshaw's structures. In conjunction with our representation of scope, *Q essentially replaces the *Wh*-Criterion (May 1985; Rizzi 1991). A language that ranks *Q higher than *t is one in which [wh] functions as a "strong feature" in the sense of Chomsky 1993; see Section 5.3.

Box 3

(5)   Notational conventions

  a.   In multiple-*wh* candidates, '+' indicates adjunction to SpecCP.

  b.   Subscripts for chains are meaningful:

      subscript i = an extracted subject,

      subscript j = an extracted direct object,

      subscript k = an extracted referential adjunct,

      subscript l = an extracted nonreferential adjunct.

  c.   Circled stars '⊛' identify constraint violations of the optimal candidate.

(Referentiality is discussed in Section 3.3.)

The constraint tableau for Chinese is given in (6a).

(6)   a.   Chinese: Multiple *wh*-questions

$[Q_i Q_j [x_i V x_j]]$	*ABSORB	*t	*Q
a. ☞ $[Q_i{+}Q_j [wh_i V wh_j]]$			⊛ ⊛
b. $[wh_i{+}wh_j [t_i V t_j]]$		*! *	
c. $[wh_{i[j]} [t_i V wh_j]]$	*	*!	

Given that, in Chinese, candidate (a) has to defeat candidate (b), and given that (a) violates *Q, a constraint not violated by the losing candidate (b), constraint *Q must be ranked lower than a constraint violated by the losing candidate (b), namely, *t. We thus obtain the basic Chinese ranking given in (6a). The relative ranking of *ABSORB doesn't matter here; absorption is irrelevant in Chinese (it is a factor only when *wh* moves — in our terms, when *Q ranks higher than *t; then it decides between candidates (b) and (c)). This situation is suggested by dotted lines separating the *ABSORB column from the others.

The constraint tableau for Bulgarian is given in (6b).

(6)   b.   Bulgarian: Multiple *wh*-questions

$[Q_i Q_j [x_i V x_j]]$	*ABSORB	*Q	*t
a. $[Q_i{+}Q_j [wh_i V wh_j]]$		*! *	
b. ☞ $[wh_i{+}wh_j [t_i V t_j]]$			⊛ ⊛
c. $[wh_{i[j]} [t_i V wh_j]]$	*!		*

For multiple fronting of *wh* to win — candidate (b) — a constraint violated by each of the suboptimal candidates (a) and (c) must be ranked higher than the constraints violated by the optimal candidate (b), namely, *t. Suboptimal candidate (a) violates *Q; comparing the pair (a) and (b) thus shows that *Q ≫ *t. Comparing (b) and (c) shows that *ABSORB must outrank *t. One violation of *t for both candidates cancels; what remains is a violation of *t for the winning parse (b) and a violation of *ABSORB for the suboptimal parse (c). Hence, *ABSORB outranks *t. The *ABSORB and *Q columns are separated by a dotted line because their relative ranking is yet to be determined.

Finally, the constraint tableau for English is given in (6c).

(6)   c.   English: Multiple *wh*-questions

$[Q_i Q_j [x_i V x_j]]$	*Q	*t	*Absorb
a. $[Q_i+Q_j [wh_i V wh_j]]$	*! *		
b. $[wh_i+wh_j [t_i V t_j]]$		* *!	
c. ☞ $[wh_{i[j]} [t_i V wh_j]]$		⊛	⊛

In English, the optimal parse is (c), which violates *Absorb and *t. Its competitors lose because candidate (b) incurs two marks against *t (versus one for candidate (c)) and candidate (a) violates *Q, which is ranked highest.

The resulting (partial) rankings for these languages are summarized in (7).[6]

(7)   Partial rankings

Chinese: *t ≫ *Q   *Absorb unranked
Bulgarian: {*Q, *Absorb} ≫ *t
English: *Q ≫ *t ≫ *Absorb

3 Long versus short movement: Government, locality, and referentiality

3.1 Government

Our representation of scope posits chains that include traces, hence the need to constrain the occurrence of these traces. We follow much standard work and in particular Rizzi 1990 and Cinque 1990 in positing that traces are constrained by head government. In English, the cost of violating head government is high; hence, the relevant constraint is high ranked. We assume with Cinque (1990) that proper head government is not sensitive to the distinction between lexical and functional categories.[7] Rather, it is sensitive to the following constraint:

(8)   Gov(t): t must be head-governed by a category nondistinct from [+V].

We only partially adopt Cinque's characterization of which categories are nondistinct from [+V]: namely, V [–N, +V], I [+V], and A [+N, +V]. In particular, we reject his assumption that C is a proper governor. Evidence that C is not a proper governor comes from the unexplained absence in (9a) of complementizer stranding in English, which otherwise allows stranding of prepositions and of I (9b).[8]

[6] The proposal made here is similar to one independently made by Billings and Rudin (1994). Note that both proposals fail to characterize languages like Italian, Irish, and Quiegolani Zapotec (Black 2000), which require fronting of one single *wh*-phrase while not allowing any others to remain in situ.
[7] Grimshaw (1997) proposes constraints requiring that *t* be head-governed (T-Gov) but distinguishes functional from lexical government (T-Lex-Gov).
[8] The claim that nouns [+N, –V] are inadequate governors is made in Kayne 1984, Rizzi 1990, and Cinque 1990: cross-clausal NP movement in passive and raising cannot take place within NPs, as in

Box 3

(9) a. *John left, we think that t.

   b. John said that he would leave and leave, he did t.

We further depart from many standard assumptions about which elements are properly head-governed. In addition to direct objects (governed by V), subjects internal to VP and adjuncts (adjoined to VP) are governed by a functional head (I for the sake of simplicity). Subjects in SpecIP are typically not properly head-governed but under certain conditions they may be governed by a matrix V (see discussion of bridge verbs below).[9] The main reason for assuming that adjuncts are properly governed comes from the crosslinguistic observation that extraction of adjuncts is possible. To mention only two cases, adjuncts can be extracted out of the complement of *think* and in multiple questions in English; in Chinese, wide scope interpretation of most adjuncts is possible out of complements of *think* as well as weak and strong islands (Tsai 1994).

We assume with Rizzi (1990) that c-command underlies head government and that a head properly governs its complement and the specifier of its complement (or adjoined position if a phrase is adjoined to the complement). Partial evidence for this definition of head government comes from *that-t* effects in English.

(10) a. *Who do you think [$_{CP}$ that [$_{IP}$ t left early]]?

    b. Who do you think   [$_{IP}$ t left early]?

In (10a), *t* is not properly head-governed — C is not a proper head governor. In (10b), *t* is head-governed by the matrix verb *think*.

3.2 Locality

A well-known generalization about *wh*-questions is that extraction is basically *local*: no "movement" can displace the extracted element too far from its previous position. Consider, for example, the extraction of adjuncts in English. ('[' is explained below.)

(11) a. How₁ did [he [fix it] t₁]?

    b. How₁ do [you [think [e₁ that [he [fixed it] t₁]]]]?

    c. *How₁ does [she [wonder [what₁ [John [fixed t₁] t₁]]]]?

The standard analysis of the contrast between (11b) and (11c) invokes successive-cyclic movement to explain the well-formedness of (11b). (11b) exploits the escape hatch in the specifier position of the embedded CP: the *wh*-chain consists of two links, joined at the intermediate trace *e₁* in SpecCP. In (11c), the specifier position of the em-

---

*John's appearance t to be sick; preposition stranding under NP movement is impossible in NPs, as in *the new law's vote for t. We assume that P is [−N] in English, hence a proper governor. P is [−N, −V] in Chinese, French, and Bulgarian, which do not allow preposition stranding; C is presumably [−V] except when it carries agreement, in which case it is, like I, [+V]. See the *qui > que* rule in French (Rizzi 1990).

[9] In this chapter, we assume that subjects are generated under VP, but nothing hinges on making this assumption rather than generating them adjoined to VP. We further assume that subjects move to SpecIP in English and Chinese (prior to extraction), but they needn't do so in Bulgarian, which doesn't show *that-t* effects (see further discussion below). To maximize the readability of English and Chinese tableaux, we systematically omit the properly head-governed *t* in SpecVP.

---

bedded CP is filled with a *wh*-phrase, with the result that movement of *how* is long, in violation of Subjacency. Any attempt to precisely characterize the intuition that shorter movement is better than longer movement must wrestle with the issue of comparing lengths, or counting units of length.[10] In OT, we can naturally distribute locality over a family of constraints, MinLink, which refers to the length of *chain links*, using Chomsky's (1986) notion of **barrier**:[11] a single link of a chain violates BAR^1 when it crosses one barrier; it violates BAR^2 when it crosses two barriers; and so on. The constraints BAR^1, BAR^2, BAR^3 are universally ranked, as shown in (13). The construction of MinLink as a **constraint power hierarchy**—including the universal hierarchy (13)—is presented in Section 4.

Like all other constraints in OT, the BAR constraints are violable: violated in well-formed structures. A preliminary list of the MinLink constraints is given in (12).

(12)   MinLink family of constraints (incomplete)

BAR^1 A single link must not cross one barrier.

BAR^2 A single link must not cross two barriers.

BAR^3 A single link must not cross three barriers.

(13)   Ranking (universal)

BAR^3 ≫ BAR^2 ≫ BAR^1

Assuming the representational equivalent of successive cyclicity, (11b) contains a *wh*-chain of two short links (how_1, e_1) and (e_1, t_1), which cross two barriers and one barrier, respectively. In contrast, (11c) contains one long link (how_1, t_1), which crosses three barriers. The full OT account requires considering the optimal output that renders (11c) suboptimal, as we will show directly. We comment first on the status of intermediate traces in our account. Each link in (11b) contains an intermediate trace *e* in the specifier of the lower CP (called *e* to differentiate it from *t* in D-Structure position). *e* is a by-product of short links and is itself constrained by GOV(t). Evidence that *e* is subject to GOV(t) comes from contexts known as strong islands out of which extraction in many languages, including English, is impossible: sentential subjects (14a), adjunct clauses (14b), and complex NPs (14c). (15) gives the corresponding declaratives.

(14)   a.   *Who$_i$ [[e$_i$ that [t$_i$ left early]]] was obvious to everyone?

b.   *Who(m)$_j$ did he get upset [e$_j$ after [he [saw t$_j$]]]?

c.   *How$_l$ did you find [a man [e$_l$ that [would fix it] t$_l$]]?

(15)   a.   [That *he* left early] was obvious to everyone.

b.   He got upset [after he saw *Mary*].

c.   I found [a man [that would fix it *fast*]].

---

[10] For a proposal within the Minimalist Program, see Collins 1994.

[11] In the tableaux, we use plain brackets ([) to represent barriers and hollow brackets ([) to represent nonbarriers, that is, L-marked maximal projections (Chomsky 1986; see Box **3**).

Box 3

Under standard assumptions, the bracketed clauses contain an escape hatch in SpecCP. Crucially, any intermediate e resulting from an attempt at forming a successive-cyclic chain fails to be properly governed. In (14a), e is not properly head-governed because there is no potential head governor for it; in (14b), e is not governed because it is not in the government domain of I (assuming CP is a sister of V'); in (14c), e is governed by the head of the relative clause, a [−V] category, in violation of the requirement that it be governed by a category nondistinct from [+V]. The fact that extraction out of these strong islands results in ill-formedness is further evidence for the earlier claim that GOV(t) ranks high in English.

GOV(t) does an important part of the work of Huang's CED, but it is a different constraint in at least four respects: (i) it is a general constraint (on all traces); (ii) it is a constraint on traces, not a constraint on some extraction domain; (iii) the level at which GOV(t) applies is not an issue, given our single level of optimization (in Huang 1982, the CED crucially does not apply at LF); and (iv) in our account, GOV(t) takes the place of the ECP as well as the CED.

Having introduced the OT versions of the main constraints needed to handle extraction facts, we now turn to the interaction of these constraints under language-particular rankings. We discuss English first.

3.2.1 English

Consider the basic case of direct object extraction out of a simple clause. To recover the relative ranking of the constraints we have proposed so far, we apply the standard OT method of systematically comparing two candidates at a time, the optimal parse and a suboptimal competitor. We compare the marks incurred by each pair of candidates, as shown in (16). Candidate (a) violates BAR^2 and *t, while candidate (b) violates BAR^2 and *Q. The violations of BAR^2 cancel. Of the two remaining constraints that are violated, *Q must outrank *t, since *t is violated by the optimal candidate.

(16) Simple questions: Direct object extraction

Input: $[Q_j [... x_j ...]]$		Violated	Comments
a. ☞ [what$_j$ did [he [fix t_j]]]		BAR^2 *t	optimal
b. [Q$_j$ [he [fixed what$_j$]]]		BAR^2 *Q	*Q ≫ *t
c. [⟨Q$_j$⟩ [he [fixed NP/⟨wh$_j$⟩]]]		PARSE(wh)	PARSE(wh) ≫ {BAR^2, *t}

The same method is applied to comparing candidate (a) and candidate (c), with the result that PARSE(wh) must outrank BAR^2 and *t, the two constraints violated by the optimal candidate. We thus obtain the following expanded partial ranking for English:

(17) {*Q, PARSE(wh)} ≫ {*t, BAR^2} ≫ *ABSORB

A more complex case is presented by extraction out of tensed *wh*-islands.

(18)   a.   ?*What/Which dish does she wonder who ate t?

          b.   *Who/Which person does she wonder what t ate?

          c.   *How/With what speed does she wonder who ate meat t?

Note first that because verbs like *wonder* subcategorize for a *wh*-complement, they provide a special competitor, one with a narrow scope interpretation, which constitutes a violation of PARSESCOPE whenever the input requires a wide scope interpretation. Consider the fact that direct objects cannot be extracted out of a tensed *wh*-island in English. We examine an input that has wide scope. Tableau (19) displays the competition between (faithful) wide scope interpretation (candidate (a)) and (unfaithful) narrow scope interpretation, which we take to be the optimal parse (candidate (b)).[12] Note that to simplify the discussion we only consider the best candidates in each tableau (it can easily be shown that all other candidates violate additional constraints and hence are suboptimal).

(19)   English: Extraction of direct object out of *wh*-island

$[Q_j\ [\text{wonder}\ [Q_i\ [x_i\ x_j]]]]$	*Q	Gv	P / wh	B / 3	P / Sc	B / 2	1	*t	*AB
a. what$_j$ do [you [wonder [who$_i$ [bought t$_j$				$*_j$!				*	
b. ☞ you [wonder [who$_{i[j]}$ [bought what$_j$					⊛				⊛

Here and in other tableaux where space constraints make it necessary, we omit closing final brackets and abbreviate constraint names as follows:

     P   = PARSE

     Sc = SCOPE

     B   = BAR

     Gv = GOV(t)

     *AB = *ABSORB

     F   = FILL

Tableau (19) shows that the optimal candidate (b) violates PARSESCOPE; suboptimal candidate (a), which contains a long link, violates BAR^3. Hence, BAR^3 must outrank PARSESCOPE in English.

     Tableau (20) displays the competition for subjects.

---

[12] In OT, one cannot simply say that a particular structure is ungrammatical. For each input and set of candidate outputs, there must be a candidate that is optimal. This optimal output is grammatical even though it may not match the input (or intended question) perfectly. It may turn out to be an indirect question or a statement rather than a direct question if that's the best the grammar can do for a given input. See Section 5 for further discussion.

Box 3

(20)   English: Extraction of subject out of *wh*-island

[Q_i [wonder [Q_j [x_i x_j]]]]	*Q	Gv	P	B	P	B		*t	*AB
			wh	3	Sc	2	1		
a. ☞ [you [wonder [who_i[j] [bought what_j]					⊛				⊛
b. who_i do [you [wonder [what_j [t_i [bought t_j]		*!		*_i		*_j		**	

In (20), the optimal candidate (a) violates PARSESCOPE and *ABSORB. Candidate (b) loses to (a) because the subject trace t_i violates GOV(t) and the subject chain violates BAR^3.[13]

The next two tableaux summarize our account of *that-t* effects in English. Under our account, structures with and without *that* compete with one another, but matrix verbs are assumed to select either an IP or a CP complement (contra Grimshaw 1997). Not all verbs allow the *that*/Ø alternation: manner-of-speaking verbs like *grieve, gloat,* and *squeal* require the complementizer *that*, and we assume they select for only one type of complement, namely, CP. Under this view, verbs like *think* have two subcategorization frames, *think*_CP and *think*_IP. This means that they correspond to different inputs. They are not distinguished in terms of government (contra Aoun et al. 1987). We assume that outputs meet subcategorization requirements embodied in a SUBCAT constraint (which for present purposes we take to be undominated).

Consider first extraction of a subject out of the complement of *think*_CP.

(21)   English: Extraction of subject out of complement of *think*_CP

[Q_i [think_CP [x_i]]]	*Q	Gv	P	B	P	B		*t	*AB
			wh	3	Sc	2	1		
a. who_i do [you [think [that [t_i [left		*!		*				*	
b. ☞ ⟨Q_i⟩ you [think [that [NP/⟨wh_i⟩ [left			⊛						

In Standard English, extraction of a subject out of the complement of *think*_CP is ungrammatical. From an OT perspective, the first question is, what does it lose to? We propose that it loses to an unfaithful parse of the input, namely, a failure to parse the [wh] feature of the [+wh] NP. The result is candidate (b), a grammatical structure, whose surface realization is a statement containing a [−wh] NP, something like *you think that someone/a person left.* (Henceforth, we adopt an abbreviation in tableaux according to which, for example, candidate (b) is denoted simply '⟨wh_i⟩'.) In other words, there is no well-formed pure information question with a *wh*-word for this particular input.[14] The winner cannot be a violation of PARSESCOPE, resulting in a narrow scope interpretation of *who*, because in the case of *think*, which does not allow an

---

[13] We assume with Grimshaw (1997) that *who* remains in SpecIP.
[14] As is well known, echo questions like *you think that WHO left?* are not requests for new information. They presuppose that the answer is already known; hence, their interpretation depends on a restricted set of values for the *wh*-variable, reminiscent of D(iscourse)-linking (see Section 3.3 for discussion). In our terms, they correspond to an input marked with a feature like [D-linked] and are the optimal output of a candidate set different from the one under discussion in (21).

indirect question as a complement, a narrow scope interpretation amounts to a violation of SUBCAT, which we assume to be undominated. Candidate (a) loses to (b) because it violates higher-ranked GOV(t).

Extraction of a subject out of the complement of *think*$_{IP}$ is possible because it does not result in a violation of GOV(t). This is shown in (22).

(22)   English: Extraction of subject out of complement of *think*$_{IP}$

[Q$_i$ [think$_{IP}$ [x$_i$]]]	*Q	GV	P wh	B 3	P Sc	B 2	1	*t	*AB
a. ☞ who$_i$ do [you [think [[t$_i$ [left						⊛		⊛	
b. ⟨wh$_i$⟩			*!						

Optimal candidate (a) violates BAR² and *t. The subject trace is properly governed by *think*. Its competitor (b) is suboptimal because it violates a higher-ranked constraint: PARSE(wh). Note how violability of constraints works in OT: a single constraint, PARSE(wh), is violated in the optimal parse in tableau (21) while it causes a competitor to lose in tableau (22).

Extraction of direct objects and adjuncts out of complements of *think*$_{CP}$ and *think*$_{IP}$ is possible because they do not involve GOV(t) violations. The OT analysis is displayed in the tableaux in (23) and (24). Note that the adjunct extraction tableaux involve constraints that are only fully introduced in Section 3.3. Adjuncts like *how* are nonreferential (in the sense of Rizzi 1990 and Cinque 1990); chains involving *how* are evaluated against the nonreferential counterparts of the BAR^k constraints, represented as BAR$^{k[-ref]}$. Universally, BAR$^{k[-ref]} \gg$ BAR^k.

In the remaining tableaux, some constraints are added while others are dropped, owing to space demands. The following abbreviations are used:

     B^{-r} = BAR$^{[-ref]}$

     SBC   = SUBCAT

     OBHD = OBLIGATORY-HEADS (Grimshaw 1993): Heads of projections must be filled.

In the case of *think*$_{CP}$ (23), the optimal parses (b) (direct object) and (f) (adjunct) take advantage of successive cyclicity, resulting in shorter links violating BAR² and BAR$^{2[-ref]}$ (ignoring violations of lower constraints); parses (c) and (g) lose to (b) and (f), respectively, because they do not take advantage of successive cyclicity, resulting in a longer link violating BAR⁴ and BAR$^{3[-ref]}$, respectively; parses (a) and (e) lose because they do not have a CP bracket, in violation of the SUBCAT constraint on *think*$_{CP}$. Candidates (d) and (h) also lose, which shows that PARSE(wh) must outrank BAR$^{2[-ref]}$ and BAR².

As shown in (24), *think*$_{IP}$ does not provide the successive cyclicity option (that is, without violating SUBCAT, as shown in candidates (b) and (e)). The optimal parses (a) for direct object and (d) for adjunct extraction violate higher BAR^k constraints. The latter are outranked by PARSE(wh), violated in suboptimal candidates (c) and (f).

Box 3

(23) English: Extraction out of complement of *think$_{CP}$*
Direct object extraction

[Q$_j$ [think$_{CP}$ [x$_j$]]]	SBC OBHD GV	B^{-r}	P	B^{-r}		B			*t
		3	wh	2	1	4	3	2	
a. what$_j$ do [you [think [he [said t$_j$	*SBC!						*		*
b. ☞ what$_j$ do [you [think [e$_j$ that [he [said t$_j$							⊛⊛		⊛⊛
c. what$_j$ do [you [think [that [he [said t$_j$				*!					*
d. ⟨wh$_j$⟩			*!						

Adjunct extraction

[Q$_l$ [think$_{CP}$ [x$_l$]]]	SBC OBHD GV	B^{-r}	P	B^{-r}		B			*t
		3	wh	2	1	4	3	2	
e. how$_l$ do [you [think [he [left] t$_l$	*SBC!						*		*
f. ☞ how$_l$ do [you [think [e$_l$ that [he [left] t$_l$				⊛		⊛			⊛⊛
g. how$_l$ do [you [think [that [he [left] t$_l$		*!							*
h. ⟨wh$_k$⟩			*!						

(24) English: Extraction out of *think$_{IP}$*
Direct object extraction

[Q$_j$ [think$_{IP}$ [x$_j$]]]	SBC OBHD GV	B^{-r}	P	B^{-r}		B			*t
		3	wh	2	1	4	3	2	
a. ☞ what$_j$ do [you [think [he [said t$_j$							⊛		⊛
b. what$_j$ do [you [think [e$_j$ [he [said t$_j$	*SBC! *OBH							**	**
c. ⟨wh$_j$⟩			*!						

Adjunct extraction

[Q$_l$ [think$_{IP}$ [x$_l$]]]	SBC OBHD GV	B^{-r}	P	B^{-r}		B			*t
		3	wh	2	1	4	3	2	
d. ☞ how$_l$ do [you [think [he [left] t$_l$							⊛		⊛
e. how$_l$ do [you [think [e$_l$ [he [left] t$_l$	*SBC! *OBH			*	*				**
f. ⟨wh$_l$⟩			*!						

Consider again the issue of competition under *think*—say, for extraction of direct object or adjunct. Suppose, as in Grimshaw 1997, that structures with and without *that* arise from the same input (no selection of IP or CP) via tying for optimality. Then, the analysis should result in two winning candidates per set (given that the presence or absence of *that* does not affect extractability). However, the number of barriers crossed in the presence or absence of *that* differs by one, with the consequence that the candidate with *that* would always lose to the candidate without *that*. Once length of chains enters the picture, it seems that grammatical structures with and without *that* cannot arise from the same candidate set.

3.2.2 A crosslinguistic prediction

Our account in terms of the interaction between a violable head government constraint and violable faithfulness constraints makes a crosslinguistic prediction: if $\text{Gov}(t)$ were ranked lower than Parse(wh) and Bar^2 were ranked higher than Parse(wh), the reverse of the well-known pattern would emerge: subjects would be extractable, direct objects would not. Such languages in fact exist, among them Bahasa Indonesia (Saddy 1991), the Wakashan language Kwakwala (Anderson 1984), Malagasy (Keenan 1976), and Tagalog (Guilfoyle, Hung, and Travis 1992). The pattern in information questions in these languages is essentially the same: subjects are extractable, but direct objects are not directly extractable; they must be passivized (or topicalized) first. While a systematic analysis of these languages is beyond our scope here, we can still sketch the following initial proposal for, say, Tagalog. We assume Guilfoyle, Hung, and Travis's (1992) analysis of Tagalog subjects or topics in SpecIP position. In our terms, object extraction is more costly than subject extraction with respect to barriers; object extraction crosses one more barrier than subject extraction.

(25)   <u>Tagalog subject extraction</u>   <u>Constraints violated</u>
   ☞ subject Bar^1 $\text{Gov}(t)$ *t
   *   ⟨wh⟩ Parse(wh)

Comparing the two candidates for subject extraction and their violations, we derive the fact that Parse(wh) must outrank all other constraints.

(26) $\text{Parse(wh)} \gg \{\text{Bar}^1, \text{Gov}(t), *t\}$

(27)   <u>Tagalog direct object extraction</u>   <u>Constraints violated</u>
   *   direct object Bar^2 *t
   ☞ ⟨wh⟩ Parse(wh)

Comparing the two candidates for object extraction and their violations, we can see that Bar^2 must outrank Parse(wh). The proposed Tagalog ranking is given in (28).

(28) $\text{Bar}^2 \gg \text{Parse(wh)} \gg \{\text{Bar}^1, \text{Gov}(t), *t\}$

3.2.3 Chinese

While Chinese has covert *wh*-extraction, it has overt topicalization. According to Huang (1982), the generalization is that covert extraction is generally possible out of

Box 3

complements of *think*, strong islands, and weak islands (except for nonreferential adjuncts), while topicalization is more constrained: it is possible out of simple clauses, complements of *think*, and *wh*-islands, but impossible out of strong islands. Legendre, Smolensky, and Wilson (1998) claim that resumptive pronouns in Chinese must appear in order to avoid an ungoverned t. Partial evidence comes from the asymmetry between subjects and direct objects with respect to some topicalizations. The t of a topicalized subject in a simple clause is obligatorily filled with a resumptive pronoun res; our informants report that the t of a topicalized direct object is only optionally filled with a resumptive pronoun. This is shown in the contrast between (29) and (30).

(29)   a.   Zhangsan$_i$, ta$_i$ xihuan kanshu.
            Zhangsan he like   reading
            'Zhangsan, he likes reading.'
       b.   *Zhangsan$_i$, t$_i$ xihuan kanshu.
            Zhangsan   like   reading
            'Zhangsan, likes reading.'

(30)   a.   Lisi$_j$, Zhangsan hen xihuan ta$_j$.
            Lisi Zhangsan very likes   him
            'Lisi, Zhangsan likes him very much.'
       b.   Lisi$_j$, Zhangsan hen xihuan t$_j$.
            Lisi Zhangsan very likes
            'Lisi, Zhangsan likes very much.'

The pattern in (30) raises the issue of optionality in an optimization framework. How can we have two optimal parses? One scenario, exemplified here, results from two equally ranked constraints,[15] *t and FILL (a faithfulness constraint that prohibits 'epenthesis' of elements not present in the input; see Prince and Smolensky 1993/2004 and Chapter 13). Tableau (31) displays the competition between (30a) and (30b). We assume that topicalization involves an operator TOp and adjunction to IP.

(31)   Chinese: Topicalization of direct object out of simple clause

[Top$_j$, [x$_j$]]	Gov(t)	...t	PARSE (top)	BAR 2	BAR 1	*TOp	FILL	*t	*Q
a. ☞ NP$_j$, [$_{IP}$ NP [$_{VP}$ V t$_j$]					⊛			⊛	
b. ☞ NP$_j$, [NP [V res$_j$					⊛		⊛		
c. TOp$_j$, [NP [V NP$_j$						*	*!		

[15] We think that a similar scenario obtains in Bulgarian multiple *wh*-questions, which display restrictions on the order of multiple *wh*-phrases. According to Rudin (1985, personal communication), subject *koj* must precede object *kakvo* 'what' and *kogo* 'whom'. Other pairs like subject *kakvo* and object *kogo* are unordered; so are pairs involving subject *kakvo* and adjuncts *koga* 'when' and *kŭde* 'where'. We propose that these patterns result from two equally ranked constraints dubbed SUBJECTFIRST and HUMANFIRST, which seem to be crosslinguistically justifiable. A very similar proposal is independently made in Billings and Rudin 1994.

Here and in the next several tableaux, '...†' abbreviates a contiguous subhierarchy of constraints, none of which are violated by the candidates under examination.

(32)   Chinese subhierarchy †

$$\text{BAR}^{3[-\text{ref}]} \gg \text{PARSE(wh)} \gg \text{BAR}^{2[-\text{ref}]} \gg \text{BAR}^{1[-\text{ref}]}$$
$$\gg \text{PARSESCOPE} \gg \text{BAR}^4 \gg \text{BAR}^3$$

(The $\text{BAR}^{N[-\text{ref}]}$ constraints will be discussed in Section 3.3.)

In tableau (31), candidates (a) and (b) incur the same pattern of constraint violations and are both optimal: they each violate BAR^1 and FILL/*t. Candidate (c), topicalization in situ, with an empty TOp operator, is suboptimal because *TOp $\gg$ {FILL, *t}. (Other candidates, not shown in tableau (31), violate higher-ranked constraints such as PARSE(top).)

The same ranking, in conjunction with higher-ranked GOV(t), yields the contrast between (29) and (30). This is shown in tableau (33).

(33)   Chinese: Topicalization of subject out of simple clause

[Top$_i$, [x$_i$]]	GOV (t)	...†	PARSE (top)	BAR 2	BAR 1	*TOp	FILL	*t	*Q
a. NP$_i$, [[$_{IP}$ t$_i$ [$_{VP}$ V NP]]	*!							*	
b. ☞ NP$_i$, [res$_i$ [V NP]]							⊛		

In tableau (33), candidate (a) loses to (b) because it contains an ungoverned subject *t*.

When topicalization occurs out of the complement of a bridge verb like *renwei* 'think', an intriguing variant of the pattern emerges: in both subject and object position, *t* and a resumptive pronoun alternate. Why should this be the case? Consider the data in (34) and the competition displayed in tableau (35).

(34)   a.   Zhangsan$_i$, wo renwei t$_i$/ta$_i$ hen congming.
             Zhangsan I   think   (he) very clever
             'Zhangsan, I think (he) is very clever.'
       b.   Zhangsan$_j$, wo zhidao ni hen xihuan t$_j$/ta$_j$.
             Zhangsan I   know you very like   (him)
             'Zhangsan, I know you like (him) very much'

Chinese does not have overt complementizers. Does *renwei* take an IP or a CP (with a null complementizer or in violation of Grimshaw's (1993) OBLIGATORY-HEADS constraint)? The answer emerges out of the competition displayed in tableau (35). Candidates (a) and (c) have IP complements; (b) and (d) have CP complements. The optimal outputs are (a) and (c); they incur equal marks (BAR^1 and FILL/*t). Candidates (b) and (d) are harmonically bounded by (a) and (c) because they incur both FILL and *t violations, besides violating BAR^1. In addition, in candidate (d) t_i is not properly governed, causing a violation of high-ranked GOV(t).[16]

---

[16] Note that this analysis entails a differentiation of two constraints barring empty elements: *t and *e.

Box 3

(35) Chinese: Topicalization of subject out of complement of *renwei* 'think'

[Topi, renwei [xi]]	Gov(t)	...†	PARSE (top)	2	1	*TOp	FILL	*t	*Q
a. ☞ NPi, [IP [VP V [IP resi						⊛	⊛		
b. NPi, [[V [CP ei [IP resi				*	*!		*	*	
c. ☞ NPi, [[V [ti						⊛			⊛
d. NPi, [[V[ei [ti	*!			*	*		*		**

Having established that complements of *renwei* are IPs, we turn to the covert *wh*-extraction facts. Note that the candidate set includes *wh*-fronting with resumptive pronoun in situ, the counterpart of the strategy for subject topicalization. Why does the latter lose to in-situ *wh* in Chinese? Consider tableau (36), where candidate (a) represents in-situ *wh*, candidate (b) represents *wh*-fronting with a resumptive pronoun in situ, and candidate (c) involves *wh*-fronting with a *t*.

The BAR² violations cancel, with the result that candidates (b) and (c) lose to candidate (a) because their violations (FILL, *t) outrank (a)'s violation (*Q). The candidate '⟨whi⟩', which fails to parse the *wh*-chain, incurs *PARSE(wh), which is high ranked in the segment of the hierarchy abbreviated to '...†' (27); it therefore is suboptimal. Here and henceforth, we omit the '⟨wh⟩' candidates (but see Footnote 17).

(36) Chinese: Covert extraction of subject out of complement of *renwei* 'think'

[Qi [renwei IP [xi]]]	Gov (t)	...†	PARSE (top)	2	1	*TOp	FILL	*t	*Q
a. ☞ Qi [IP [VP V [IP whi				⊛					⊛
b. whi [[V [resi				*			*!		
c. whi [[V [ti				*				*!	

Chinese permits covert extraction from *wh*-islands of subjects, direct objects, and some adjuncts (corresponding to *where*, *when*, instrumental *how*, purpose *why*) (Tsai 1994).

(37) a. Ni xiang-zhidao [shei zai nali   gongzuo]?
     you wonder   who at where   work
     'Who do you wonder where works?'
     'Where do you wonder who works?'

    b. Ni xiang-zhidao [Lisi   shenmeshihou mai-le   shenme]?
     you wonder   Lisi   when   buy-ASP   what
     'What do you wonder when Lisi bought?'
     'When do you wonder what Lisi bought?'

This is because violations of *e by intermediate traces do not license resumptive elements in Chinese: FILL ≫ *e. Languages like Irish, Chamorro, and Kinande, which register successive-cyclic movement in CP morphologically, may turn out to be languages in which a violation of *e licenses a resumptive element: relative to FILL, *e is equally or higher ranked.

The structure corresponding to the covert extraction in (37b) is given in (38).

(38) $[Q_j [_{IP} ni [_{VP} xiang-zhidao [[_{CP} Q_k [_{IP} Lisi [_{VP} shenmeshihou_k mai-le shenme_j]]]]]]]$

Consider direct object extraction, shown in tableau (34). (The omitted subhierarchy '‡' here is $BAR^{3[-ref]} \gg PARSE(wh) \gg BAR^{2[-ref]} \gg BAR^{1[-ref]} \gg PARSESCOPE.$)

(39)   Chinese: Covert extraction of direct object out of *wh*-island

$[Q_j [xiang-zhidao [Q_i [x_i x_j]]]]$	GOV (t)	...‡	BAR 4	BAR 3	P (top)	BAR 2	BAR 1	*TOp	F	*t	*Q
a. ☞ $Q_j [[V [Q_i+e_j [wh_i [wh_j$						$\circledast_j\circledast_j$	$\circledast_i$		⦂	$\circledast$	$\circledast\circledast$
b. $Q_j [[V [Q_i \quad [wh_i [wh_j$			$*_j!$				$*_i$		⦂		$**$
c. $Q_j [[V \quad\quad [wh_i [wh_j$				$*_j!$					⦂		$*$

The optimal parse (a) violates BAR^2, BAR^1, *t, *Q. The fact that indirect questioning of *shei* 'who' is covert is instantiated by an empty Q_i in the specifier of the embedded CP, with the result that the chain corresponding to the wide scope interpretation of the direct object 'what' (Q_j, wh_j) can be successive cyclic, that is, composed of short links; candidate (b) (instantiating a non-successive-cyclic chain) loses to candidate (a) because the chain (Q_j, wh_j) violates BAR^4, universally higher ranked than BAR^2. Candidate (c) differs from (b) in lacking vacuous covert movement of the subject. Recall that the chains produced by *Gen* have a Q-operator in the highest specifier of a clause containing the corresponding variable; here, we have a variable in SpecIP in a clause with no CP, so the variable is already in a legitimate scope position for its Q. Thus, the minimal licit chain contains a single element that is simultaneously Q_i and x_i. This single element is overtly realized as wh_i in candidate (c).

Extraction of a subject out of a *wh*-island receives essentially the same account, since in the absence of traces, GOV(t) is irrelevant. The only thing that matters is the number and type of BAR constraints violated. Where GOV(t) is irrelevant, shorter links (instantiated by successive cyclicity) always win over longer links. The tableau for subject extraction is given in (40).

(40)   Chinese: Covert extraction of subject out of *wh*-island

$[Q_i [xiang-zhidao [Q_j [x_i x_j]]]]$	GOV (t)	...‡	BAR 4	BAR 3	P (top)	BAR 2	BAR 1	*TOp	F	*t	*Q
a. ☞ $Q_i [[V [Q_j+e_i [wh_i [wh_j$						$\circledast_i\circledast_j$	$\circledast_i$		⦂	$\circledast$	$\circledast\circledast$
b. $Q_i [[V [Q_j \quad [wh_i [wh_j$				$*_i!$		$*_j$			⦂		$**$

The one complication in Chinese has to do with adjuncts: the counterparts to *when*, *where*, instrumental *how*, and purpose *why* behave like direct objects in being covertly extractable out of all islands, while the counterparts to manner *how* and reason *why* are covertly extractable out of simple clauses and complements of bridge verbs, but not out of complements of nonbridge verbs and islands (Tsai 1994). Covert man-

Box 3

ner and reason *wh*-extractions are exemplified in simple clauses (41a), complements of *renwei* 'think' (41b), *wh*-islands (41c), and sentential subjects (41d).

(41) a.   Lisi zenmeyang chuli   zhe-jian shi?
             Lisi how   handle this-CL   matter
             'By what means/In what manner did Lisi handle this matter?'

      b.   Ni renwei [Lisi   yinggai zenmeyang chuli   zhe-jian shi]?
             you think   Lisi   should how   handle this-CL   matter
             'How (means/manner) do you think that Lisi should handle this matter?'

      c.   Ni   xiang-zhidao [shei zenmeyang chuli   zhe-jian shi]?
             you wonder   who how   handle this-CL   matter
             *'How (manner) do you wonder who handled this matter?'
             'You wonder who handled this matter how.'

      d.   *[Women weishenme chuli   zhe-jian shi]   bijiao hao?
             we   why   handle this-CL   matter more appropriate
             'Why (reason) is it more appropriate for us to handle this matter?'

Assuming that the distinction is one of referentiality, as has often been proposed (e.g., Rizzi 1990; Cinque 1990; Tsai 1994), we show in Section 3.3 how referentiality can be incorporated into the MINLINK family of constraints.

3.3 Referentiality

Under 'referentiality', many linguists have subsumed distinct properties that affect extractability in similar ways. The two most common sources of referentiality discussed in the literature are thematic roles and discourse linking. Rizzi (1990) and Cinque (1990) distinguish "referential" from nonreferential thematic roles, which we may interpret along a hierarchy of participants to an event with central participants (agent, patient) at one end and exterior conditions at the other (manner, reason).

The grammar of a particular language selects a cutoff point on the hierarchy that divides it into two parts, which syntax treats differently. In Chinese, for example, the cutoff point is between adjuncts: locative, temporal, means, and purpose *wh*-phrases pattern with agent and patient *wh*-phrases—they allow wide scope interpretation out of all context islands—while manner and reason *wh*-phrases (homophonous with means and purpose *wh*-phrases, respectively) allow wide scope interpretation out of a restricted set of contexts (see (41a–d) above). In English, as Rizzi (1990) discusses, the distinction shows up for example in extraction out of *wh*-islands with ambiguous verbs like *weigh*.

(42)   ?What did John wonder how to weigh t?

Rizzi comments that (42) can only be properly answered with a patient phrase like *apples* and not with a measure phrase like *200 lbs*. The former is characterized as a referential thematic role, the latter as a quasi-argumental nonreferential thematic role

(Rizzi 1990, 86). Rizzi's analysis in terms of a binding relationship is by definition sensitive to this distinction.

Pesetsky (1987) invokes discourse (D-) linking to handle the absence of expected superiority effects in English, such as the contrast exemplified in (43).

(43) a. *Mary asked what$_j$ who read t$_j$?

     b. Mary asked which book$_j$ which man read t$_j$?

In (43a), there is no presupposition that either speaker or hearer has a particular set of objects and readers in mind: *what* and *who* are non-D-linked. In (43b), the range of answers is limited by the particular set of books and readers both speaker and hearer have in mind: *which book* and *which man* are D-linked. Rudin (1988) discusses contrasts in Bulgarian extractions out of *wh*-islands that seem to fall squarely under D-linking (see (44) below). Comorovski (1989) discusses additional examples in Bulgarian. Pending a fully specified OT theory of referentiality, we simply adopt the distinctions proposed in the literature and integrate them into our OT account.

If our family of MINLINK constraints includes constraints on the length of chains containing nonreferential elements, then we can account for these patterns in a straightforward fashion. A proper treatment of the referentiality hierarchy, and typological variation in the cutoff point, should be naturally handled by OT (much as is the sonority hierarchy in Prince and Smolensky 1993/2004). But for the purposes of this chapter, we assume that what counts as referential is specific to a language and that the constraints refer only to [−ref].

(44) Family of MINLINK constraints (expanded)

    BAR^1 A single link must not cross one barrier.

    BAR^2 A single link must not cross two barriers.

    BAR^3 A single link must not cross three barriers.

    BAR$^{1[-ref]}$ A single [−ref] link must not cross one barrier.

    BAR$^{2[-ref]}$ A single [−ref] link must not cross two barriers.

    BAR$^{3[-ref]}$ A single [−ref] link must not cross three barriers.

We propose that BAR$^{k[-ref]}$ universally outranks BAR^k because of the additional markedness a link has in virtue of being nonreferential. (This issue is addressed further in Section 4.) For readability of the tableaux, we keep the name 'BAR^1', but henceforth intend it to be interpreted as BAR$^{1[+ref]}$.

We now turn to a MINLINK analysis of Chinese and Bulgarian referentiality contrasts in *wh*-islands.

3.3.1 Chinese

Examples like (45)—with a nonreferential adjunct—are possible in Chinese, but they are not interpreted as having wide scope. Rather, they have a narrow scope interpretation, as Aoun et al. (1987) point out.

Box 3

(45) Ni xiang-zhidao shei weishenme mai-le   shu?
      you wonder   who why   buy-ASP book
      'You wonder who bought books why.'
      (Aoun et al. 1987)

Tableau (46) displays the competition between the two interpretations and the role played by constraints on nonreferential links.

(46) Chinese: Extraction of adjunct [−ref] out of *wh*-island

[Q₁ [xiang-zhidao [Qᵢ [xᵢ x₁]]]]	B⁻ʳ	P	B⁻ʳ		P	BAR		P	BAR			*TOp	F	*t	*Q
	Gv	3	wh	2	1	Sc	4	3	top	2	1				
a. Q₁ [IP[VP V [CP Qᵢ+eₗ [IP whᵢ whₗ				*ₗ!	*ₗ					*ᵢ					*
b. ☞ V [Q₁+Qᵢ [whᵢ whₗ				⊛ₗ	⊛ₗ					⊛ᵢ					

The optimal parse (b) includes a nonreferential chain (Q_l, wh_l) that violates PARSESCOPE: both *wh*-forms are paired in the embedded clause. We can ignore the referential chain (Q_i, wh_i), as its violations in (a) and (b) cancel. In parse (a), one link in the nonreferential chain (Q_l, e_l) violates BAR$^{2[-ref]}$ while the only MINLINK constraint that parse (b) violates is BAR$^{1[-ref]}$.

It is worth examining the interplay of violations: a middle-length link of type BAR$^{2[+ref]}$ is better than a failure to parse scope, but a middle-length link of type BAR$^{2[-ref]}$ is worse than a failure to parse scope.[17] It is not the case that Chinese equally disprefers middle-length links across the board. This shows that not all instances of locality can be analyzed in terms of one single constraint stating that shorter chains are better than longer chains. We need two families of constraints that are interrupted by unrelated constraints — like PARSESCOPE — on the hierarchy.

3.3.2 Bulgarian

We turn finally to Bulgarian, where extractions of *koj* (subject) and *kakvo* (direct object) out of a *wh*-island are equally bad, as shown in (47).[18]

(47) a. *Koj se čudiš   kude e   otišul?
          who REFL wonder-2s where AUX gone
          'Who are you wondering where has gone?'
      b. *Kakvo pitaš koj e   čel?
          what   ask-2s who AUX read
          'What are you asking who has read?'

---

[17] And a longer link violating BAR$^{3[-ref]}$ is worse than a failure to parse [wh]. Recall that extracting a nonreferential adjunct out of a sentential subject is ungrammatical (41d). The successive-cyclic parse corresponding to (41d) violates GOV(t); its non-successive-cyclic counterpart violates BAR$^{3[-ref]}$. For that input, failure to parse [wh] is optimal.

[18] Our informant provided the examples in (47) and (48) and noted that (47a) is acceptable under an echo reading. Our discussion here and below pertains only to neutral, nonecho readings.

When *kakvo* is replaced by a D-linked *wh*-phrase like 'which of these books', the result is basically fine. The same contrast is observed with *koj* 'who'.

(48) a.   ?Koj   student se   čudiš   kakvo e   napisal?
           which student REFL wonder-2S what AUX written
           'Which student are you wondering what has written?'

      b.   Koja   kniga pitaš koj   e   čel?
           which of these books ask-2S who AUX read
           'Which of these books are you asking who has read?'

In our terms, (47b) and (48b) are not in competition with each other since they have different discourse properties and hence are outputs of different inputs. For an input containing a non-D-linked *wh*-phrase, the optimal output does not faithfully parse the input as a direct question (there is no grammatical way of directly asking (47b)); rather, it fails to parse the intended scope of the input. The optimal output is thus a narrow scope (rather than wide scope) interpretation of the input.

(49)   Bulgarian: Extraction of non-D-linked direct object $x_j^{[-dl]}$ out of *wh*-island

$[Q_j [V [Q_i [x_i x_j^{[-dl]}]]]]$	SBC GV *AB	B^{-r} 4	P wh	B^{-r} 3	P 2	Sc	BAR 4	3	2	$\text{B}^{\pm r}$ 1	*t
a. $wh_j^{[-dl]} [_{IP}[_{VP} [_{CP} wh_i+e_j\quad [_{IP}[_{VP} t_i\ t_j$				*j!	*j				*i		***
b. ☞ $[\ [\ [wh_i+wh_j^{[-dl]} [\ [\ t_i\ t_j$						⊛					⊛ ⊛

The optimal parse (b) violates PARSESCOPE. Focusing strictly on the *wh_j* chain, we note that competitor (a) loses to (b) because it violates $\text{BAR}^{2[-ref]}$ twice.[19]

    This situation contrasts with tableau (50) for an input containing a D-linked direct object *wh*-phrase.

(50)   Bulgarian: Extraction of D-linked direct object $x_j^{[+dl]}$ out of *wh*-island

$[Q_j [V [Q_i [x_i\ x_j^{[+dl]}]]]]$	SBC GV *AB	B^{-r} 4	P wh	B^{-r} 3	P 2	Sc	BAR 4	3	2	$\text{B}^{\pm r}$ 1	*t
a. ☞ $wh_j^{[+dl]} [_{IP}[_{VP}[_{CP} wh_i+e_j [_{IP}[_{VP} t_i\ t_j$									⊛j⊛j⊛i		⊛ ⊛ ⊛
b. $[[[wh_i+wh_j^{[+dl]} [\ [\ t_i\ t_j$						*!			*j *i		**

The optimal parse (a) violates BAR^2, which is lower ranked than the highest constraint violated by competitor (b), PARSESCOPE. The Bulgarian pattern shows that the BAR constraints are interrupted by an unrelated constraint, PARSESCOPE. Locality is distributed over the hierarchy of constraints: longer chains are better than not parsing intended scope if they are referential, but worse than not parsing intended scope if they are nonreferential. Note again the violability of constraints at work here:

---

[19] We follow Rudin in assuming that neutral interpretations of *koj* correspond to location in SpecCP. Rudin (1985, 84–5) gives data showing that *wh*-phrases in SpecIP or in postverbal position can only have an echo interpretation: *kazvat če KOJ e došŭl? / kazvat če e došŭl KOJ?* 'they say that WHO came?'.

Box 3

PARSESCOPE is violated in an optimal parse (49) but is active (i.e., its violation is fatal) in a suboptimal parse in (50).

Turning to subjects, we note first that Bulgarian shows no *that-t* effects in non-*wh* complements, despite the presence of an obligatory complementizer *če*.

(51)   Koj misliš   če e   došŭl?
       who think-2s that has come
       'Who do you think that came?'
       (Rudin 1985)

The relatively free word order of Bulgarian discussed in Rudin 1985 suggests that the subject is free to remain under VP; the absence of *that-t* effects supports this hypothesis because VP-internal subject traces are, in our terms, properly head-governed (by I).[20] Extraction of subjects then looks like extraction of direct objects; no violation of GOV(t) occurs. Tableau (52) represents extraction of a (non-D-linked) subject out of a *če* 'that' complement.

(52)   Bulgarian: Extraction of subject out of *če*-complement

$[Q_i [V [\text{če} [x_i^{[-dl]}]]]]$	SbC Gv $*AB$	B⁻ʳ 4	P wh	B⁻ʳ 3	P 2	BAR Sc	4	3	2	1	*t
a. $wh_i [_{IP}[_{VP} V [_{CP} \text{čc} [_{IP}[_{VP} t_i$			*!								*
b. ☞ $wh_i [\ [\ V [\ e_i \text{ če } [\ [\ t_i$									⊛⊛		⊛⊛
c. $\langle wh_i \rangle$					*!						

The optimal output in (52) is (b) because, compared with its competitors, it incurs the least costly violation (BAR$^{2[-\text{ref}]}$); it involves two successive-cyclic links.

Finally, consider the analysis of ungrammatical subject extractions out of a *wh*-island (neutral interpretation). Example (47a) is repeated here for convenience.

(53)   *Koj se   čudiš   kude e   otišul?
       who REFL wonder-2s where AUX gone
       'Who are you wondering where has gone?'

In (54), candidate (a) loses as a combined effect of two factors: (i) the chain (wh_i, t_i) consists of a long link and (ii) *koj* 'who' is non-D-linked; hence, MINLINK violations involve long nonreferential links or BAR$^{4[-\text{ref}]}$ violations. Candidate (b) involves shorter links, but as they are nonreferential, the candidate is still suboptimal. The optimal output is (c), which fails to parse the intended scope of the input. Failing to parse [wh], candidate (d), is a less harmonic unfaithful option.

---

[20] The absence of *that-t* effects is of course consistent with extraction out of a postverbal position given that subjects can appear postverbally (Rudin 1985). In that case, the subject might be extracted out of an adjoined position that still qualifies for proper head government. We are not aware of any arguments that distinguish the two analyses and hence choose the minimal one.

(54)   Bulgarian: Extraction of subject $x_i^{[-dl]}$ out of *wh*-island

$[Q_i\ [V\ [Q_k\ [x_i^{[-dl]}\ x_k]]]]$	SBC GV *AB	B^{-r} 4	P wh	B^{-r} 3	P 2	BAR Sc	4	3	2	$B^{\pm r}$ 1	*t
a. $wh_i\ [_{IP}[_{VP}\ V\ [_{CP}\ wh_k\quad [_{IP}[_{VP}\ t_i]\ t_k]$		$*_i$!								$*_k$	**
b. $wh_i\ [\ [\ V\ [wh_k{+}e_i\ [\ [\ t_i]\ t_k]$					$*_i*_i$!					$*_k$	***
c. ☞ $[\ [\ V\ [wh_i{+}wh_k\ [\ [\ t_i]\ t_k]$					$\circledast_i$	$\circledast$				$\circledast_k$	$\circledast\circledast$
d. $\langle wh_i\rangle$			$*_i$!							$*_k$	

4 CONSTRAINTS ON *WH*-CHAINS

Having shown examples of MINLINK in action, we turn to MINLINK's formal structure: how it formalizes 'Shortest Link'. The starting point is the simple locality constraint (55).

(55)   BAR: A chain link may not cross a barrier.

In an important sense, BAR alone is too weak. For example, ceteris paribus, chains that are cyclic should be more harmonic; it is to satisfy locality constraints that movement is sometimes cyclic—made up of several short links rather than one long link. So a proper characterization of locality must disfavor noncyclic chains—but BAR does not.

(56)   Cyclic versus noncyclic chains: Equally marked, according to BAR (β = barrier)

	BAR
a. Cyclic, 2 links ☞ $[X_i \cdots \beta \cdots \beta \cdots t_i \cdots \beta \cdots Y_i]$	** *
b. Noncyclic, 1 link *☞ $[X_i \cdots \beta \cdots \beta \cdots\ \cdots \beta \cdots Y_i]$	***

A ('cyclic') chain consisting of two shorter links (56a) will violate BAR to the same degree as a ('noncyclic') chain with only one link (56b); this will not do, given contrasts between environments offering intermediate landing sites and those without, the former broadly tending to better afford extraction.

The natural solution to this problem is provided by a general OT mechanism; we now derive the **local conjunction power hierarchy** of constraints, constructed from the single fundamental constraint BAR (see (Chapter 12 (43); Box 14:3)).

Given two constraints $\mathbb{C}_1$ and $\mathbb{C}_2$, their **local conjunction** (with respect to a domain type $\mathcal{D}$), $\mathbb{C}_1 \&_{\mathcal{D}} \mathbb{C}_2$, is a new constraint that is violated when two distinct violations of $\mathbb{C}_1$ and $\mathbb{C}_2$ occur *within a single domain of type $\mathcal{D}$*. (This was proposed for phonological applications in Smolensky 1993; see Chapter 14.) As a further part of the definition of local conjunction, we have these *universal* rankings:

$$\mathbb{C}_1 \&_{\mathcal{D}} \mathbb{C}_2 \gg \{\mathbb{C}_1, \mathbb{C}_2\}.$$

The local conjunction of BAR with itself (with domain $\mathcal{D}$ = link) is a new constraint, BAR $\&_{\mathcal{D}}$ BAR $\equiv$ BAR^2, which is violated when a link has two distinct violations

Box 3

of BAR—that is, when it crosses two barriers.

(57)   BAR^2: A single link must not cross two barriers.

Thus, we have derived from more fundamental elements the constraint BAR^2.

By definition of the local conjunction operation, this ranking holds *universally*:

(58)   BAR^2 ≫ BAR

Recursion then produces the hierarchy in (59).

(59)   **Universal BAR power hierarchy ≡ MINLINK**

       ⋯ ≫ BAR^3 ≫ BAR^2 ≫ BAR^1

       BAR^k: A chain link must not cross k barriers.[21]

Now note that, unlike BAR alone, the BAR power hierarchy—our MINLINK—correctly favors cyclic chains.

(60)   Cyclic ≻ noncyclic chains, according to BAR power hierarchy: MINLINK

		MINLINK			BAR
		BAR^3	BAR^2	BAR^1	
a. Cyclic	☞ $[X_i \cdots \beta \cdots \beta \cdots t_i \cdots \beta \cdots Y_i]$		*	*	** *
b. Noncyclic	$[X_i \cdots \beta \cdots \beta \cdots \ \cdots \ \cdots \beta \cdots Y_i]$	*!			***

The MINLINK constraint hierarchy establishes a Harmony scale of chains that can be loosely summarized as 'A chain is as weak as its longest link', where link length is measured in barriers. More precisely: (i) If the longest link of chain C is longer than that of chain C′, then C is less harmonic than C′; that is, C ≺ C′. (ii) If the longest links of C and C′ are the same length, but C has *more* longest links, then C ≺ C′. (iii) If the longest links in C and C′ are equal in length and number, so they *tie* with respect to longest links, which chain is less harmonic is recursively determined by ignoring the longest links and comparing the chains with respect to the remaining links.

This evaluative structure is provided directly by OT. Universal constraint sub-hierarchies like MINLINK were developed in Prince and Smolensky 1993/2004; their importance for universal grammar was argued on the basis of the roles of the sonority hierarchy in syllabification and of coronal unmarkedness in segmental phonology (see Chapter 14 of this book).

Why construct a power hierarchy from BAR but not from the other constraints? Consider the *local* conjunction of other constraints with themselves: for example, GOV(t)^2 = ('A trace must be head-governed')^2. Now *locally*—at the same trace—there can't be multiple distinct violations of head government: either the trace is head-

---

[21] Does a link that crosses three barriers violate BAR^2? Yes, but Box 14:3 shows:
  Theorem. If each violation of a higher-ranked constraint logically entails a separable set of violations of lower-ranked constraints, the lower-ranked violations cannot affect the results of optimality computation.
Therefore, we may ignore violations of BAR^2 by links crossing more than two barriers, and take BAR^k to be violated only by links crossing exactly k barriers.

governed or it isn't. So the entire power hierarchy thus collapses to just GOV(t) itself. For *t, the same story holds; the power hierarchy generated by *t is just *t itself, because there can't be multiple violations of 'No trace' at a single trace.

As noted earlier, more referential elements tend to be more extractable; but the notion of referentiality at work here is complex. In the ultimate OT theory, a family of constraints pertaining to different aspects of referentiality must be developed, and crosslinguistic variation in referentiality effects explained by reranking of these constraints relative to others. (For an OT analysis of related effects, see Bakovic 1998.) In the work reported here, we have adopted the provisional assumption that a language makes a binary [±ref] distinction based on either of these dimensions:

> Event structure peripherality: Argument ⋯ adjunct [Here: English, Chinese] (Rizzi 1990; Cinque 1990), or

> D(iscourse)-linking [In our analysis: Bulgarian; in reality, English also] (Pesetsky 1987; Cinque 1990).

The basic constraint at work here is then simply this:

(61)   REF: Chains are referential.

Crosslinguistically, the interaction between REF and MINLINK has a general character nicely illustrated by Chinese:

> 1.   Nonreferential chains are acceptable, if short.
> 2.   Long chains are acceptable, if referential.
> 3.   Chains violating both MINLINK and REF are unacceptable.

This chain inventory 'bans the worst of the worst' (Prince and Smolensky 1993/2004, Sec. 9.1.2); generally, this implicates local conjunction (see Chapter 14 of this book). So we posit the following in UG:

(62)   MINLINK & REF ≡ MINLINK$^{[-ref]}$

This is a universal subhierarchy built of the following constraints:[22]

(63)   BAR^{k} & REF ≡ BAR$^{k[-ref]}$: A link in a nonreferential chain does not cross k barriers.

The universal constraint subhierarchy MINLINK$^{[-ref]}$ derived by conjunction is thus as follows:

(64)   ⋯ ≫ BAR$^{3[-ref]}$ ≫ BAR$^{2[-ref]}$ ≫ BAR$^{1[-ref]}$

The definition of local conjunction also entails these universal relative rankings:

(65)   BAR$^{k[-ref]}$ ≫ BAR^{k}

---

[22] Does a [−ref] chain violate the more general BAR^{k} constraints, in addition to BAR$^{k[-ref]}$? The same analysis as for BAR^{3} and BAR^{2} above (Footnote 21) applies. The theorem given there ensures that we can ignore violations of the lower-ranked, more general constraint BAR^{k} that are incurred by nonreferential chains, recording only violations of BAR$^{k[-ref]}$. Thus, BAR^{k} can be treated as though it were BAR$^{k[+ref]}$.

Box 3

Thus, our theory of *wh*-chains can be schematically summarized as in (66).

(66)   Summary of proposed constraints on *wh*-chains

	BAR, REF	Two general constraints on chains
+	local conjunction	+ a general, independent OT mechanism
	MINLINK $^{([-ref])}$	"Shortest Move"
	MINLINK $^{([-ref])}$	"Shortest Move"
+	*t, GOV(t), *Q	+ three general constraints on traces, operators
	our proposed theory of *wh*-chains	

5   GENERAL ISSUES: INEFFABILITY AND FAITHFULNESS IN SYNTAX

The basic ideas underlying our analysis of *wh*-extraction can be summarized as follows. MINLINK is a universal subhierarchy of constraints establishing a scale on which longer links are less harmonic (more marked) than shorter links. Inputs to the OT grammar specify *target scopes* for operators; FAITHFULNESS constraints require output chains to realize these targets. (These constraints are violable, of course.) Extraction patterns result from the interleaving of MINLINK and FAITHFULNESS constraints in a language's constraint hierarchy. Crosslinguistic variation in extraction patterns results from the reranking of these constraints (and others).

Perhaps the most important result of the analysis is this. In this account, there is no need to stipulate that "Shortest Move" is measured in terms of Relativized Minimality violations; the Relativized Minimality effect is a consequence of a MINLINK constraint in which link length is assessed simply in terms of barriers crossed. None of our constraints require "relativized" distance measurements, or "minimality" of any kind. Minimality effects arise purely from the constraint *interaction* automatically provided by OT, so the constraints themselves do not (*must* not; Prince 1997) refer to "minimality." And as we have just shown, relativization effects (e.g., *wh* is harder to extract over *wh*) are also a derived *consequence* of competition and constraint interaction. A configuration such as *wh*-over-*wh* sets up a special competitive environment, the inner *wh* providing a potentially more local binder for an embedded variable. Otherwise, this is a competition like any other in OT, a framework with minimality built into its very foundations (see Chapter 12 (24)).

5.1   The input of the question, and the question of the input

Our analysis has not yet faced an important question: given that every OT competition has an optimal output, how can we account for the existence of languages (Irish, Italian, and others) that do not allow multiple questions?

As usually conceived, an OT grammar is a device that takes an input and produces an output, the correct structural description or 'parse' of the input. In phonology, an input is canonically taken to be the underlying form of a word, and the output, when phonetically interpreted, the pronunciation of that word.[23] A crucial job of the input is to determine what structures compete: given an input *I*, the competing parses are the set *Gen*(*I*)—all possible parses *of I*. That forms with different phonetic interpretations compete is a consequence of the fact that not all the parses of *I* in *Gen*(*I*) are faithful to *I*; the phonetic interpretation of such parses may include material not in *I*, or fail to include material present in *I*. Such unfaithful parses are optimal only when the faithfulness violations they incur are outranked by other violations arising from faithful parsing. Faithfulness violations, visible as 'deep/surface' disparities between the *target phonetics* in an underlying form *I* and the actual phonetic interpretation of *I*'s optimal parse, are readily apparent in phonology via surface alternations, where the same morpheme undergoes faithful parsing in one environment and unfaithful parsing in another.

Much of this structure is not readily apparent in syntax, however; the questions of the input, and of what structures compete, and of the role of faithfulness, all seem rather more opaque. In phonology, the question of the surface form of a given morpheme provides a sound theoretical base, supporting a view of the grammar as a device for mapping a particular underlying form deriving from a lexicon into its correct structural description. In syntax, we believe, this is the wrong view of the grammar. The alternative view, however, was also developed in phonology in Prince and Smolensky 1991, 1993/2004, for example, in the analysis of basic CV syllable structure (Chapter 13). There, the question of interest is not, "What is the structural description of a *particular* input (say, /VCVC/)?" The question is more global: "What is the *inventory of all possible* output syllable shapes, as the input is allowed to range over all possible input strings of Cs and Vs?" Correspondingly, the question of interest in *wh*-theory, we claim, is not, "Given some *particular* input structure, what is its particular output structure?" Rather, it is, "What is the *inventory of all possible* questions in a given language, deduced by considering all possible inputs?" So, in particular, in a language that allows no extractions from *wh*-complements, our concern is to show that, given our proposed OT grammar, no matter what input we consider, the optimal output structure never contains an extraction from a *wh*-complement. It is not of central concern what the output happens to be given a *particular* input—for example, one that *would* produce a *wh*-complement extraction in another language whose question inventory includes such extractions.

To summarize, for syntax we adopt the *inventory* perspective within OT (Prince and Smolensky 1993/2004, Chap. 9), rather than the perhaps more familiar *particular input-output mapping* perspective. In any event, we do *not* construe an OT grammar itself as an account of the 'production' system, responsible to the question "Given an intention to utter *X*, what does the speaker do?" Rather, we take OT to answer the question "What is the inventory of grammatical structures in a language?" It is the job of OT performance theories to explain how speakers manage to deploy the structures made available by the grammar (see Section 12:2 and Chapter 19).

[23] For a comparative, violable-constraint approach to phonology with no such concept of input, see Burzio 1994.

Box 3

5.2 The problems of language-particular ineffability and marked output

In the inventory perspective on OT, the job of the input *I* is to determine what competes: for a given *I*, the structures in the set *Gen*(*I*) compete. Usually, *I* can be thought of as the substructure two candidates must share in order to be competitors. Thinking of it this way, we might call *I* the **Index** of its particular candidate set; henceforth, we replace 'input' with 'Index' in order to suppress the 'particular input-output perspective' on OT, and to avoid the baggage the term 'input' inappropriately brings to syntax.[24]

For studying S-Structure forms, an attractive hypothesis is that the Index consists of a pair [D-Structure, LF]; that is, two S-Structure forms compete if and only if they derive from the same D-Structure form and yield the same structure at LF (Grimshaw 1993). The interpretive information of D-Structure and LF is fixed among competitors; syntax determines the S-Structure realization of this interpretive information.[25]

This attractive approach brings us to our first problem, that of **language-particular ineffability**. There are questions that can be realized in some languages but not others; for example, 'who ate what' can be realized in English, but not in languages such as Irish and Italian. Such a question must be generable by *Gen* since it is realized in some languages, and *Gen* is universal. This question is part of a candidate set that is also universal. It is optimal in English. The problem is, *What in this candidate set is optimal in Irish?* In an OT syntax, the optimal candidate must be *grammatical*. Yet the optimal candidate must mean 'who ate what', since *everything* in the candidate set means 'who ate what', by hypothesis. But in Irish and Italian, there is no grammatical form that means 'who ate what'.

So something must give. One option is to abandon OT's equation *optimal = grammatical*, so that in the 'who ate what' candidate set, the optimal structure in Irish would not be grammatical. This might be done by adding language-particular inviolable constraints to an otherwise-OT syntax. Or it might be achieved by sending the optimal parse out of the syntax, but having it "crash" at interpretation; but since, by

---

[24] The sense of 'index' intended here is exactly the mathematical usage in which each member of a collection is *indexed* — uniquely labeled — by a member of an 'index set'. Here, a member of the collection in question is a particular candidate set, and its Index uniquely specifies it. Two structures compete — are in the same candidate set — exactly when they are co-Indexed.

[25] An approach within the Minimalist Program that assumes that only LF-equivalent derivations compete (e.g., Fox 1998) would be viewed from our perspective as having an Index = [numeration, LF]: derivations that compete share the substructure specified by the Index; *Gen*(Index) is the set of derivations using the Index's numeration and having the Index's LF. Faithfulness to the Index is inviolable in such a Minimalist Program approach (as in OT approaches like that of Grimshaw 1993); for us, such faithfulness is crucially violable. Another difference, that the numeration is an unstructured list of featurally rich lexical items while its counterpart in our Index is a predicate-argument structure, amounts to less than it might appear; the LF roles of lexical items and their features (e.g., case) in the numeration together constrain the structural roles of items to a high degree, so it is quite unclear how crucial are the differences between the information in this Minimalist Program Index and that in our predicate-argument-structure-plus-operator-variable Index.

Another reason we adopt 'Index' in lieu of 'input' is that only part of the Index — the numeration — serves as the *input* to the derivation. The other part — the LF — is, however, an equally important part of the Index: the structure that determines which derivations compete.

---

hypothesis, all competitors have a valid interpretation, 'who ate what', it's not clear how this would work. To say that the Irish winner crashes at interpretation while the English winner does not would seem to say that the competitors are not all interpretively equivalent after all. Which is the second option: abandon the requirement that competitors must have the same LF interpretation. As we will show, once this option is adopted, there is no need to appeal to anything beyond a strictly OT syntax.

Thus, the solution we adopt to the first problem, language-particular ineffability, is this: competitors need not have the same LF structure (hereafter, simply 'LF'). An LF unrealizable in a language is a structure such that every syntactic output with that LF interpretation is less harmonic in that language than a competitor with a different LF.

To take a concrete example, consider again Chinese adjunct extractions from *wh*-islands (41), the data for which are schematically summarized in (67).

(67)   Chinese: Adjunct extractions from *wh*-islands (Tsai 1994)

Referentiality	Scope	
	Narrow	Wide
+	✓	✓
−	✓	*

What does the one ungrammatical form, wide scope [−ref] extraction, lose to? In our analysis, it loses to the *narrow* scope [−ref] structure, which is grammatical. This possibility, open once we let LF-inequivalent structures compete, is a particularly natural one in Chinese, since the winning structure with narrow scope interpretation and the losing one with wide scope interpretation are homophonous.

But this immediately raises our second problem: if the wide and narrow scope structures compete, how can *both* be optimal in the case of [+ref] extraction? On a level playing field, narrow scope will always win, preferred by "Shortest Move." This is a special case of the general problem faced by any optimization-based theory: *How can marked structures ever be optimal — why don't they always lose to unmarked structures? Why doesn't everything surface as the one perfect syllable/word/sentence (perhaps 'ba')?* The general OT answer to this problem of marked outputs is simply *faithfulness* (see Chapter 12 (59)). The input, or 'Index' as we are calling it, contains *targets* for the output, and (violable) faithfulness constraints require that the output hit these targets. What competitors are competing for is the title of optimal compromise between hitting the target, on the one hand, and general structural well-formedness constraints, on the other. Marked outputs arise just when faithfulness constraints outrank those markedness-defining constraints that must be violated in order to be faithful to some Index.

Thus, our solution, a special case of the general OT solution, has two parts.

Box 3

(68)   Solution to the problem of marked outputs

    a.   An Index contains *target scopes* for operators.

        For example, a schematic input with narrow target *wh*-scope (marked by *wh*-operator Q) might be

$$\text{Index}_1: \text{ you wonder } [Q_i\, Q_j\, x_i \text{ ate } x_j]$$

        (faithfully rendered in English as 'you wonder who ate what'); a schematic input with wide target scope for subject x_i might be

$$\text{Index}_2: \ Q_i \text{ you wonder } [Q_j\, x_i \text{ ate } x_j]$$

        (faithfully: 'who [do] you wonder what ate', not optimal in English).

    b.   A constraint PARSESCOPE of the faithfulness family of constraints requires that output structures realize the target scopes of the Index;

        for example, 'you wonder who ate what' is an unfaithful parse of Index$_2$: it violates PARSESCOPE for x_i.

In sum, *outputs with different LFs compete, but not on a level playing field:* each Index contains a target LF, and outputs that are not faithful to it suffer constraint violations.[26] Unfaithful outputs are crucial and often optimal; they are essential to our explanation of how sentences can be ungrammatical in the absence of a grammatical alternative realization of the same LF (a situation not explicitly treated in most OT syntax work to date).[27] Note that the LF in the optimal *output* determines its interpretation — the target LF in its Index does not (just as in phonology, where the material in the output parse determines its phonetic interpretation, not the material in the 'phonetic target': the input/underlying form).

[26] Of course, when constraints requiring faithfulness to the target LF are undominated, outputs that are not faithful to the LF in the Index cannot be optimal, and their presence in the candidate set has no consequences.

[27] Another approach to ineffability in OT (McCarthy and Prince 1993; Prince and Smolensky 1993/2004) employs the *null parse* Ø; when this is the optimal candidate in *Gen(I)*, the Index *I* has no realization (see Ackema and Neeleman 2000 for an example in syntax). Of course, Ø does not share an LF with any nonempty structure, so to allow it in the candidate set is already to abandon the principle that only LF-equivalent structures compete. We have found it unworkable to use Ø as the winner for every case of ineffability, for the following general reason. Since Ø occurs in every candidate set, it determines a fixed Harmony threshold for the *entire* language: Ø wins every competition in which the best alternative has lower Harmony. The Harmony of Ø is governed by the ranking of PARSE, in the simplest analysis: this is the constraint violated by Ø. PARSE must be ranked so that *every* parse of every ineffable Index violates a constraint higher than PARSE (and loses to Ø); PARSE must also be ranked so that *some* parse of every effable Index violates no constraint higher than PARSE (and bests Ø). This has not proved possible: it is imperative that the relative Harmonies of Index-specific faithful and unfaithful parses be decisive. Our solution, in essence, is to use *mini* 'null parses' to *selectively* unparse just the most problematic aspects of an Index. Rather than a single unfaithful parse (Ø) in all candidate sets, we employ multiple Index-specific unfaithful parses in which just an operator scope, or just a [wh] feature, is not parsed.

    Our interpretation of an LF-unfaithful winner is that it surfaces as a grammatical sentence, but with a different LF interpretation. But it seems that little or nothing would change if instead we gave LF-unfaithful winners no interpretation at all, like Ø — no realization of the Index; this, because every LF-*unfaithful* winner can also be obtained as an LF-*faithful* winner for another Index. What is crucial is that LF-inequivalent structures compete, that LF targets be present in the Index, and that LF-unfaithful candidates win for ineffable LFs; it does not seem crucial whether these unfaithful structures are given their natural interpretation, or none at all.

5.3 On the relation to the Minimalist Program

In Chapter 12, it was emphasized that OT is not inherently committed to simultaneously evaluating entire output representations with all constraints—as in *parallel* OT. While all empirical analyses in this book, and most of those in the literature, are framed within parallel OT, we speculate in this section how our *wh*-analysis might be reformulated as an OT account employing derivations, with specific attention to the Minimalist Program as presented in Chomsky 1995 (see also Chapter 12(60) and Müller, to appear). (Readers not familiar with the Minimalist Program may want to go directly to Section 6.)

While some see a major divide between the derivationally oriented Minimalist Program and OT, we do not. Of course, there are likely to be differences of empirical import between the nonderivational, chain-based theory of "Shortest Move" developed here—MINLINK—and a particular derivational Minimalist Program proposal, but such differences seem comparable to those between different approaches to syntax within OT, or to those between different proposals within the Minimalist Program; they do not seem to follow from some major divide between the OT and Minimalist Program frameworks. In fact, derivational theories can be naturally formalized within OT, in at least two ways. **Harmonic Serialism** is a derivational version of OT developed in Prince and Smolensky 1993/2004 in which each step of the derivation produces the optimal next representation. Under another approach, seemingly needed to formalize the Minimalist Program within OT, *Gen* produces *derivations;* it is these that are evaluated by the constraints, the optimal derivation being determined via standard OT evaluation. Thus, on our view, while the issue of derivations is an important one, it is largely orthogonal to OT: any evidence there may be *for* derivations is not ipso facto evidence *against* OT. (See Müller 1998, 1999, and Hale and Legendre 2004 for a comparison of analyses of German remnant movement within parallel OT and Harmonic Serialism.)

Another such issue is the feature-checking theory of movement embodied in the Minimalist Program. Any putative evidence for the feature-checking theory is also evidence for OT theories with constraints governing chains (or movement) such as

> CHECK(F): specifier-head F-agreement with overt chain element ≻
> specifier-head F-agreement with empty chain element ≻
> no F-agreement.

That is, agreement with an overt element (overt movement to check F) is best; agreement with an empty chain element like our Q (covert movement) is next best; no chain (movement) is worst. (CHECK(wh) is essentially our *Q.) CHECK(F) conflicts with *t, essentially PROCRASTINATE. When CHECK(F) ≫ *t, F is a strong feature, and overt movement to check F is optimal; when *t ≫ CHECK(F), F is a weak feature and covert movement is optimal. Crosslinguistic variation arises from reranking the CHECK(F) features (this is also observed in Grimshaw 1997). To analyze a language with a ranking in which

Box 3

{CHECK(F_1), CHECK(F_2), ..., CHECK(F_n)} $\gg$ *t,

we can encapsulate the constraints {CHECK(F_1), CHECK(F_2), ..., CHECK(F_n)} into a constraint CHECKSTRONGF whose content is defined by the language-specific set of strong features {F_1, F_2, ..., F_n}.

So neither the use of derivations nor the feature-checking theory of movement conflicts with the commitments of OT. Those commitments are (i) grammatical = optimal; (ii) optimal = most harmonic; (iii) Harmony is computed from ranked violable constraints as formally specified in OT; (iv) crosslinguistic variation = alternative rankings of universal constraints (*only*; no functional parameters in the lexicon). None of these commitments is obviously inconsistent with the Minimalist Program— even (iv), in light of the preceding observation that the strong/weak distinction can be naturally formalized in OT in terms of whether a constraint CHECK(F) is literally stronger or weaker than a constraint amounting to PROCRASTINATE. And as we have argued above, OT's Harmony calculation affords formalizations of economy principles such as "Shortest Link" that are natural, explanatory, and empirically powerful. Further explanatory purchase arises from violable versions of noneconomy constraints such as the ECP, and from faithfulness, integral to OT competition.

In our view, the OT approach developed here offers several attractive "minimizing" features for linguistic theory. For example, it employs a single, unitary syntactic representation that serves both the phonological and interpretive interfaces. And it opens the door to a grammatical theory in which a single theoretical framework serves both the phonological and syntactic components of grammar. As we have occasionally illustrated in this chapter, OT phonology and OT syntax have enjoyed considerable cross-fertilization, and they are now jointly contributing to the development of OT's characterization of UG.

6 CONCLUSION

When expressed in the violable constraint framework of OT, simple government, locality, and referentiality constraints account for a rich set of *wh*-extraction patterns in three typologically distinct languages. That the same constraints are used to build these grammars explains the crosslinguistic commonalities in the extraction patterns; differential rankings of the constraints explain the crosslinguistic contrasts.

The constraints we have proposed are these:

(69)   Constraints:
  a.   Faithfulness family
          PARSE family: PARSE(wh), PARSE(top), PARSESCOPE
          FILL
  b.   MINLINK family
          BAR^1 $\ll$ BAR^2 $\ll$ BAR^3 $\ll$ ...
          BAR$^{1[-ref]}$ $\ll$ BAR$^{2[-ref]}$ $\ll$ BAR$^{3[-ref]}$ $\ll$ ...

    c.   Government

          Gov(t)

    d.   Operator family

          *Q, *TOp, *Absorb

    e.   Economy

          *t

    f.   Subcat

Our main claims are that (i) OT allows such a strong but flexible MinLink to be constructed directly from general principles, and (ii) the resulting MinLink explains a broad range of crosslinguistic (overt and covert) extraction facts.

    In addition, we argue for certain general solutions to fundamental questions for comparison-based syntactic formalisms.

(70)   Competition in syntax

    a.   *What structures compete?* Those that share a common target LF.

    b.   *What is the 'input'?* (More properly, the 'Index'.) By definition, it is that which is shared among competitors: a target LF, including target scopes for quantifiers, target features such as [+wh] on variables, and so on.

    c.   *How is language-particular ineffability possible?* The optimal candidate for a target LF may have a different LF. (This violates faithfulness constraints, but may still be optimal.) If there is no optimal structure with a given LF, then that LF is ineffable. Whether this happens is ranking dependent, hence language particular.

    d.   *How are marked outputs possible?* Each Index (target LF) determines a candidate set in which all candidates are required by faithfulness constraints to match that target LF. With faithfulness ranked sufficiently highly, the optimal candidate will match the target LF, which will typically entail that it is not the least marked structure.[28]

---

[28] For most helpful conversations, we thank Luigi Burzio, Robert Frank, Jane Grimshaw, and Alan Prince; for useful comments, audiences at the Society for Philosophy and Psychology, the Association for Computational Linguistics, the University of Toronto, Johns Hopkins University, the University of Delaware, Brown University, and Georgetown University. For help with the Bulgarian facts, we thank Tzvetelina Ganeva and Catherine Rudin; the Chinese facts, Yi-ching Su and Ningsheng Liu.

Box 3

References

ROA = Rutgers Optimality Archive, http://roa.rutgers.edu

Ackema, P., and A. Neeleman. 2000. Absolute ungrammaticality. In *Optimality Theory: Phonology, syntax, and acquisition*, eds. J. Dekkers, F. van der Leeuw, and J. van de Weijer. Oxford University Press.

Anderson, S. R. 1984. Kwakwala syntax and the Government-Binding Theory. In *Syntax and semantics*. Vol. 16, *The syntax of Native American languages*, eds. Eung-Do Cook and Donna B. Gerdts. Academic Press.

Aoun, J., N. Hornstein, D. Lightfoot, and A. Weinberg. 1987. Two types of locality. *Linguistic Inquiry* 18, 537–77.

Aoun, J., and Y.-h. A. Li. 1993. *Wh*-elements in situ: Syntax or LF? *Linguistic Inquiry* 24, 199–238.

Baker, C. L. 1970. Notes on the description of English questions: The role of an abstract question morpheme. *Foundations of Language* 6, 197–219.

Baković, E. 1998. Optimality and inversion in Spanish. In *Is the best good enough? Optimality and competition in syntax*, eds. P. Barbosa, D. Fox, P. Hagstrom, M. McGinnis, and D. Pesetsky. MIT Press and MIT Working Papers in Linguistics.

Billings, L., and C. Rudin. 1994. Optimality and superiority: A new approach to overt multiple *wh* ordering. In *Symposium on Formal Approaches to Slavic Linguistics*.

Black, C. A. 2000. *Quiegolani Zapotec syntax: A principles and parameters account*. SIL International and University of Texas at Arlington.

Burzio, L. 1994. *Principles of English stress*. Cambridge University Press.

Chomsky, N. 1973. Conditions on transformations. In *A festschrift for Morris Halle*, eds. S. R. Anderson and P. Kiparsky. Holt, Rinehart and Winston.

Chomsky, N. 1981. *Lectures on government and binding*. Foris.

Chomsky, N. 1986. *Barriers*. MIT Press.

Chomsky, N. 1993. A minimalist program for linguistic theory. In *The view from Building 20*, eds. K. Hale and S. J. Keyser. MIT Press.

Chomsky, N. 1995. *The Minimalist Program*. MIT Press.

Cinque, G. 1990. *Types of Ā-dependencies*. MIT Press.

Cole, P., and G. Hermon. 1994. Is there LF *wh*-movement? *Linguistic Inquiry* 25, 239–62.

Collins, C. 1994. Economy of derivation and the Generalized Proper Binding Condition. *Linguistic Inquiry* 25, 45–61.

Comorovski, I. 1989. Discourse-linking and the *Wh*-Island Constraint. In *Proceedings of the North East Linguistic Society 19*.

Fox, D. 1998. Locality in variable binding. In *Is the best good enough? Optimality and competition in syntax*, eds. P. Barbosa, D. Fox, P. Hagstrom, M. McGinnis, and D. Pesetsky. MIT Press and MIT Working Papers in Linguistics.

Georgopoulos, C. 1985. Variables in Palauan syntax. *Natural Language and Linguistic Theory* 3, 59–94.

Georgopoulos, C. 1991. *Syntactic variables: Resumptive pronouns and A' binding in Palauan*. Kluwer.

Grimshaw, J. 1993. Minimal projection, heads, and optimality. Technical report RuCCS-TR-4, Rutgers Center for Cognitive Science, Rutgers University. ROA 68.

Grimshaw, J. 1997. Projection, heads, and optimality. *Linguistic Inquiry* 28, 373–422.

Guilfoyle, E., H. Hung, and L. Travis. 1992. Spec of IP and Spec of VP: Two subjects in Austronesian languages. *Natural Language and Linguistic Theory* 10, 375–414.

Hale, J., and G. Legendre. 2004. Minimal links, remnant movement, and (non-)derivational grammar. In *Minimality effects in syntax*, eds. A. Stepanov, G. Fanselow, and R. Vogel. Mouton de Gruyter.

Higginbotham, J., and R. May. 1981. Questions, quantifiers and crossing. *The Linguistic Review* 1, 41–80.

Huang, C.-T. J. 1982. Logical relations in Chinese and the theory of grammar. Ph.D. diss., MIT.

Kayne, R. S. 1984. *Connectedness and binary branching*. Foris.

Keenan, E. L. 1976. Remarkable subjects in Malagasy. In *Subject and topic*, ed. C. Li. Academic Press.

Lasnik, H., and M. Saito. 1992. *Move α: Conditions on its application and output*. MIT Press.

Legendre, G., P. Smolensky, and C. Wilson. 1998. When is less more? Faithfulness and minimal links in *wh*-chains. In *Is the best good enough? Optimality and competition in syntax*, eds. P. Barbosa, D. Fox, P. Hagstrom, M. McGinnis, and D. Pesetsky. MIT Press and MIT Working Papers in Linguistics. ROA 117.

Legendre, G., C. Wilson, P. Smolensky, K. Homer, and W. Raymond. 1995. Optimality in *wh*-chains. In *University of Massachusetts occasional papers in linguistics 18: Papers in Optimality Theory*, eds. J. Beckman, L. Walsh Dickey, and S. Urbanczyk. Graduate Linguistic Student Association, University of Massachusetts at Amherst.

Manzini, M. R. 1992. *Locality*. MIT Press.

May, R. 1985. *Logical Form: Its structure and derivation*. MIT Press.

McCarthy, J. J., and A. Prince. 1993. Prosodic Morphology I: Constraint interaction and satisfaction. Technical report RuCCS-TR-3, Rutgers Center for Cognitive Science, Rutgers University, and University of Massachusetts at Amherst. ROA 482, 2001.

Müller, G. 1998. *Incomplete category fronting: A derivational approach to remnant movement in German*. Kluwer.

Müller, G. 1999. Shape conservation and remnant movement. In *Proceedings of the North East Linguistic Society 30*. ROA 365.

Müller, G. 2003. Local vs. global optimization in syntax: A case study. In *Proceedings of the Stockholm Workshop on Variation within Optimality Theory*. ROA 598.

Pesetsky, D. 1987. *Wh*-in-situ: Movement and unselective binding. In *The representation of (in)definiteness*, eds. E. J. Reuland and A. G. B. ter Meulen. MIT Press.

Prince, A. 1997. Endogenous constraints on OT constraints. Talk presented at the Hopkins Optimality Theory Conference/Maryland Mayfest.

Prince, A., and P. Smolensky. 1991. Notes on connectionism and Harmony Theory in linguistics. Technical report CU-CS-533-91, Computer Science Department, University of Colorado at Boulder.

Prince, A., and P. Smolensky. 1993/2004. *Optimality Theory: Constraint interaction in generative grammar*. Technical report, Rutgers University and University of Colorado at Boulder, 1993. ROA 537, 2002. Revised version published by Blackwell, 2004.

Reinhart, T. 1976. The syntactic domain of anaphora. Ph.D. diss., MIT.

Rizzi, L. 1990. *Relativized Minimality*. MIT Press.

Rizzi, L. 1991. Residual verb second and the *Wh*-Criterion. Technical Reports in Formal and Computational Linguistics 2, University of Geneva.

Ross, J. R. 1967. Constraints on variables in syntax. Ph.D. diss., MIT.

Ross, J. R. 1986. *Infinite syntax!* Ablex.

Rudin, C. 1985. *Aspects of Bulgarian syntax: Complementizers and wh constructions*. Slavica Publishers.

Rudin, C. 1988. On multiple questions and multiple *wh*-fronting. *Natural Language and Linguistic Theory* 6, 445–501.

Saddy, D. 1991. *Wh* scope mechanisms in Bahasa Indonesia. In *More papers on* wh-*movement*. eds. L. L.-S. Cheng and H. Demirdache. MIT Working Papers in Linguistics.

Smolensky, P. 1993. Harmony, markedness, and phonological activity. Handout of talk presented at the Rutgers Optimality Workshop–1. ROA 87.

Srivastav, V. 1991. Subjacency effects at LF: The case of Hindi *wh*. Linguistic Inquiry 22, 762–9.

Tsai, W.-T. D. 1994. On nominal islands and LF extraction in Chinese. *Natural Language and Linguistic Theory* 12, 121–75.

Wahba, W. A. B. 1991. LF movement in Iraqi Arabic. In *Logical structure and linguistic structure*, eds. C.-T. J. Huang and R. May. Kluwer.

17 Optimality in Language Acquisition I: The Initial and Final States of the Phonological Grammar

Lisa Davidson, Peter Jusczyk,
and Paul Smolensky

As emphasized in Chapters 1 and 12, the research program of the Integrated Connectionist/Symbolic Cognitive Architecture (ICS) places grammar squarely at the center of the cognitive science of language. The responsibilities of grammatical theory in ICS are not limited to those that the generative grammar tradition has circumscribed as the purview of competence theory. The duties of a theory of grammar also include explaining how language is acquired, how it is used during performance, and how it is biologically instantiated. In this chapter, we examine the value of ICS's highest-level grammatical theory, Optimality Theory, for understanding the course of acquiring English phonology, through performance studies of processing speech input and producing speech output. In the bigger picture, this work contributes to Section 8.7 of the ICS map in Chapter 2. For relevant background material concerning phonological theory, see Box 12:2.

We explore here the implications of a fundamental but subtle principle of OT—Richness of the Base—for the initial and final states of linguistic knowledge. Via explicit hypotheses linking grammatical properties to observable language behavior, these predictions of Richness of the Base are tested experimentally: we ask infants to attend to phonological stimuli that either satisfy or violate universal well-formedness principles, and ask adults to produce forms that are illegal according to their knowledge of English phonology.

* A version of this chapter appeared as Davidson, Jusczyk, and Smolensky 2004.

Contents

In this chapter, we present the initial stages of work that attempts to assess the "psychological reality" of one of the more subtle grammatical principles of Optimality Theory (OT; Prince and Smolensky 1993/2004), Richness of the Base. Within the OT competence theory, we develop several of this principle's empirical predictions concerning the grammar's final state (Section 1) and initial state (Section 2). We also formulate linking hypotheses that allow these predictions concerning competence to yield predictions addressing performance. We then report and discuss the results of experiments testing these performance predictions with respect to linguistic processing in infants (Section 2) and adults (Section 3).

1 INTRODUCTION

OT is a highly output-oriented grammatical theory. The strongest hypothesis is that *all* systematic, language-particular patterns are the result of output constraints — that there is no other locus from which such patterns can derive. In particular, the *input* is not such a locus. Thus, for example, the fact that English words never begin with the velar nasal *ŋ* cannot derive from a restriction on the English lexicon barring *ŋ*-initial morphemes. Rather, it must be the case that the English grammar *forces* all its outputs to obey the prohibition on initial *ŋ*. This requirement amounts to a counterfactual: *even if there were* an *ŋ*-initial lexical entry in English, providing an *ŋ*-initial *input*, the corresponding *output* of the English grammar would *not* be *ŋ*-initial. Thus, the absence of *ŋ*-initial words in English must be explained within OT by a grammar — a ranking of constraints — with the property that *no matter what the input*, the *output* of the grammar will not be *ŋ*-initial. That is, the OT analysis of English must consider a set of inputs to the grammar — the **base** — that is as *rich* as possible: the base contains all universally possible inputs, including those that are *ŋ*-initial, those that contain clicks, those that consist of 17 consecutive consonants, and so on.

This principle — **Richness of the Base** (Section 12:1.6) — means that it is not sufficient that the ranking constituting the English grammar derive the correct outputs from inputs drawn from a putative English lexicon of underlying forms. The grammar must also ensure that any hypothetical input at all, even one that violates the systematic patterns of English, produces an output that obeys these patterns.

This constitutes the first 'prediction' of Richness of the Base relevant here: an English learner's final ranking must filter out initial *ŋ*s as well as, say, consonant clusters that are not legal in English. Thus, for example, when subject to the English constraint ranking, the input /ktobi/ must be mapped to an output such as [kətobi] that lacks the English-illegal onset [kt].

This prediction resides in the OT competence theory: it is a claim about an abstract input-output mapping. In order to use this prediction to assess the "psychological reality" of Richness of the Base — that is, its role in performance — we need a working hypothesis linking competence to performance. For example: if auditorily presented with [ktobi] — produced fluently by a Polish speaker, for example — and asked to employ this "place name" fluently in a sentence, adult monolingual native speakers of English will produce [kətobi] or some other form respecting English phonotactic patterns. We seek experimental confirmation of this prediction in Section 3. Clearly, a naturalistic approximation to this situation occurs in loanwords, and the broad empirical generalization is that indeed foreign words are adapted to conform to native patterns. However, this adaptation is often only partial: loanwords frequently contain structures illegal in the borrowing language. The experimental results we report below display this incomplete nativization as well, with outputs exhibiting deviations from English that show interesting regularities. In Section 3, we will attempt an extension of Richness of the Base that recognizes particular propensities for partial nativization as an integral part of the final state of a native grammar.

The second prediction from Richness of the Base that we exploit is more subtle and concerns not the final but the initial state of the grammar. In Section 2, we develop a learnability argument leading to this prediction, which is simply stated: in the initial state, markedness constraints must dominate faithfulness constraints— otherwise, the final state demanded by Richness of the Base could not be achieved in certain problematic cases. The assumption here is that OT grammars consist of only two types of constraints: faithfulness constraints, which compare the input and output and demand that they be equal, and markedness constraints, which examine only the output and penalize universally dispreferred or **marked** structures (Chapter 12 (14)).

Like the derivation of the prediction MARKEDNESS ≫ FAITHFULNESS concerning the initial state, the linking hypothesis connecting this prediction to performance is somewhat complex; we take it up in Section 2.3. The result is an experimental paradigm designed to test whether infants behave in accordance with the 'MARKEDNESS dominates FAITHFULNESS' prediction. The outcomes of such experiments are presented in Section 2.3.

2 LEARNABILITY AND THE INITIAL STATE

How does the adult language-specific grammar—constraint ranking—come about? There are two aspects of this grammar to consider: the origin of the constraints themselves, and the determination of their relative ranking. Since the ranking is language particular, it must be learned; we turn to this matter shortly. But since the constraints themselves are universal, it is not necessarily the case that they are learned from experience: it is logically possible that they are somehow innately specified (see Chapter 21), and OT makes no commitment on this issue. The research summarized in this section extracts a theoretical prediction from the hypothesis that knowledge of universal constraints in OT is innate; the research summarized in the next section attempts to put this prediction to an experimental test.

According to the learning theory for OT proposed in Tesar and Smolensky 1993, 1998a, b, 2000, the language learner reranks constraints in the face of learning data. When the learner's current grammar declares that the optimal output for a word is an erroneous pronunciation, constraints are minimally demoted so that the correct pronunciation is declared optimal by the revised grammar. The learning algorithm for a stochastic version of OT proposed in Boersma 1998 performs more gradual reranking, but it is also driven by the errors made by the learner's current grammar.

2.1 The initial state

What is the initial ranking of constraints, prior to the reranking induced by the data of the language to be learned? Adopting the working hypothesis that the universal OT constraints are innate and thus present in the initial state, and elaborating an argument originally from Alan Prince (personal communication, 1993), Smolensky (1996a) developed a learnability argument showing that as a class, *markedness constraints must outrank faithfulness constraints in the initial state*; otherwise, certain languages would not be learnable. This characterization of the initial ranking is consistent with a body of work analyzing data from child phonology within the OT framework (Demuth 1995; Gnanadesikan 1995; Levelt 1995; Levelt and Van de Vijver 1998; Pater and Paradis 1996). Broadly speaking, with MARKEDNESS dominating FAITHFULNESS in the initial ranking, the child's productions will contain only unmarked forms: violations of markedness constraints can only be optimal if higher-ranked faithfulness constraints require them, and in this initial state there *are no* higher-ranked faithfulness constraints.

Smolensky (1996b) exhibited a perhaps surprising consequence of the assumption that in the initial state, markedness constraints are present and dominate faithfulness constraints: this assumption can broadly explain the discrepancy observed in language learners' early production and comprehension abilities. In particular, perceptual capacities that infants display in speech processing contrast with the inaccuracies that are apparent in their speech production. On the surface, the skill that infants show in comprehension appears to demand that faithfulness constraints be ranked high, whereas their difficulties in producing speech seem to require that faithfulness constraints be ranked low. However, Smolensky (1996b) argued that what distinguishes production from comprehension is only which structures compete: in production, it is structures sharing the same underlying form, whereas in comprehension, it is structures sharing the same surface form. Once this difference in competition is taken into account, a single ranking—with markedness dominating faithfulness—accounts for both highly unfaithful child production and relatively faithful child comprehension. (See Section 4:4; cf. Hale and Reiss 1998; Pater 2004.)

We now quickly sketch the learnability argument showing that markedness must outrank faithfulness initially, illustrating with the example of word-initial η. The question facing the learner here is, what is the correct ranking of the relevant markedness and faithfulness constraints? The markedness constraint is violated by η-initial words; for expository purposes, we'll take it to be a constraint against syllable-initial η, and simply call it M_η. The relevant faithfulness constraints, which we'll call F_η, require that an underlying initial η be faithfully mapped to an initial η in the output. Again, the learner's problem is to determine the relative ranking of M_η and F_η.

There are three cases to consider. The first is the easiest, the case illustrated by Vietnamese. Here, some words of the language are pronounced with an initial η in violation of M_η. This violation must be forced by a higher-ranking constraint $\mathbb{C}$: $\mathbb{C} \gg M_\eta$. $\mathbb{C}$ cannot be a markedness constraint: there is no universal constraint *favoring* initial η. So $\mathbb{C}$ must be a faithfulness constraint, F_η. Thus, the presence of η-initial words in this type of language immediately informs the learner that the ranking must be $F_\eta \gg M_\eta$. Only under this ranking can an η-initial underlying lexical form actually be pronounced with an initial η. This first case will be called a **marked inventory**: the language's inventory of allowed sound structures includes the marked element in question—initial η.

In the remaining two cases, the target ranking is the reverse, $M_\eta \gg F_\eta$; these are **unmarked inventories**. One such case is English, but first we take up the easier case, a hypothetical language we will call English'. English' contains words like *sing* taking a suffix -*er* to form *singer*. The pronunciations of these two forms in English' are [sɪŋ] and [sɪ.nə] (the period marking a syllable boundary): *sing* is pronounced as in real English, with η in the syllable coda, but in *singer*, the nasal is pronounced n (as in *sinner*)—because now it is in syllable-initial (onset) position. The English' pronunciation of *singer* violates the faithfulness constraint F_η: the underlying form has a velar nasal, while the pronounced form has a coronal nasal. This alternation of a sound between η and n tells the child learning English' that in this language, F_η is lower ranked than the markedness constraint M_η that prohibits η in onset position. Thus, when a language exhibits alternations of this sort, the child has explicit evidence for the language-particular ranking $M \gg F$; this case will be called an **unmarked inventory with alternation**.

But such evidence is not always present. The third case—an **unmarked inventory without alternation**—is illustrated by real English: there is no alternation between η and n like that found in English'. Nonetheless, the adult speaker of English must, according to Richness of the Base, rank $M_\eta \gg F_\eta$. Since the lexicon of English only places η where it can be syllabified faithfully into the coda, the pronunciation of English words never forces the child to choose between satisfying M_η and satisfying F_η: because each underlying η in coda position is always faithfully pronounced, both M_η and F_η are always satisfied. Regardless of how M_η and F_η may be ranked, the learner will make no errors in pronunciation. Therefore, there will be no evidence of the sort used in the learning algorithm to drive constraint reranking. Thus, if the learner's constraints are to end up—as Richness of the Base requires—with the ranking $M_\eta \gg F_\eta$, then these constraints *must start off with this ranking*.

Because this same argument can apply to any pair of potentially conflicting markedness and faithfulness constraints, the conclusion is quite general: in the initial state, markedness constraints must outrank faithfulness constraints. Only if the language provides overt evidence contradicting this ranking—the case of a marked inventory—will the reverse ranking come to be posited by the learner.

It is worth noting that what is crucial to the learnability argument is that the M-constraint is *contrast neutralizing* and the F-constraint is *contrast inducing*. The force of M is to restrict the output to the unmarked pole of a dimension of possible variation (e.g., to prevent ŋ-initial words rather than to allow words to be either ŋ-initial or not). The force of F is to require that input differences along this dimension be maintained in the output. So the argument's conclusion might be generally stated in these terms: neutralization-inducing constraints must dominate contrast-inducing constraints. Thus, it is not actually critical to any of the analyses in this chapter whether the phonological phenomenon in question is literally a contest between markedness and faithfulness; 'M' and 'F' should be taken to refer to the relevant contrast-suppressing and -inducing constraints, whatever their formal character. Thus, the conclusion of the learnability argument can in fact be stated in rather theory-neutral terms: in the initial state, the grammar favors neutralizations to the unmarked, and only under pressure of observed marked forms does the grammar change to allow marked structures to surface.

As pointed out by Hayes (2004) and Prince and Tesar (1999), the pressure that Richness of the Base exerts toward the ranking MARKEDNESS ≫ FAITHFULNESS is not limited to the initial state. Through interaction with other constraints, reranking that occurs during learning can disturb the initial ranking M ≫ F even in a language lacking marked structures, where this ranking must prevail in the end. These authors propose various mechanisms by which the pressure toward MARKEDNESS ≫ FAITHFULNESS can be continually imposed by a learning algorithm, reinstating this aspect of the initial state, except where this pressure is overcome by positive evidence that F ≫ M—evidence from the presence of marked structures in the target language.

Opposing the line of argument we have just summarized is another intuition. From the perspective of a developmental psychologist, one might have expected something entirely different: that, at the outset, faithfulness constraints should dominate markedness constraints (see also Hale and Reiss 1997). According to this alternative point of view, the simplest assumption an infant might make is that surface forms faithfully mirror their underlying structure. Only in the face of evidence to the contrary would the learner assume there is a more complicated relationship between surface forms and their underlying representations. The assumption that surface forms faithfully mirror underlying forms amounts to the assumption that faithfulness constraints outrank markedness constraints; this would then be the initial state as infants begin to acquire a native language. In this alternative theory, inaccuracies in the earliest productions of words would be ascribed not to grammar, but to difficulties that infants have in coordinating the actions of the articulators.

As a new source of evidence to complement these theoretical arguments concerning the character of the initial state, we have conducted experiments to evaluate the relative ranking of MARKEDNESS and FAITHFULNESS in the earliest grammars.

2.2 Nasal place assimilation

To date, our experiments addressing the relative rankings of MARKEDNESS and FAITHFULNESS in the initial state have focused on a single phonological phenomenon, nasal place assimilation (see Box 12:2 and Section 14:5.2). For now, we will assume that nasal place assimilation is driven by a markedness constraint requiring that every nasal that is followed by a consonant must have the same place of articulation as that consonant; we will call this constraint $M_{NASALPL}$ or simply M_{NP}. This markedness constraint potentially conflicts with the faithfulness constraint F_{NP} requiring that the place of articulation of a consonant in the input be preserved in the output. At issue will be the relative ranking of M_{NP} and F_{NP}.

Since the experiments we report here involve English-learning infants, it is relevant to consider the status of nasal place assimilation in English, which is somewhat complex. Within a single morpheme, it is almost always respected; for example, English has words like *bend*, *bump*, and *bank* [bæŋk], but no words like hypothetical **bemd*, **bunp*, or **bamk*. However, when a nasal at the end of one morpheme contacts a consonant at the beginning of a following morpheme, two outcomes are possible, depending on whether the morpheme boundary is the 'inner' type characteristic of Level 1 affixation, or the 'outer' type of Level 2.[1] For the inner type, the nasal behaves as if it were in the same morpheme as the following consonant: it assimilates. An example of this type is the prefix *in-*, meaning 'not', as in *inaudible* and *inexpensive*. The nasal consonant of this prefix is pronounced [n] before a coronal stop such as [t, d] (*intolerable, indefinite*), but [m] before a labial stop, [p, b] (*imperfect, imbalance*).[2] An affix of the second, outer type will not alternate in this way and does not exhibit assimilation. For example, the outer affix *in-* (a different morpheme, meaning 'directed inward' rather than 'not') gives *input, inbound*.

Thus, the situation confronting the learner of nasal place assimilation in English is in fact a composite of the three cases illustrated above for word-initial *ŋ*. Considering only simple, monomorphemic words, English clusters are assimilated, that is, unmarked with respect to M_{NP}: English has an unmarked inventory without alternations. This is the hard case for learning, where the initial ranking must rank M_{NP} above F_{NP} in order for the language to be learnable. For morphologically complex words with inner, Level 1, affixation, clusters are still unmarked: here, English has an unmarked inventory *with* alternations, as exhibited by *in-* 'not'. Finally, for morphologically complex words with Level 2 affixation, English does allow unassimilated clusters violating M_{NP}, so now the inventory appears to be marked.

This heterogeneous pattern is of course quite familiar in morphophonology, where, to grossly oversimplify, morpheme junctions at an inner level look like morpheme-internal environments, whereas junctions at an outer level look like the sim-

---

[1] According to Lexical Phonology (Kiparsky 1982 et seq.), English affixes divide broadly into two classes. Level 1 affixes are attached first, derivationally; Level 2 affixes attach only after all Level 1 affixes are in place. Thus, Level 1 affixes are interior to (closer to the word root than) Level 2 affixes.

[2] This morpheme *in-* 'not' fails to assimilate to other following consonants, however: for example, *incompetent, ingratitude, informal, involuntary*.

ple concatenation of separate words with little or no influence on one another. Although there are several theoretical proposals for handling this general pattern within OT and other phonological frameworks, here we will adopt a highly simplified approach adequate to our limited needs. We will assume that the markedness constraint M_{NP} requires that a nasal consonant have the same place of articulation as a following consonant if these two consonants are in the same **stem**. On this simplified view, inner, Level 1 morpheme junctions lie within the stem, while more superficial, Level 2 junctions lie outside the stem. Thus, in *imperfect* the (Level 1) prefix *in-* 'not' falls within the same stem as the root *perfect*, so M_{NP} applies, requiring assimilation. In *input*, however, the (Level 2) prefix *in-* 'directed inward' falls outside the stem containing the root *put*, so M_{NP} does not apply, just as it fails to apply (in careful speech) between the two words in the compound *pinpoint* or the two words in the phrase *in perpetuity*.

On this analysis, the adult English ranking is $M_{NP} \gg F_{NP}$. There is evidence in the language for this ranking from alternations, but these are highly limited, applying to *in-* 'not' (before labial stops only) and perhaps also to *con-* 'together' (*contemporary, compatriot, congruence*). It seems reasonable to assume that children cannot exploit this evidence during their first two years, the period of time we examine in the experiments discussed below. So for all intents and purposes, for infants, English nasal assimilation presents the difficult case of an unmarked inventory without alternations—the case for which learnability requires that the initial ranking be MARKEDNESS ≫ FAITHFULNESS. Furthermore, at the age of the youngest children we tested (4.5 months), the literature shows no evidence of the acquisition of language-particular phonotactics (Jusczyk et al. 1993; Jusczyk, Luce, and Charles Luce 1994; Mattys and Jusczyk 2001). Thus, it is unlikely that any behavior we see in these infants is the result of statistical analysis of English consonant clusters. Any evidence we find that these youngest infants rank MARKEDNESS above FAITHFULNESS would seem to support the nativist learnability argument that this is knowledge encoded in the initial state.

Thus, we ask the experimental question: do infants show evidence of the ranking MARKEDNESS ≫ FAITHFULNESS? Focusing on nasal place assimilation, our goal then is to determine whether the youngest English learners give evidence of observing each type of constraint, and if so, to determine how they rank these two types of constraints with respect to one another.

2.3 Experimental explorations of the initial state

We argued above that under the nativist hypothesis, Richness of the Base, a principle fundamental to OT, entails that in order for languages with unmarked inventories to be learnable, the initial state must be characterized by the schematic ranking MARKEDNESS ≫ FAITHFULNESS. In this section, we assess this conclusion experimentally.

2.3.1 Experimental methods, hypotheses, and predictions

The work discussed here attempts to assess the hypotheses stated in (1).

(1)   The central grammatical hypotheses (initial state)

Insight into infants' processing of linguistic input can be gained from the assumptions that, in the infants' grammars,

    a.   markedness constraints are present;

    b.   faithfulness constraints are present;

    c.   MARKEDNESS ≫ FAITHFULNESS.

The technique we employ for observing the linguistic processing of infants is the headturn preference procedure, a computer-automated method used extensively in infant speech research (Kemler Nelson et al. 1995; Jusczyk 1998). The dependent variable is the length of time infants listen to two types of spoken stimuli designed to differ significantly only along the linguistic dimension of interest—the independent variable. In this procedure, each infant sits on a caregiver's lap in a chair in the center of a three-sided enclosure. A test trial begins with the flashing of a light on the center panel. When the infant fixates the center light, it is extinguished, and a light on one of the side panels begins to flash. When the infant makes a headturn of at least 30 degrees in the direction of the flashing light, the experimenter initiates a speech sample from the loudspeaker on the same side as the light and begins recording the infant's looking time by pressing a button on the response box. If the infant turns away from the loudspeaker by 30 degrees for less than 2 consecutive seconds and then reorients in the appropriate direction, the trial continues, but the time spent looking away from the loudspeaker is eliminated from the total orientation time on that particular trial (the experimenter presses another button on the response box to stop the timer). If the infant looks away for more than 2 consecutive seconds, the trial is terminated. Both the experimenter and the caregiver wear sound-insulated headphones and listen to loud masking music to prevent them from hearing the stimulus materials throughout the experiment.

To link OT principles concerning the competence grammar to the performance of infants, we adopt the working hypotheses given in (2).

(2)   Linking hypotheses, initial state: Higher Harmony ⇒ longer listening time

    a.   Infants will attend longer to stimuli that conform better to their current grammar, all else being equal.

    b.   Phonologically unrelated stimuli presented as isolated words 'conform to a grammar' if each is a possible output of the grammar.

Relative version: Given two such stimuli A and B, A 'conforms better' to a grammar if, treated as isolated outputs and evaluated by the grammar, A has higher Harmony than B. Underlying forms for these outputs are assumed to be chosen to maximize Harmony (as in the lexicon optimization of Prince and Smolensky 1993/2004, Chap. 9, or the Robust Interpretive

Parsing of Smolensky 1996b and Tesar and Smolensky 1996, 1998b, 2000; see Chapter 12 of this book).

c. Phonologically related stimuli presented in a potentially grammatically related configuration 'conform to a grammar' if they are in fact so related by the grammar. In particular, consider a set of spoken items presented as a list of triads consisting of three prosodic words of the form

> X ... Y ... XY',

where XY' is a concatenation of X and Y in which some sound changes may have possibly occurred (e.g., *on...pa...ompa*). Such a triad 'conforms to a grammar' if there is a choice of inputs /x/ and /y/ such that X, Y, and XY' are respectively the output of the grammar for the three inputs /x/, /y/, and /xy/, in which /xy/ is literally the concatenation of x and y (possibly separated by a morphological boundary). (Thus, depending on the ranking of FAITHFULNESS in the grammar, the conforming XY' may be a faithful concatenation of X and Y, or an unfaithful concatenation reflecting phonology.)

Relative version: One set of such stimuli *A* 'conforms better' to a grammar than another set *B* if *A* has higher Harmony according to the grammar. The inputs /x/ and /y/ are presumed chosen to maximize Harmony. (Thus, *on...pa...ompa* conforms better to a grammar than does *on...pa...onpa* if the grammar assigns higher Harmony to the input-output mapping /onpa/ → *ompa* than it does to the mapping /onpa/ → *onpa*.)

Hypothesis (2b) suffices for evaluating the hypothesis (1a) that markedness constraints are evidenced in the initial state, because markedness constraints involve only outputs. The more complex hypothesis (2c) is necessary, however, for assessing FAITHFULNESS and its ranking relative to MARKEDNESS, since inputs as well as outputs of the grammar must be involved. Use of triad stimuli of the form described in (2c) will be referred to as the **X/Y/XY paradigm**.

The core of the linking hypothesis, (2a), is the simple supposition that infants will attend longer to more language-like stimuli, that is, stimuli that conform better to their grammar. In fact, studies using the headturn preference procedure provide considerable support for this hypothesis. For example, infants have been shown to listen significantly longer to passages in which pauses are inserted at clausal or phrasal boundaries than at inappropriate locations within clauses or phrases (Hirsh-Pasek et al. 1987; Jusczyk et al. 1992). Similarly, investigations have shown that infants listen longer to lists of words that conform to native than to nonnative phonotactic patterns (Friederici and Wessels 1993; Jusczyk et al. 1993), and to those that conform to predominant word stress (Jusczyk, Cutler, and Redanz 1993; Turk, Jusczyk, and Gerken 1995) and phonotactic (Jusczyk, Luce, and Charles Luce 1994) patterns of native-language words. In general, when infants are presented with highly varied sets of speech stimuli, they display listening preferences for ones that conform to familiar patterns in the language they are acquiring (Jusczyk 1997). (Situations for which infants have been reported to display preferences for novel patterns are generally those that involve a long prior exposure period to a very limited set of stimuli with little variation (e.g., Saffran, Aslin, and Newport 1996; Echols, Crowhurst, and Childers 1997; Saffran et al. 1999; Johnson and Jusczyk 2001) — a situation that seems likely to result in infants habituating to the familiarization stimuli (Hunter and Ames 1989).)

This section reports the initial results of a general research program with a wide range of potential applications within grammatical theory. If the proposed linking hypotheses (2) — including the X/Y/XY paradigm — bear up under experimental investigation, listening times can be used to investigate many aspects of the grammars of infants. The initial work reported here involves two dimensions of phonological markedness: syllable structure and nasal place assimilation. The corresponding markedness constraints are respectively ONSET/NOCODA and M_{NP}, a constraint (introduced in Section 2.2) requiring that the place of articulation of a nasal consonant agree with that of a following consonant.

With respect to syllable structure, we examine a prediction of the Basic CV Syllable Theory (Prince and Smolensky 1993/2004, Chap. 6 (Chapter 13 here)),: a single intervocalic consonant will universally be parsed into the onset of the following syllable rather than the coda of the preceding syllable. That is, ···VCV··· will always be parsed ···V.CV··· rather than ···VC.V···, where the period marks the syllable boundary. Thus, all else being equal, stimuli with the syllable structure ···V.CV··· (such as *ba.di to.ma ...*) will conform better to any grammar than those with the structure ···VC.V··· (*bad.i tom.a ...*). The reason is as follows. These forms may well violate many markedness constraints — for example, *toma* violates a constraint prohibiting nasals — but the two matched lists will fare equally well with respect to all constraints except those sensitive to the only difference between the lists, the location of the syllable boundary. And here, both the constraints ONSET ('Syllables have onsets') and NOCODA ('Syllables do not have codas') are violated by all the forms in the second list and satisfied by all those in the first. Regardless of where these markedness constraints may be ranked in the infant's current grammar, this entails that the first list is more harmonic than the second, and by hypothesis (2b), infants are thus predicted to attend longer to the first list — if ONSET or NOCODA is indeed present in their grammars.

The case of syllable structure was chosen for the initial study in part because the competing alternatives — different syllabifications (e.g., *to.ma* vs. *tom.a*) — are equally faithful to any underlying form.[3] There can therefore be no question of conflict between the markedness constraints ONSET/NOCODA and faithfulness constraints. This allows for a relatively simple experiment, but does not allow us to test the hypothesis

---

[3] We are assuming here that syllabification is not present in underlying forms. This is commonly assumed to account for the strong crosslinguistic generalization that syllable structure is not lexically contrastive. If syllable structure were present in underlying forms, the predictions stated in the text would still follow, but now because of the ranking structure of the initial state: faithfulness to underlying syllable structure would be dominated by markedness. See the discussion of nasal assimilation below for an experimental approach to testing such a ranking.

concerning the relative ranking in the initial state of MARKEDNESS and FAITHFULNESS. For this purpose, we turned to a different markedness constraint, $M_{NASALPL}$: satisfying this constraint can require changing the place of articulation of a consonant, violating FAITHFULNESS and thereby setting up a conflict of the desired type.

The experimental study of M_{NP} (Jusczyk, Smolensky, and Allocco 2002) tested all three hypotheses in (1). First, to test the hypothesis that FAITHFULNESS is present in the infants' grammars and relevant to their behavior in the way hypothesized in (2c), we compared a list of items of the form *om...pa...ompa ɪn...du...ɪndu* ... with a matched list of items of the form *om...pa...ɪndu ɪn...du...ompa* ....[4] The lists were designed to fare equally well on all constraints except FAITHFULNESS, which is satisfied in the first list and violated in the second. In particular, note that the lists were constructed so that the XY forms do not violate M_{NP}: the final nasal in X always agrees in place with the initial stop in Y. Thus, if FAITHFULNESS is present in the infants' grammars and relevant to their behavior in the way hypothesized in (2c), infants should attend longer to lists of the first—faithful—type.

Next, to test whether M_{NP} is in fact present in infants' grammars, we compared lists such as *ompa ... ɪndu ...* with matched lists such as *omdu ... ɪnpa ....* The first list satisfies M_{NP} while the second list violates it, and the matching of syllables employed in the two lists means that the two lists fare equally with respect to other constraints. Thus, if M_{NP} is present in the initial state, then, according to (2b), infants should attend longer to the first type of list.

For direct comparison with the faithfulness experiment, it is actually preferable to design the markedness experiment using lists of triads comparable to those used for studying faithfulness. The first type of list includes triads of the form *om...pa...ompa ɪn...du...ɪndu* ..., while the second type of list is a matched list of items of the form *ɪn...pa...ɪnpa om...du...omdu* .... Both lists satisfy FAITHFULNESS because each 'XY' bisyllable is a faithful concatenation of the 'X' and 'Y' monosyllables. But the consonants coming into contact in XY were selected so that nasal place assimilation was satisfied in the first list and violated in the second. Again, according to (2c), infants should attend longer to the first type of list. This is the paradigm actually employed in the experiments described below.

Finally, to test whether MARKEDNESS ≫ FAITHFULNESS, we must pit F_{NP} against M_{NP}. Now the first list consists of triads of the form *on...pa...ompa*, while the second list contains matched items of the form *on...pa...onpa*. The first list violates F_{NP} but satisfies M_{NP}, and the reverse is true of the second list. The prediction from the Richness of the Base argument in Section 2 is that infants will attend longer to lists of the first type.

---

[4] There were six lists of each of the two types in each experiment. The X items had the form VC or CVC, where the initial C was an obstruent and the final C one of the nasals *n*, *m*, or *ŋ*; in each list of eight triads, all X forms had the same nasal. The Y items had the form CV, where C was a voiced or unvoiced obstruent and V a vowel occurring word-finally in English. X, Y, and XY' were each naturally produced (by a female native speaker of English) as a single prosodic word; XY' was produced with initial stress and was not an English word. Triads were separated by 1 s, and items within each triad were separated by 0.5 s. The total duration of each list was approximately 25 s.

Clearly, if the overall research program enabled by the linking hypotheses (2) is viable, experiments of this general sort can be used to address virtually any putative markedness constraint. The approach may even extend to syntax in older children.

2.3.2   Experimental results: Youngest infants

In determining the age groups to test, we took into consideration experimental results showing that although 9-month-old infants show significant listening preferences for sound patterns that observe the phonetics and phonotactics of English, 6-month-olds do not (Jusczyk et al. 1993; Jusczyk, Luce, and Charles Luce 1994; Jusczyk, Houston, and Newsome 1999; Mattys and Jusczyk 2001). We thus felt it important to test infants no older than 6 months in order to better access the initial state, prior to acquisition of significant language-particular knowledge of phonology. The youngest age at which infants have sufficient head and neck control to be tested in the headturn preference procedure is about 4.5 months.

The experimental results are summarized in Table 1. Each row corresponds to a single experiment. The column labeled 'MARKEDNESS' indicates whether a given experiment addressed markedness of syllable structure or nasal place of articulation. The ages of infants participating in these experiments are indicated as well: 6 and 4.5 months, respectively. In each experiment, we tested the prediction that infants will attend longer to stimuli with greater Harmony, according to the hypothesized initial grammar. In the experiments labeled 'Markedness' in the 'Constraints' column, the stimuli presented differed only in that the forms with lower Harmony violated the markedness constraint(s) in question ('∗M'), while the forms with higher Harmony satisfied the markedness constraint(s) ('✓M'). In the 'Faithfulness' experiment, the higher-Harmony stimuli satisfied FAITHFULNESS ('✓F') while the lower-Harmony stimuli did not ('∗F'). In the 'Markedness versus Faithfulness' experiment, the higher-Harmony triads respected MARKEDNESS but violated FAITHFULNESS, while the reverse was true of the lower-Harmony triads. In all other respects, the two types of stimuli were matched in each experiment.

The infants' listening times to the two types of stimuli presented in each experiment are shown in the columns headed 'Higher Harmony' and 'Lower Harmony'. The mean times are shown in boldface, and beneath them are the standard deviation (SD) and standard error (SE). The difference in listening times for each experiment is assessed by several measures in the final column. The proportion of infants preferring the higher-Harmony stimuli is shown as a fraction with denominator 20 or 16, depending upon whether the data from 20 or 16 infants were used in the experiment. In boldface, the p value of the significance of the difference in mean listening times is shown, according to a paired t test; the t value is shown beneath the p value.

As shown in Table 1, the results of Experiment 1 provide evidence that at 6 months infants' grammars include a markedness constraint on syllable structure (either ONSET or NOCODA). Since natural production of the marked syllable structure

VC.V is problematic, these stimuli were created by splicing together two separately recorded syllables. The V.CV forms were also produced by splicing, in order to minimize differences other than syllable structure between the two types of stimuli. As a check on the results of Experiment 1, in Experiment 2 we tested infants' preference between lists of simple CV and VC forms; these stimuli involved no splicing, although it is no longer as obvious that they equally well satisfy FAITHFULNESS. Nonetheless, hypothesis (2b) implies that infants should attend longer to the CV forms than the matched VC forms, since the latter but not the former violate ONSET/NO-CODA, while the two types of forms fare equally well with respect to markedness constraints evaluating individual segments. The results shown in Table 1 confirm the presence of syllable markedness constraints in the grammar of 6-month-old infants.

Table 1. Results of experiments addressing the initial state

	MARKED-NESS	Age (mo)	Con-straints	Higher Harmony *Example* **Mean time** SD / SE (sec)	Lower Harmony *Example* **Mean time** SD / SE (sec)	Difference Proportion *p* *t*
1	ONSET/ NOCODA	6	Marked-ness	*V.CV* **10.99** 2.77 / 0.62	*VC.V* **9.35** 2.98 / 0.67	14/20 .007 2.996
2	ONSET/ NOCODA	6	Marked-ness	*CV* **10.63** 1.64 / 0.37	*VC* **9.50** 1.94 / 0.43	14/20 .017 2.63
3	M$_{\text{NASALPL}}$	4.5	Faithful-ness	*ɪm...po...ɪmpo* ✓M ✓F **15.36** 3.89 / 0.97	*ɪm...po...uŋkə* ✓M *F **12.31** 4.55 / 1.14	11/16 .006 3.22
4	M$_{\text{NASALPL}}$	4.5	Marked-ness	*ɪm...po...ɪmpo* ✓M ✓F **15.23** 4.49 / 1.12	*ɪn...po...ɪmpo* *M ✓F **12.73** 4.80 / 1.20	11/16 .044 2.21
5	M$_{\text{NASALPL}}$	4.5	Marked-ness vs. faithful-ness	*ɪn...po...ɪmpo* ✓M *F **16.75** 4.58 / 1.14	*ɪn...po...ɪmpo* *M ✓F **14.01** 4.01 / 1.00	12/16 .001 4.21

The table further displays the results of Experiments 3 and 4, which provide evidence for the presence of FAITHFULNESS and MARKEDNESS with respect to nasal place, respectively. The relative ranking of these constraints was examined in Experiment 5, which provides evidence confirming the nativist learnability argument's prediction that MARKEDNESS $\gg$ FAITHFULNESS in the grammars of 4.5-month-old infants, the youngest age at which the headturn preference procedure can be employed.[5]

2.3.3 Markedness and faithfulness in older infants

Experiments 3–5 are presented in full in Jusczyk, Smolensky, and Allocco 2002, which also presents seven other experiments. These additional experiments examine nasal place markedness in infants at ages 10, 15, and 20 months. A faithfulness experiment at 10 months confirms the presence of FAITHFULNESS as assessed in the X/Y/XY paradigm, as Experiment 3 did at 4.5 months. Markedness experiments at 10 and 15 months confirm the presence of M_{NP}, as Experiment 4 did at 4.5 months. The results of the markedness versus faithfulness experiments are more complex. At 10 months, infants show the same result as the 4.5-month-olds did in Experiment 5: they favor markedness over faithfulness. At 15 months, however, infants show no preference: there is no significant difference between listening times for the two types of stimuli. This experiment was repeated with 16 different 15-month-olds, with precisely the same results. But this state of indeterminate ranking is short lived. By 20 months, infants return to a clear preference for forms obeying MARKEDNESS at the expense of FAITHFULNESS.

What factors are responsible for the absence of any clear ranking of these markedness and faithfulness constraints in 15-month-olds? The fact that two separate groups of infants at this age displayed exactly the same pattern of results indicates that the absence of any consistent ranking of these constraints should be taken seriously. Daniel Dinnsen (personal communication, 1998) has suggested a possible explanation for the uncertainty in the ranking at 15 months. In particular, it is at this age that infants show the first signs of learning about morphology in their comprehension of language. For example, Shady (1996) found that neither 12- nor 14-month-old English-learning infants showed significant listening preferences for passages with function words (functor morphemes) in the proper position (natural passages) over passages with function words in improper positions (unnatural passages). However, by 16 months, English learners are sensitive to the phonetic and distributional properties of function words and listen longer to the natural passages. Similarly, Santelmann and Jusczyk (1998) explored English learners' sensitivity to the relationship between the auxiliary verb *is* and the verb suffix *-ing*. The *-ing* morpheme is one of the earliest-acquired morphemes in children's productions of English (Brown 1973; de Villiers and de Villiers 1973). Santelmann and Jusczyk found that sensitivity to the basic dependency between the function morpheme *is* and the morpheme *-ing* develops between 15 and 18 months of age. Together, these studies provide evidence

---

[5] In each of Experiments 3–5, 16 infants (7 males, 9 females), from monolingual English-speaking homes, were tested. The average age of the infants for each experiment fell between 4 months, 16 days and 4 months, 20 days, with ages of individual infants ranging from 4 months, 2 days to 5 months, 8 days. Additional infants (6 for Experiments 3 and 4, 14 for Experiment 5) were tested but not included because of excessive fussiness or crying, failing to orient properly to the test apparatus, experimenter error, or parental interference. See Jusczyk, Smolensky, and Allocco 2002.

Table 1

that, beginning around 15 months, infants are becoming sensitive to the presence of morphemes in the speech around them.

As Laura Benua has pointed out (personal communication, 2000), the beginnings of morphology pose difficulties for the child's analysis of nasal assimilation in English. Presented with a single-syllable item like *ım* in a stimulus triad of the experiment, 15-month-old infants may now explore the new possibility that this is a prefix, combining with the following root *po* to form a morphologically complex word *ımpo*. Now under this analysis, it is unclear whether a prefix-final nasal should assimilate to a following consonant: the evidence available from English is mixed. As mentioned earlier, an 'inner' (Level 1), affix like *in-* 'not' will assimilate; an 'outer' (Level 2), affix like *in-* 'directed inward' will not. Until the child's morphology becomes sophisticated enough to sort out such subtleties, the evidence will provide conflicting information about whether it is MARKEDNESS or FAITHFULNESS that should dominate here. The result might well be indefiniteness of ranking of the sort exhibited by the 15-month-olds in our study.

By 20 months, it may be that children are no longer treating the hypothetical forms in the experiment as novel affixes. Perhaps their receptive lexicons are now substantial enough that the complete absence of recognizable lexical items suggests to them that, while the sound patterns they are hearing are highly English-like, these are not actually English lexical items. Thus, perhaps the 20-month-olds are not attempting lexical and morphological analysis, just as an adult presumably would not. The forms are being treated as morphologically simple items, subject to the basic patterns of English phonology, which demand that nasals assimilate. The constraints that are being applied to the experimental stimuli are the most basic ones, where nasal place markedness dominates faithfulness.

2.3.4 Extensions

We have discussed initial work in an experimental research program that attempts to rather directly observe the presence and ranking of grammatical constraints in infants too young to be producing any linguistic utterances. If this research program proves successful, it may become possible for such experimental observation to directly inform theory development, even with respect to some of the most theoretically intricate issues in linguistic theory.

Take nasal place assimilation, for example. It can be exploited to examine a deep theoretical question concerning OT: must the type of optimization used in OT to date be modified to allow constraints to be highly selective in the forms they compare? Wilson (2000) proposes such a fundamental modification of the theory in order to address what he argues to be a fundamental problem in standard OT (see Footnote 12:14). While the problem is much more general, it is nicely illustrated by nasal place assimilation. (Here we apply Wilson's general approach to the particular case of nasal assimilation; this is not a case Wilson treats explicitly.) It appears to be a strong empirical generalization that when a nasal comes in contact with a following consonant with a different place of articulation, if place assimilation occurs, *it must be the nasal that assimilates*. Within standard OT, an output constraint like M_{NP} that requires a nasal consonant N to agree in place with a following consonant C *can* be satisfied by changing the place of C, and, as Wilson shows in a number of such cases, this entails that in the typology predicted by standard OT, there are languages in which it is C, not N, that assimilates under certain general conditions. In Wilson's proposed modification of OT, the markedness constraint M_{NP} is replaced with a different type of constraint, which we will call $^{\rightarrow}M_{NP}$. Now M_{NP} asserts that a form in which a nasal fails to agree in place with a following consonant is less harmonic than *any* form lacking such agreement failure. But $^{\rightarrow}M_{NP}$ is a **targeted constraint**: it asserts only that a form *S* in which a nasal fails to agree in place with a following consonant is less harmonic than the single form *S'*, which is exactly like *S* except that the nasal's place has changed to agree with that of the following consonant.

Targeted constraints solve this and many other important problems for standard OT. But the formal definition of optimization required in the new theory—called TCOT ('TC' for 'targeted constraints')—must be made significantly more complex in order to deal with the new possibility that constraints can be targeted, because such constraints refuse to assert a Harmony relationship between all but a small set of closely related pairs of forms (like *S* and *S'*).

A new type of evidence that a move from OT to the more formally complex TCOT is empirically warranted might be provided by experiments like those discussed above. According to standard OT, triads like *on…ba…onda* should satisfy M_{NP} and thus be preferred to their faithful counterparts *on…ba…onba*. But according to TCOT, the opposite is the case. In TCOT, being unfaithful to the place of a nasal in order to achieve agreement with a following consonant will raise Harmony when markedness outranks faithfulness. But unfaithfulness to the consonant's place cannot raise Harmony: the agreeing form is *not* declared more harmonic by the *targeted* constraint $^{\rightarrow}M_{NP}$—it is merely unfaithful. The studies reported here are neutral concerning the difference between OT and TCOT: since the triads used in the experiment always altered the place of the nasal, OT and TCOT both hold that the resulting unfaithfulness will increase Harmony when markedness outranks faithfulness. Thus, empirical light of a new sort might be directed toward fundamental theoretical questions in phonology by further experiments examining unfaithfulness in the postnasal consonant, and potentially many other theoretically important contexts as well.[6]

[6] Three follow-up experiments conducted by Karen Arnold and Elliott Moreton give a complex pattern of results. Infants 4.5 months old showed no significant preference between *on…ba…onda* and faithful *on…ba…onba* ($p < .4$); OT and TCOT would seem to each predict a difference, although in opposite directions. They also showed no preference between *on…ba…onda* and *on…ba…omba* ($p < .3$). They did, however, prefer *on…ba…omba* to faithful *om…ba…omba* ($p < .05$). It is as though the former's positive evidence for the grammar MARKEDNESS ≫ FAITHFULNESS makes it of greater interest than the latter, which offers no evidence on the relative ranking of MARKEDNESS and FAITHFULNESS because both are satisfied. Yet in Experiment 4 of the text, infants preferred *om…ba…omba* to *on…ba…onba*; while the former may give no ranking evidence, the latter flatly contradicts the grammar MARKEDNESS ≫ FAITHFULNESS. These four experiments, plus Experiment 5 of the text, can be synopsized as follows: If stimulus list *A* is consistent with MARKEDNESS ≫ FAITHFULNESS and *B* is consistent with FAITHFULNESS ≫ MARKEDNESS, then *A* is preferred to *B*; otherwise, there is no reliable

Table 1

3 EXPERIMENTAL EXPLORATIONS OF THE FINAL STATE

In Section 2.3, we discussed experimental evidence suggesting that, at the earliest time they can be tested (4.5 months), infants possess markedness and faithfulness constraints and rank them MARKEDNESS ≫ FAITHFULNESS, as predicted for the initial state by Richness of the Base in a nativist interpretation of OT. We now turn to experimental exploration of the *final* state. In Section 3.1, we consider theoretical implications that partial nativization of loanwords has for Richness of the Base; this leads to the concept of hidden rankings and an extended formulation of Richness of the Base itself. In Section 3.2, we formulate hypotheses linking Extended Richness of the Base to phonological performance, and we present the design of our primary experimental condition. In Section 3.3, we present the experimental results, which reveal hidden strata among the onset clusters illegal in English. In Section 3.4, we analyze the experimental results, introducing the crucial notion of local conjunction of constraints. In Section 3.5, we discuss the other experimental conditions we examined and their implications for our proposed analysis. Finally, in Section 3.6 we briefly consider alternative possible explanations for the experimental findings, and, in Section 3.7, possible explanations for the origin of hidden rankings.

As explained in Section 1, a prediction concerning the final state of the grammar follows immediately from Richness of the Base, and might even be taken as defining it: the constraint ranking of an adult who has mastered English always outputs a form consistent with the general patterns of English, regardless of the input given to the grammar. To probe this aspect of the final state, we wish to induce adult English speakers to give as inputs to their phonological grammars underlying forms that, if faithfully parsed, would be illegal in English. Under such conditions, if Richness of the Base is correct, the grammar must "repair" these "defects", producing an English-legal output.

3.1 Covert grammars

The actual situation must, however, be more complex. We know that when foreign words are borrowed into a language in which their phonological form would be illegal, many types of defects are repaired, but often some types of defects are systematically left untouched (e.g., Saciuk 1969; Kiparsky 1973; Holden 1976; Yip 1993; Itô and Mester 1995b). It is as though the final grammar does not treat all illegal structures equally: some it simply will not tolerate, others it will let pass. As a case in point, consider the well-studied loanword phenomena of Japanese, where, roughly speaking, the established lexicon provides a kind of archaeological slice through time, in which forms that were borrowed at different points in time display different regularities. Itô and Mester (1995a, b, 1999) present an extensive OT analysis that allows us to state this precisely; this has been the point of departure for further work in OT (e.g.,

---

preference. The latter situation arises if *A* or *B* is inconsistent with universal grammar, that is, with *no* ranking between FAITHFULNESS and MARKEDNESS.

Davidson and Noyer 1996; Fukazawa 1998; Fukazawa, Kitahara, and Ota 1998; Katayama 1998).

The truly native or **Yamato** vocabulary of Japanese can be characterized by a certain constraint ranking that sharply divides all forms into the legal and the illegal. But among forms borrowed from Chinese, some of the constraints observed by all Yamato forms are seen to be imposed on the foreign forms, while others are not. Itô and Mester exploit the markedness/faithfulness structure of OT to provide an elegant formal analysis of this mixed situation. According to their analysis, among the constraints obeyed by Yamato forms, some have stronger force than others: they are higher ranked. Schematically, the ranking in (3) holds among the constraints in (4).

(3)　　$M_1 \gg M_2 \gg F \gg M_3$

(4)　　Constraints relevant to Japanese lexical stratification
   a.　M_1　　No voiced geminates.
   b.　M_2　　No unvoiced obstruents following a nasal.
   c.　F　　IDENT([voice]): Voicing of input segments is preserved in the output.
   d.　M_3　　NoCoda

According to this ranking, in native words, the markedness constraint M_3 can be violated, but both M_1 and M_2 must be respected because they dominate a relevant faithfulness constraint F. In the Yamato lexicon, there is no evidence for the relative ranking of M_1 and M_2; their relative ranking might just as well be reversed, as in (5).

(5)　　$M_2 \gg M_1 \gg F \gg M_3$

Alternatively, we could say that the Yamato lexicon provides evidence only for the partial ranking in (6).

(6)　　$\{M_1 , M_2\} \gg F \gg M_3$　　　　—base form of grammar

But when a Japanese speaker processes a Chinese loan input, suppose some faithfulness constraints are allowed to move up in rank, as in (7).

(7)　　$M_1 \gg M_2 \gg F \gg M_3$

This means that the Chinese borrowings will be "repaired" to satisfy M_1, but violations of M_2 will now be tolerated. Such is actually the case in Sino-Japanese forms with the constraints in (4).

We propose to explore what we believe to be a new interpretation of this state of affairs: at the time when the Chinese forms were being borrowed, the base adult Japanese grammar actually *was* (3). The ranking $M_1 \gg M_2$ was a **hidden ranking**: there was no evidence for it in the Japanese lexicon at that time. The forms violating M_1 and those violating M_2 define two **hidden strata** of Japanese, a covert distinction among Japanese-illegal forms.

Suppose furthermore that at the time of borrowing, the ranking of F was somewhat variable: it was a **floating constraint** (Reynolds 1994; Zubritskaya 1994, 1997;

Table 1

Nagy and Reynolds 1997; Anttila 1998; Boersma 1998; Legendre et al. 2000; Boersma and Hayes 2001). Schematically:

(8)　　$M_1 \gg \underline{M_2} \gg M_3$　　　　— covert form of grammar
　　　　　　F

Each time a form is pronounced, the position of a floating constraint is fixed somewhere in its range. Thus, rather than the ranking (3), sometimes the following ranking will apply:

(9)　　$M_1 \gg F \gg M_2 \gg M_3$

When F occupies the lowest ranking in its range, we will say it is in its **base position**, and we will refer to the resulting grammar as the **base ranking**, (3). In both of the total rankings generated by the floating constraint — (3) and (9) — M_1 will be respected in all outputs; but M_2 will be respected only by the outputs of the base grammar. Suppose we assume, as a mutual constraint between the lexicon and the grammar, that a native vocabulary item must be assigned a consistent pronunciation by the grammar: the output must be the same for both rankings (3) and (9). The native forms, then, must all obey M_2. Therefore, considering only native lexical forms, there is no evidence for the true full ranking (8) — only for the partial ranking (6).

But the nonnative inputs provided by Chinese allow us to see the hidden rankings in the final state. Suppose that, perhaps with the commitment of additional cognitive resources, the speaker can sometimes push the ranking of F up to its elevated position. This allows for a more faithful pronunciation of the foreign input, although not generally a fully faithful pronunciation, as there remain markedness constraints like M_1 that are ranked still higher than elevated F. The result is that the foreign input will be partially nativized. And the character of the partial nativization in the output provides information about the adult Japanese grammar that could not be extracted by considering native forms alone: it shows that the grammar possesses the hidden rankings in (8) and that the description in (6) is inaccurate.

Over time, the incorporation of a large number of borrowed Chinese forms into the Japanese lexicon presumably led to the establishment of a standardized elevated 'docking' position for F, with the now-partially-nativized Sino-Japanese lexical items marked in the lexicon as forming a distinct **stratum** corresponding to this elevated FAITHFULNESS position. At this point, learning Japanese includes learning the different positions for F, so no special cognitive effort is involved in employing the Sino-Japanese vocabulary.

The ultimate fate of loanwords in a language is not our direct concern here. What is relevant to our discussion is only the initial point in the borrowing process, a point at which a foreign input is being processed by a grammar that was learned in a linguistic environment in which such forms were absent. Our interest in this arises because of its potential to reveal the structure of the final state of a native grammar.

These considerations lead to the following extension of Richness of the Base to grammars with floating FAITHFULNESS.

(10)   **Extended Richness of the Base**

    a.   The final state of the grammar is in general a partial ranking containing floating faithfulness constraints.

    b.   The location of a faithfulness constraint within its range is probabilistic. For any given input, this range of total rankings yields a set of outputs (possibly a singleton); the probability of each output in this set equals the probability of the collection of all total rankings yielding that output.

    c.   Marginally, this may lead to variation in the surface forms of the language.

    d.   Abstracting away from surface variation, the core generalizations exhibited in the (nonvarying) surface forms of a language arise because its lexical items are subject to the metaconstraint that their outputs must be constant over the grammar, that is, constant over the floating range of faithfulness constraints. Underlying forms are otherwise unconstrained.

    e.   Thus, for a native input, the output of the grammar is invariable and therefore equal to the single output of the base grammar (with faithfulness constraints at the bottom of their floating range). For native inputs, only the base grammar need be considered; floating can be ignored.

    f.   Inputs that are *not* drawn from the native lexicon will in general yield variable outputs; with FAITHFULNESS elevated from the base grammar, outputs of nonnative inputs will in general violate the surface generalizations of the language.

    g.   It follows that the base grammar satisfies standard Richness of the Base: it generates only outputs respecting the surface generalizations of the language, given any input whatever.

An argument for the crucial final point (10g) goes as follows. Suppose there were some possible input I, which the base grammar mapped to an output O, which violated a surface generalization. This case would arise because the relevant markedness constraints were outranked by relevant faithfulness constraints in their base position. But then I would also yield O with FAITHFULNESS elevated from its base position. Thus, I would yield O consistently across the full grammar with floating constraints, so I would be a potential underlying form. Since there are no other constraints on underlying forms, there is nothing to bar such an I from the lexicon, thereby destroying the observed surface generalization.[7] Therefore, such an I cannot exist.

An important feature of Extended Richness of the Base (10) is that it subsumes previous work in OT under standard Richness of the Base: this work is now taken to be the study of base grammars, which are determined by the inventory of native forms. The consequences of floating FAITHFULNESS only arise when analyzing the partial nativization evident in actual outputs from nonnative inputs, or the residue of

---

[7] This abbreviated argument assumes a simplified situation like that discussed above, in which a single faithfulness constraint is floating. An argument considering the fully general case with multiple faithfulness constraints that may change their relative ranking by floating is beyond the scope of the present discussion.

Table 1

such partial nativization in borrowing-induced lexical strata. It is precisely for such analysis that floating FAITHFULNESS has been previously invoked.

Knowing the articulated final ranking provided in the covert form displayed in (9)—rather than the less informative base form illustrated in (6)—is important not only to precisely account for the partial nativization of foreign words, but also to account for second language (L2) acquisition. It is commonly assumed in the L2 literature that for adults learning a second language, the initial state for L2 acquisition is the final state of their native language, L1 (Broselow and Finer 1991; Archibald 1993; Broselow and Park 1995; Pater 1997; Broselow, Chen, and Wang 1998; Hancin-Bhatt and Bhatt 1998). But the unarticulated base form of the grammar of L1 is generally silent on distinctions that are important in L2. For inputs from the L1 vocabulary, the base form suffices to determine the optimal output, but for the foreign inputs of L2, other rankings can be crucial. And in order to account for early L2 productions and the influence of L1 on the initial course of L2 acquisition, the ability of L1 speakers to elevate faithfulness constraints in the face of foreign inputs needs to be precisely specified, as it is in the covert form of the ranking.

Because ultimate application to L2 was a primary motivation for the work reported below, the phonological domain we chose to explore in our experiments was one frequently studied in the L2 literature: consonant clusters. Previous work has focused on cases in which L2 is English and L1 is a language whose inventory of clusters is impoverished relative to that of English (Broselow 1983; Anderson 1987; Tropf 1987; Broselow and Finer 1991; Eckman and Iverson 1993; Archibald 1998; Carlisle 1998; Hancin-Bhatt and Bhatt 1998). Because English speakers were most readily available as experimental participants, we chose English for L1 and tested the production of clusters that are illegal in English. As a convenient way to get a large number of fluently produced English-illegal clusters, we asked a Polish speaker to generate the experimental stimuli. While our results have implications for English-speaking learners of Polish, that was not the topic of this research. Rather, our goal was to examine the consonant cluster component of the final state of the English grammar.

3.2 Experimental design

In the experimental work we now summarize, our goal is to determine the degree to which phonological theory in OT can contribute to an understanding of performance. To this end, we adopt the following strong working hypotheses linking competence and performance, with the intention of backing off from these hypotheses only as compelled by the performance data.

(11) Linking hypotheses, final state: Probability of production = probability of grammar output

    a. In the face of nonnative inputs, speakers can, when sufficient cognitive resources are allocated, elevate a faithfulness constraint from its base posi-

tion to a higher position within its floating range. Increasing the probability of greater deviation from the base position requires allocating greater
cognitive resources at the time of production.

b.   Given a nonnative form to pronounce, the probability that a speaker will
actually produce a given output is the probability assigned to that output
by the grammar, where the input to the grammar is the underlying form
faithful to the given form. This assumes the speaker has sufficient cognitive resources to correctly perceive the form and retain it in memory until
the time of production.

Later, we will examine these hypotheses in light of our experimental results; for now,
we simply adopt it in order to see how much insight into performance can be directly
provided by grammatical theory.

A task that makes ample cognitive resources available is simple repetition of a
foreign form. This is the condition under which FAITHFULNESS can best be elevated,
sometimes resulting in quite faithful rendering of forms that violate multiple surface
generalizations of the native language. We will discuss experimental results concerning the repetition task in Section 3.5. Our primary concern, however, is to design an
experimental condition that best reveals the base grammar of the language, which,
according to Richness of the Base, forces any input to meet the surface generalizations of English.

In our experimental design, 16 monolingual adult native English speakers were
asked to produce forms with initial clusters illegal in English. The procedure is schematically shown in Figure 1. (For full details, see Davidson 2001.)

Figure 1. Experimental procedure

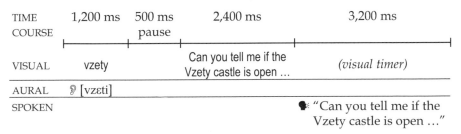

TIME COURSE	1,200 ms	500 ms pause	2,400 ms	3,200 ms
VISUAL	vzety		Can you tell me if the Vzety castle is open ...	*(visual timer)*
AURAL	𝔇 [vzɛti]			
SPOKEN				🔊 "Can you tell me if the Vzety castle is open ..."

The target item — *vzety* in the example of Figure 1 — was presented in both aural and
written form; the orthography was English-like (not IPA or Polish). The written
forms were intended to decrease the probability of misperceiving the consonants in
the cluster; it is likely that the combined aural and visual presentation also produced
a stronger representation in memory, decreasing the probability of memory errors.
Speakers were asked to produce the target item in the middle of a carrier sentence
that was presented visually; this was intended to increase the probability that the
"normal" English grammar was employed during production of the target item.

Figure 1   *Table 1*

Three further aspects of the design were also intended to minimize deviations from English. First, during production, the written form of the sentence was not available, so speakers could not simply read the target item; they had to generate it, along with the rest of the sentence, from a representation in memory. Second, a visual timer provided pressure for a slightly speeded response, again with the intention of minimizing opportunities for shifting out of the English grammar. Third, to further discourage speakers—at a conscious level—from deviating from "normal" English in order to produce the foreign item, were told to imagine themselves as American spies in a foreign country. They were told that to avoid raising suspicion, they were to act like "typical American tourists": if they were too accurate with their pronunciations of the foreign words, they would be uncovered as American spies.

In the terms of the linking hypotheses (11), the experiment was designed to strike a delicate balance with respect to the cognitive resources available to the speakers at the time they produced the target item. Combined visual and aural presentation of the target item was intended to provide an accurate, robust representation of the target, so the task demands would not be so great as to induce errors in what we analyze as the *input* to the grammar. The other factors were intended to make the task sufficiently demanding at production time that speakers would not have ample resources available to elevate faithfulness constraints. Below, we will compare performance in this experimental condition with performance in other conditions that presumably allowed greater allocation of cognitive resources to elevating FAITHFULNESS; as we will show, the propensity to nativize the input then reduces substantially.

The particular initial consonant clusters used in the experimental materials were chosen to meet several criteria: they must be present in Polish; they must be absent in English but involve no non-English segments; they must be sufficiently few to enable all trials of the experiment to be completed in a sufficiently short time; they should vary along multiple phonetic dimensions and sample clusters with varying sonority distances. The last criterion reflects a hypothesis discussed below that a substantial factor in performance on a target cluster is whether English permits the sonority distance between its segments. The experimental materials contained 15 clusters, each used as the onset of four different disyllabic pseudo-Polish words; there were 30 carrier sentences, each used twice.

3.3 Experimental results

The results of the experiment are displayed in Figure 2, which also shows the particular target clusters employed. Plotted is the mean proportion correct over all speakers and all tokens of a given cluster.

The clusters fall into four rather distinct groups. Performance was above 90% on all English-legal clusters (*šl, sn, šr, sm, fl*), assuming *šl* to be legal at least in the East Coast American dialect predominating among our experimental participants. Performance dropped to 63% for what we will call the **easy** non-English clusters, *zm* and *zr*. Performance dropped again to 34–39% for the **intermediate** clusters *kt, pt, kp, čk*.

The cluster *tf* falls halfway between the intermediate and easy clusters; it is convenient for analysis to group it with the intermediate clusters, which can then be characterized as the voiceless-stop-initial clusters. (Obviously, more extensive and systematic follow-up experiments will be needed for a more definitive classification of clusters of this type.) Lowest in terms of performance were the **difficult** clusters *vn, vz,*
and *dv*, at 11–20% correct.

Figure 2. Experimental results

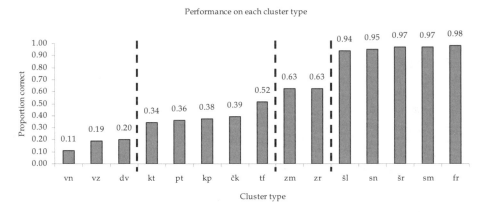

While the labels easy/intermediate/difficult are transparent, we emphasize that
the dependent measure in the experiment is *accuracy*, not *difficulty* per se.

Pairwise comparison of performance on individual clusters shows statistical justification for the post hoc three-way grouping of the English-illegal clusters. In Figure
3, we summarize the significance levels of performance differences, taking $p < .1$ as
our criterion. The grayed cells correspond to comparisons of clusters in the same
class; these should not show significant differences, and they do not. The white cells
correspond to comparisons of clusters in different classes; these should show significant differences, and they do. The only exceptions are indicated by the numbers in
Figure 3, which give p levels too high to satisfy the criterion. We have listed only one
cluster in the English-legal class, since all these clusters behave alike statistically.

At the boundary between the intermediate and difficult classes, the comparison
kt versus *dv* barely fails the criterion of significance ($p < .12$). The other exceptions all
involve *tf*. Performance on *tf* fails to differ significantly from performance on either
member of the easy class (*zr, zm*); while it differs significantly from performance on
the two members of the intermediate class on which scores were lowest (*pt* and *kt*), it
fails to differ significantly from performance on the other two (although with *kp* it is
close). (While there may be some indication here that *tf* is better classified as easy, we

Figure 2   *Table 1*

will await more significant results before complicating the analysis proposed below to account for such a classification.)[8]

Figure 3. Pairwise cluster differences (where not indicated otherwise, white: $p < .1$; gray: $p \geq .1$)

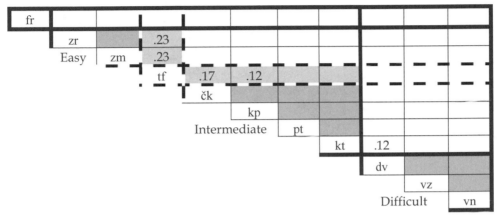

As a final, within-speaker means for confirming our grouping of clusters, we tested the following prediction implicit in the grouping: each subject should produce more correct forms for clusters of the easy class than for clusters of the intermediate class, and similarly more for the intermediate than for the difficult class.

In the scatter plots shown in Figure 4, each point represents the performance of a single speaker. In the first plot, proportion correct on easy clusters is plotted on the y-axis, while intermediate cluster performance is plotted on the x-axis. All points are predicted to lie above the principal diagonal ($y = x$), that is, in the upper left triangle. This prediction is confirmed ($p < .002$), with only two speakers failing to meet it. Exactly the same result holds in the intermediate/difficult comparison shown in the second scatter plot.

The experimental results seem to suggest that the illegal initial clusters are divided by the grammar of English into 'hidden strata', each group of clusters defining a stratum. Inputs with clusters from the easy stratum are most likely to produce faithful, English-illegal outputs, with no nativization. Inputs with clusters in the intermediate and difficult strata are successively less likely to surface faithfully, that is, more likely to undergo nativization.

---

[8] A natural direction for refining the analysis would be to consider *tf* to occupy its own stratum between easy and intermediate, and analyze it by extending the hierarchy proposed below for consonant release: *$S_{\bar{A}} \gg {}^*C_C$ (14)–(15). Introducing a new constraint in this family, ranked above the other two, *$S_{[-cont]}$ ('A stop must not release into a noncontinuant'), would distinguish *tf*, which satisfies the new constraint, from the intermediate clusters, which violate it. (Although the status of the affricate in *čk* is a complexity we systematically ignore here, simply treating it like a stop.)

Figure 4. Performance comparisons between accuracy classes

Intermediate vs. difficult

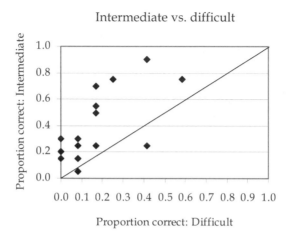

Proportion correct: Difficult

Easy vs. intermediate

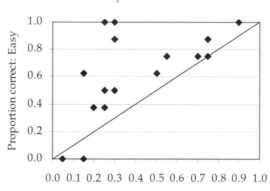

Proportion correct: Intermediate

The "repairs" performed when English-illegal inputs failed to surface faithfully overwhelmingly took the form of epenthesis, as shown in Figure 5.

Figure 4   *Table 1*

Figure 5. Error types

Error categories

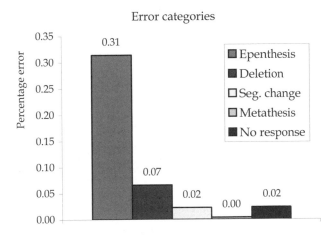

3.4 Analysis

We now examine whether phonological theory can shed light on the hidden strata revealed by the experiment. One hypothesis already proposed in the literature, which in fact guided the selection of the clusters used, is that a primary role is played by sonority distance—the difference in sonority levels of the consonants (see Box 12:2). English allows some clusters with a sonority distance of 1 (e.g., *sn*) but none with sonority distance of 0 (e.g, **pk*). This hypothesis predicts, then, that speakers should produce English-illegal clusters with a legal sonority distance (1 or more) more accurately than those with the illegal sonority distance 0. As shown in Table 2, however, this is not the case.

Table 2. Sonority distance versus cluster accuracy

Sonority distance	Difficult			Intermediate					Easy	
	vn	vz	dv	kt	kp	pt	čk	tf	zm	zr
0		•		•	•	•	•			
≥ 1	•		•					•	•	•

In Table 2, the clusters are listed in order of increasing proportion correct; there is little correlation between this sequence and the distinction between sonority distances. The lack of performance difference between the two sonority-distance categories was evident in a one-way repeated-measures analysis of variance (ANOVA) across the mean proportion correct for each category; among English-illegal clusters, there was no significant effect either by subjects ($F_1(1, 15) = 2.65$, $p > .12$) or by items ($F_2(1, 38) = 1.75$, $p > .19$). (There was a significant effect of English-legal vs. English-illegal among the clusters with nonzero sonority distance; $p < .0001$ by both subjects and items.)

Given that sonority distance appears to distinguish clusters too coarsely, we turn to a more fine-grained analysis in terms of phonological features, many of which in fact provide the substrate for sonority conditions on onset well-formedness (Section 14.6). Can the markedness of different feature combinations, suitably formalized, account for the hidden strata? Table 3 is suggestive.

Table 3. Featural analysis of clusters
(S = stop; F = fricative; A = approximant; Ā = nonapproximant)

English-legal clusters	(−voi S)A	pl, pr, tr, kl, kr	
	(−voi F)A	fl, fr, sl, šl, šr	
	(−voi, cor F)Ā	sm, sn, šn, šm, sv, sf	
	(**+voi** S)A	bl, br, dr, gl, gr	
English-illegal clusters (from experiment)	(**+voi**, cor F)A	zr	Easy
	(**+voi**, cor F)Ā	zm	
	(−voi, cor <u>S˺</u>)Ā	tf, čk	Intermediate
	(−voi, *¬cor* <u>S˺</u>)Ā	kt, kp, pt	
	(**+voi**, cor <u>S˺</u>)Ā	dv	Difficult
	(**+voi**, *¬cor* F)Ā	vn, vz	

What the table shows is that as as performance on the clusters gets worse, the clusters themselves get more and more *marked*. In Table 3, marked feature values along various dimensions have been highlighted; the basic markedness constraints involved are given in (12). The markedness of [+voi(ce)] for obstruents is indicated by highlighting this feature in boldface; the markedness of noncoronal place, by highlighting [¬cor] in bold italics. The markedness of [+continuant] for obstruents (or perhaps for onsets) is indicated by boldface on F = fricative. And underlining highlights the markedness of a stop followed by a nonapproximant (Ā); in this environment, the stop is marked because it is unreleased, as indicated by S˺. We return to this dimension of markedness in a moment.

(12)   Segmental markedness constraints

	a.	*F	*[+continuant, −sonorant]	No fricatives.
	b.	*VOL_SON	*[+voice, −sonorant]	No voiced obstruents.
	c.	*COR	*PL/{[labial], [dorsal]}	No noncoronal place.

What Table 3 suggests is that, if the compounding of markedness with decreasing accuracy can be properly formalized, it should allow an explanation of the hidden strata. But the strong interaction of markedness dimensions evidenced here requires a technical device that allows a special type of inventory: one that 'bans only the worst of the worst' (Prince and Smolensky 1993/2004, Chap. 9). As a simple example, consider the interaction of voicing and continuancy, both of which are marked in obstruents. As the initial member of a cluster, a voiced obstruent is marked—but the inventory of English clusters nonetheless includes voiced-obstruent-initial clus-

Figure 5   *Table 3*

ters (e.g., *bl*). Similarly, continuant obstruents (fricatives) are marked—but as an initial consonant, they are allowed in the English cluster inventory (e.g., *fl*). However, an initial obstruent that is both voiced and continuant—the worst of the worst—is excluded from the inventory (e.g., **vl*). Such an inventory—one that bans only the worst of the worst—cannot be achieved by simply ranking the relevant faithfulness constraints with the relevant markedness constraints *F and *VOL$_\text{SON}$. For allowing any fricatives at all requires that *F be outranked by all relevant faithfulness constraints (e.g., MAX); otherwise, optimal outputs would be unfaithful to avoid violating *F. The same must be true of *VOL$_\text{SON}$ since voiced obstruents are allowed in the inventory. But now it must be that the inventory also contains obstruents that are both continuant and voiced—voiced fricatives—because all relevant faithfulness constraints must outrank both *F and *VOL$_\text{SON}$.

Not only are inventories that bar only the worst of the worst common, they are, it would seem, a type of inventory for which OT ought to provide a natural account, since they are readily understood in terms of banning sufficiently marked elements. (More formally, these inventories have the central OT property of **harmonic completeness**—they are, in fact, necessary in general to fill out OT typologies sufficiently to achieve **strong harmonic completeness**; Prince and Smolensky 1993/2004, Chap. 9.) As discussed in detail in Chapter 14, there is a simple, general means for admitting worst-of-the-worst inventories and achieving strong harmonic completeness in OT typologies. (In fact, the complex problem of Lango vowel harmony analyzed at length in Chapter 14 displays considerable formal similarity to the problem posed here by cluster inventories.) The proposal is that, besides interacting via domination, constraints in OT interact via the **local conjunction operator**, & (Smolensky 1993, 1995, 1997). We illustrate with the current example in tableau (13). *F & *VOL$_\text{SON}$ is a constraint violated by a segment that is *both* a fricative *and* a voiced obstruent. This constraint makes it possible to strengthen the interaction between *F and *VOL$_\text{SON}$ beyond that which arises by mere domination; it now becomes possible for OT to yield the desired inventory banning only the worst of the worst. In addition to the rankings discussed above, which admit into the inventories obstruents that are either continuant or voiced but not both, we add the local conjunction *F & *VOL$_\text{SON}$ to the grammar, ranking it above all relevant faithfulness constraints. Now, while the markedness incurred by either *F or *VOL$_\text{SON}$ alone is *not* sufficient to render an unfaithful output optimal, the markedness incurred by both together *is*. (In this chapter, individual violations of basic constraints (e.g., *F and *VOL$_\text{SON}$) are marked by '⊙' when they combine to trigger a violation of their conjunction (*F & *VOL$_\text{SON}$). We consider here only the special case of a cluster-initial consonant; how this restriction is achieved in the actual proposed analysis—via further local conjunction—will be evident shortly.)

In general, the conjunction of a constraint $\mathbb{C}_1$ with another constraint $\mathbb{C}_2$ local to a domain type $\mathcal{D}$, written $\mathbb{C}_1 \&_{\mathcal{D}} \mathbb{C}_2$, is a new constraint that is violated if and only if there is both a violation of $\mathbb{C}_1$ and a violation of $\mathbb{C}_2$ within a single domain of type $\mathcal{D}$.

The relevant domain is frequently the segment, as it is in the analysis we propose here.[9]

(13)   Local conjunction enables inventories that ban only the worst of the worst

	*F & *VOL$_{SON}$	MAX	*F	*VOL$_{SON}$
/blik/				
☞ blik				*
lik		*!		
/flik/				
☞ flik			*	
lik		*!		
/vlik/				
vlik	*!		❂	❂
☞ lik		*		

Before showing how local conjunction provides the necessary means of combining markedness dimensions to account for the hidden strata in the English cluster grammar, we return to a dimension of markedness particular to the cluster environment, one involving consonant release.

According to Steriade (1993), a plain, released stop is a plosive (total absence of oral airflow) followed by an approximant (maximum degree of oral aperture): a liquid, glide, or vowel. In English onsets, stops can only appear before approximants; unreleased stops are prohibited. In medial and final positions, on the other hand, this prohibition does not hold (*apt, aptitude*). The following constraint expresses the markedness of a stop that is followed by a nonapproximant:[10]

(14)   *S$_{\bar{A}}$ A stop must release into an approximant in onsets (no S before Ā).

*S$_{\bar{A}}$ is related to the following constraint, which prefers CV syllables:

(15)   *C$_C$ A consonant must release into a vowel in onsets (no C before C).

Any violation of *S$_{\bar{A}}$—a stop followed by a nonapproximant, hence nonvowel—will entail a violation of *C$_C$. Hence, *S$_{\bar{A}}$ is in a Pāṇinian relation with the more general constraint *C$_C$. And so, by Pāṇini's Theorem, in order for *S$_{\bar{A}}$ to be active, it must be ranked above *C$_C$ (Prince and Smolensky 1993/2004, Chap. 5). That SĀ clusters are banned in English, but not all clusters are, is due to the existence of a relevant faithfulness constraint ranked between the two constraints *S$_{\bar{A}}$ and *C$_C$; this admits into

---

[9] Local conjunction has been employed for a variety of purposes in OT phonology and syntax; see the multiple references in Chapter 14.

[10] Related results are reported by Davidson (2003), who showed that when asked to produce *f*-initial, *z*-initial, and *v*-initial clusters, speakers are reliably more accurate on *f*C than *z*C than *v*C. These data are also treated as evidence for hidden strata, but the analysis of the results differs slightly from that presented here in that the constraints are formulated to incorporate insights both from Steriade's (1997) Licensing-by-Cue framework and from Articulatory Phonology (Browman and Goldstein 1986 et seq.).

Figure 5   *Table 3*

the inventory FĀ and SA clusters (which both satisfy *S$_{\bar{A}}$), but bars SĀ clusters. For concreteness of exposition, we will assume that the specific faithfulness constraint relevant here is DEP, since epenthesis was the most common simplification strategy used by participants in the experiment.[11] Since there were few errors of deletion or segment change, MAX and IDENT evidently outrank DEP (Section 12:1.4).

With these tools in place, we can posit a ranking to account for the hidden strata in the English grammar. In Table 4, Table 3 has been expanded to show the constraint violations of legal English clusters and the illegal clusters used in the experiment. Each cell in the final column shows the local conjunctions that render each class of clusters more marked than those appearing higher in the table; the violations of the individual constraints in these conjunctions are marked with '✪'.

Table 4. Decreasing accuracy with increasing markedness, constraints unranked

			*S$_{\bar{A}}$	*C$_C$	*VOL$_{-SON}$	*F	*COR	Crucial violated constraints
English	(−voi S)A	tr,pl,pr,kl,kr		*			(*)	
	(−voi F)A	sl,šl,šr,fl,fr		*		*	(*)	
	(−voi, cor F)Ā	sm,sn,šn,šm,sv,		*		*		
		sf,dr,bl,br,gl,gr		*	*		(*)	
	(**+voi** S)A							
Easy	(**+voi**, cor F)C	zr, zm		✪	✪	✪		*VOL$_{-SON}$ & *F & *C$_C$
Int.	(−voi, cor S̲)Ā	tf, čk	✪	*				*S$_{\bar{A}}$
	(−voi, ¬cor S̲)Ā	kt, kp, pt	✪	*			*	
Diff.	(**+voi**, cor S̲)Ā	dv	✪	*	✪			*VOL$_{-SON}$ & *S$_{\bar{A}}$
	(**+voi**, ¬cor F)Ā	vn, vz		✪	✪	✪	✪	*COR & *VOL$_{-SON}$ & *F & *C$_C$

The interpretation of Table 4 may be illustrated as follows. The clusters *zr, zm* are more marked than legal English clusters because the initial segment is the locus of *three* simultaneous constraint violations, namely, *VOL$_{-SON}$, *F, and *C$_C$; the three marks '✪' incurred by the initial *z* in these clusters entail violation of the local conjunction *VOL$_{-SON}$ & *F & *C$_C$. Note that violating any *two* of these constraints in the same segment does not generate sufficient markedness to result in exclusion from English. Violating *F and *C$_C$ in the same segment is permitted, as in the cluster *fl*;

---

[11] In fact, experimental results from ultrasound imaging of the tongue during production of nonnative clusters suggest that epenthesis of a schwa is probably not how speakers repair the phonotactically illegal sequences (Davidson 2003). Instead, these results indicate that speakers are failing to coordinate the consonants with sufficient overlap, resulting in production of a transitional schwa between the two consonants. For a formal analysis of this repair within a gestural coordination framework, see Davidson 2003.

violating *VOL$_{SON}$ and *C$_C$ is likewise acceptable (*bl*). And both *VOL$_{SON}$ and *F are violated in all voiced fricatives (*z*).

Note that all clusters violate *C$_C$, which functions like *COMPLEX in Prince and Smolensky 1993/2004, except that it explicitly localizes its violation to the initial C of a CC cluster. Thus, to violate a *local* conjunction $\mathbb{C}$ & *C$_C$, the violation of $\mathbb{C}$ must occur in the *initial* segment of a CC cluster (or, more generally, in a C that is not the final segment of a cluster).

To take one more example from Table 4: like the easy clusters, the difficult clusters *vn*, *vz* violate the third-order conjunction [*VOL$_{SON}$ & *F & *C$_C$]. In addition, however, the initial consonant *v* has marked place; that is, it violates *COR. Thus, the increased markedness of these difficult clusters is registered by their violation of the fourth-order conjunction *COR & [*VOL$_{SON}$ & *F & *C$_C$].

It is clear in Table 4 that constraint ranking plays an important role in distinguishing the hidden strata. The cluster *tf*, like many English legal clusters, violates only two of the listed constraints, yet it falls in the intermediate stratum, while the cluster *zr*, violating three constraints, falls in the easy stratum. Unlike *zr*, the cluster *tf* violates *S$_Å$, a constraint that is unviolated among the English-legal clusters. The high rank of *S$_Å$ is responsible for its strong impact, single-handedly separating the easy clusters, which satisfy it, from the intermediate clusters, which do not.

The formal definition of each conjunctive constraint in Table 4 follows automatically from the general definition of constraint conjunction, together with the substantive definitions of the basic constraints that are conjoined, given above in (12), (14), and (15). It is useful, however, to provide an English paraphrase of the *effect* of these conjunctions; this is given in (16).

(16) Exegesis of local conjunctions (within onset clusters)

	Conjunction	Violated by:
a.	___ *VOL$_{SON}$ & *F & *C$_C$	a voiced fricative before any C
b.	*COR & *VOL$_{SON}$ & *F & *C$_C$	a noncoronal voiced fricative before any C
c.	*VOL$_{SON}$ & *S$_Å$	a voiced stop before an obstruent or nasal

The ranking implicit in Table 4 is made explicit in Figure 6. The floating range of DEP is indicated, with four positions indicated by the circled digits. The base position ❶ defines the base grammar of English, which admits only those clusters appearing in English lexical items. Elevating DEP to the next higher position ② adds to the inventory the group of easy clusters. Elevating DEP still further, to position ③ and then to ④, incrementally adds the intermediate and then the difficult clusters.

To explicitly relate this grammar to the dependent variable observed in the experiment, proportion correct, first consider the simplest assumption, **uniform floating** (Anttila 1998). On this assumption, all positions ❶–④ are visited with equal probability under the conditions of the experiment. The predicted values for percentage correct production in the four strata are given in Table 5. For a cluster in the difficult stratum (last row) to be correctly produced, DEP must float to its highest position (④),

Figure 5 *Table 4*

which, under the uniform floating hypothesis, occurs on 25% of productions. For the intermediate stratum, floating to ④ entails correct production, but so does floating to ③. Thus, the predicted percentage correct production is now 50%. And so forth up to the English-legal stratum, where correct production is predicted to be 100%.

Figure 6. English grammar: Hidden constraint rankings and hidden cluster strata

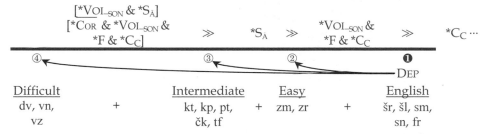

It is important that the theory correctly accounts for the qualitative ordering of the strata, regardless of the quantitative assumptions concerning the probability DEP will float to each of the four positions. Each position that yields correct production in one stratum *s* also yields correct production in the strata listed above *s* in Table 5. Thus, whatever the quantitative value of the probabilities of visiting different positions, the predicted percentage correct will increase up the table. (This would be true even if the visitation probability were greatest for ④ and least for ❶.)

Table 5. Proportion correct across hidden strata

	EXPERIMENT	THEORY	Uniform floating		Empirically fit floating	
Cluster stratum	Observed correct	FAITH position	Visitation probability	Predicted correct	Visitation probability	Predicted correct
šr, šl, sm, sn, fr	96%	❶	25%	100%	33%	96%
zm, zr	63%	②	25%	75%	23%	63%
kt, kp, pt, čk, tf	40%	③	25%	50%	24%	40%
dv, vn, vz	16%	④	25%	25%	16%	16%

Using the observed percentage correct values, it is easy to fit the data with assumed values for visitation probabilities, as shown in the portion of Table 5 headed 'Empirically fit floating'. Thus, the experimental results suggest that the probability of elevating DEP to different positions decreases as the degree of elevation increases: most probable is the base position ❶ (33%); least probable, the highest ④ (16%).

The values for visitation probabilities in Table 5 are fit to average accuracy values over all subjects. The scatter plots in Figure 4—with a separate point for each speaker—show considerable variance across speakers. On the analysis we are proposing, this variance may be attributed to differences across speakers and trials of the effectiveness of cognitive resources allocated to the elevation of FAITHFULNESS. The relative rankings of markedness constraints, however, are what define the hidden strata, and the evidence is consistent with a common underlying hidden ranking of MARKEDNESS across speakers. While one speaker might be unusually successful at elevating FAITHFULNESS, a shared hidden MARKEDNESS ranking entails that, no matter how good that speaker's performance may be on difficult clusters, that same speaker's performance on intermediate clusters must be better, and on easy clusters, better still. Averaging within speakers over the clusters in each hidden stratum, Figure 4 shows that this prediction is strikingly borne out, holding for all but 2 of 16 speakers.

3.5 Other experimental conditions

As explained in Section 3.2, the experimental condition we have discussed so far was designed to minimize the cognitive resources allocated to elevating FAITHFULNESS in response to a clearly foreign input, without overly taxing the resources required to accurately perceive and recall that input. According to the linking hypotheses (11), if greater resources are made available, the probability of elevating FAITHFULNESS should increase, predicting higher proportions of faithful pronunciations.

The same speakers who participated in the experimental condition reported above also participated in two other conditions. The first of these — the 'foreign condition' — was just like the one reported above (the 'English condition'), except that the instructions were different (the stimuli were identical). Now speakers were asked to imagine themselves as tourists traveling in a foreign country. While they did not know the language of this country, they would find themselves having to ask natives for directions to different places, or how to buy different products. They could assume that the natives spoke some English, but they were warned to pronounce the foreign word as carefully as possible, since if they did not, the natives might misunderstand them.

The intent in this manipulation was to probe the conscious, metalinguistic component of the task. In the English condition, speakers were discouraged at a conscious level from making special efforts to faithfully pronounce the foreign words; in the foreign condition, speakers were explicitly encouraged to make such efforts.

In the third, 'repetition' condition, subjects heard two repetitions of one token of a word and were then asked to repeat it. The English-like orthographic representation of the word was available throughout the trial, during both perception and production. The same pseudo-Polish words were used as in the other two conditions.

We assume that, in the terms of the linking hypotheses (11), the cognitive resources available for elevating FAITHFULNESS were greatest in the repetition condition, least in the English condition, and intermediate in the foreign condition. Accordingly, these hypotheses predict that the proportion of faithful productions should increase from the English to the foreign and again to the repetition condition. More specifi-

Figure 6   *Table 5*

cally, they predict that the same hidden strata should be evident in all three conditions: these strata are defined by the relative rankings of markedness constraints, which are unaffected by the across-condition manipulations.

The experimental results are shown in Figure 7. As the graph shows, there is a very strong correlation between the performance ordering of clusters across the three conditions. In fact, the rank correlations between the English and repetition conditions is 0.97, that between the English and foreign conditions is 0.91, and that between the foreign and repetition conditions is 0.89 (all p < .001).

There is some evidence for discrete strata in the foreign condition, and while these correlate with those of the English condition, the boundaries of the intermediate stratum seem to shift: *čk* approaches the difficult group, while the others approach the easy group. Evidence for strata in the repetition condition is even murkier, perhaps because a ceiling effect is starting to set in: as performance starts to approach 100%, there is less variation across the majority of clusters and so achieving statistically significant differences requires more experimental power.

As far as the manipulation concerning instructions is concerned, there is little evidence that conscious attempts to "sound foreign" (rather than "sound American") affect the *relative* accuracy of the clusters, although the proportion of faithful utterances increases for nearly all clusters. The only exceptions are *sn*, *sm*, where speakers displayed a tendency to produce *šn*, *šm* in their attempts to "sound foreign."

Figure 7. Experimental results: English, foreign, and repetition conditions

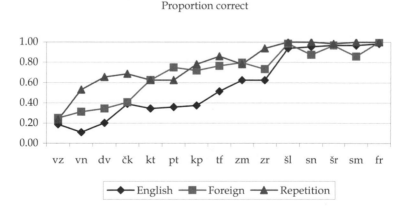

Proportion correct

3.6 Alternative hypotheses

In this section, we briefly consider a few alternative approaches to explaining the experimental findings.

3.6.1   Final grammar = base grammar

In our basic hypothesis (10), we have assumed that the final state of the grammar includes floating FAITHFULNESS, with the lowest positions of faithfulness constraints defining the base grammar. The native lexicon is constrained to yield consistent outputs from the full grammar, and as a consequence floating FAITHFULNESS has no effect on the outputs from native inputs. With nonnative inputs, however, we can see the effects of floating FAITHFULNESS, revealing the full grammar, including covert rankings.

An obvious alternative is to simply assume that the final state of the grammar is the base grammar, with no floating FAITHFULNESS (leaving aside the flotation responsible for variation in native outputs, which we have been neglecting in our general discussion). Faced with a nonnative input, the speakers in our experiment simply depart from their English grammar, "artificially" elevating FAITHFULNESS in some way driven by the particular demands of the artificial tasks we ask them to perform.

The differences between this interpretation and the one presented in (10) are subtle, and we take no strong stance. We presented (10) as our initial hypothesis because it is the grammatically strongest one, in the sense of making the grammar responsible for explaining the greatest range of data. It appears necessary for OT grammars to admit floating constraints in order to deal with multiple types of variation: synchronic adult variation in phonology (Nagy and Reynolds 1997; Anttila 1998) and syntax/semantics (Anttila and Fong 2000), diachronic variation (Zubritskaya 1997; Anttila and Cho, 1998), variation in child language (Legendre et al. 2000), and (under our interpretation here) variation across lexical strata (Itô and Mester 1995a, b, 1999). With this mechanism already introduced within grammatical theory, the grammatically strongest hypothesis would appear to be that floating accounts for any other type of variation. The type of variation observed in our speakers' productions appears to be one for which the floating constraint mechanism provides insight. If the adult speakers' grammar encodes their knowledge of phonology, part of that knowledge—according to Richness of the Base—concerns the pronunciations of nonnative inputs, and, as far as we have been able to determine experimentally, that part of their knowledge of phonology can be usefully formalized with floating constraints.

3.6.2   Statistics

We just considered backing off—very slightly—from the point of view we have advocated, that the grammar should encode the knowledge speakers display in our experiments. On the slightly grammatically weakened view, as on the view we have favored, covert rankings of markedness constraints are responsible for the relative accuracy of nonnative clusters; but the FAITHFULNESS elevation necessary to account for non-English outputs is not seen as part of the final state per se. A much more severe weakening of the grammatical perspective would in addition deny that covert MARKEDNESS rankings are responsible for relative accuracy—that relative accuracy is not a consequence of the grammar that, say, treats all nonnative forms equally. In-

Figure 7   *Table 5*

stead, explanation of relative accuracy might be sought in the statistics of English, with greater frequency predicting greater accuracy. Of course, in onset position, the frequency of the non-English clusters is nominally zero, by definition. But one might look to the relative frequency of heterosyllabic and coda clusters for explanation.

Figure 8. Statistical status of relative cluster accuracy

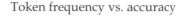

Token frequency vs. accuracy

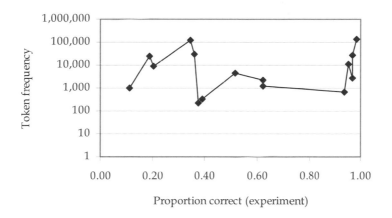

Type frequency vs. accuracy

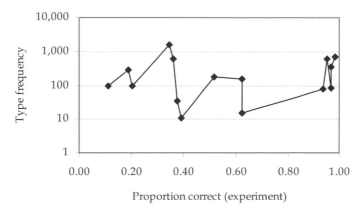

A frequency count from the CELEX 2 lexical database is not encouraging for the statistical perspective, however.[12] As Figure 8 indicates, whereas a statistical explana-

[12] We are extremely grateful to Matt Goldrick for his assistance with these counts.

tion would require that accuracy be a monotonically increasing function of frequency, there is in fact essentially no correlation between the orders of relative accuracy and relative frequency, whether of tokens or types. The rank correlation coefficient between frequency and accuracy in the experiment is only 0.14 ($p < .3$) for tokens, 0.06 ($p < .4$) for types.

The poor rank correlation between frequency and accuracy is also shown in (17). In (17a), the clusters are listed from lowest to highest accuracy in the experiment, with boldface marking the difficult stratum, bold italics marking the intermediate stratum, italics marking the easy stratum, and regular typeface indicating English-legal clusters. In (17b–c), the clusters are listed in order of increasing token and type frequencies.

(17)   Orderings of clusters by frequency and accuracy
    a.   Accuracy ordering (experiment)
        vn vz dv *kt pt kp čk tf* zm zr šl sn šr sm fr
    b.   Token frequency ordering
        kp čk šl **vn** *zr zm* šr *tf* **dv** sn **vz** sm *pt kt* fr
    c.   Type frequency ordering
        čk zr kp šl šr **vn dv** *zm tf* **vz** sm sn *pt* fr *kt*

Of course, it is impossible to prove the impossibility of a statistical account, given the potential infinity of statistics that might be computed. For example, it is possible that an extremely careful analysis of casual and fast speech would reveal that vowel deletion yields onset clusters that are nominally illegal in English, with statistical distributions that might mirror the accuracy data. We return to this line of thought shortly.

3.7 Origin of hidden rankings

We have attempted to contrast explanations of relative cluster accuracy based on phonological, statistical, and phonetic distinctions. A fundamental challenge in this regard is the inherent connectedness of these factors. Phonological markedness constraints can often be seen as the grammaticalization of articulatory difficulty (e.g., Archangeli and Pulleyblank 1994; Jun 1995; Steriade 1999; Boersma 1998; Kirchner 1998; Hayes 1999), so distinctions based on articulatory difficulty in a phonetic explanation will necessarily correlate with distinctions based on markedness in a phonological explanation. If the speakers' grammars contain constraints militating against marked structures, all else being equal, the frequency with which structures surface should be inversely correlated with their markedness. Further, if grammars include floating constraints with probabilistic positions, grammatical structure manifests itself in the statistics of output distributions, as shown in Table 5.

This tight coupling of phonology, phonetics, and surface statistics is at play not only in the final, adult state, but also in the learning process. As a final issue, we briefly consider how the covert rankings could be learned. The case of interest arises

Figure 8   *Table 5*

when there are few nonnative forms in the learner's environment, so sufficient direct evidence of the sort elicited in the experiment is not available.

Future research will assess the degree to which the covert rankings uncovered in the experiment reflect universal markedness tendencies. Such tendencies would raise the possibility of nativist grammatical explanations of covert rankings, encoded perhaps in the initial state. And these tendencies might well reflect factors of articulatory difficulty.

How might language-particular covert rankings be learned? One possibility, first suggested to us by Rochelle Newman (personal communication, 1999), is that the frequency with which an 'illegal' onset cluster arises in rapid speech might reflect its hidden stratum. As mentioned, if empirically substantiated, this proposal might suggest a statistical mode of explanation, or perhaps a phonetic one (Kohler 1990).

In general, Davidson (2003) showed that in fact English speakers do not typically produce 'well-formed' illegal initial clusters (such as [pt] for *potato*) in fast speech. Instead, detailed acoustic analysis of English speakers' productions of words with word-initial pretonic schwa indicates that at the very least, significant aspiration is produced between voiceless consonants (e.g., *potato* or *Topeka*), and often a voiced schwa is found between consonants, regardless of voicing (e.g., *developers*). The sequences most likely to undergo total deletion of the schwa were those that began with fricatives (including both /s/- and /f/-initial sequences, as in *photographer*) and those with /l/ as the second member (e.g., *malaria*).

Nevertheless, to account for the sequences that permit occasional schwa deletion, a grammatical line of explanation might also be developed by extending our linking hypotheses (11). In this extension, the degree of elevation of a constraint $\mathbb{C}$ from its base position determines the extent of reduction for rapid speech. The constraint $\mathbb{C}$ is, however, not the faithfulness constraint DEP-V, but a conceptually related markedness constraint in the family *STRUC banning structure (Prince and Smolensky 1993/ 2004). Epenthesis of schwa into a cluster creates additional structure, in particular, a weak syllable (an open syllable headed by a reduced vowel, perhaps one problematic for metrical foot parsing). Let us call the constraint violated by such syllables '*ŏ'.

(18) *ŏ   No weak syllables. (*STRUC family)

Replacing DEP-V by *ŏ above does not affect the analysis, since for the inputs of interest, which possess an initial CC cluster, the two constraints are violated by the same candidates. But if we turn to reduction of native forms in rapid speech, what is at issue is not whether to epenthesize a reduced vowel, but whether to delete one, and here *ŏ is no longer equivalent to DEP-V.

In its base position, *ŏ must be dominated by MAX-V so that the base English grammar retains weak syllables; this is illustrated in tableau (19), which shows a range of relevant hypothetical inputs. The base grammar allows the initial, weak vowel in inputs like /C_1C_2ant/ to surface faithfully, for any pair of consonants C_1 and C_2. This grammar also allows the initial cluster *pl* to surface faithfully, but not the illegal clusters *pt* (intermediate stratum) and *dv* (difficult stratum); as in the analysis above, these clusters are broken up by epenthesis. In this tableau, the unfaithful candidates are italicized, and a preceding '*' marks faithful candidates that are nonoptimal; these flag the clusters banned by this ranking. Weak vowels in candidates are marked V̌ to distinguish them from other vowels, marked V́. The rankings in the markedness constraint subhierarchy *VOL$_{SON}$ & *S$_Å$ ≫ *S$_Å$ ≫ *C$_C$ are the hidden rankings proposed above that separate the hidden strata including *dv*, *pt*, and *pl*.

(19)   Exposing covert rankings 1: English base grammar

	*VOL$_{SON}$ & *S$_Å$	*S$_Å$	MAX-V	*ŏ̆	DEP-V	*C$_C$
/pɪlant/						
☞ pĭlánt				*		
plánt		*!				*
/plant/						
☞ plant						*
pŏ̆lánt				*!	*	
/pɪtant/						
☞ pĭtánt				*		
ptánt		*!	*			
/ptant/						
* ptánt		*!				
☞ *pŏ̆tánt*				*	*	
/dɪvant/						
☞ dĭvánt				*		
dvánt	*!		*			
/dvant/						
* dvánt	*!					
☞ *dŏ̆vánt*				*	*	

Now elevating *ŏ̆ just above MAX-V enables some weak vowels to be deleted for rapid speech. Such deletion typically creates consonant clusters, and these are subject to the hierarchy of constraints with the covert rankings in question. With minimal elevation of *ŏ̆, deletion of weak vowels occurs if this creates an English-legal cluster, but is blocked if an illegal cluster would result. This is illustrated in tableau (20).

When the ranks of the constraints violated by illegal clusters are infiltrated by floating *ŏ̆, their relative rankings are exposed. Tableau (21) illustrates a degree of elevation in which *ŏ̆ still ranks below the constraints violated by clusters in the difficult stratum, but ranks above those violated by clusters in the intermediate stratum. Now weak vowels delete when this creates a cluster that is either English-legal (*pl*) or within the first two (easy; intermediate: *pt*) hidden strata of the illegal clusters. However, weak vowel deletion is blocked when an illegal cluster in the third (difficult: *dv*) hidden stratum would result.

Figure 8

Table 5

(20)   Exposing covert rankings 2: Rapid speech, English-legal clusters only

	$*\mathrm{VOL_{SON}}$ & $*\mathrm{S_{\bar{A}}}$	$*\mathrm{S_{\bar{A}}}$	$*\breve{\sigma}$	MAX-V	DEP-V	$*\mathrm{C_C}$
/pɪlant/						
* pĭlánt			*!			
☞ *plánt*				*		*
/plant/						
☞ plant						*
pŏlánt			*!		*	
/pɪtant/						
☞ pĭtánt			*			
ptánt		*!		*		
/ptant/						
* ptánt		*!				
☞ *pŏtánt*			*		*	

(21)   Exposing covert rankings 3: Rapid speech, English+easy+intermediate clusters

	$*\mathrm{VOL_{SON}}$ & $*\mathrm{S_{\bar{A}}}$	$*\breve{\sigma}$	$*\mathrm{S_{\bar{A}}}$	MAX-V	DEP-V	$*\mathrm{C_C}$
/pɪlant/						
* pĭlánt		*!				
☞ *plánt*				*!		*
/plant/						
☞ plant						*
pŏlánt		*!			*	
/pɪtant/						
* pĭtánt		*!				
☞ *ptánt*			*	*		
/ptant/						
☞ ptánt			*			
pŏtánt		*!			*	
/dɪvant/						
☞ dĭvánt		*				
dvánt	*!			*		
/dvant/						
* dvánt	*!					
☞ *dŏvánt*		*			*	

Just as in the analysis of the experimental results developed above, floating *ŏ̃ exposes the hidden strata by rendering reduction increasingly less probable as the resulting clusters enter hidden strata increasingly distant from base English.

We hasten to repeat that it remains for future research to evaluate the empirical soundness of any line of explanation based in rapid speech. Our intent here is only to suggest that, while such an explanation might invite an agrammatic, simply statistical interpretation, it appears that there is in fact at least one grammatical approach that may offer a unified explanation of the patterns exhibited in rapid speech and in the pronunciation of nonnative inputs.

4 GRAMMAR IN PERFORMANCE

In this chapter, we have attempted to formulate working hypotheses that place the greatest demands on phonological theory to explain phonological performance. The theory is asked to make a prediction about the phonological knowledge initially present in infants, and it does so with the help of a nativist hypothesis: universal constraints are present and ranked broadly as MARKEDNESS ≫ FAITHFULNESS. The theory is next asked to predict the phonologically relevant behavior of infants, and it does so, with the help of linking hypotheses claiming that one of the few reliably measurable behaviors of infants, orientation time, will positively correlate with the degree to which phonological stimuli conform to their knowledge—their phonological grammars. The theory is finally asked to characterize the expected behavior of adults producing forms that violate their phonological knowledge, and it does so with the help of the previously developed notion of probabilistically floating constraints. When experiments are conducted to test all these theoretical predictions, we find that the theory indeed brings the experimental data into sharp focus. We have identified several respects in which the experimental program needs strengthening in future work. The experiments reported here are the first we have conducted. Our hope is only to have made the case that such a program of research—directly confronting OT phonological theory with performance data—is worth pursuing further. We hope also to have shown how Richness of the Base—a subtle, inherently counterfactual principle of OT that might have been thought to have only abstruse theoretical import—may in fact have a surprisingly important role to play in the explanation of human linguistic performance.

Figure 8   *Table 5*

References

ROA = Rutgers Optimality Archive, http://roa.rutgers.edu

Anderson, J. 1987. The markedness differential hypothesis and syllable structure difficulty. In *Interlanguage phonology: The acquisition of a second language sound system*, eds. G. Ioupo and S. Weinberger. Newbury House.

Anttila, A. 1998. Deriving variation from grammar. In *Variation, change, and phonological theory*, eds. F. Hinskens, R. van Hout, and W. L. Wetzel. Benjamins.

Anttila, A., and V. Fong. 2000. The partitive constraint in Optimality Theory. ROA 416-09100.

Anttila, A., and Y.-m. Y. Cho. 1998. Variation and change in Optimality Theory. *Lingua* 104, 31–56.

Archangeli, D., and D. Pulleyblank. 1994. *Grounded Phonology.* MIT Press.

Archibald, J. 1993. *Language learnability and L2 phonology.* Kluwer.

Archibald, J. 1998. *Second language phonology.* Benjamins.

Boersma, P. 1998. *Functional phonology: Formalizing the interactions between articulatory and perceptual drives.* Holland Academic Graphics.

Boersma, P., and B. Hayes. 2001. Empirical tests of the gradual learning algorithm. *Linguistic Inquiry* 32, 45–86. ROA 348.

Broselow, E. 1983. Nonobvious transfer: On predicting epenthesis errors. In *Language transfer in language learning*, eds. S. Gass and L. Selinker. Newbury House.

Broselow, E., S. Chen, and C. Wang. 1998. The emergence of the unmarked in second language phonology. *Studies in Second Language Acquisition* 20, 261–80.

Broselow, E., and D. Finer. 1991. Parameter setting in second language phonology and syntax. *Second Language Research* 7, 35–59.

Broselow, E., and H. B. Park. 1995. Mora conservation in second language prosody. In *Phonological acquisition and phonological theory*, ed. J. Archibald. Erlbaum.

Browman, C. P., and L. Goldstein. 1986. Towards an articulatory phonology. *Phonology Yearbook* 3, 219–52.

Brown, R. 1973. *A first language: The early stages.* Harvard University Press.

Carlisle, R. 1998. The acquisition of onsets in a markedness relationship: A longitudinal study. *Studies in Second Language Acquisition* 20, 245–60.

Davidson, L. 2001. Hidden rankings in the final state of the English grammar. In *RuLing papers II*, eds. G. Horwood and S.-K. Kim. Department of Linguistics, Rutgers University.

Davidson, L. 2003. The atoms of phonological representation: Gestures, coordination and perceptual features in consonant cluster phonotactics. Ph.D. diss., Johns Hopkins University.

Davidson, L., P. W. Jusczyk, and P. Smolensky. 2004. The initial and final states: Theoretical implications and experimental explorations of Richness of the Base. In *Constraints in phonological acquisition*, eds. R. Kager, J. Pater, and W. Zonneveld. Cambridge University Press. ROA 428.

Davidson, L., and R. Noyer. 1996. Loan phonology in Huave: Nativization and the ranking of faithfulness constraints. In *Proceedings of the West Coast Conference on Formal Linguistics 15.*

Demuth, K. 1995. Markedness and the development of prosodic structure. In *Proceedings of the North East Linguistic Society 25.* ROA 50.

de Villiers, J. G., and P. A. de Villiers. 1973. A cross-sectional study of the acquisition of grammatical morphemes in child speech. *Journal of Psycholinguistic Research* 2, 267–73.

Echols, C. H., M. J. Crowhurst, and J. B. Childers. 1997. The perception of rhythmic units in speech by infants and adults. *Journal of Memory and Language* 36, 202–25.

Eckman, F., and G. Iverson. 1993. Sonority and markedness among onset clusters in the interlanguage of ESL learners. *Second Language Research* 9, 234–52.

Friederici, A. D., and J. M. I. Wessels. 1993. Phonotactic knowledge and its use in infant speech perception. *Perception and Psychophysics* 54, 287–95.

Fukazawa, H. 1998. Multiple input-output faithfulness relations in Japanese. Ms., University of Maryland at College Park. ROA 260.

Fukazawa, H., M. Kitahara, and M. Ota. 1998. Lexical stratification and ranking invariance in constraint-based grammars. Ms., University of Maryland at College Park, Indiana University, and Georgetown University. ROA 267.

Gnanadesikan, A. 1995. Markedness and faithfulness constraints in child phonology. Ms., University of Massachusetts at Amherst. ROA 67.

Hale, M., and C. Reiss. 1997. Grammar optimization: The simultaneous acquisition of constraint ranking and a lexicon. Ms., Concordia University. ROA 231.

Hale, M., and C. Reiss. 1998. Formal and empirical arguments concerning phonological acquisition. *Linguistic Inquiry* 29, 656–83. ROA 233.

Hancin-Bhatt, B., and R. Bhatt. 1998. Optimal L2 syllables: Interactions of transfer and developmental effects. *Studies in Second Language Acquisition* 19, 331–78.

Hayes, B. 1999. Phonetically-driven phonology: The role of Optimality Theory and inductive grounding. In *Functionalism and formalism in linguistics*. Vol. 1, *General papers*, eds. M. Darnell, E. Moravscik, M. Noonan, F. Newmeyer, and K. Wheatly. Benjamins.

Hayes, B. 2004. Phonological acquisition in Optimality Theory: The early stages. In *Constraints in phonological acquisition*, eds. R. Kager, J. Pater, and W. Zonneveld. Cambridge University Press. ROA 327.

Hirsh-Pasek, K., D. G. Kemler Nelson, P. W. Jusczyk, K. Wright Cassidy, B. Druss, and L. Kennedy. 1987. Clauses are perceptual units for young infants. *Cognition* 26, 269–86.

Holden, K. 1976. Assimilation rates of borrowings and phonological productivity. *Language* 52, 131–47.

Hunter, M. A., and E. W. Ames. 1989. A multifactor model of infant preferences for novel and familiar stimuli. *Advances in Infancy Research* 5, 69–95.

Itô, J., and R. A. Mester. 1995a. The core-periphery structure of the lexicon and constraints on reranking. In *University of Massachusetts occasional papers in linguistics 18: Papers in Optimality Theory*, eds. J. Beckman, L. Walsh Dickey, and S. Urbanczyk. Graduate Linguistic Student Association, University of Massachusetts at Amherst.

Itô, J., and R. A. Mester. 1995b. Japanese phonology. In *Handbook of phonological theory*, ed. J. A. Goldsmith. Blackwell.

Itô, J., and R. A. Mester. 1999. The phonological lexicon. In *Handbook of Japanese linguistics*, ed. N. Tsujimura. Blackwell.

Johnson, E. K., and P. W. Jusczyk. 2001. Word segmentation by 8-month-olds: When speech cues count more than the statistics. *Journal of Memory and Language* 44, 548–67.

Jun, J. 1995. Perceptual and articulatory factors in place assimilation: An optimality theoretic approach. Ph.D. diss., UCLA.

Jusczyk, P. W. 1997. *The discovery of spoken language*. MIT Press.

Jusczyk, P. W. 1998. Using the headturn preference procedure to study language acquisition. In *Advances in infancy research*. Vol. 12, eds. C. Rovee-Collier, L. P. Lipsitt, and H. Hayne. Ablex.

Jusczyk, P. W., A. Cutler, and N. J. Redanz. 1993. Preference for the predominant stress patterns of English words. *Child Development* 64, 675–87.

Jusczyk, P. W., A. D. Friederici, J. M. I. Wessels, V. Y. Svenkerud, and A. M. Jusczyk. 1993. Infants' sensitivity to the sound patterns of native language words. *Journal of Memory and Language* 32, 402–20.

Jusczyk, P. W., K. Hirsh-Pasek, D. G. Kemler Nelson, L. Kennedy, A. Woodward, and J. Piwoz. 1992. Perception of acoustic correlates of major phrasal units by young infants. *Cognitive Psychology* 24, 252–93.

Jusczyk, P. W., D. M. Houston, and M. Newsome. 1999. The beginnings of word segmentation in English-learning infants. *Cognitive Psychology* 39, 159–207.

Jusczyk, P. W., P. A. Luce, and J. Charles-Luce. 1994. Infants' sensitivity to phonotactic patterns in the native language. *Journal of Memory and Language* 33, 630–45.

Jusczyk, P. W., P. Smolensky, and T. Allocco. 2002. How English-learning infants respond to markedness and faithfulness constraints. *Language Acquisition* 10, 31–73.

Katayama, M. 1998. Optimality Theory and Japanese loanword phonology. Ph.D. diss., University of California at Santa Cruz.

Kemler Nelson, D. G., P. W. Jusczyk, D. R. Mandel, J. Myers, A. Turk, and L. A. Gerken. 1995. The headturn preference procedure for testing auditory perception. *Infant Behavior and Development* 18, 111–6.

Kiparsky, P. 1973. How abstract is phonology? In *Three dimensions of linguistic theory*, ed. O. Fujimura. TEC.

Kiparsky, P. 1982. Lexical phonology and morphology. In *Linguistics in the morning calm*, ed. I. S. Yang. Hanshin.

Kirchner, R. 1998. An effort-based approach to consonant lenition. Ph.D. diss., UCLA. ROA 276.

Kohler, K. J. 1990. Segmental reduction in connected speech in German: Phonological facts and phonetic explanations. In *Speech production and speech modelling*, eds. W. J. Hardcastle and A. Marchal. Kluwer.

Legendre, G., P. Hagstrom, A. Vainikka, and M. Todorova. 2000. An optimality theoretic model of acquisition of tense and agreement in French. In *Proceedings of the Cognitive Science Society 22*.

Levelt, C. 1995. Unfaithful kids: Place of articulation patterns in early child language. Talk presented at the Department of Cognitive Science, Johns Hopkins University.

Levelt, C., and R. van de Vijver. 1998. Syllable types in cross-linguistic and developmental grammars. ROA 265.

Mattys, S. L., and P. W. Jusczyk. 2001. Phonotactic cues for segmentation of fluent speech by infants. *Cognition* 78, 91–121.

Nagy, N., and W. Reynolds. 1997. Optimality Theory and variable word-final deletion in Fætar. *Language Variation and Change* 9, 37–55.

Pater, J. 1997. Metrical parameter missetting in second language acquisition. In *Focus on phonological acquisition*, eds. S. J. Hannahs and M. Young-Scholten. Benjamins.

Pater, J. 2004. Bridging the gap between perception and production with minimally violable constraints. In *Constraints in phonological acquisition*, eds. R. Kager, J. Pater, and W. Zonneveld. Cambridge University Press.

Pater, J., and J. Paradis. 1996. Truncation without templates in child phonology. In *Proceedings of the Boston University Conference on Language Development 20*.

Prince, A., and P. Smolensky. 1993/2004. *Optimality Theory: Constraint interaction in generative grammar*. Technical report, Rutgers University and University of Colorado at Boulder, 1993. ROA 537, 2002. Revised version published by Blackwell, 2004.

Prince, A., and B. B. Tesar. 1999. Learning phonotactic distributions. Ms., Rutgers University. ROA 353.

Reynolds, W. 1994. Variation and phonological theory. Ph.D. diss., University of Pennsylvania.

Saciuk, B. 1969. The stratal division of the lexicon. *Papers in Linguistics* 1, 464–532.

Saffran, J. R., R. N. Aslin, and E. L. Newport. 1996. Statistical learning by 8-month-old infants. *Science* 274, 1926–8.

Saffran, J. R., E. K. Johnson, R. N. Aslin, and E. L. Newport. 1999. Statistical learning of tone sequences by human adults and infants. *Cognition* 70, 27–52.

Santelmann, L. M., and P. W. Jusczyk. 1998. Sensitivity to discontinuous dependencies in language learners: Evidence for limitations in processing space. *Cognition* 69, 105–34.

Shady, M. E. 1996. Infants' sensitivity to function morphemes. Ph.D. diss., State University of New York at Buffalo.

Smolensky, P. 1993. Harmony, markedness, and phonological activity. Handout of talk presented at the Rutgers Optimality Workshop–1. ROA 87.

Smolensky, P. 1995. On the internal structure of the constraint component *Con* of UG. Talk presented at the UCLA Linguistics Department. ROA 86.

Smolensky, P. 1996a. The initial state and 'Richness of the Base' in Optimality Theory. Technical report JHU-CogSci-96-4, Cognitive Science Department, Johns Hopkins University. ROA 154.

Smolensky, P. 1996b. On the comprehension/production dilemma in child language. *Linguistic Inquiry* 27, 720–31. ROA 118.

Smolensky, P. 1997. Constraint interaction in generative grammar II: Local conjunction (or, random rules in Universal Grammar). Talk presented at the Hopkins Optimality Theory Conference.

Steriade, D. 1993. Closure, release, and nasal contours. In *Nasals, nasalization, and the velum*, eds. M. Huffman and R. Krakow. Academic Press.

Steriade, D. 1997. Phonetics in phonology: The case of laryngeal neutralization. In *UCLA Working Papers in Linguistics 2*, ed. M. K. Gordon.

Tesar, B. B., and P. Smolensky. 1993. The learnability of Optimality Theory: An algorithm and some basic complexity results. Technical report CU-CS-678-93, Computer Science Department, University of Colorado at Boulder. ROA 2.

Tesar, B. B., and P. Smolensky. 1996. Learnability in Optimality Theory (long version). Technical report JHU-CogSci-96-3, Cognitive Science Department, Johns Hopkins University. ROA 156.

Tesar, B. B., and P. Smolensky. 1998a. Learnability in Optimality Theory. *Linguistic Inquiry* 29, 229–68.

Tesar, B. B., and P. Smolensky. 1998b. Learning optimality-theoretic grammars. *Lingua* 106, 161–96.

Tesar, B. B., and P. Smolensky. 2000. *Learnability in Optimality Theory*. MIT Press.

Tropf, H. 1987. Sonority as a variability factor in second language phonology. In *Sound patterns in second language acquisition*, eds. A. James and J. Leather. Foris.

Turk, A. E., P. W. Jusczyk, and L. A. Gerken. 1995. Do English-learning infants use syllable weight to determine stress? *Language and Speech* 38, 143–58.

Wilson, C. 2000. Targeted constraints: An approach to contextual neutralization in Optimality Theory. Ph.D. diss., Johns Hopkins University.

Yip, M. 1993. Cantonese loan word phonology and Optimality Theory. *Journal of East Asian Linguistics* 2, 261–92.

Zubritskaya, K. 1994. Markedness and sound change in OT. Talk presented at the 25th meeting of the North East Linguistic Society.

Zubritskaya, K. 1997. Mechanism of sound change in Optimality Theory. *Language Variation and Change* 9, 121–48.

18

Optimality in Language Acquisition II: Inflection in Early French Syntax

Géraldine Legendre, Paul Hagstrom,
Anne Vainikka, and Marina Todorova

Turning from phonology to morphosyntax, in this chapter we continue the exploration of Optimality Theory's potential for shedding light on language acquisition (Section 8.7 of Chapter 2's Integrated Connectionist/Symbolic Cognitive Architecture (ICS) map). We present a novel theoretical model of multiple stages in the acquisition of verbal inflection for tense and agreement in child French. First, we show that tense and agreement inflection follow independent courses of acquisition. Over the three stages of development attested in the data, tense production starts and ends at near-adult levels, but suffers a dip in production at the second stage. Agreement develops linearly, going roughly from 0% to 100% over the same time. This profile suggests a *competition* between tense and agreement at the second stage—naturally formalized in terms of Optimality Theory's output optimization, constraint violability, and constraint reranking. The proposed theory incorporates the further mechanism of partial rankings of constraints: for the three stages observed, the analysis successfully accounts for not only the qualitative variability in production, but also the quantitative frequencies with which children use tensed, agreeing, and uninflected verb forms.

This chapter is a slight revision of parts of Sections 1–4 of Legendre et al. 2002.

Contents

1 INTRODUCTION

In this chapter, we reanalyze production data from three French children and make two basic points. First, we show that inflection for tense (past and future) and agreement (first and second person singular) follow independent courses of acquisition in child French. Tense production starts and ends at near-adult levels, but suffers a dip in production in the intermediate stage. Agreement develops linearly, going roughly from 0% to 100% over the same time. This profile suggests an analysis in which tense and agreement *compete* at the intermediate stage. Second, using a mechanism of grammatical development based on partial rankings of constraints (in terms of Optimality Theory; Prince and Smolensky 1993/2004), our analysis successfully predicts, over three stages, the frequency with which children use tensed, agreeing, and nonfinite verbs.

As our results in Section 2 show, there are systematic and independent progressions in the development of tense and of agreement in child French, which we were able to identify by analyzing our data in stages. The stages we use are defined not by mean length of utterance (Brown 1973) but by a measure that we claim correlates better with syntactic development. We outline this measure (the predominant length of utterance) in Section 2.2 and refer the reader to Vainikka, Legendre, and Todorova 1999 for further discussion.

Viewed from the perspective of Optimality Theory (OT), a grammar consists of structural markedness constraints pitted against conflicting faithfulness constraints. Adult grammars differ from one another not in the constraints involved (which form the core of universal grammar (UG)), but in the relative rankings between them. Thus, children's acquisition of syntax must in large part involve learning the relative rankings of the constraints. In this chapter, we propose a particular view of the reranking of constraints in child language acquisition that can explain not only the *existence* of the observed child forms, but also the *frequency* with which these forms appear, something that has not been substantially addressed in previous formal work on syntactic acquisition.

As discussed in more detail below, the key to our approach is **partial ordering of constraints** (a concept borrowed from synchronic and diachronic studies on variation, primarily from the phonological literature; see Kiparsky 1993; Reynolds 1994; Anttila 1997; Boersma 1997; Boersma and Hayes 2001). One or more partially ordered constraints will give rise to a *set* of totally ordered rankings, containing one ranking for each position the partially ordered constraints could take with respect to the other constraints. Given a single input form, each of these rankings will yield a single optimal output form for that input, but not every pair of rankings will pick distinct outputs; a given output form might be optimal under several distinct rankings (extrapolating from this, the number of possible languages is not the same as the number of possible rankings; see Legendre, Raymond, and Smolensky 1993; Legendre 2001).

Turning the picture around and considering the set of possible output forms given by these several rankings, we can observe what proportion of the rankings result in any given output form being optimal. Under a model of grammatical variation in which each of these rankings is equally available to evaluate input forms, we can predict the probability of that output's occurrence. Concretely, our model allows us to predict how often, for example, the verb is realized without tense in child speech at a given stage of development. Traditional syntactic analyses do not lend themselves to even a description of the actual proportions attested (let alone to an explanation), whereas the partial ordering analysis presented here provides an account of (what gives rise to) them. [1]

In a nutshell, our analysis pits structural realization of tense features and of agreement features (both faithfulness constraints) against constraints on the maximal complexity of the syntactic structure (markedness constraints). In the first stage examined here, the mandate to realize tense features is roughly on a par with the constraint limiting structure, both taking priority over realizing agreement features. The result is an alternation between tensed and nonfinite forms, none of which are agreeing. The second stage sees an increased priority for agreement features, but at the expense of the realization of tense; observationally, we see a drop in the production of tensed forms corresponding to the increase in the production of agreeing forms. In the third stage, the faithfulness constraints overcome the markedness constraints, resulting in constant production of both tense and agreement (in appropriately complex structures). Our particular implementation of the grammar of variation allows us to predict the observed proportions at each stage, as discussed in Section 3.

In Section 2.1, we provide some general background to the crosslinguistic acquisition of grammatical phenomena under study: finite and nonfinite verb forms in child language. In the remainder of Section 2, we describe our data from child French on finite and nonfinite verbs. Finally, in Section 3 we present our analysis of these data. (For technical terminology, refer to Box 12:1.)

2   THE ACQUISITION OF TENSE AND AGREEMENT IN FRENCH

2.1   Root infinitives and other nonfinite root forms

In addition to producing adult-like finite verbs with tense and agreement marking, young children often produce sentences with a nonfinite (i.e., uninflected) verb form in a main clause, which are ungrammatical in the adult language. These 'root infinitives' (Wexler 1994) have posed a challenging problem for current research on the early acquisition of syntax, especially if one assumes that UG is innate, therefore already in place (as Wexler does). We will use the term **nonfinite root forms** (**NRFs**) to

---

[1] This is of course not to say that one could not graft a system to predict proportions onto a traditional analysis; yet it would be an independent module. Under our analysis, the proportional predictions follow naturally from the syntactic system, from elements that are needed independently to predict the existence of the forms in the first place.

refer to nonfinite verbs in root contexts because it explicitly encompasses both infinitives (e.g., *to go*) and other nonfinite forms (such as bare participles like *gone*) that are used as main verbs. Some examples of NRFs from child French are provided in (1), obtained from the CHILDES database (MacWhinney and Snow 1985; see also Vainikka, Legendre, and Todorova 1999).

(1) Nonfinite forms

    a. Cabinets ouvrir.   (Grégoire 1;9.28)
        restroom open-INF
        '(I will) open the restroom (door).'

    b. Ranger   Christian.   (Grégoire 1;10.20)
        clean.up-INF Christian
        'Christian cleans up.'

    c. Assis   Grégoire.   (Grégoire 1;10.20)
        sit.down-PART Grégoire
        'Grégoire is sitting down.'

Robust occurrences of NRFs (specifically infinitives) have been attested in many languages, including French (Pierce 1992; Ferdinand 1996); for surveys, see Phillips 1995; Wexler 1998. On the other hand, in the Romance languages Italian, Spanish, and Catalan, NRFs are reportedly rare (Grinstead 1994; Guasti 1994); but see Davidson and Legendre 2003.

Drawing on the well-studied infinitive NRFs in German, Dutch, French, and the Scandinavian languages, we can synthesize a list of common properties, and we make the plausible assumption that these properties carry over to noninfinitive NRFs. A very thorough overview of (infinitive) NRFs provided by Phillips (1995) concludes with the findings summarized in (2).

(2) Summary of widely accepted findings on properties of (infinitive) NRFs

    a. The word order of utterances containing (infinitive) NRFs provides evidence that verbs are within VP on the surface (cf., e.g., Poeppel and Wexler 1993; Rohrbacher and Vainikka 1994).

    b. Auxiliary verbs do not occur as (infinitive) NRFs (De Haan and Tuijnman 1988; Wexler 1994).

    c. (Infinitive) NRFs are very likely to co-occur with a null subject (Krämer 1993).

    d. (Infinitive) NRFs decline gradually with age (Miller 1976).

    e. The richer the inflectional paradigm of the adult language, the less common (infinitive) NRFs are (Phillips 1995).

The analyses proposed to account for the NRF phenomenon can be divided into two categories: (i) those assuming a null modal or auxiliary (e.g., Miller 1976; Boser et al. 1992; Ferdinand 1996) and (ii) those involving missing (or underspecified) functional projections (e.g., Radford 1990; Pierce 1992; Rizzi 1993/1994; Wexler 1994, 1998;

Hyams 1996). Approaches of either type can account for properties (2a–c), while neither approach accounts for properties (2d–e).

The analysis of child French developed in this chapter follows this second general approach: our proposal entails that NRFs lack certain functional projections. Unlike previous analyses, however, ours offers a way to approach property (2d) and in fact allows us to predict how the gradual decline in NRFs interacts with the other aspects of syntactic development. The last property, (2e), does not follow directly from our approach, although it stands to reason that the primary linguistic data in languages with richer inflection provide the child with more abundant evidence for the rankings of the constraints concerned with tense and agreement, which in turn could accelerate the acquisition process in this domain. If this is true, we might expect to find NRFs in the child data for languages with rich inflectional paradigms, but only earlier in development and for a shorter time (making them more difficult to detect) (see also Crago and Allen 2001; Davidson and Legendre 2003).

2.2 Predominant-length-of-utterance stages in early syntax

To analyze syntactic development, it is important to be able to measure a child's stage of development using a metric that is comparable across children and independent of particular syntactic constructions. Age and MLU (mean length of utterance; Brown 1973) are well known to be unreliable (see, e.g., Klee and Fitzgerald 1985), but the PLU (predominant length of utterance) measure developed elsewhere (Vainikka, Legendre, and Todorova 1999) has been very effective in isolating qualitative shifts in development. The stages represented in our data are defined below. PLU stages are defined over two dimensions, the primary stage reflecting the number of words in the majority of a child's utterances, and the secondary stage reflecting the proportion of utterances containing a verb.

(3)   PLU stages in our data
    a.   Stage 3: "Two-word" stage[2]
        ♦   Over 40% of the utterances contain more than one word.
        ♦   Yet utterances still tend to be very short, with one-word and two-word utterances predominating over multiword utterances (i.e., utterances of more than two words).
    b.   Stage 4: Predominantly multiword stage
        ♦   Multiword utterances predominate over both one-word and two-word utterances.

(4)   Secondary PLU stages in our data
    Secondary stage b: 11–60% of all utterances contain a verb
    Secondary stage c: more than 60% of all utterances contain a verb

---

[2] Stage 3 is intermediate between Stage 2, not discussed here, and Stage 4. Stage 3 most closely corresponds to the traditional "two-word" stage.

Previous research on the PLU as a measure of syntactic development has shown that the proportion of verbs in the data is indicative of the child's developmental stage. Given the crucial status of verbs in adult syntax, this measure perhaps most reliably gets at the status of syntactic development in the child's mental grammar. The PLU metric has also been used successfully to differentiate qualitatively different stages in several other languages, clearly a crucial component of analyzing the course of syntactic development (see Davidson and Legendre 2003 for Catalan; Legendre et al. 2004 for Mandarin).

Figure 1. MLUs and NRFs at PLU Stage 4b (Grégoire, Philippe)

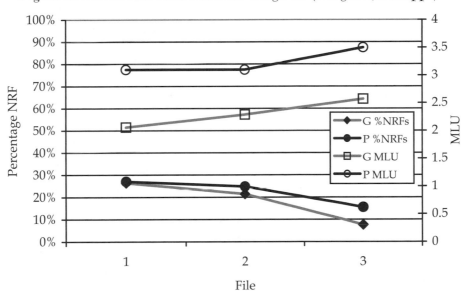

This PLU-based approach to identifying stages of syntactic development has its conceptual grounding in the traditional observation that children progress through one-word, two-word, and multiword stages; the PLU measure reveals these stages directly. Another advantage is its generality. The PLU measure can classify child data reliably into syntactic stages much more accurately than a simple MLU cutoff would allow. Although, roughly speaking, higher MLUs correlate with more advanced PLU stages, it is clear that a direct mapping from MLU to PLU stage is not possible. This point is demonstrated clearly in Figure 1, which shows three files each from Grégoire and Philippe, all at PLU Stage 4b. We have plotted the percentage of NRFs and each file's MLU measure. Note that the percentage of NRFs is about the same for both children, indicating that we are looking at the same stage of syntactic development, but the MLU measures are quite far separated. We can conclude from this that it is not possible to simply compute the PLU stage from the MLU measure across children.

2.3 Subject profiles

We have examined the spontaneous speech production data from three French-learning children, Grégoire, Philippe, and Stéphane, whose early files are available in the CHILDES database (MacWhinney and Snow 1985). All files were analyzed by hand and classified into PLU stages by the first author. The data obtained from Grégoire's and Stéphane's files had the greatest developmental spread, spanning PLU Stages 3b, 4b, and 4c. Philippe's data were found to instantiate Stages 4b and 4c.[3] The profile for each child is given in Table 1.

The files were further analyzed with respect to the development of finite inflection in the verbal system and the occurrence of NRFs. Before presenting our findings, we give a brief overview of the verb inflection paradigm of French to illustrate the specific challenges it presents to the researcher interested in the development of finiteness and to point out the methodological decisions we have made in analyzing the data.

Table 1. Children, files, and ages included in this study

Child	Corpus	Files	Age	PLU stage	Total # of utterances
Grégoire	Champaud	1–4	1;9–1;10	3b	874
		5–7	2;0–2;3	4b	732
		8–10	2;5	4c	1,038
Stéphane	Rondal 1985	1–3	2;2–2;3	3b	644
		6a/6f/8a	2;6–2;8	4b	688
		25b	3;3	4c	257
Philippe	Suppes, Smith and Leveillé 1973	1–3	2;1–2;2	4b	898
		11	2;6	4c	387

2.4 Coding tense and agreement in French

Determining the status of a French verb with respect to tense and agreement is complicated by the fact that many agreeing forms of the regular verbal paradigm are homophonous. Pierce (1992), assuming (as we do here) that the presence of a clitic subject in French indicates subject-verb agreement,[4] found that agreement in French is

---

[3] We have analyzed one file (the first) from Philippe's Stage 4c, Philippe 11, but there are several later files that have not been analyzed here. We also looked at Philippe 10, not included above; it appears to be intermediate between Stages 4b and 4c (see also Footnote 26 for additional brief comments). As for Stéphane, the corpus contains only one file that was classified as being Stage 4c. Given the difficulty of analyzing Stéphane's transcripts (due to phonological problems that Stéphane exhibits), we chose a representative sample of his transcripts rather than attempting to analyze them all.

[4] 'Clitic subject' refers to a subtype of subject pronoun found in French. These are phonologically weak elements (i.e., they cannot be stressed) that immediately precede finite verbs. They can only be separated from their verbal 'host' by another clitic, typically a clitic object: *les garçons aiment les filles* 'boys like girls' > *ils* (clitic subject) *les* (clitic object) *aiment* 'they like them'. Clitic subjects always agree in person and number with their verbal host. French also has a set of strong pronouns that can stand

acquired very early, possibly before age 2.[5] However, Pierce's analysis often collapses data spanning several months, making it impossible to discern the relative order of acquisition between tense and agreement. Ferdinand (1996), using the same data set,[6] provides a better description of the acquisition of tense and agreement in early French, although she too considers tense and agreement together. Our analysis of the French data reveals clearly that tense is acquired before agreement.

The overwhelming majority of French verbs (90%; Dietiker 1978) belong to the regular conjugation whose infinitive ends in *-er*. The present tense agreement paradigm for this conjugation is illustrated in (5) for the verb *danser* 'to dance'.[7]

(5)   The *-er* conjugation (French)

		Singular	Phonetic		Plural	Phonetic
1.	(je)	**dans**e	[dãs]	(on)	**dans**e	[dãs]
2.	(tu)	**dans**es	[dãs]	(vous)	**dans**ez	[dãse]
3.	(il, elle, on)	**dans**e	[dãs]	(ils, elles)	**dans**ent	[dãs]

As the phonetic transcriptions indicate, all present tense forms of the verb except the second person plural are homophonous; despite its misleading spelling conventions, French has a highly impoverished agreement paradigm in these regular *-er* verbs. This means that except for the second person plural, and in the absence of an overt subject, it cannot be determined whether a verb form produced by the child indeed carries correct agreement. Worse, the identifiable form in the plural is usually the last to appear during acquisition, which renders it relatively uninformative for studying the earliest stages of development. Fortunately, agreement in French is not only realized in the verbal endings; subject clitics also appear to be overt instantiations of agreement, as a number of analyses have argued (e.g., Lambrecht 1981; Roberge 1990; Miller 1992; Auger 1994). In the acquisition literature, studies have been unanimous in interpreting both nominative and accusative clitics in French as agreement markers (e.g., Meisel 1990; Kaiser 1994; Ferdinand 1996; Jakubowicz and Rigaut 1997). Pierce (1992) reports that over 95% of the subject clitics produced by the four children she studied occurred with finite verbs, while this correlation does not hold for strong (nonclitic) subject pronouns or lexical NP subjects.[8] In addition, several studies have

on their own, which are used (among other things) to answer questions and to stress a referent: first person singular *moi*, third person masculine singular *lui*, and so on. Unlike French, most other Romance languages do not have clitic subjects; rather, distinctions in tense, person, and number appear as audible suffixes on the verb. These languages typically (i.e., in the proper context where a referent is known) make use of null subjects. English subject pronouns are not clitics. For example, in *he ate the whole pizza*, *he* can be stressed to refer to a specific person while excluding others present in the context (linguistic or nonlinguistic).

[5] Pierce's data come from the following four children: Nathalie (1;9–2;3) and Daniel (1;8–1;11) from the Lightbown corpus (Lightbown 1977); Grégoire (1;9–2;3) and Philippe (2;1–2;3) from the CHILDES database. The data from the latter two children will be discussed at length here.

[6] Ferdinand's analysis covers Philippe's data over a longer period of time (from 2;1 to 2;6).

[7] The absence of the first person plural (*nous*) form from (5) is intentional; in modern spoken French (the primary linguistic data for the children), *on* has completely replaced the more formal *nous*.

[8] Pierce also reports that subject clitic pronouns were never dislocated, a finding she attributes to their fixed attachment to the left of an inflectional (Infl) head—further evidence for the contingency between subject clitics and finiteness.

reported that nominative clitics are typically acquired earlier than accusative clitics (e.g., Clark 1985; Hamann, Rizzi, and Frauenfelder 1995; Ferdinand 1996). This order of acquisition parallels that of subject and object agreement in languages that uncontroversially have both (such as Basque; see Meisel and Ezeizabarrena 1996). Accordingly, we take subject clitics to be an overt realization of agreement, a reliable diagnostic for finiteness. This also implies that adult French sentences where the only indication of the subject is a subject clitic should be analyzed as in fact having a null subject (the clitic instantiating subject agreement).[9]

Irregular verbs, including the auxiliaries *être* 'to be', *aller* 'to go', and *avoir* 'to have', display greater diversity in inflectional endings and are used frequently both as main verbs and in the periphrastic tenses discussed shortly. The agreement paradigms for these verbs contain four distinct forms (the second and third person singular forms are homophonous with the first person plural *on* form), which can be easily identified.

We turn now to tense inflection. French has two past and two future tenses. Of these, two are periphrastic: the *passé composé*, or perfect past, and the *future proche*, or near future, are formed with an auxiliary verb (*avoir/être* 'to have/be' and *aller* 'to go', respectively) combined with a nonfinite form of the verb (the past participle or the infinitive, respectively). Agreement in these tenses is carried on the auxiliary verb.[10] (6) gives the periphrastic past and future tense paradigms for the verb *danser* 'to dance'.

(6)   Passé composé, 'danced'

		Singular	Phonetic		Plural	Phonetic
1.	(j')	**ai dansé**	[e dãse]	(on)	**a dansé**	[a dãse]
2.	(tu)	**as dansé**	[a dãse]	(vous)	**avez dansé**	[ave dãse]
3.	(il, elle)	**a dansé**	[a dãse]	(ils, elles)	**ont dansé**	[õ dãse]

(7)   Future proche, 'going to dance'

		Singular	Phonetic		Plural	Phonetic
1.	(je)	**vais danser**	[ve dãse]	(on)	**va danser**	[va dãse]
2.	(tu)	**vas danser**	[va dãse]	(vous)	**allez danser**	[ale dãse]
3.	(il, elle)	**va danser**	[va dãse]	(ils, elles)	**vont danser**	[võ dãse]

It is worth pointing out that a difficulty in coding tense arises from the widespread tendency of young children to omit auxiliaries in their early production. A past participle without an auxiliary can have an adjectival use in adult French, and in the absence of an auxiliary in a child utterance it is nearly impossible to determine which use the child intended (adjective, main verb, or past tense). Similarly, some

---

[9] In all of the (3,000+) utterances we examined, we found only three cases that are at least arguably nonfinite forms with clitic subjects, forms like *je lav[e]* 'I wash-nonfinite'. We have excluded these from our analysis.

[10] The remaining finite tenses, the imperfective past and the simple future, are synthetic. The periphrastic tenses are more frequent in spoken French and are the first to be used by the child acquiring the tense system of French. Accordingly, we focus on the periphrastic tenses here.

Figure 1   *Table 1*

bare infinitives might be instances of the future tense lacking an auxiliary, or they might be true NRFs.

Only forms of the verb consisting of both the auxiliary and the participle/infinitive were coded as instantiations of a future or past tense form. Participles and infinitives used without the auxiliary were coded as nonfinite forms.[11]

2.5 Development of tense and agreement

It is well known that the third person singular (3sg) and present tense forms are the first to appear in child productions, and for a time may be the only finite forms produced by the child. Furthermore, young children tend to overuse 3sg and present tense forms, in contexts where a different form of inflection would be appropriate. This suggests that these 3sg forms and present tense forms serve as **default** forms, causing a complication in coding 3sg verbs with 3sg subjects. Such cases are ambiguous; one cannot tell whether the 3sg verb is truly *agreeing* with the 3sg subject or whether it instead simply lacks agreement and is taking on an "elsewhere" form (see also Ferdinand 1996 for discussion). There is no way to tell the difference empirically (in French); hence, we counted only non-3sg and nonpresent forms as unambiguously showing the presence of agreement and tense. Taking these to indicate true agreement and tense is essentially in accord with Meisel's (1990) definition of acquisition of an inflectional paradigm, according to which a paradigm cannot be considered to have been acquired until the child uses at least two distinct affixes from that paradigm productively. Given that the first affixes are clearly 3sg agreement and present tense, non-3sg and nonpresent tense forms will constitute the second and beyond. Examples from the actual corpus (specifically, Grégoire's) of each finite type are given in (8)–(10).[12]

[11] There were a very small number (3) of examples like *vais partir* 'go to leave' (Grégoire 2;3.0) that unambiguously show first person singular (1sg) agreement yet lack the expected subject clitic. Similarly, there were also rare (we found 9 instances out of 649 agreeing verbs in Grégoire's Stage 4b data) examples like *je va jusqu'ici* 'I goes until here' (Grégoire 2;5.1) where a 1sg subject clitic is paired with a verb showing third person singular (3sg) agreement. Both of these types of utterances were counted as 'agreeing', although their effect on the total number of agreeing verbs is small. We coded any other form of 3sg as potentially default agreement. At Stage 3b, we found no instances of *ce* (*c'*) or *ça* 'this' (as in 'this is mine'), and we counted the few instances of *elle* (3sg feminine) the same as we counted *il* (3sg masculine), as a potential 3sg default. It is possible that only 3sg masculine *il* is a potential default, in which case we might have been able to count 3sg feminine *elle* as truly agreeing, in the same way we took 1sg subject agreement to be truly agreeing. However, because we compared the number of non-3sg forms produced by children with the non-3sg adult targets, and because the number of instances of *elle* subjects was relatively small (Grégoire used *elle* 14/874 times in Stage 3b, 15/732 in Stage 4b, and 49/1,038 in Stage 4c; Philippe used *elle* 29/898 times in Stage 4b and 23/387 in Stage 4c), we believe that we have not introduced any significant error by viewing the 3sg default as we did.

[12] Examples are typically drawn from Grégoire's corpus because Grégoire seems to have a greater spread of forms than Philippe, and Stéphane's utterances are very difficult to code because of the transcription method used in his files.

(8) Marked for both tense and agreement (passé composé, 1sg clitic)

Et   moi **j'ai** roulé sur moi la belle   voiture.   (Grégoire 2;3.0)
and I   I've run   over me the beautiful car
'I have run the beautiful car all over me.'

(9) Tensed but not agreeing (future, but 3sg form of *aller* 'go')[13]

Va assis.   (Grégoire 2;1.25)
go sit.down
'Go sit down. = I am going to sit down.'

(10) Agreeing but not tensed (1sg clitic, but present tense)

Je peux pas.   (Grégoire 2;3.0)
I   can not
'I can't.'

Tables 2 and 3 summarize our findings relating to the use of tense and agreement, respectively, by each child.[14] We make use of several measures in our analysis. Verbs that are 'marked for tense' are verbs that are marked for any tense at all, including present tense.[15] This number includes some verbs that display default present tense (as discussed above), but does not include NRFs. Similarly, verbs that are 'marked for agreement' exclude NRFs but include some verbs marked with default 3sg agreement instead of true agreement.

Table 2 indicates how many of the verbs showing tense marking definitely showed *true* (i.e., nonpresent) tense marking. Table 3 indicates how many verbs showing agreement definitely showed *true* (i.e., non-3sg) agreement marking.

Table 2. Verbs with nonpresent tense inflection (out of tensed verbs)

Child	Stage 3b	Stage 4b	Stage 4c
Grégoire	34% (66/194)	21% (44/212)	32% (205/646)
Stéphane	37% (19/52)	10% (17/179)	25% (34/135)
Philippe		13% (44/334)	30% (74/246)
Weighted average	35% (85/246)	15% (105/725)	31% (313/1,027)

---

[13] While the third person singular form *va* 'goes' and second person singular *vas* 'go' are homophonous, it is clear from the context that a second-person form is not intended.
[14] The data in Tables 2–4 exclude imperative verbs from consideration, but we include questions because many of the child uses of 2sg forms (true agreement) occurred in questions (excluding questions would not have accurately reflected the children's knowledge of agreement).
[15] The present discussion focuses on the acquisition of forms rather than their semantic interpretation. Hence, we do not go into the issue of whether the so-called tensed forms express tense (the external temporal structure of an event) or aspect (the internal structure or unfolding of the event).

Figure 1   *Table 2*

Table 3. Verbs with non-3sg agreement inflection (out of agreeing verbs)

Child	Stage 3b	Stage 4b	Stage 4c
Grégoire	3% (5/156)	19% (33/172)	34% (221/649)
Stéphane	5% (2/43)	12% (13/109)	38% (51/133)
Philippe		15% (44/303)	40% (98/246)
Weighted average	4% (7/199)	15% (90/584)	36% (370/1,028)

Of course, in adult speech (i.e., in the target language), most of the verbs are in the present tense or show 3sg agreement, so these measures of the child data in Tables 2–3 do not hold much meaning until they are compared with the rate of adult non-3sg and nonpresent tense usage.[16] We therefore performed a similar count on the adult utterances in two of the CHILDES files (Philippe 11 and Grégoire 9) in order to get at least a reasonable estimate of the adult use of non-3sg and nonpresent forms. The results are given in Table 4. The combined results from Tables 2–4 are graphed in Figure 2, to illustrate the development of tense and agreement across the attested PLU stages.

Table 4. Adult usage of non-3sg and nonpresent tense

Adults from file	Nonpresent	Non-3sg
Grégoire 9	28% (184/661)	35% (231/659)
Philippe 11	34% (173/507)	41% (206/506)
Stéphane (25b)	31% (61/197)	32% (63/197)
Average	31% (418/1,365)	37% (500/1,362)

Assuming that adults *always* produce finite verbs and observing that they produce nonpresent tense verbs roughly 31% of the time, we can reasonably take the 35% production of nonpresent tense (of tensed verbs) at Stage 3b to be an adult-like level of production. On the other hand, we can also reasonably suppose that the 4% production of non-3sg (of agreeing verbs) at Stage 3b indicates that the children are not realizing agreement and are using a default (3sg) form.

As Tables 2 and 3 and Figure 2 indicate, tense and agreement undergo distinct patterns of development. At Stage 3b, the proportion of (truly) agreeing forms in the children's speech is negligible—it is clear that they are not yet using agreement. At the same time, the proportion of tensed forms is sufficiently high to allow us to conclude that tense is already in regular use. At the subsequent stage, 4b, agreement emerges at a significant, though not yet adult-like, level.

---

[16] The data files are recordings of spontaneous speech between one or more grown-ups and a child playing with toys and dropping them, looking at books, running to the bathroom, refusing to eat, and so on. The context is clearly about the here and now. Yet the use of passé composé and near future by all participants is completely appropriate because activities change through the course of a single recording. For example, the child becomes suddenly hungry and says (while running to the kitchen) that he is going to eat; the child returns to the playroom and looks for the toy car that he previously hid behind a teddy bear; and so on.

Notice that at Stage 4b, tense suffers a dip in production compared with Stage 3b. This interesting correlation between increased use of agreeing forms and decreased use of tensed forms suggests a temporary *competition* between the two before they both stabilize at the subsequent stage, 4c. We expand on this idea further in our analysis of the tense and agreement data in Section 3.

Figure 2. Tense and agreement

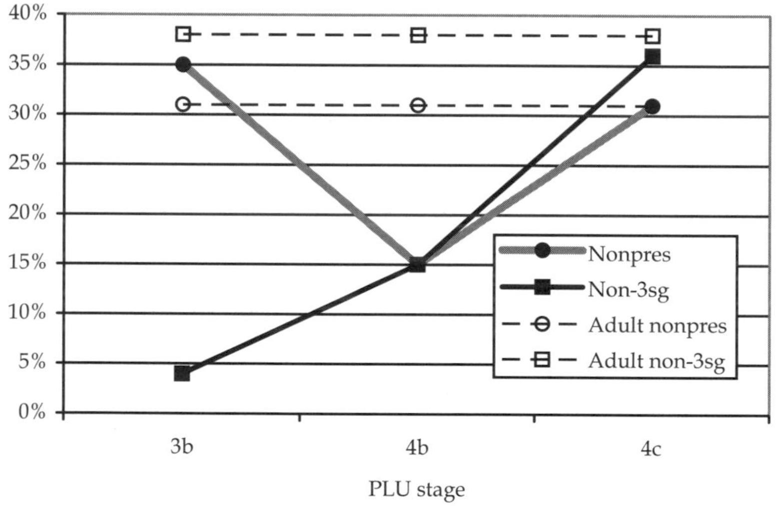

PLU stage

The dissociation between tense and agreement is especially striking in the children's production of periphrastic tenses. Throughout Stage 3b, Grégoire and Stéphane produce numerous instances of the past and future tenses; however, the auxiliary that appears in these utterances is always 3sg.

(11) a. Est tombé puzzle.   (Grégoire 1;9.18)
          is   fallen puzzle
          'The puzzle has fallen down.'

      b. Papa et   Maman est parti.   (Grégoire 2;0.5)
          Father and Mother is gone
          'Father and Mother have gone.' (lit. 'Father and Mother has gone.')

Broadly speaking, our results are consistent with previously reported data from child French. However, we cannot directly compare our findings with those in the existing literature for two reasons. First, we see a fine-grained course of development through stages delimited by the PLU measure, with systematic differences between stages; yet previous research with which we could otherwise have compared our results has generally analyzed data collapsed over two or more PLU stages, or even over the entire corpus (e.g., Pierce 1992; Ferdinand 1996).

Figure 2   *Table 4*

Second, previous work on the acquisition of French has used 'finiteness' as a cover term encompassing both tense and agreement inflection, precluding any systematic study of the development of these inflections individually. However, we have shown that tense and agreement do follow different courses of development: agreement develops in an incremental linear fashion, not acquired at Stage 3b but controlled by Stage 4c, while tense develops in a U-shaped curve, controlled at Stages 3b and 4c yet often omitted at Stage 4b. Our findings from French thus strongly indicate that these two grammatical categories are independent. This conclusion is also strongly bolstered by the results from the acquisition of Catalan reported by Davidson and Legendre (2003), which also show tense and agreement developing independently, but in the reverse order, with agreement becoming productive before tense (see also Grinstead 1994).

2.6 Nonfinite root forms

Turning now to NRFs, we found that children produce steadily fewer as their age/PLU stage increases. Our findings are illustrated in Table 5 and the accompanying graph, Figure 3.[17] Table 5 displays the proportion of NRFs out of all verbs, excluding questions. Some of these verbs were not clearly determinable as either NRFs or tensed/agreeing forms; such verbs were excluded from the count of NRFs, although not from the count of all verbs. This means that the proportions in Table 5 are conservative and might be underestimates.

Table 5. Proportion of nonfinite root forms of all verbs

Child	Stage 3b	Stage 4b	Stage 4c
Grégoire	28% (82/297)	16% (46/287)	1% (6/711)
Stéphane	48% (51/106)	12% (25/205)	2% (3/152)
Philippe		21% (102/476)	4% (11/260)
Weighted average	33% (133/403)	18% (173/968)	2% (20/1,123)

Comparing Figure 3 with the graph of agreement (Figure 2), we note that the reduction in the use of NRFs over time appears to be inversely correlated with the development of agreement: in a sense, the NRF pattern is the mirror image of the pattern we found for agreement (recall Table 3). By contrast, the decrease in NRFs does not appear to correlate with the development of tense; compare Figure 3 with the graph of tense (Figure 2). Put another way, if there is a connection between the occur-

---

[17] It is likely that an earlier stage (PLU Stage 2) can be observed, where the proportions of NRFs are much higher (and those of tensed and agreeing forms much lower) than the ones attested in our data. Although Stage 2 was not instantiated in our French data, we have observed such a stage in the utterances of the Swedish-learning children Harry and Markus, who produced 68% NRFs at that stage. Furthermore, the French-learning child Nathalie, whose production was studied by Pierce (1992) and Ferdinand (1996), is reported to produce only 4% finite verbs and almost no overt subjects in her earliest file (age 1;9.3). It is possible that Nathalie's production reflects the syntax at Stage 2; however, we have been unable to study this child's speech since her files are not publicly available.

rence of NRFs and the development of either tense or agreement, the connection is between NRFs and agreement, not tense.

Figure 3. Proportion of nonfinite root forms of all verbs

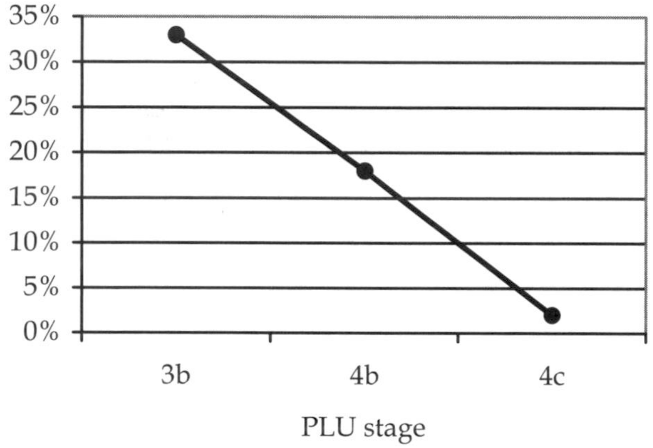

PLU stage

3 An Optimality Theory analysis of the development of finiteness

In this section, we argue that an analysis that exploits three formal properties of OT — (i) competition (for a single projection), (ii) constraint reranking, and (iii) partial ordering of constraints at any stage of the developing grammar—straightforwardly accounts for the developmental course outlined above as well as the observed percentages summarized in Sections 2.5–2.6.

3.1 Development of finiteness: General analysis

Informally, the main idea is this. At Stage 3b, constraints requiring realization of finiteness compete with constraints on economy of structure, sometimes resulting in finite verbs and sometimes resulting in NRFs. At Stage 4b, tense and agreement compete for a single structural position, a functional projection that can realize the features either of tense or of agreement (but not both).[18] At Stage 4c, two positions and therefore two projections become available, allowing both tense and agreement features to be realized without competition. Formally, the constraints that require realization of the functional features (tense, agreement) rise in the ranking relative to a

---

[18] The categories tense and agreement are implemented as functional projections following the X′ Theory schema: the Inflectional Phrase (IP) has simply been split into two projections, TP and AgrP, headed by Tense and Agreement, respectively (Pollock 1989; Belletti 1990; see Box 12:1). While alternative representations of inflectional/functional categories presumably can be developed, we do not think they would alter the basic claims of this chapter. The functional projection approach is a convenient way to express structure building, and it allows a comparison with numerous related studies using the same kind of representation but making radically different claims.

Figure 3   *Table 5*

fixed hierarchy of constraints penalizing structure (*STRUCTURE, Prince and Smolensky 1993/2004; Chapter 12 (40a) of this book). Variation in the optimal outcome arises from a constraint's ranking being specified by a range (Reynolds 1994; Nagy and Reynolds 1997).

The constraints requiring realization of functional features are faithfulness constraints. They ensure that what is expressed (the output of the grammar) differs minimally from what is intended (the input to the grammar, which we assume does contain functional features like tense and agreement). Constraints prohibiting structure, on the other hand, are economy constraints belonging to the family of markedness constraints. The present study supports the general picture emerging from studies of acquisition of phonology (e.g., Levelt 1994; Demuth 1995; Gnanadesikan 1995; Pater and Paradis 1996; Stemberger and Bernhardt 1998). Empirically speaking, it appears that in adult grammars, faithfulness constraints often dominate markedness constraints, whereas in early child grammars, the reverse often holds, with markedness constraints dominating faithfulness constraints (resulting in "simplified" (less marked) structures). In fact, Smolensky (1996) shows that, assuming children's underlying representations (or "inputs" to the optimality evaluation system) are the same as adults', for unmarked structures to be learnable, the markedness constraints must outrank the faithfulness constraints in the initial state of the grammar (see Chapters 4 and 17). From this perspective, the process of acquisition consists in reranking the constraints such that some faithfulness constraints outrank markedness constraints (see Tesar and Smolensky 1998, 2000 for discussion of constraint demotion as a learning procedure in strict domination hierarchies; Hayes 2004 and Prince and Tesar 1999 on maintaining the dominance of markedness during learning; and Boersma 1997 and Boersma and Hayes 2001 for discussions of learning partial rankings statistically).[19] The present study contributes evidence that this proceeds via constraints **floating** over a certain range (i.e., yielding a partial constraint ordering), rather than through abrupt and absolute constraint reranking.

Our analysis uses the economy-of-structure constraints defined in (12).

(12)   Economy-of-structure constraints (*STRUCTURE family)

   *F   No functional heads.

   *F^2 No pairs of functional heads.

The constraint *F is violated by any candidate structure that has a functional projection, be it Tense or Agreement. *F is satisfied only by nonfinite verbs, which, by assumption, have no functional projections realizing tense or agreement features. *F^2 is violated by any structure that has two functional projections—that is, by structures in which both tense and agreement features are realized.[20]

---

[19] While inventories of entirely unmarked structures would presumably be easiest to process in production and comprehension, they do not allow for the range of distinctions that adult language expresses. Therefore, learning a target grammar rich enough to express such distinctions requires interleaving faithfulness constraints among structural markedness constraints. On this view, reranking is driven by the cognitive and functional role of grammars, that is, the need to express distinctions.

[20] *F^2 is not a basic constraint; rather, it is the local conjunction of two instances of *F (*F^2 ≡ *F&*F) (see

The faithfulness constraints relevant to our analysis are given in (13). PARSET is violated by any untensed form, and PARSEA by any nonagreeing form.

(13)   Faithfulness constraints (PARSE family; Prince and Smolensky 1993/2004)

   PARSET   Parse Tense (i.e., realize input Tense).

   PARSEA   Parse Agreement (i.e., realize input Agreement).

We assume that the input to every evaluation has tense and agreement features subject to these faithfulness constraints. There are four candidate structures relevant to this analysis; they are given in (14) along with examples and the constraints each satisfies and violates.

(14)   Candidates for input containing past tense and 1sg agreement features

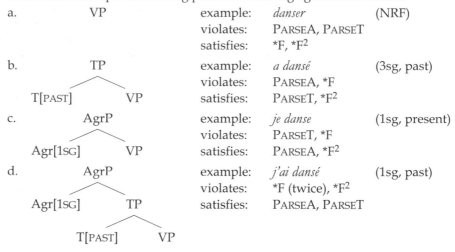

		example:	*danser*	(NRF)
a.	VP	violates:	PARSEA, PARSET	
		satisfies:	*F, *F^2	
b.	TP	example:	*a dansé*	(3sg, past)
	T[PAST] VP	violates:	PARSEA, *F	
		satisfies:	PARSET, *F^2	
c.	AgrP	example:	*je danse*	(1sg, present)
	Agr[1SG] VP	violates:	PARSET, *F	
		satisfies:	PARSEA, *F^2	
d.	AgrP	example:	*j'ai dansé*	(1sg, past)
	Agr[1SG] TP	violates:	*F (twice), *F^2	
	T[PAST] VP	satisfies:	PARSEA, PARSET	

The four candidate structures are evaluated against a strictly ranked set of constraints, meaning that for any two constraints, one has priority over the other. We interpret this as a requirement on each *evaluation* rather than on each *grammar*, however. By allowing a single grammar to encode several possible rankings (by allowing

Section 12:1.8 and Chapter 14). That is, *F^2 is a constraint formed from two (identical) more basic constraints. *F^2 is necessarily ranked above *F, because they are part of a power hierarchy (Chapters 12, 14, 16); a local conjunction universally outranks the individual conjoined constraints. This formalizes the intuition we wish to capture, that having two functional heads is qualitatively more costly than having one, which results in the fixed ranking *F^2 ≫ *F. Where no constraints intervene between two universally ranked constraints, they can be 'encapsulated' as if a single constraint in the hierarchy (see Davidson and Legendre 2003; Prince and Smolensky 1993/2004, Chap. 8; and Box 13:1). As we will show, constraints can be ranked between *F^2 and *F, which therefore have to be separated into two distinct constraints. Even in a theory with floating constraints, constraints are strictly ranked with respect to one another in any given evaluation, and therefore it is not possible for two violations of *F to overpower a higher-ranked constraint. Finally, note that constraints against structure (like *F and *F^2) have been argued to play a role in the adult language as well (see, e.g., Grimshaw 1994), as we would expect, given the claim of OT that the inventory of constraints is universal. For a similar idea, not couched in OT terms, see Speas's (1994) Economy of Projection in adult grammars and an application to early child English in Roeper and Rohrbacher 1994.

Figure 3   *Table 5*

partial rankings in the grammar, which are fixed in some possibly different strict order before each evaluation), we gain a means to explain variation: for example, across sociolects, throughout the evolution of a language, or—as is particularly relevant here—over the course of language acquisition. Others have pursued this idea in studying variation in phonology, morphology, and learnability (Kiparsky 1993; Reynolds 1994; Anttila 1997; Boersma 1997; Nagy and Reynolds 1997; Boersma and Levelt 1999; Boersma and Hayes 2001). Behind this approach is the recognition that (grammar-level) partial constraint rankings determine sets of strict rankings (consistent with Prince and Smolensky 1993/2004), each of which can potentially yield a different optimal output.

The key to our proposal is the ability of the faithfulness constraints to 'float' over a certain range in the ranking (unlike the *STRUCTURE constraints discussed above, which remain fixed in their universal relative ranking) during development. This is illustrated in (15), where PARSET ranges from below *F to above *F. A partial ordering like (15a) translates into the set of two rankings in (15b).

(15)   a.   Partial ordering
            Fixed: $*F^2 \gg *F$
            Floating: PARSET   ——————— $\Rightarrow$

          b.   Set of total rankings
              i. $*F^2 \gg *F \gg$ PARSET winning candidate: (14a) yields: untensed verb
             ii. $*F^2 \gg$ PARSET $\gg *F$ winning candidate: (14b) yields: tensed verb

A different candidate structure wins under each of the rankings in (15b): under ranking (15b.i), a candidate with a nonfinite verb wins; under ranking (15b.ii), a candidate with a tensed verb (i.e., with a functional projection to realize tense features). For any given evaluation, a grammar with the partial ordering in (15a) will use one of the rankings, either (15b.i) or (15b.ii), to determine the optimal candidate. Thus, in any given evaluation, either a tensed verb or an untensed verb will win the competition. We adopt the further assumption that, randomly, *either of the two rankings has an equal chance of being called upon during an evaluation* (Anttila 1997, 1998). This means there is a 50% chance that ranking (15b.i) will be used, yielding an untensed verb as the optimal candidate. To put it another way, we expect to see the untensed candidate 50% of the time (and to see the tensed candidate the other 50% of the time). Under this hypothesis, the model allows us to predict not only *that* we will see variation between output forms *A* and *B* in the developing grammar, but also *with what frequency* we will see each.[21]

---

[21] An alternative way to interpret floating constraints of this sort would be to suppose that, while various rankings are possible given the range over which the constraints float, some are more likely than others. For example, it might be that a constraint is more likely to be evaluated in the ranking at the center of its range than near the edges of its range (a version of such an approach is developed in Boersma 1997). We have not explored this alternative in any detail, but it is also not clear that either interpretation can lay claim to being the obvious null hypothesis. We therefore pursue the view that all possible rankings are equally probable, with the understanding that a view based on a normal distribution over a range might also be tenable.

This example illustrates well the nature of the conflict underlying the development of finiteness. Functional features can only be parsed (satisfying the faithfulness constraints PARSET and/or PARSEA) if the economy-of-structure constraints (*F and possibly *F^2) are violated. The conflict is resolved by the ranking. If economy of structure dominates faithfulness, then functional features cannot be realized and the optimal candidate will be a nonfinite form acting as a main verb (an NRF). If faithfulness dominates economy of structure, then functional features will be parsed into a functional head, yielding a finite form as the optimal candidate (recall that *either* tensed *or* agreeing forms count as 'finite' under our terminology). The actual course of development of finiteness we propose here is an expanded version of this basic reranking schema. We will show that the PARSE constraints advance separately, with PARSET invariably outranking PARSEA at one point (Stage 3b), with the result that the observed finite forms are tensed, but nonagreeing. In the following section, we present our analysis of the development of finiteness stage by stage.

3.2 Development of finiteness: A stage-by-stage analysis

We begin with Stage 3b, where the rankings are as in (16), yielding the three rankings given in (17).

(16)   Stage 3b partial ordering
       Fixed: *F^2 ≫ *F
       Floating: PARSET   ——————————
                PARSEA   ——

(17)   Stage 3b total rankings
    a.   PARSET ≫ *F^2 ≫ *F ≫ PARSEA   yields: tensed
    b.   *F^2 ≫ PARSET ≫ *F ≫ PARSEA   yields: tensed
    c.   *F^2 ≫ *F ≫ PARSET ≫ PARSEA   yields: NRF

At Stage 3b, PARSET spans a range allowing it to sometimes outrank *F^2, and sometimes be outranked by *F. PARSEA is always outranked by both PARSET and *F.[22]

Of the three rankings in (17), only (17c) results in an NRF; under this ranking, it is better not to have a functional projection (satisfying *F) than to realize tense (which

---

A second point about the partial rankings is that we take them to be simply *orderings*, without any further mathematical structure, an assumption we would only want to depart from in the face of convincing evidence that further complication is required (although, for a possible instance of such evidence, see Davidson and Goldrick 2003). If rankings are viewed as orderings, there is no meaningful way to say that constraint A is ranked "more above than below" another constraint B; constraint A either overlaps constraint B or it doesn't. This significantly narrows the range of possible predictions our system can make, which is clearly desirable. As we will show, our assumptions yield a tight match between predicted and observed percentages of alternative child forms.

[22] The fact that PARSET outranks PARSEA does not follow from our analysis; it could as easily have been the other way around. The evidence from French indicates that PARSET initially outranks PARSEA, but evidence from Catalan (Davidson and Legendre 2003) appears to show PARSEA initially outranking PARSET. The difference is presumably a function of the primary linguistic data the child receives, but we will not pursue this question further here.

Figure 3   *Table 5*

would satisfy PARSET) or agreement (which would satisfy PARSEA). This means that we expect NRFs to comprise one-third of a child's utterances at Stage 3b.

The other two rankings yield a tensed form, but without agreement. Under these two rankings, PARSET outranks *F, making it more important to realize tense in a functional projection than to avoid functional projections. Neither ranking yields a form that also agrees because this would require two functional projections, and PARSEA is outranked by $*F^2$ under both rankings. Thus, we expect tensed forms (lacking agreement) to comprise the other two-thirds of a child's utterances at Stage 3b.[23]

What we actually observed (recall Table 5) was 33% NRFs and 67% finite forms, exactly our prediction. Of the finite forms, we counted only nonpresent forms, and found 35% such forms (Table 2). Recall that when this is compared with the adult production of 31% nonpresent forms (Table 4), it appears that all finite utterances the children produce at Stage 3b are tensed. For agreement (Table 3), we found very few (4%) non-3sg forms, compared with an adult rate of 38%. So, idealizing a little, we find that all finite child utterances at Stage 3b are tensed but nonagreeing, as predicted.

In Stage 4b, illustrated in (18), PARSEA advances to a position equal to PARSET; both now sometimes outrank $*F^2$ and can sometimes be outranked by *F. Moreover, in some rankings PARSET outranks PARSEA, while in others PARSEA outranks PARSET. These ranges yield the 12 rankings in (19).[24]

(18)   Stage 4b partial ordering
       Fixed: $*F^2$ $\gg$ *F
       Floating: PARSET   ————————————
                   PARSEA   ————————————

---

[23] Although we have not investigated this systematically here, our analysis also predicts that if negation introduces a functional projection of its own that violates *F, it should similarly compete with tense and agreement, predicting that we should see more default forms and NRFs in negative utterances than in nonnegative ones. Existing studies on the interaction of negation and NRFs (e.g., Levow 1995) have not differentiated default from nondefault tense and agreement, leaving the question open, although this prediction clearly runs counter to Rizzi's (1993/1994) prediction that negation should entail tense. It is perhaps suggestive that in a brief review of Grégoire's Stage 3b and 4b files, we indeed found only present tense (potential default) verbs in negative contexts, although Grégoire was producing nondefault tensed verbs otherwise. In his Stage 4c files, on the other hand, he used several nonpresent finite verbs with negation.

[24] To avoid confusion, a word about the "psychological reality" of this system may be in order. Although a higher degree of constraint overlap results in a larger number of possible rankings for each evaluation, this does not in any way mean that the child must "exert more effort to choose" when there is a large number of possible rankings than when there is a small number of possible rankings. We could use the metaphor of choosing a random number for each constraint, to determine at which point in its range it will fall for the purposes of the ranking (Boersma 1998). Under this metaphor, the child's task is to choose a random position for each constraint before each evaluation, a task that doesn't change no matter how much or how little constraints overlap with one another. Knowing the constraint ranges, we can predict which rankings could result and compute the individual likelihood of each, but the number of possibilities we determine this way has no effect on the procedure required to fix a ranking; for 4 constraints, there are always 4 random positions to choose, whether these choices could result in 2, 3, or 12 different possible rankings.

(19)   Stage 4b total rankings

     a.   PARSET $\gg$ PARSEA $\gg$ *F^2 $\gg$ *F   yields: tensed and agreeing

     b.   PARSEA $\gg$ PARSET $\gg$ *F^2 $\gg$ *F   yields: tensed and agreeing

     c.   *F^2 $\gg$ *F $\gg$ PARSET $\gg$ PARSEA   yields: NRF

     d.   *F^2 $\gg$ *F $\gg$ PARSEA $\gg$ PARSET   yields: NRF

     e.   *F^2 $\gg$ PARSET $\gg$ PARSEA $\gg$ *F   yields: tensed

     f.   *F^2 $\gg$ PARSEA $\gg$ PARSET $\gg$ *F   yields: agreeing

     g.   PARSET $\gg$ *F^2 $\gg$ PARSEA $\gg$ *F   yields: tensed

     h.   PARSEA $\gg$ *F^2 $\gg$ PARSET $\gg$ *F   yields: agreeing

     i.   PARSET $\gg$ *F^2 $\gg$ *F $\gg$ PARSEA   yields: tensed

     j.   PARSEA $\gg$ *F^2 $\gg$ *F $\gg$ PARSET   yields: agreeing

     k.   *F^2 $\gg$ PARSET $\gg$ *F $\gg$ PARSEA   yields: tensed

     l.   *F^2 $\gg$ PARSEA $\gg$ *F $\gg$ PARSET   yields: agreeing

First, notice that two of these rankings, (19a–b), yield verb forms that are both tensed and agreeing (i.e., essentially adult forms), since under those rankings it is more important to realize both tense and agreement than it is to avoid having two functional projections. Another two rankings, (19c–d), yield NRFs, since under these rankings it is more important not to have any functional projections than it is to realize either tense or agreement. The remaining rankings (19e–l) yield finite forms that are either tensed (when PARSET outranks PARSEA) or agreeing (when PARSEA outranks PARSET), but not both.

This predicts, then, that only 17% (2 out of 12) of the verb forms uttered at Stage 4b should be NRFs. We observed (Table 5) 19% NRFs, very close to the prediction. Of the remaining verbs, all finite, 20% are predicted to be adult-like (with both tense and agreement), the remaining forms having only one or the other (40% with only tense, 40% with only agreement). To compute the predictions we make for the child data, we must scale the percentages by the expected proportion of nonpresent forms and non-3sg forms, on the basis of the observed adult speech (Table 4). Concretely, our analysis predicts 60% of finite forms will be tensed (there are 10 finite rankings, 4 of which result in tense alone, and 2 of which result in both tense and agreement), and adults produce 31% nonpresent forms, so we expect to find 60% × 31% = 19% nonpresent forms in the children's (finite) utterances. Similarly, since adults produce 38% non-3sg forms, we expect to find 60% × 38% = 23% non-3sg forms in the children's (finite) utterances. Again, the predictions line up well with the observations. Among the finite verbs, we predict 19% nonpresent forms and observe 15% (Tables 2 and 4), and we predict 23% non-3sg forms and observe 15% (Tables 3 and 4).

Compare Stage 4b and Stage 3b with respect to the realization of tense. Notice that, while at Stage 3b, 100% of the finite forms are tensed, at Stage 4b only 60% (6 out of 10) are tensed. In other words, we predict (and in fact observe) a dip in the child's production of tensed forms. If children were simply "learning tense" (speaking vaguely), we would not have expected them to get *worse* at any point during development.[25] The proposed analysis provides an explanation for this otherwise puzzling fact. Back in Stage 3b, PARSEA was ranked so low as to ensure that tense features were realized in the single functional projection allowed. What has happened at Stage 4b is that the tense features and agreement features now *compete* for realization in the single functional projection available. Since tense sometimes (in fact, half the time) loses to agreement, we predict the observed dip in the proportion of tensed forms, which coincides with an increase in the proportion of agreeing forms.

In the last stage covered in our data, Stage 4c, PARSET and PARSEA together move to a position high enough in the hierarchy to invariably outrank *F^2.[26] This yields two rankings, but both produce the same optimal candidate, a finite form that realizes both tense and agreement. At this stage, we predict no NRFs, and we observed only 2% NRFs in child speech (Table 5). We also expect the children's production of non-present forms and non-3sg forms to match the proportion in adult speech, which it does quite well; we observed (Tables 2–4) 31% nonpresent tense forms compared with 31% for adults, and 36% non-3sg forms compared with 37% for adults.

(20) Stage 4c partial ordering
   Fixed: *F^2 ≫   *F
   Floating: PARSET ——
                   PARSEA ——

(21) Stage 4c total rankings
   a.   PARSET ≫ PARSEA ≫ *F^2 ≫ *F   yields: tensed and agreeing
   b.   PARSEA ≫ PARSET ≫ *F^2 ≫ *F   yields: tensed and agreeing

We have now illustrated our analysis of the development of finiteness in child language acquisition, whose predictions match the observed figures quite closely.

3.3 Summary of the predictions and results

We have outlined the framework of partial rankings and floating constraints in OT and have given a specific analysis for three stages of child language in terms of the

---

[25] Note that this does not appear to be a traditional "U-shaped curve" attributed to the use of memorized forms early on, followed by a learned but overgeneralized rule, and finally followed by a reduction in the domain of application for the rule. In Grégoire's transcripts, for example, he uses several verb stems in both present and past forms (including *tourner* 'turn', *monter* 'go up', *passer* 'drive by', *manger* 'eat', and *voir* 'see'), and most verbs appear in both finite and nonfinite (often the past participle) variants. The existence of these verbs in the transcripts suggests that the observed dip in tense production is not simply due to early memorization.

[26] There are discontinuous jumps in the rankings between Stages 3b and 4b and between Stages 4b and 4c. Given that, we might expect to find intermediate stages as well; for example, between Stages 3b and 4b we might expect a Stage 3b' in which PARSEA has advanced partway, but is still always ranked below *F^2, and between Stages 4b and 4c we might expect a Stage 4b' in which PARSEA and PARSET are no longer ever outranked by *F. While we do not have much evidence on this issue, we did find one file (Philippe 10) between Stage 4b and Stage 4c that shows roughly the proportions we would expect for a stage with 4b' rankings. It has been harder to find a convincing case of Stage 3b' in the data we have examined. More thorough investigation of these intermediate stages must await future research.

rankings of the two faithfulness constraints PARSET and PARSEA and the two markedness constraints *F and *F². We end this chapter by showing the close match between the predictions of the system and the observed rates of tense and agreement marking over the course of acquisition.

In Figures 4–6, we compare graphically the observed and predicted results for nonpresent tense, non-3sg agreement, and NRFs for each stage.

We wish again to highlight the fact that the predictions made here are not made (either correctly or incorrectly) by existing analyses of the acquisition of tense and agreement. Given our results from Section 2, showing that the course of acquisition is systematic and grammatical in nature (as shown by the differential rates of tense and agreement use), it is clear that these facts require explanation. While previous analyses in the literature have concentrated on predicting the *existence* of different forms at different points during acquisition, this analysis goes a step further and predicts *how often* the forms will occur.

Figure 4. Predictions of the analysis versus observed data: Nonfinite root forms

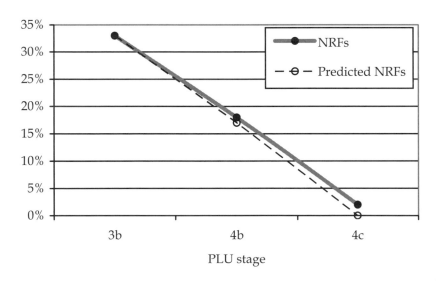

Figure 4   *Table 5*

Figure 5. Predictions of the analysis versus observed data: Non-3sg forms

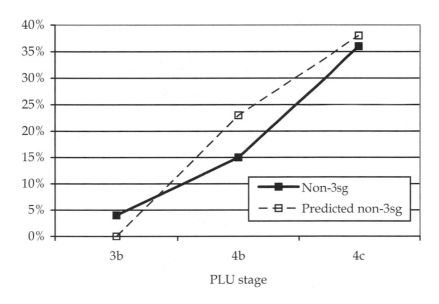

PLU stage

Figure 6. Predictions of the analysis versus observed data: Nonpresent tense form

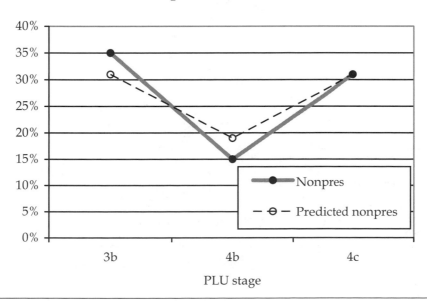

PLU stage

References

ROA = Rutgers Optimality Archive, http://roa.rutgers.edu

Anttila, A. 1997. Variation in Finnish phonology and morphology. Ph.D. diss., Stanford University.

Anttila, A. 1998. Deriving variation from grammar. In *Variation, change, and phonological theory*, eds. F. Hinskens, R. van Hout, and W. L. Wetzel. Benjamins.

Auger, J. 1994. Pronominal clitics in Québec colloquial French: A morphological analysis. Ph.D. diss., University of Pennsylvania.

Belletti, A. 1990. *Generalized verb movement*. Rosenberg and Sellier.

Boersma, P. 1997. How we learn variation, optionality, and probability. In *Proceedings of the Institute of Phonetic Sciences of the University of Amsterdam 21*.

Boersma, P. 1998. *Functional phonology: Formalizing the interactions between articulatory and perceptual drives*. Holland Academic Graphics.

Boersma, P., and B. Hayes. 2001. Empirical tests of the gradual learning algorithm. *Linguistic Inquiry* 32, 45–86. ROA 348.

Boersma, P., and C. Levelt. 1999. Gradual constraint-ranking learning algorithm predicts acquisition order. In *Proceedings of the Child Language Research Forum 30*.

Boser, K., B. C. Lust, L. Santelmann, and J. Whitman. 1992. The syntax of CP and V-2 in early child German: The strong continuity hypothesis. In *Proceedings of the North East Linguistic Society* 23.

Brown, R. 1973. *A first language: The early stages*. Harvard University Press.

Clark, E. 1985. The acquisition of Romance, with special reference to French. In *The crosslinguistic study of language acquisition*. Vol. 1, *The data*, ed. D. I. Slobin. Erlbaum.

Crago, M. B., and S. E. M. Allen. 2001. Early finiteness in Inuktitut: The role of language structure and input. *Language Acquisition* 9, 59–111.

Davidson, L., and M. Goldrick. 2003. Tense, agreement and defaults in child Catalan: An optimality theoretic analysis. In *Linguistic theory and language development in Hispanic languages*, eds. S. Montrul and F. Ordóñez. Cascadilla Press.

Davidson, L., and G. Legendre. 2003. Defaults and competition in the acquisition of functional categories in Catalan and French. In *A Romance perspective on language knowledge and use: Selected papers from the 2001 Linguistic Symposium on Romance Languages (LSRL)*, eds. R. Nuñez-Cedeño, L. López, and R. Cameron. Benjamins.

De Haan, G. R., and K. Tuijnman. 1988. Missing subjects and objects in child grammar. In *Language development*, eds. P. Jordens and J. Lalleman. Foris.

Demuth, K. 1995. Markedness and the development of prosodic structure. In *Proceedings of the North East Linguistic Society 25*. ROA 50.

Dietiker, S. 1978. *En bonne forme: Révision de grammaire française*. D. C. Heath.

Ferdinand, A. 1996. *The development of functional categories: The acquisition of the subject in French*. Holland Institute of Generative Linguistics.

Gnanadesikan, A. 1995. Markedness and faithfulness constraints in child phonology. Ms., University of Massachusetts at Amherst. ROA 67.

Grimshaw, J. 1994. Minimal projection and clause structure. In *Syntactic theory and first language acquisition*, eds. B. Lust et al. Erlbaum.

Grinstead, J. 1994. Tense, agreement, and nominative case in child Catalan and Spanish. Master's thesis, UCLA.

Guasti, M. 1994. Verb syntax in Italian child grammar: Finite and nonfinite verbs. *Language Acquisition* 3, 1–40.

Hamann, C., L. Rizzi, and U. Frauenfelder. 1995. On the acquisition of the pronominal system in French. *Recherches Linguistiques* 24, 83–101.

Hayes, B. 2004. Phonological acquisition in Optimality Theory: The early stages. In *Constraints in phonological acquisition*, eds. R. Kager, J. Pater, and W. Zonneveld. Cambridge University Press. ROA 327.

Hyams, N. 1996. The underspecification of functional categories in early grammar. In *Generative approaches to first and second language acquisition*, eds. H. Clahsen and R. Hawkins. Benjamins.

Jakubowicz, C., and C. Rigaut. 1997. L'acquisition des clitiques nominatifs en français. In *Les pronoms: Syntaxe, morphologie et typologie*, ed. A. Zribi-Hertz. Presses Universitaires de Vincennes.

Kaiser, G. 1994. More about INFL-ection and agreement: The acquisition of clitic pronouns in French. In *Bilingual first language acquisition: French and German grammatical development*, ed. J. Meisel. Benjamins.

Kiparsky, P. 1993. Variable rules. Talk presented at the Rutgers Optimality Workshop-1.

Klee, T., and M. D. Fitzgerald. 1985. The relation between grammatical development and mean length of utterances in morphemes. *Journal of Child Language* 12, 251–69.

Krämer, I. 1993. The licensing of subjects in early child language. In *Papers on case and agreement II*, ed. C. Phillips. MIT Working Papers in Linguistics, MIT.

Lambrecht, K. 1981. *Topic, antitopic and verb agreement in nonstandard French*. Benjamins.

Legendre, G. 2001. An introduction to Optimality Theory in syntax. In *Optimality-theoretic syntax*, eds. G. Legendre, J. Grimshaw, and S. Vikner. MIT Press.

Legendre, G., P. Hagstrom, J. Chen-Main, L. Tao, and P. Smolensky. 2004. Deriving output probabilities in child Mandarin from a dual-optimization grammar. *Lingua* 114, 1147–85.

Legendre, G., P. Hagstrom, A. Vainikka, and M. Todorova. 2002. Partial constraint ordering in child French syntax. *Language Acquisition* 10, 189–227.

Legendre, G., W. Raymond, and P. Smolensky. 1993. An optimality-theoretic typology of case and grammatical voice systems. In *Proceedings of the Berkeley Linguistics Society 19*. ROA 3.

Levelt, C. 1994. *On the acquisition of place*. Holland Institute of Generative Linguistics.

Levow, G.-A. 1995. Tense and subject position in interrogatives and negatives in child French: Evidence for and against truncated structure. In *Papers on language acquisition and processing*, eds. C. Schütze, J. Ganger, and K. Broihier. MIT Working Papers in Linguistics.

Lightbown, P. 1977. Consistency and variation in the acquisition of French. Ph.D. diss., Columbia University.

MacWhinney, B., and C. Snow. 1985. The Child Language Data Exchange System. *Journal of Child Language* 12, 271–96.

Meisel, J. 1990. INFL-ection: Subjects and subject-verb agreement. In *Two first languages: Early grammatical development in bilingual children*, ed. J. Meisel. Foris.

Meisel, J., and M. Ezeizabarrena. 1996. Subject-verb and object-verb agreement in early Basque. In *Language acquisition: Empirical findings, theoretical considerations, cross-linguistic comparisons*, ed. H. Clahsen. Benjamins.

Miller, M. 1976. *Zur Logik der frühkindlichen Sprachentwicklung*. Klett.

Miller, P. 1992. *Clitics and constituents in phrase structure grammar*. Garland.

Nagy, N., and W. Reynolds. 1997. Optimality Theory and variable word-final deletion in Fætar. *Language Variation and Change* 9, 37–55.

Pater, J., and J. Paradis. 1996. Truncation without templates in child phonology. In *Proceedings of the Boston University Conference on Language Development 20*.

Phillips, C. 1995. Syntax at age two: Cross-linguistic differences. In *Papers on language acquisition and processing*, eds. C. Schütze, J. Ganger, and K. Broihier. MIT Working Papers in Linguistics.

Pierce, A. 1992. *Language acquisition and syntactic theory: A comparative analysis of French and English child grammars*. Kluwer.

Poeppel, D., and K. Wexler. 1993. The full competence hypothesis of clause structure in early German. *Language* 69, 1–33.

Pollock, J.-Y. 1989. Verb movement, Universal Grammar, and the structure of IP. *Linguistic Inquiry* 20, 365–424.

Prince, A., and P. Smolensky. 1993/2004. *Optimality Theory: Constraint interaction in generative grammar*. Technical report, Rutgers University and University of Colorado at Boulder, 1993. ROA 537, 2002. Revised version published by Blackwell, 2004.

Prince, A., and B. B. Tesar. 1999. Learning phonotactic distributions. Ms., Rutgers University. ROA 353.

Radford, A. 1990. *Syntactic theory and the acquisition of English syntax*. Blackwell.

Reynolds, W. 1994. Variation and phonological theory. Ph.D. diss., University of Pennsylvania.

Rizzi, L. 1993/1994. Some notes in linguistic theory and language development: The case of root infinitives. *Language Acquisition* 3, 371–93.

Roberge, Y. 1990. *The syntactic recoverability of null arguments*. McGill-Queen's University Press.

Roeper, T., and B. Rohrbacher. 1994. Null subjects in early child English and the theory of economy of projection. Ms., University of Massachusetts at Amherst and University of Pennsylvania.

Rohrbacher, B., and A. Vainikka. 1994. On German verb syntax under age 2. IRCS Technical report 94-24, Institute for Research in Cognitive Science, University of Pennsylvania.

Rondal, J. A. 1985. *Adult-child interaction and the process of language understanding*. Praeger.

Smolensky, P. 1996. The initial state and 'Richness of the Base' in Optimality Theory. Technical report JHU-CogSci-96-4, Cognitive Science Department, Johns Hopkins University. ROA 154.

Speas, M. 1994. Null arguments in a theory of economy of projections. In *University of Massachusetts occasional papers in linguistics 17: Functional projections*, eds. E. Benedicto and J. Runner. Graduate Linguistic Student Association, University of Massachusetts at Amherst.

Stemberger, J. P., and B. H. Bernhardt. 1998. *Handbook of phonological development from the perspective of constraint-based nonlinear phonology*. Academic Press.

Suppes, P., R. Smith, and M. Leveillé. 1973. The French syntax of a child's noun phrases. *Archives de Psychologie* 42, 207–69.

Tesar, B. B., and P. Smolensky. 1998. Learning optimality-theoretic grammars. *Lingua* 106, 161–96.

Tesar, B. B., and P. Smolensky. 2000. *Learnability in Optimality Theory*. MIT Press.

Vainikka, A., G. Legendre, and M. Todorova. 1999. PLU stages: An independent measure of early syntactic development. Technical report JHU-CogSci-99-10, Johns Hopkins University.

Wexler, K. 1994. Optional infinitives, head movement, and economy of derivation. In *Verb movement*, eds. N. Hornstein and D. Lightfoot. Cambridge University Press.

Wexler, K. 1998. Very early parameter setting and the Unique Checking Constraint: A new explanation of the optional infinitive stage. *Lingua* 106, 23–79.

19

Optimality in Sentence Processing

Suzanne Stevenson and Paul Smolensky

To what extent can Optimality Theory—the highest-level, symbolic grammatical theory of the Integrated Connectionist/Symbolic Cognitive Architecture (ICS)—advance our understanding of online language processing? Chapter 17 considers phonological production; this chapter, syntactic comprehension. We explore the possibility that within OT, a single syntactic grammar can directly yield not only competence-theoretic results on the grammatical distributions of elements, but also performance-theoretic results on relative preferences when processing sentences with various syntactic ambiguities. Whereas the competence theory applies the grammar at the level of an entire sentence, the performance theory incrementally optimizes interpretation one word at a time. Rankings of syntactically motivated constraints yield correct predictions for a number of ambiguities in English sentence processing and account for a range of crosslinguistic variation in parsing preferences for a widely studied class of ambiguities. The chapter contributes to ① and ② of Figure 6 in Chapter 2's ICS map.

Contents

Aprimary focus of research in sentence processing is to determine how, in the face of pervasive ambiguity, the human parser chooses the best interpretation of a sentence. That such decisions result from a process of simultaneously satisfying multiple violable constraints of differing strengths is a familiar idea. In the past, this conception of online parsing—"linguistic performance"—has been at odds with conceptions of grammar in theoretical linguistics—"linguistic competence" (see Box 23:9). This has created a fundamental problem: connecting the competence grammar to the online parser.

Several approaches (e.g., Gibson 1991; Stevenson 1994b) reinterpret the discrete, inviolable conditions from syntactic theory (Chomsky 1981; Rizzi 1990; Boxes 12:1, 15:1, 16:1–3) as weighted, violable constraints in parsing, with the result that grammar and parser, while sharing underlying constraint knowledge, are based in different computational frameworks. Phillips (1996) takes an alternative approach of redefining grammar itself as a process of incremental structure-building, but this view does not connect with the notion of multiple constraint satisfaction in parsing. Thus, the linkage between grammar and parser remains unclear, while grammatical influences on parsing are simply deemphasized in the prevailing constraint-based models of sentence understanding (among many others, MacDonald, Pearlmutter, and Seidenberg 1994; Trueswell and Tanenhaus 1994).

This situation has changed profoundly with the advent of Optimality Theory (OT) as a framework for competence grammars (Prince and Smolensky 1993/2004; Hendriks, de Hoop, and de Swart 2000; Legendre, Vikner, and Grimshaw 2001; Blutner and Zeevat 2003): both the parser and the grammar are in the business of simultaneously satisfying conflicting violable constraints. The possibility arises that the parser uses both the same underlying knowledge and the same computational mechanism of constraint optimization as the grammar. Specifically, in our work, we explore the idea that the disambiguation mechanism of the human parser—the component that chooses the best interpretation of a sequence of words—is in fact the grammar itself.

How exactly does the nature of OT enter into this proposal? Within the prevailing view of sentence processing, words are integrated one at a time as they are received. During this process, various ambiguities arise as the sentence unfolds over time. The incremental nature of online interpretation entails that preferences in resolving those ambiguities are determined on the basis of sentence fragments. Yet processing a sentence fragment is fundamentally impossible within a grammatical framework of inviolable constraints, or serial rule derivation: fragments simply cannot meet inviolable constraints and simply have no derivation. This is what has made it difficult in the past for a model to directly use grammatical principles to guide the ambiguity resolution process. By contrast, in OT, *any* input receives an analysis, by a uniform mechanism. Thus, an OT grammar can be asked to determine the optimal structural description of a sentence fragment, just as it can an entire sentence. In the former case, the grammar is functioning as an online parser.[1] In the latter case, it is functioning like a traditional competence grammar. The only difference lies in the completeness of the input.

In this chapter, we examine this possibility by asking whether an OT grammar that is well motivated from the perspective of theoretical syntax can explain online parsing preferences of comprehenders, as evidenced by empirical data on the processing of sentences that, at intermediate positions, have various structural ambiguities. We focus on English but also consider some crosslinguistic evidence.

The first work exploring this possibility was Gibson 1995 (see Gibson and Broihier 1998). Gibson examined several plausible constraint systems and concluded that none of them was satisfactory when implemented in an OT grammar. Using a different set of constraints, we will conclude that an OT grammar can explain a wide range of sentence-processing facts, including those examined by Gibson. Despite our different conclusions, we wish to clearly acknowledge the debt our work owes to Gibson's original idea and its thoughtful development.

In addition to forming a clearer connection between linguistic competence and performance, we argue that the OT approach has a further advantage: it provides a relatively restrictive framework within which to interpret the empirical data. Specifically, we show that, with regard to an important set of structural ambiguities, the restrictions entailed by the OT framework do not permit unattested preference patterns, at least some of which a system of numerical constraints would allow.

1 THE THEORY

The key idea is expressed in (1) as a hypothesis linking grammar and performance; we will test it in the empirical domain of structural ambiguity resolution.

(1)   Linking hypothesis

    a.   Processing word w_i means building the tree structure that has $w_1 w_2 \ldots w_i$ as its terminal string and that is optimal according to the OT grammar.

    b.   Processing difficulties occur when the optimal parse at word w_i is not consistent with the optimal parse at word w_{i-1}.

The goal here is not to offer a general algorithm for OT parsing—that is, a procedure, composed of primitive computational operations, for constructing candidate representations for an input and selecting the optimal one (see Section 12:2). Rather, as noted above, we propose to use the grammar to specify the disambiguation decisions of the parser—that is, to identify among a set of possible candidate structures the one that is preferred. We focus here on modeling initial preferences in parsing, as indicated in (1a). We will not address in detail the problem of predicting the degree of difficulty induced if later input proves a preference wrong, forcing the parser to **re-**

---

[1] More precisely, the grammar specifies the output of the disambiguation component of an online parser; the grammar is not itself a processing algorithm for *computing* the preferred parse (Chapter 12 (11)).

analyze the originally preferred structure. For now, we simply assume the informal notion suggested by (1b), that processing difficulty is proportional to the degree to which an earlier preferred structure diverges from what subsequent input requires. We return to this question in Section 4, laying out an initial proposal for determining the cost of reanalysis in our framework.

Given hypothesis (1), we should find that, at each step of the incremental parsing process, the *preferred* parse is the *optimal* parse. Our technique for testing whether this goal can be achieved is as follows:

(2)   General method

    a.   Empirically determine the preferred structure from the set of candidate structures for each of a set of example ambiguities.

    b.   Rank the constraints so that the preferred parse is optimal at the point of ambiguity in each case.

    c.   Verify that the ranking holds across additional example ambiguities.

This approach depends on several assumptions about preferences, candidate structures, and constraints, which we motivate here.

The first assumption concerns what constitutes the preferred parse. We follow standard practice in adopting as the preferred structure for an ambiguous input the structure that corresponds to the preferred interpretation as determined through psycholinguistic experimentation or accepted intuitions discussed in the sentence-processing literature. Typically, these are revealed by inferring back from processing difficulty to preferences in ambiguity resolution: if a particular sentence induces processing difficulty at some disambiguating word w_i, it must be because the parse needed at w_i is not consistent with the previously established preferred structure for that ambiguity (1b). For example, in processing the sentence *John put the candy on the table into his mouth*, people experience difficulty at the PP *into his mouth*. Since this PP must be the locative argument of *put* ('put x into his mouth'), the perceived difficulty indicates an earlier preference to interpret the PP *on the table* as the locative argument of *put* ('put x on the table').

The second assumption concerns the candidate parse structures. Our theory employs the extension of OT presented in Chapter 12 that incorporates not just production- (or generation-) directed optimization, but also comprehension- (or interpretation-) directed optimization. For interpretation-directed optimization, candidate parses are provided by a function *Int*, the counterpart of *Gen* in generation-directed optimization. Both *Gen* and *Int* establish a relationship between an underlying interpretation and an overt string, which is mediated by a structured representation. In our domain, an interpretation is a predicate-argument structure that incorporates and interrelates the lexical specifications of the words employed. As spelled out in Chapter 12, for *Gen*, an 'input' is such a predicate-argument structure, and an 'output' is a structured syntactic representation (a parse tree) and its corresponding (pronounced) string. In contrast, for *Int*, the 'input' is a string of overtly pronounced words, and the 'output' is a parse tree and its corresponding predicate-argument structure, including all relevant lexical specifications.[2]

The candidate parses provided by *Int* are, we assume, syntactic trees each of which has as its (overt) yield the 'input' thus far (the sequence of words w_1 through w_i). We assume that all such trees are candidates subject to evaluation by our grammar. As discussed in Section 12:2, a symbolic parsing algorithm would never actually generate more than a small set of these trees. The incremental nature of human parsing could be naturally modeled by algorithms that generate a small number of potentially optimal candidates as they proceed left to right through the input string. But here we are not proposing a parsing algorithm per se; rather, we are examining the proposal that the grammar can distinguish the best candidate from the entire logically possible set. We leave it to future work to determine how, in the human sentence processor, the grammar and parsing algorithm interact at an earlier stage of structure building to exclude most suboptimal parses. In a subsymbolic, connectionist parser, it could well be that no actual parse would be constructed aside from the optimal parse (see Box 2:3; Sections 2:8.5, 10:2, 20:3.7, and 21:3).

We assume furthermore that each candidate tree provided by *Int* satisfies X′ Theory (Box 12:1) and thus each candidate structure is a fully connected tree with a single root node, like all trees. However, we do not assume that the trees *Int* produces are all rooted in S (i.e., a sentence node; also labeled as IP or CP in X′ representation). If the initial words of the sentence are parsed as an NP, for example, the parse tree is rooted in NP; later, this NP may be embedded as, say, the subject of a matrix clause, at which point the tree will be rooted in S.

Faithfulness concerns the relation between a paired interpretation and a structured representation (Chapter 12). In our model, a candidate output for an overt word string $w_1w_2...w_i$ contains a parse tree p and a corresponding predicate-argument structure. The tree may be *unfaithful* to the predicate-argument structure, so long as the yield of p matches the string $w_1w_2...w_i$. (Recall that the predicate-argument structure incorporates the lexical specifications of $w_1w_2...w_i$.)

As in generation-directed OT, there are two general ways in which a tree may be unfaithful. The first is **overparsing**, in which the parse tree p contains "extra" structure not specified by the lexical properties of the input thus far — specifically, phrases that have no head. (By comparison, in generation-directed phonology, overparsing amounts to the addition or epenthesis of material not present in an underlying form.) The second type of unfaithful output involves **underparsing**. Here, the parse tree lacks structure needed to meet the lexical specifications of the words in the predicate-argument structure; for example, the predicate-argument structure may include a verb V, but the parse tree may fail to include all of V's required arguments. (In generation-directed phonology, underparsing is deletion of underlying material.) Examples of over- and underparsing in our framework are presented after our constraints.

---

[2] In this chapter, we present the parse tree part of the output of *Int* and assume that the corresponding predicate-argument structure can be read off from the tree.

Our final, and perhaps most crucial, assumption concerns what constitutes the set of constraints that we apply to these candidate structures in determining the optimal form. Since our goal is to bring together the grammar and the parser, as far as possible we want to adopt existing grammatical constraints from OT work on syntax. But numerous constraints have been proposed, and we risk having a large number of constraints that are irrelevant to the structural ambiguity phenomena under investigation. On the other hand, the particular ambiguities we look at may necessitate constraints on aspects of syntax that have not yet been explored in OT research. Because of this potential mismatch, we look to work in sentence processing to guide us in focusing on a subset of grammatical constraints relevant to the phenomena of interest.

Our approach is to work simultaneously from OT grammar and from an established computational model of sentence processing, the **competitive attachment (CA)** model (Stevenson 1994b), itself formulated as a grammar-based parser in which inviolable grammatical constraints are translated into weighted influences on activation levels in a connectionist framework. We proceed as follows. First, we analyze the CA parser to reveal the primary influences on activation (or strength) levels, which are the determinants of preferences in the model. Then we translate those numeric influences into discrete but violable OT constraints. In each case, we find a direct correlate either to an existing OT constraint or to a well-established condition of grammar proposed in another grammatical framework.

We motivate our constraints by presenting a numeric influence on preferences in the CA model, and its motivation (in (a) of (3)–(6)), and the corresponding grammatical (violable) constraint that we adopt (in (b)). Note that the numeric influences in (a) are not absolute; rather, they should be read as 'All else being equal, configuration X gains more activation (is stronger or more preferred) than configuration Y'.

(3) a. Hypothesized phrases (phrases projected in the parse without explicit input to serve as the head of the phrase) have less activation than structure headed by overt input.

> Hypothesized phrases are created when an overt phrase cannot be directly connected to the rest of the parse tree, as for example in English when the parser processes the subject of a complement clause but has not yet processed the embedded verb. Essentially, input words are the source of activation in the model, so hypothesized structure entails that the same amount of activation must be shared among a greater number of phrases. Specifically, a hypothesized phrase must share activation with the overt phrase that triggers it.

  b. **ObHd** (Obligatory-Heads): The head of a phrase must be filled (Grimshaw 1997).

> Note that the head of the phrase may be filled by a word in the input, or by a coindexation relationship between the phrase and another element in the sentence, as with a trace of movement (Box 12:1).

(4)   a.   Argument attachments have higher activation than adjunct attachments.

Arguments are phrases that have an essential relation to a predicate, while adjuncts provide more peripheral modifying information (Box 15:1). To capture their different properties, the CA model must encode these relationships differentially. Argument and adjunct attachment sites exhibit differing competitive behavior, in that argument sites compete more strongly for attachment to a potential argument phrase (see Stevenson 1995).

       b.   ASSIGN-θ: A predicate must assign all of its thematic roles (Chomsky 1981; Box 15:1).

We adopt this "half" of the Theta Criterion as a violable constraint.

(5)   a.   More recent attachment sites have higher activation than less recent sites.

This is due to decay of activation of attachment sites over time, a typical behavior of connectionist models (see Stevenson 1994a).

The result of this, in terms of preferred attachment configurations, is that low right attachment for a phrase XP is preferred over a higher attachment in which XP would c-command (Box 16:3) material intervening between it and its attachment site.

       b.   LOCALITY: If XP asymmetrically c-commands YP, then XP precedes YP (the **Linear Correspondence Axiom**, or **LCA** (Kayne 1994); see also Phillips 1996 for a similar principle within grammar and processing).

By definition, X **asymmetrically c-commands** Y if and only if X c-commands Y but Y does not c-command X. (That is, X does not dominate Y, the parent node of X dominates Y, and the parent node of Y does not dominate X. This is a standard variant of the c-command definition of Box 16:3.)

Again, we adapt an inviolable constraint from another grammatical framework as a violable constraint within our OT approach.

(6)   a.   Attachments that satisfy grammatical constraints have higher activation than those that do not.

This derives from reinterpretation in the CA model of inviolable grammatical constraints on a complete sentence as weighted violable constraints within an incremental parse.

The constraints of interest here are thematic and agreement requirements. Assignment of thematic requirements is covered by (4b), so here we are concerned with agreement, and we focus on **(abstract) case** (Box 15.1) because of its observed role in ambiguity resolution (Bader 1996; Meng and Bader 1997).

       b.   *CASE **hierarchy:** *GEN ≫ *DAT ≫ *ACC ≫ *NOM

This is a universal markedness hierarchy (Section 12:1.8.2) that ranks possible case assignments to NPs, genitive being the most and nominative the least marked case (Grimshaw 2001; Woolford 2001).[3]

We assume that nominative is assigned to the subject position, accusative to the object of a verb, dative to the object of a preposition (or to the indirect object of a verb), and genitive to the possessive (i.e., to *Sara* in either *Sara's servant* or *the servant of Sara*).[4]

c. **AGRCASE:** A relative pronoun must agree in case with the NP that its relative clause modifies (Sauerland and Gibson 1998; Fanselow et al. 1999; Artstein 2000).

This is a constraint with grammatical motivation, as observed by Fanselow et al. (1999); it has been proposed as a violable constraint in each of the frameworks cited above.[5]

We assume that AGRCASE applies whatever the overt expression of the relative pronoun (as in *the woman who/ whom/ that I saw*), or even when it is not overtly expressed (as in *the woman I saw*).

The five constraints we have adopted fall into the two broad categories seen throughout OT work, faithfulness and structural markedness (Chapter 12 (14)). OBHD and ASSIGN-θ enforce faithfulness between a candidate's predicate-argument structure and its parse tree. LOCALITY, *CASE, and AGRCASE are markedness constraints on the morphosyntactic properties of the parse tree. We discuss them briefly in turn.

OBHD penalizes overparsing: the parse tree created by *Int* contains structure that is unspecified by the lexical properties of the observed sequence of words. For example, consider processing the input *James donated his ~~books to the library~~*, at the word *his*. (Overstrikes mark words not yet received in the input.) The parser must posit an XP phrase in which *his* fills the specifier position. At this point in the parse, the head X of this XP projection is unfilled since the input word *books*, which will head the phrase, has not yet been reached. Thus, at *his*, there is a mismatch between the lexical specifications of the input string and the parse tree: a violation of OBHD.

Later examples will show an OBHD violation in candidates in which a noun phrase is parsed as the specifier of an embedded clause whose verb has not yet been processed, as in *Mary knows Jane ~~left~~* (14b); the relevant portion of the associated parse tree is shown in (7). The violating head is underlined.

---

[3] Woolford (2001, 513) advocates *DAT ≫ *ACC ≫ *NOM; Grimshaw (2001, 226) employs *DAT ≫ *ACC; Aissen (2001, 65) proposes thematic and relational hierarchies aligned with Nom > Acc. Thomas Wasow (personal communication) calls the ranking *ACC ≫ *NOM into question, citing evidence that accusative is the default case in English. Woolford (2001, 538n9) explicitly considers this concern, although an actual account of the relevant English facts does not seem available at this time.

[4] 'Gen' or '*GEN' refers to genitive case. 'Gen' refers to the candidate generator, not truly relevant to the interpretation-directed optimization studied here; its role is played by *Int*, as discussed above.

[5] This constraint is motivated by sentence-processing phenomena involving the attachment of relative clauses, which we discuss in Section 3, as well as by grammatical and processing properties of relative clauses observed previously. In the CA model, this idea has been developed as a general agreement process between a relative pronoun and the modified noun (Stevenson, in preparation), but here we focus on the more widely studied contributions of case.

ASSIGN-θ, on the other hand, penalizes underparsing: the parse tree created by *Int* lacks structure that is specified by the lexical properties of the input words. ASSIGN-θ is violated any time the thematic requirements of a word, as specified in its lexical entry, are not realized in the parse tree. As a violable constraint, it applies equally to obligatory and optional thematic roles. The example above, *James donated his ~~books to the library~~*, has an instance of underparsing as well: the second argument of *donate* has not been processed yet, leading to an ASSIGN-θ violation. Note that we assume that a lexical head can assign a thematic role to a phrase as soon as that phrase is projected, even if the head of the recipient phrase is as yet unfilled — that is, even in the case of an OBHD violation, discussed in the previous paragraph. Thus, in this example, there is a violation of ASSIGN-θ for the goal argument of *donate* (*~~to the library~~*) but not for the theme argument (*his books*), even though *~~books~~* has not been processed yet.

(7)   OBHD violation

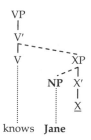

knows **Jane**

The remaining constraints assess structural markedness. As is standard in OT, a structural constraint may be elaborated as a **universal markedness hierarchy** of related but more finely distinguished constraints (Section 12:1.8.2). For example, the *CASE constraint we adopt from morphosyntactic OT research is specified as such a markedness hierarchy in (6b), which asserts, for example, that it is worse for an NP to have genitive case than to have dative case, nominative case being the least marked. AGRCASE could similarly be further discriminated according to the particular case features being matched, but for our purposes it is sufficient to consider it as a single constraint that is violated whenever a relative pronoun does not agree with the case of the modified NP, whatever that case is.

LOCALITY, another structural constraint (our violable version of the LCA), admits of a slightly different type of hierarchy. We assume LOCALITY violations apply to an XP that asymmetrically c-commands but follows (in linear precedence) a phrase YP. We have no evidence, at least as yet, that any difference in markedness results from the syntactic properties of the phrase YP that causes the LOCALITY violation. However, LOCALITY is a *gradiently* violable constraint; that is, if a phrase XP asymmetrically c-commands and follows multiple phrases, $YP_1 \ldots YP_n$, in a particular candidate structure, then LOCALITY will be violated n times by XP in that candidate.

Following Legendre et al. (1995) and Legendre, Smolensky, and Wilson (1998) (see Chapter 16), we assume that gradiently violable constraints may also lead to a hierarchical family of constraints, a **power hierarchy** generated by multiple local conjunction of a gradiently violable constraint with itself (see Sections 12:1.8.3 and 14:6.1). Such a hierarchy is ordered by number of violations; for LOCALITY (LOC), the power hierarchy is

$$(8) \quad \cdots \gg \mathrm{Loc}^k \gg \mathrm{Loc}^{k-1} \gg \cdots \gg \mathrm{Loc}^2 \gg \mathrm{Loc}$$

where Loc^k is violated if a single XP suffers k violations of LOCALITY. If no other constraints are ranked between the members of this hierarchy, the family of constraints can be collapsed into a single gradiently violable constraint. However, if there is evidence that some constraint $\mathbb{C}$ dominates k violations of LOCALITY but is dominated by $k+1$ violations, then the LOCALITY constraint must be formulated as a power hierarchy with $\mathrm{Loc}^{k+1} \gg \mathbb{C} \gg \mathrm{Loc}^k$. As in all power hierarchies, in this one the universal ranking $\mathrm{Loc}^{k+1} \gg \mathrm{Loc}^k$ holds for all values of k. Initially, we will assume the simpler formulation in which LOCALITY is a single constraint, although later we will present evidence that it indeed must be formulated as a power hierarchy.

2 THE ENGLISH CONSTRAINT RANKING

Recall that our technique is to observe the empirically preferred structure of a set of candidate structures at the point of an ambiguity, and then rank the constraints so that the preferred parse is in fact the optimal candidate. We first do this for two types of ambiguity, deriving a hierarchy of the above constraints. We then verify that this ranking makes correct predictions for six other types of ambiguities. (In these examples, we follow the standard approach of ignoring the influence of prosody, not because prosody plays no role in ambiguity resolution, but simply to try to isolate the structural factors that also play a role. Since most sentence-processing experiments use textual stimuli, we can be assured of robust preference effects with no prosody.)

Here, we focus on the ranking of OBHD, ASSIGN-θ, LOCALITY, and the *CASE constraints; we return to AGRCASE in Section 3.[6]

2.1 Two ambiguities that fix the primary constraint ranking

We begin with data pertinent to ranking OBHD, ASSIGN-θ, and LOCALITY. Consider the example in (9), which illustrates the general preference to attach a PP as an argument of a preceding verb, rather than as a modifying adjunct of the object NP (Frazier 1978; Gibson 1991). (In this and all remaining examples, the less and more difficult continuations are respectively marked '✓' and '#'.)

Tableau (9) shows the two structures possible when processing the word *on*, shown in boldface. In the first (preferred) tree, the PP headed by *on* is attached as an argument of the verb *put*. This is the tree that is consistent with the less difficult con-

---

[6] Some example sentences in this section, (17)–(20), contain relative clauses, but in none of them does AGRCASE play a role in determining the preference, since the attachment of the relative clause is not at issue. AGRCASE can only influence the choice between two or more relative clause attachments.

tinuation given in brackets: *the table* (9a). In the second (dispreferred) tree, the PP headed by *on* is attached as a modifier (adjunct) of the preceding NP, *the candy*. This tree is consistent with the more difficult continuation: *the table into his mouth* (9b). (Attachments formed to parse the most recent word are shown with dashed lines; attachments to previous words, with solid lines. All strictly vertical lines, like that between VP and V' or between V and *put* in (9), will be omitted for readability.) The preferred parse violates LOCALITY because the PP (in boldface) asymmetrically c-commands the direct object NP (underlined) but does not linearly precede it. (The LOCALITY violation mark '*' bears a subscript identifying the c-commanded phrase.) The dispreferred interpretation violates ASSIGN-θ because the locative thematic role of *put* has not been assigned: no phrase has been projected in the position of the missing locative argument. The position of the absent locative argument is marked in our trees by *e*, attached with a dotted line: there is no actual phrase at this location in the parse tree. (The violation arises even if the locative argument is optional, as in *Sara brought the letter to Mary*, since ASSIGN-θ applies equally to obligatory and optional roles.)

(9)   John put the candy on

    a.   ✓   the table.
    b.   #   the table into his mouth.

PP argument/NP adjunct		OBHD	ASSIGN-θ	LOCALITY
John put the candy **on** [✓ the table.]	☞ VP V' - - - - - **PP** V ⌐ NP on put the candy			*NP
[# the table into his mouth.]	VP V' .... *e* V ⌐NP put NP ⌐ **PP** the candy on		*e	

Given the indicated violations, it must be that

(10)   ASSIGN-θ ≫ LOCALITY

for the preferred structure to be optimal. Note that the constraint OBHD is satisfied by both candidates (the NP and PP both have their heads filled overtly); thus, these competitors provide no information concerning the ranking of OBHD.[7]

Next consider example (11), which illustrates the preference to group a second

---

[7] Information concerning OBHD can be obtained by considering another candidate, one just like the second candidate in (9) except that in the argument position marked by *e*, a phrase XP has been projected. Since the head of this phrase has not (yet) appeared in the input, OBHD is violated. The conclusion is that, like ASSIGN-θ, OBHD must dominate LOCALITY. This follows from the stronger result (12) obtained in the next example.

noun following a verb with a preceding noun, if possible, rather than to interpret the second noun as the subject of a forthcoming embedded clause. (This example is similar to ones in Pritchett 1992, showing an analogous structural ambiguity with *convince*.)

At the word *committees*, an NP may be formed from *department* and *committees*, of which *committees* is the head, as in the preferred interpretation. This structure violates Assign-θ because *told* is (at this point) missing its sentential complement (again, the missing argument is indicated by e, in the first tree). The sentential argument is provided in the alternative (dispreferred) parse: a phrasal complement is hypothesized, of which *committees* is the specifier (subject). This phrase is denoted 'XP' because its head X (underlined) is not (yet) filled; this produces an ObHd violation. There is also a Locality violation because XP asymmetrically c-commands NP_1 (underlined; *the department*) but does not precede it.

(11)   I told the department committees

    a. ✓   that budgets were cut.

    b. #   would be formed.

Compound noun/sentential complement		OBHD	ASSIGN-θ	LOCALITY
I told the department **committees** [✓ that budgets were cut.] ☞	VP / V' $\cdots e$ / V ‑ NP_2 / told NP_1 N' / the N / department **committees**		$*_e$	
[# would be formed.]	VP / V' ‑ XP / V $\underline{NP_1}$ NP_2 X' / told the dept. **comm.** $\underline{X}$	$*_X$		$*_{NP_1}$

We already know that ASSIGN-θ ≫ LOCALITY (10); thus, in order for the dispreferred candidate in (11) to lose, the following ranking must hold:

(12)   OBHD ≫ ASSIGN-θ

Combining this with the earlier ranking (10) yields the hierarchy (13).

(13)   OBHD ≫ ASSIGN-θ ≫ LOCALITY

2.2 Predictions of the account

The hierarchy (13) has been derived by considering two candidate parses of each of two strings. The following examples illustrate that this hierarchy correctly accounts for a number of other structural preferences — in other words, that the grammar correctly generalizes well beyond the two examples from which it was deduced. The annotated tableaux are self-explanatory.

(14)   Mary knows Jane
    a. ✓   well.
    b. #   left.

NP/S complement (minimal attachment)	OBHD	ASSIGN-θ	LOCALITY
Mary knows **Jane** ☞ VP / V′ / V ⎯ NP (knows Jane) [✓ well.]			
[# left.] VP / V′ / V ⎯ XP / NP X′ / X (knows Jane)	*X		

(15)   While Mary was mending the socks
    a. ✓   she sang.
    b. #   fell.

Direct object/Main subject (late closure)	OBHD	ASSIGN-θ	LOCALITY
While Mary was mending **the socks** ☞ CP / C′ / C ⎯ IP / while NP I′ (Mary) I VP / was V′ / V ⎯ NP (mending the socks) [✓ she sang.]			
[# fell.] XP / CP ⎯ XP / C′ NP X′ / C ⎯ IP (the socks) X / while NP I′ (Mary) I VP / was V′ / V ⎯ e (mending)	*X	*e	*IP *VP

(16)   The hippie from the tenement on
    a.   ✓   Haight died.
    b.   #   drugs died.

Modifier attachment	OBHD	ASSIGN-θ	LOCALITY
The hippie from the tene- ment **on** ☞ NP₁ / N′ / N ＼PP / hippie P′ / P ＼NP / from NP₂ ⸍PP / the tenement on [✓ Haight died.]			
[# drugs died.] NP ⋯ / NP₁ ⸍⸍⸍⸍⸍ PP / N′ on / N ＼PP / hippie P′ / P ＼NP₂ / from the tenement			*PP *NP₂

(17)   The computer companies
    a.   ✓   failed.
    b.   #   buy stinks. [*The computer (that) companies buy...*]

Compound noun/Relative clause	OBHD	ASSIGN-θ	LOCALITY
The com- puter **com-** **panies** ☞ NP₂ ⸍⸍⸍ / NP₁ N′ / N′ N / N companies / computer [✓ failed.]			
[# buy stinks.] NP / NP₁ ＼XP / N′ X′ / N X ⸍⸍⸍XP / computer **NP₂** X′ / X / companies	*X₁ *X₂		

(18)   John gave the child the dog

     a.   ✓   for Christmas.
     b.   #   bit medicine. [*the child (that) the dog bit ...*]

Double object / Relative clause		OʙHᴅ	Assɪɢɴ-θ	Lᴏᴄᴀʟɪᴛʏ
John gave the child **the dog** [✓ for Christmas.] ☞ VP V' ⸱⸱⸱NP₂ / V ⟍NP₁ the dog / gave the child				*NP₁
[# bit medicine.] VP V' ⸱⸱⸱ₑ / V ⟍NP / gave NP₁ XP / the child X' / X ⸱⸱⸱XP / NP₂ X' / the dog X		*ₓ*ₓ	*ₑ	

(19)   Mary told the doctor that

     a.   ✓   she had fainted.
     b.   #   examined her that she felt fine.

Sentential complement / Relative clause		OʙHᴅ	Assɪɢɴ-θ	Lᴏᴄᴀʟɪᴛʏ
Mary told the doctor **that** [✓ she had fainted.] ☞ VP V' ⸱⸱⸱CP / V ⟍NP that / told the doctor				*NP
[# examined her that she felt fine.] VP V' ⸱⸱⸱ₑ / V ⟍NP / told NP ⸱⸱⸱CP / the doctor that			*ₑ	

Note that some examples depend only on the *existence* of the constraints we propose, rather than their specific ranking. This arises when the preferred structure violates a subset (possibly empty) of the constraints violated by the dispreferred structure; the former **harmonically bounds** the latter and must therefore win under any ranking of the constraints (Section 12:1.6). Also, some dispreferred continuations are easy for people to process (as in (14b)), and others are quite difficult (as in (17b) or (18b)). Here we consider only initial preferences, returning briefly in Section 4 to the issue of reanalysis difficulty — how hard a dispreferred continuation is to process.

The preference judgments in (14)–(19) are based on experimental or intuitive evidence from, among others, Frazier 1978, (14); Frazier and Rayner 1982, (15); Gibson 1991, (17); Pritchett 1992, (18), (19); Traxler, Pickering, and Clifton 1996, (16). In relative clauses, there is an understood empty operator in the specifier position of the highest phrase XP, which may have an unfilled head position (it is labeled 'CP' when headed by *that*, as in (19)–(20)).

2.3 LOCALITY as a power hierarchy

Consider the example in (20), in which the PP headed by *on* can be attached as the second argument of the verb *put* or as an adjunct (modifier) of the verb *seen*.

(20)　I put the biscuits that Jane had seen on

　　　a.　✓　　　　　　　　　　　　　the table back in the tin.
　　　b.　#　　　　　　　　　　　　　the table.

PP argument/NP adjunct	Loc²	Assign-θ	Loc
I put the biscuits that Jane had seen **on** [✓ the table back in the tin.]		$*_e$	$*NP_2$
[# the table.]	$*$		$*NP_1$ $*CP$ $*IP$ $*VP$ $*NP_2$

In the account developed so far, even with the numerous LOCALITY violations engendered by the argument attachment, it should be preferred here exactly as in (9), *John put the candy on* ..., because ASSIGN-θ ≫ LOCALITY. However, evidence indicates that with a greater distance between the argument site and the phrase to be attached, a more recent adjunction site may prevail (Kamide 1998). We suggest that this is a case of a gradiently violable constraint for which multiple violations (by a single entity) have a stronger effect than merely more marks at a single level in the hierarchy. As mentioned above, the device of a power hierarchy has been employed in formally similar situations in other OT analyses (e.g., Chapters 8, 14, and 16), and we propose to use it here. Multiple violations of LOCALITY by a single attachment cause a violation of higher-ranked constraints in the universal power hierarchy (8), repeated here.

(21) $\cdots \gg \text{Loc}^k \gg \text{Loc}^{k-1} \gg \cdots \gg \text{Loc}^2 \gg \text{Loc}$

We make the minimal assumption permitted by these data, that it is Loc^2 that is at work in example (20). (The losing candidate violates not only Loc^2, but also Loc^3 – Loc^5. Until we are forced to deploy higher constraints, we will employ Loc^2.) With Loc^2 dominating ASSIGN-θ as indicated in tableau (20), the correct preference is obtained. Thus, while a slightly nonlocal attachment (with a single XP violating LOCALITY) is preferable to a violation of ASSIGN-θ, a more highly nonlocal attachment (with two or more XPs violating LOCALITY, yielding a violation of Loc^2) is not preferable to a violation of ASSIGN-θ.

2.4 *CASE rankings

In the examples thus far, constraints from the *CASE subhierarchy play no role in determining preferences. Interestingly, one area where they appear to play a visible role is in filler-gap ambiguities—that is, in determining the preferred association of a filler (*wh*-phrase) with its *gap* or trace *t*, an empty element with which it is coindexed (Box 12:1) (Artstein and Stevenson 1999; Artstein 2000).

For example, at the point of processing the verb *give* in (22), the *wh*-phrase *which dog* may be (a) interpreted as the object of the verb (receiving accusative case, compatible with the continuation in (22a)); (b) interpreted as the indirect object of the verb (receiving dative case, compatible with the continuation in (22b)); or (c) unassociated with either complement position (compatible with the continuation in (22c)).

(22)   Which dog$_i$ did John give ...

   a. t_i to Mary? [The trace receives the theme role and accusative case.]
   b. t_i a bone? [The trace receives the recipient role and dative case.]
   c.   a bone to t_i? [There is no trace when the verb is processed, so the thematic role is unassigned.]

Artstein and Stevenson (1999) find that the preferred continuation is (a): it is better to associate a filler with an argument position that is assigned accusative case (a) than to leave it unassociated (c). (The preference for (a) over (b) is given by the *CASE hierarchy: *DAT ≫ *ACC.) If the filler is associated with an argument position, as in (a) (or (b)), then the verb can assign a thematic role to that position and avoid an ASSIGN-θ violation. If the filler is left unassociated, as in (c), then it cannot. This indicates the ranking in (23).

(23)   ASSIGN-θ ≫ *ACC

Continuing this example, however, reveals that it is better to leave a filler unassociated (and a thematic role unassigned) than to associate it with an argument position that is assigned dative case. Consider the situation arising if the partial input in (22) is continued with *a bone*, compatible with one of the dispreferred continuations in (22b) or (22c); which of those possibilities will then be preferred? The filler *which dog$_i$* may be associated with a trace in the dative-receiving indirect object position (as in (24a)) or may be left unassociated (as in (24b)).

(24)   Which dog$_i$ did John give a bone …

      a.   Which dog$_i$ did John give t$_i$ a bone? [trace receives dative case]

      b.   Which dog$_i$ did John give a bone *e*? [second argument not filled]

      c.   Which dog$_i$ did John give a bone to t$_i$? [continuation of (b): second argument filled with subsequent PP]

The preferred continuation is of (24) is (c), indicating that (b) must have been preferred over (a) given the input in (24); a dative-receiving trace incurs a worse violation than does leaving the filler unassociated. Here, the *CASE violation is worse than the ASSIGN-θ violation; that is, the ranking in (25) holds.

(25)   *DAT ≫ ASSIGN-θ

From these kinds of preferences in the incremental interpretation of a filler, Artstein and Stevenson (1999) derive the subranking in (26).

(26)   *DAT ≫ ASSIGN-θ ≫ *ACC

The general idea behind the analysis is that a tension arises from binding a gap by a filler: on the one hand, the binding eliminates a violation of ASSIGN-θ (because the filler-gap chain serves as the expected argument of a verb); on the other hand, it induces a *CASE violation (because the bound gap — the coindexed empty element $t_{i\_}$ receives case from the verb). The upshot of ranking (26) is that if the gap is in a position that receives accusative case, then it is better to bind it by the filler, but if the gap is in a dative-receiving position, it is better to leave it unbound.

When we incorporate the *CASE subhierarchy into our earlier analysis, we also determine the following ranking from example (18), in which the preferred interpretation has an additional *DAT violation (not shown in the earlier tableau):

(27)   OBHD ≫ *DAT

That is, the high rank of OBHD entails that it is not possible to avoid a *DAT or *ACC violation by positing an empty phrase to allow restructuring of NPs to achieve lower-ranked case violations.

These observations lead to the hierarchy in (28), merging our earlier rankings with the new *CASE rankings. Note that the examples thus far provide no evidence about the relative ranking of the *CASE and LOCALITY constraints.

(28)   OBHD ≫ {LOC^2, *DAT} ≫ ASSIGN-θ ≫ {LOC^1, *ACC} ≫ *NOM

3 RELATIVE CLAUSE ATTACHMENT TYPOLOGY

A relatively well-studied ambiguity is the attachment of a relative clause when there is more than one NP that it could modify, as in (29) (Cuetos and Mitchell 1988).

(29)   The servant of the actress who ...

The relative clause introduced by the relative pronoun *who* could modify either *the servant* ('high attachment') or *the actress* ('low attachment'). Further embedding of NPs within PP modifiers can occur, making even more than two NPs possible attachment sites (as in *the servant of the actress with the director who...*). Experimental studies have investigated the preferences in two- and three-NP attachment site cases, revealing that high or low attachment preference varies with number of attachment sites, type of preposition, and language.

Our goal here is to determine, under the varying conditions, both the possible and impossible patterns of attachment preferences (i.e., high vs. middle vs. low attachment). We propose an account of the syntactic contribution to these patterns (as distinct from the contributions of prosody and discourse—see Fodor 1998; Hemforth, Konieczny, and Scheepers 2000). Our proposal resembles those of Gibson et al. (1996) and Hemforth, Konieczny, and Scheepers (2000) in relying on two factors; it differs, though, by involving no "processing" principles distinct from the syntactic constraints proposed as elements of the competence grammar.

Specifically, we propose to explain relative clause attachment preferences as the result of the interaction of two classes of constraint introduced above: the LOCALITY constraints (5b), (8), and the case constraints (6), the latter consisting of AGRCASE (6c) and the universal case markedness hierarchy *GEN ≫ *DAT ≫ *ACC ≫ *NOM (6b). Clearly, the LOCALITY constraints are sensitive to the relative height of the alternative NPs to which the relative clause can attach. Because the relative pronoun (e.g., *who*, *which*, *that*) must agree in case with the noun the relative clause modifies (according to AGRCASE (6c)), the case constraints are sensitive to type of preposition, as prepositions vary in the case they assign to their complement NPs.

Conflict arises among the case and LOCALITY constraints when the head of the complex NP (the 'highest' NP, such as *the servant* in (29)) is assigned nominative or accusative case, and the prepositions assign the more marked cases dative or genitive. In such configurations, the case markedness hierarchy favors high attachment; LOCALITY always favors low attachment. This is illustrated in (30), which shows three candidate attachments for *who* in (29). Two 'low' attachment candidates are shown, one with nominative case, the other genitive case. The latter satisfies AGRCASE because it agrees with the genitive case of the NP to which it attaches (*the actress*). But this candidate has the most marked case, violating *GEN. The low-attached candidate with the least marked case, nominative, improves the *CASE violation to *NOM, but incurs a violation of AGRCASE. The high attachment can satisfy AGRCASE and still have the least marked case: the highest NP bears nominative case. But this violates LOCALITY, specifically, LOC^2: with the high attachment, *who* asymmetrically c-commands a PP (*of*) and an NP (*actress*) that precede it.

Which attachment is preferred—that is, optimal? If LOCALITY is dominated by the case constraints—{*GEN, AGRCASE} ≫ LOC^2—the high attachment wins; otherwise—if LOC^2 ≫ *GEN or LOC^2 ≫ AGRCASE—one of the low attachments is optimal. The possibilities are richer when we consider prepositions that assign other cases, and when we consider three nested NPs, where attachment to the highest NP will violate LOC^4, and attachment to the middle NP will violate LOC^2, as shown in (31).

(30)   The servant of the actress who …

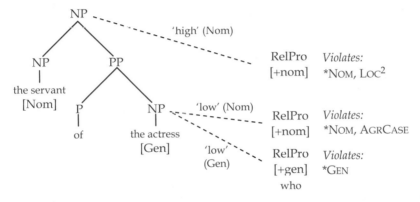

(31)   LOCALITY power hierarchy violations

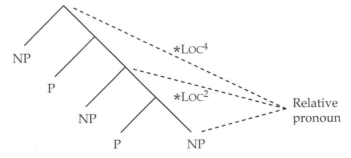

We now explore the typology of attachment preferences that results from reranking the proposed constraints. In this analysis, we consider the portion of the full typology in which the following conditions hold:

(32)   Conditions of analyzed structures

   a.   The highest NP has nominative or accusative case (i.e., is the subject or object of a verb, and not itself the object of a preposition).

   b.   The prepositions employed assign genitive case (*of*) or dative case (all other prepositions).

   c.   The relative pronoun is case-ambiguous (i.e., *who*, *which*, or *that*, each of which is compatible with any case).

Under these conditions, the following conclusion holds:

(33)   Attachment of a relative clause to the complement of a preposition requires violation of at least one of the following constraints:

   AGRCASE, *GEN, or *DAT.

Agreeing in case violates either *GEN or *DAT because those are the cases assigned by a preposition; disagreement in case (presumably to avoid a higher-ranked case constraint) violates AGRCASE.

3.1 Three attested attachment preference patterns

As mentioned above, our initial goal is to derive from the competence grammar a typology of possible (and impossible) patterns of relative clause attachment preferences. Several types of patterns have been proposed to describe the observed preferences in various languages. For example, it has been suggested that English and Brazilian Portuguese consistently show low attachment preference (Gibson et al. 1996; Miyamoto 1998). A number of languages, Spanish and German among them, appear to exhibit high attachment in two-site cases and low attachment in three-site cases (Cuetos and Mitchell 1988; Gibson et al. 1996; Hemforth, Konieczny, and Scheepers 2000). Finally, it has been proposed that, at least for some two-site cases in some languages (English and Spanish), high attachment is preferred after some prepositions (*of*) but not others (Gilboy et al. 1995; Frazier and Clifton 1996). In this section, we explain how each of these attested patterns results from a relative ranking of case and LOCALITY constraints in our framework.

   A simple system is described in (34): (a) gives the ranking conditions, and (b) the resulting preference pattern.

(34)   LOCALITY strictly dominates case

   a. $\text{LOC}^2 \gg \text{AGRCASE}$ or $\text{LOC}^2 \gg \text{*GEN}$

   b.   Low attachment is optimal in every configuration.

In this type of language, it is more important to attach to the most recent (lowest) NP than to satisfy a case-based condition (i.e., than to ensure that the case of the relative pronoun matches the case of the NP it attaches to, or that it avoids the marked cases genitive and dative).

More precisely, if $\textsc{Loc}^2 \gg \textsc{AgrCase}$, then any high attachment is dispreferred to low attachment with nominative case. If the relative pronoun in the high attachment candidate has nominative case, then high attachment violates *NOM and at least $\textsc{Loc}^2$, while low attachment violates *NOM and $\textsc{AgrCase}$. Since $\textsc{Loc}^2 \gg \textsc{AgrCase}$, low attachment is preferred. A high attachment with a nonnominative case can only make the high attachment even worse, so any high attachment is worse than low attachment with nominative case. (There may be an even better low attachment candidate—that is, one with agreeing case C, if $\textsc{AgrCase} \gg {}$*C—but in any event, a low rather than high attachment will be optimal.)

Similarly, if $\textsc{Loc}^2 \gg {}$*GEN, then any high attachment is dispreferred to low attachment with case agreeing with that NP. Whatever this case may be, the worst violation it can incur is *GEN, universally ranked highest on the *CASE hierarchy; and even a *GEN violation is preferred to the LOCALITY violation that results from attaching to any higher NP, which is at least $\textsc{Loc}^2$. Since $\textsc{AgrCase}$ is satisfied by this low attachment, its ranking is irrelevant. Thus, no high attachment can be optimal. (Again, there may be a better low attachment candidate: low attachment with nominative case will be optimal if *C $\gg \textsc{AgrCase}$, where C is the agreeing case. But either way, similarly to the situation above, a low attachment is best.)

Thus, under either subcase of the rankings (34a), low attachment is optimal.

A more complex pattern is described in (35).

(35)   Severe, but not mild, LOCALITY violations are worse than case violations.

    a. $\textsc{Loc}^4 \gg \textsc{AgrCase}$ or   *$\textsc{Loc}^4 \gg {}$*GEN
         and $\{\textsc{AgrCase}, {}^*\textsc{Gen}, {}^*\textsc{Dat}\} \gg \textsc{Loc}^2$

    b.   High attachment is preferred in two-site cases; low attachment in three-site cases where both prepositions assign the same case, or the higher preposition assigns a "worse" case (genitive) than the lower preposition (dative). (That is, low attachment obtains with three sites when the case assigned to the middle NP is the same as or worse than that assigned to the lowest NP. The alternative situation—in which the middle NP is assigned a less-marked case than the lowest NP—is described in (40) below.)

In this class of language, a case-based condition is more important than a low-ranked LOCALITY constraint, but less important than a high-ranked LOCALITY constraint.

More precisely, with two attachment sites, high attachment with agreeing case (nominative or accusative) violates $\textsc{Loc}^2$, but satisfies the higher constraints, $\textsc{AgrCase}$, *GEN, and *DAT; low attachment violates at least one of those higher-ranked constraints (33).

Recall that, with three attachment sites, high attachment violates $\textsc{Loc}^4$, intermediate attachment violates $\textsc{Loc}^2$, and low attachment incurs no LOCALITY violations (31). Given the rankings in (35a), high attachment with three sites cannot be optimal because of the $\textsc{Loc}^4$ violation: if $\textsc{Loc}^4 \gg \textsc{AgrCase}$, a lower attachment with nominative case has higher Harmony, as it will at worst violate $\textsc{AgrCase}$; if $\textsc{Loc}^4 \gg {}$*GEN, a lower attachment that agrees in case will have higher Harmony because it will at worst violate *GEN. This is parallel to case (34): LOC^4 here plays the role of LOC^2 there.

Also, with three sites, intermediate attachment cannot be optimal when an intermediate NP is assigned the same case as or a more marked case than the lower NP. By (33), both violate one of AGRCASE, *GEN, or *DAT, with the case violation of the middle NP no better than that of the lowest NP. The lowest NP is then preferred: it does not incur the additional LOC^2 violation arising with intermediate attachment.

With three sites, then, low attachment is optimal, except in the single configuration discussed below in (40). This establishes (35).

A third, still more complex pattern is given in (36).

(36)   The relative importance of LOCALITY and case depends on the particular case being assigned.

    a.   LOC^4 ≫ AGRCASE   or   LOC^4 ≫ *GEN
       and   {AGRCASE, *GEN} ≫ LOC^2 ≫ *DAT

    b.   High attachment in two-site cases with a genitive-assigning preposition (*of*), low attachment in two-site cases with a dative-assigning preposition, and low attachment in three-site cases where both prepositions assign the same case, or the higher preposition assigns a "worse" case (genitive) than the lower preposition (dative). (Compare (35b).) In this type of language, the importance of LOCALITY relative to a case-based condition varies according to the identity of the *CASE constraint involved.

The ranking here is the same as in (35a), except for the domination of *DAT by LOC^2. The resulting pattern is thus the same as in (35b), except when the preposition in a two-site structure assigns dative case. In that situation, it is optimal, under the ranking (36), to attach low with dative case and avoid the now higher-ranked LOC^2 violation. Thus, for example, the ranking (36a) yields a distinction in preference between *the sweater with sleeves that* ... and *the sweaters of wool that* ..., the former yielding a low attachment preference (*the sweater with sleeves that are too short*), and the latter a high attachment preference (*the sweaters of wool that are too expensive*). (See Gilboy et al. 1995; Frazier and Clifton 1996.)

3.2 Typologically excluded systems

The proposed constraints predict that certain patterns are impossible, given certain properties of the grammatical system: the universal rankings of the LOCALITY power hierarchy and of the *CASE markedness hierarchy, and their limited interactions in constraint reranking. We discuss two such examples in (37) and (38).

(37)   Predicted impossible: low attachment in all two-site configurations and high attachment in a three-site configuration.

For low attachment to be preferred in all two-site configurations, LOC^2 must dominate either AGRCASE or both *GEN and *DAT (see (30), which illustrates the situation for a genitive-assigning preposition). Since universally $\text{Loc}^4 \gg \text{Loc}^2$, this entails that Loc^4 also dominates either AGRCASE or both *GEN and *DAT; and by the same logic low attachment is preferred with three sites, contrary to (37).

(38) Predicted impossible: with two sites, high attachment after a dative-assigning preposition and low attachment after a genitive-assigning preposition.

For high attachment to be favored after a dative-assigning preposition, both AGRCASE and *DAT must dominate Loc^2. Since *GEN $\gg$ *DAT universally, this entails that *GEN also dominates Loc^2. Thus, low attachment with genitive case (or with disagreeing nominative case) is less harmonic than high attachment with nominative case, so high attachment is required for genitive- as well as dative-assigning prepositions.

The impossibility of these two patterns in our OT system is interesting because, while the "reverse" of each has been proposed to correspond to behavior in some language (i.e., high attachment in two-site configurations and low in three-site configurations, or high attachment after a genitive assigner and low after a dative assigner), the patterns in (37) and (38) have not, to our knowledge, been empirically observed.

3.3 Typologically predicted systems

Two patterns are predicted possible by our analysis but have not, so far as we know, been documented in the literature: (39) and (40).

(39) Case extremely high ranked relative to LOCALITY

  a. *AGRCASE, *GEN, *DAT $\gg$ Loc^4

  b. High attachment with three (and two) sites

In this type of language, case constraints are so much stronger than LOCALITY that attachment to the highest NP that has agreeing nominative or accusative case is compelled even when this incurs four simultaneous violations of LOCALITY. Thus, NPs embedded in PPs are simply unavailable for modification by a relative clause (at least in two- and three-site cases). We are not aware of a language uniformly showing high attachment in three-site cases. If in fact such languages do not exist, their absence might suggest some grammatical or functional factor limiting the constraint interaction involving the LOCALITY and *CASE hierarchies, to prevent a ranking like (39a). This factor may correspond to a limitation on the case constraints, prohibiting a situation in which both (i) *GEN and *DAT are very highly ranked, and (ii) AGRCASE is very highly ranked. Condition (i) makes the use of such cases difficult in general. Condition (ii) is in direct tension with (i): by forcing case agreement between a relative pronoun and the modified NP, it strongly restricts the use of less-marked cases for relative pronouns. Alternatively, the factor in question may correspond to limitations on the LOCALITY power hierarchy, prohibiting its domination by certain classes of constraints. We leave further investigation of such restrictions to future work.

(40)   Intermediate attachment with three sites

    a.   Rankings of (35) or (36)

    b.   Intermediate attachment with three sites when the intermediate-level PP assigns dative case, and the lower-level PP, genitive. Otherwise, low attachment with three sites.

The relevant situations here are those, alluded to in (35) and (36), in which the lowest NP is assigned a worse case than the middle NP in the three-site configuration. The Harmony benefit of *DAT over *GEN arising from intermediate rather than low attachment, with agreeing case, exceeds the Harmony cost of incurring LOC^2. This is similar to the two-site situation described for (36), in that a worse case violation (*GEN) on the lowest NP can force higher attachment, whereas a lesser case violation (*DAT) cannot. But in the three-site instance, attachment is forced to the middle NP, because the additional benefit of *NOM over *DAT that derives from highest attachment is exceeded by the cost of LOC^4.

    Thus, the typology derived from the above constraints predicts the existence of languages for which intermediate attachment is possible in a phrase such as *the thread from the sweater of wool that was hand-dyed* …. To our knowledge, this situation has not been experimentally investigated, but it seems a plausible result for English, for which it has been proposed that the genitive-assigning *of* does not block higher attachment.

    Obviously, at this time, psycholinguistic investigation of such questions is sufficiently limited that the empirical status of this prediction, and that of (39), remain to be determined.

4 REANALYSIS

Thus far, we have developed a theory of initial preferences—that is, we explain the preferred interpretation for an ambiguity as the candidate structure that is optimal according to our OT constraints: (1a). The other class of data that a theory of ambiguity resolution must account for is what happens when an ambiguity is (later) disambiguated and the result is inconsistent with the initial preference: (1b). At this point, the parser must abandon its initial preference and adopt a different structure as its newly preferred interpretation—a phenomenon known as **reanalysis**.[8]

    Any theory of reanalysis must address the questions in (41) and (42).

(41)   What qualifies as reanalysis?

Since the simple act of integrating each new word into the developing parse tree constitutes a change to the preferred parse, we must define what qualifies as a genuine

---

[8] We use the term 'reanalysis' to mean any change in the parser's representation of what is the preferred interpretation of the input. The actual operation may be one of reparsing, modifying the current parse, selective backtracking, or (in a parallel framework) adopting an alternative structure that was previously computed but not the preferred choice.

alteration in the preferred interpretation.

(42)   What determines the degree of difficulty induced by any particular reanalysis?

Difficulty in changing a preferred interpretation lies on a continuum from mild influences on processing (e.g., if the sentence fragment *Mary knows Jane* is continued with the verb *left*) to severe garden path effects (e.g., if *Jane gave the child the dog* is continued with *bit a Band-Aid*). A theory of reanalysis must therefore specify the relation between the parse tree changes identified in (41) with a measure of processing difficulty.

Regarding question (41), we assume, following Stevenson (1998), that *any* change to the parse constitutes a reanalysis. That is, every incremental step in parsing is a process of revising the prior interpretation, either by "filling in" empty structure (the elements of the parse indicated by '*e*' or 'XP' in our tree diagrams) or by actually changing earlier attachment relations. This is the simplest assumption that can be made about reanalysis: there is no special set of reanalysis operations; rather, *Int* uniformly provides candidates for each and every sentence fragment.

Not only is this the most parsimonious approach, it is also most consistent with our OT framework, which treats all sentence fragments (partial or complete sentences) uniformly: candidates for each incremental step in the input string are constructed uniformly, without singling out particular *Int* operations that qualify as reanalysis operations. Similarly, there are no constraints in the evaluation mechanism that compare types of changes from the previously preferred parse to the candidate being evaluated. This contrasts with other approaches to reanalysis in which certain incremental parsing (reanalyzing) operations are distinguished as more costly (see, e.g., Weinberg 1995; Sturt and Crocker 1996; Lewis 1998). Here, each candidate is produced with the same set of operations and evaluated solely according to the constraints provided by the grammar.

Given that every incremental incorporation of an input word is 'reanalysis', and therefore there are no special reanalysis operations or constraints, how do we determine the *difficulty* of reanalysis as required by (42)? Again, we are guided by the simplest assumption under our OT framework: the degree of difficulty at each stage in processing is determined by the pattern of constraint violations incurred by the optimal candidate — that is, its Harmony. Specifically, processing difficulty at word w_i is measured by the *change in Harmony* (or 'unmarkedness') from the preferred parse at word w_{i-1} to the preferred (optimal) parse at word w_i. Note that here we depart from standard practice in OT by comparing two structures that correspond to two different inputs: that is, we compare the optimal structure for words w_1 to w_{i-1} with the optimal structure for words w_1 to w_i. If the pattern of constraint violations worsens (from one preferred interpretation to the next) owing to additional violations of low-ranked constraints, there will be only mild effects, while additional violations of high-ranked constraints can cause significant processing difficulty.

To illustrate this range of processing difficulty, we consider the dispreferred continuations of three of our earlier preference examples. In these examples, the following subhierarchy of our English ranking will play a role in the account of relative difficulty:

(43)   OBHD $\gg$ LOC^2 $\gg$ ASSIGN-θ $\gg$ {LOC^1, *ACC} $\gg$ *NOM

In example (14), the preferred interpretation of the input *Mary knows Jane* violates only *CASE constraints (*NOM and *ACC), with *Jane* attached as an argument of *knows*. If this fragment is continued with the verb *left*—giving *Mary knows Jane left*—people experience little processing difficulty. (This difficulty is generally below the level of conscious awareness, but it has been observed experimentally by Frazier and Rayner (1982).). In our framework, the new parse will have a single violation of ASSIGN-θ (due to the missing optional object argument of the verb *left*) and two violations of *NOM. Thus, the Harmony decreases, but only by the additional violation of a constraint intermediate in our hierarchy (and in fact one *CASE constraint has been replaced by a lower-ranked one).

Compare the dispreferred continuation of example (9) in which the initial fragment *John put the candy on the table* violates LOC^1 (since *on* attaches above the NP *the candy* as the second argument of *put*), as well as *NOM, *ACC, and *DAT for the cases assigned to the NPs. The dispreferred continuation, *John put the candy on the table into*, causes noticeable difficulty for the human sentence processor (Gibson 1991). In our model, the new parse violates the same constraints as the previous parse, with the addition of a LOC^2 violation for the new PP (which c-commands and follows *the candy on the table*). Thus, here the change in markedness is more severe than above, as it involves the added violation of a higher-ranked constraint, LOC^2.

Finally, the preferred interpretation of example (18), *John gave the child the dog*, similarly violates LOC^1 and the three *CASE constraints *NOM, *ACC, and *DAT. The dispreferred continuation, *John gave the child the dog bit*, causes a severe garden path effect in people (Pritchett 1992). This parse incurs one violation each of OBHD,[9] ASSIGN-θ, and *ACC, and two violations of *NOM. Note that although this parse fares better on the *CASE constraints, the violation of the very highly ranked OBHD decreases the Harmony greatly, accounting for the difficulty.

We conclude, then, that a promising notion for building a theory of reanalysis difficulty is the change in Harmony between the optimal structures determined successively during incremental parsing. The approach has the advantage of applying a uniform mechanism for initial preferences and reanalysis difficulty, and strengthens the evidence for the grammar-parser relation we hypothesized in (1).

5 CONCLUSION

The OT approach to sentence processing outlined here has, in our view, three primary advantages over other types of theories.

---

[9] The OBHD violation is due to the highest phrase XP of the relative clause, which has an (understood) empty operator in specifier position, but whose head has no lexical material. The parse is the tree for (18b), with the lowest head X now filled by *bit*.

(44)   Advantages of the OT approach

    a. *Basis in grammar.* The OT approach looks directly to the grammar for the cause of preferences. The assumption is that surface-level phenomena that seem to influence processing (such as word order flexibility; see Gibson et al. 1996; Miyamoto 1998) are themselves a reflex of grammar (likely the case system, which we exploit here).

    b. *Uniformity.* All the constraints proposed here have grammatical motivation and play a role in both grammar and processing. This is possible in part because we adopt a grammaticalized notion of locality that captures effects that have typically been cast as extrasyntactic in other work (e.g., Gibson 1991; Stevenson 1994b; Gibson et al. 1996; Hemforth, Konieczny, and Scheepers 2000).

    c. *Restrictiveness.* The theory has the flexibility to yield general preference patterns observed crosslinguistically (because of constraint reranking), at the same time formally generating a restricted typology that excludes unattested patterns (because of the general grammatical structure of OT—such as universal markedness hierarchies and strict domination, rather than numerical weighting). We have demonstrated this behavior for one important class of ambiguities (relative clause attachment), and future work will investigate the generality of this result.

Of course, fundamental conceptual questions remain open. How do the rankings employed here for a performance theory relate to those of the ordinary competence grammar? It appears that, very generally speaking, the ranking needed for the performance theory of a language will be more constrained than that needed for the competence grammar. For instance, in the competence theory, it makes no difference how the grammar ranks two constraints $\mathbb{C}$ and $\mathbb{C}'$ that are both unviolated in the surface forms of the language. Both constraints can be simultaneously satisfied given a *complete* sentence. But prior to completion of a sentence, it may not be possible to satisfy both $\mathbb{C}$ and $\mathbb{C}'$, so their relative priority may guide the preference among competing incremental analyses. Thus, these same constraints may need to be ranked in a particular way to make the right predictions concerning online processing.

Now if the hierarchy needed for the processing theory has more specified rankings than the hierarchy needed for the competence theory, how does the learning process determine not only the rankings of the competence grammar, but also the additional rankings relevant to processing? We will not speculate on this intriguing question here. We note, however, that there are suggestive parallels between this question, pertaining to syntactic comprehension, and the problem discussed in Chapter 17 of learning the 'hidden rankings' implicated in phonological production.

The preliminary empirical results reported here suggest that the general approach may be a fruitful one. OT provides a conception of grammar that incorporates one of the central computational insights of sentence-processing theories, competitive optimization. It thus raises the possibility of a unified theory in which a single grammar can explain both the competence data of theoretical linguistics and the performance data of psycholinguistics.

References

ROA = Rutgers Optimality Archive, http://roa.rutgers.edu

Aissen, J. 2001. Markedness and subject choice in Optimality Theory. In *Optimality-theoretic syntax*, eds. G. Legendre, S. Vikner, and J. Grimshaw. MIT Press.

Artstein, R. 2000. Case constraints and empty categories in Optimality Theory parsing. Ms., Rutgers University.

Artstein, R., and S. Stevenson. 1999. Case constraints and empty categories in Optimality Theory parsing. Talk presented at the Conference on Architectures and Mechanisms for Language Processing (AMLaP-1999).

Bader, M. 1996. Reanalysis in a modular architecture of the human sentence processing mechanism. Poster presented at the CUNY Conference on Human Sentence Processing.

Blutner, R., and H. Zeevat, eds. 2003. *Pragmatics in Optimality Theory*. Palgrave Macmillan.

Chomsky, N. 1981. *Lectures on government and binding*. Foris.

Cuetos, F., and D. Mitchell. 1988. Cross-linguistic differences in parsing: Restrictions on the use of the late closure strategy in Spanish. *Cognition* 30, 73–105.

Fanselow, G., M. Schlesewsky, D. Cavar, and R. Kliegl. 1999. Optimal parsing: Syntactic parsing preferences and Optimality Theory. Ms., University of Potsdam. ROA 367.

Fodor, J. D. 1998. Learning to parse? *Journal of Psycholinguistic Research* 27, 285–319.

Frazier, L. 1978. On comprehending sentences: Syntactic parsing strategies. Indiana University Linguistics Club.

Frazier, L., and C. Clifton. 1996. *Construal*. MIT Press.

Frazier, L., and K. Rayner. 1982. Making and correcting errors during sentence comprehension: Eye movements in the analysis of structurally ambiguous sentences. *Cognitive Psychology* 14, 178–210.

Gibson, E. 1991. A computational theory of human linguistic processing: Memory limitations and processing breakdown. Ph.D. diss., Carnegie-Mellon University.

Gibson, E. 1995. Optimality Theory and human sentence processing. Talk presented at the MIT Conference on Optimality and Competition in Syntax.

Gibson, E., and K. Broihier. 1998. Optimality Theory and human sentence processing. In *Is the best good enough? Optimality and competition in syntax*, eds. P. Barbosa, D. Fox, P. Hagstrom, M. McGinnis, and D. Pesetsky. MIT Press and MIT Working Papers in Linguistics.

Gibson, E., N. Pearlmutter, E. Canseco-Gonzalez, and G. Hickok. 1996. Recency preference in the human sentence processing mechanism. *Cognition* 59, 23–59.

Gilboy, E., J.-M. Sopena, C. Clifton, and L. Frazier. 1995. Argument structure and association preferences in Spanish and English complex NPs. *Cognition* 54, 131–67.

Grimshaw, J. 1997. Projection, heads, and optimality. *Linguistic Inquiry* 28, 373–422.

Grimshaw, J. 2001. Optimal clitic positions and the lexicon in Romance clitic systems. In *Optimality-theoretic syntax*, eds. G. Legendre, S. Vikner, and J. Grimshaw. MIT Press.

Hemforth, B., L. Konieczny, and C. Scheepers. 2000. Syntactic attachment and anaphor resolution: Two sides of relative clause attachment. In *Proceedings of the Conference on Architectures and Mechanisms for Language Processing (AMLaP-2000)*, eds. M. Crocker, M. Pickering, and C. Clifton. Cambridge University Press.

Hendriks, P., H. de Hoop, and H. de Swart, eds. 2000. Special issue on the optimization of interpretation. *Journal of Semantics* 17, 185–314.

Kamide, Y. 1998. The role of argument structure requirements and recency constraints in human sentence processing. Ph.D. diss., University of Exeter.

Kayne, R. S. 1994. *The antisymmetry of syntax*. MIT Press.

Legendre, G., P. Smolensky, and C. Wilson. 1998. When is less more? Faithfulness and minimal links in *wh*-chains. In *Is the best good enough? Optimality and competition in syntax*, eds. P. Barbosa, D. Fox, P. Hagstrom, M. McGinnis, and D. Pesetsky. MIT Press and MIT Working Papers in Linguistics. ROA 117.

Legendre, G., S. Vikner, and J. Grimshaw, eds. 2001. *Optimality-theoretic syntax*. MIT Press.

Legendre, G., C. Wilson, P. Smolensky, K. Homer, and W. Raymond. 1995. Optimality in *wh*-chains. In *University of Massachusetts occasional papers in linguistics 18: Papers in Optimality Theory*, eds. J. Beckman, L. Walsh Dickey, and S. Urbanczyk. Graduate Linguistic Student Association, University of Massachusetts at Amherst.

Lewis, R. L. 1998. Reanalysis and limited repair parsing: Leaping off the garden path. In *Reanalysis in sentence processing*, eds. J. D. Fodor and F. Fernanda. Kluwer.

MacDonald, M. C., N. Pearlmutter, and M. S. Seidenberg. 1994. Lexical nature of syntactic ambiguity resolution. *Psychological Review* 101, 676–703.

Meng, M., and M. Bader. 1997. Syntax and morphology in sentence parsing: A new look at German subject-object ambiguities. Ms., University of Jena.

Miyamoto, E. 1998. A low attachment preference in Brazilian Portuguese relative clauses. Talk presented at the Conference on Architectures and Mechanisms for Language Processing (AMLaP-98).

Phillips, C. 1996. Order and structure. Ph.D. diss., MIT.

Prince, A., and P. Smolensky. 1993/2004. *Optimality Theory: Constraint interaction in generative grammar*. Technical report, Rutgers University and University of Colorado at Boulder, 1993. ROA 537, 2002. Revised version published by Blackwell, 2004.

Pritchett, B. 1992. *Grammatical competence and parsing performance*. University of Chicago Press.

Rizzi, L. 1990. *Relativized Minimality*. MIT Press.

Sauerland, U., and E. Gibson. 1998. How to predict the relative clause attachment preference. Talk presented at the CUNY Conference on Human Sentence Processing.

Stevenson, S. 1994a. Competition and recency in a hybrid network model of syntactic disambiguation. *Journal of Psycholinguistic Research* 23, 295–322.

Stevenson, S. 1994b. A competitive attachment model for resolving syntactic ambiguities in natural language parsing. Ph.D. diss., University of Maryland.

Stevenson, S. 1995. Arguments and adjuncts: A computational explanation of asymmetries in attachment preferences. In *Proceedings of the Cognitive Science Society 17*.

Stevenson, S. 1998. Parsing as incremental restructuring. In *Reanalysis in sentence processing*, eds. J. D. Fodor and F. Ferreira. Kluwer.

Stevenson, S. In preparation. Agreeing to attach: Structure building and feature processing. Ms., University of Toronto.

Sturt, P., and M. Crocker. 1996. Monotonic syntactic processing: A cross-linguistic study of attachment and reanalysis. *Language and Cognitive Processes* 11, 449–94.

Traxler, M., M. Pickering, and C. Clifton. 1996. Architectures and mechanisms that process prepositional phrases and relative clauses. Talk presented at the Conference on Architectures and Mechanisms for Language Processing (AMLaP-96).

Trueswell, J., and M. K. Tanenhaus. 1994. Toward a lexicalist framework for constraint-based syntactic ambiguity resolution. In *Perspectives on sentence processing*, eds. C. Clifton, L. Frazier, and K. Rayner. Erlbaum.

Weinberg, A. 1995. Licensing constraints and the theory of language processing. In *Japanese sentence processing*, eds. R. Mazuka and N. Nagai. Erlbaum.

Woolford, E. 2001. Case patterns. In *Optimality-theoretic syntax*, eds. G. Legendre, S. Vikner, and J. Grimshaw. MIT Press.

20

The Optimality Theory –
Harmonic Grammar Connection

Géraldine Legendre, Antonella Sorace,
and Paul Smolensky

Harmonic Grammar plays a key role in the overall Integrated Connectionist/Symbolic Cognitive Architecture (ICS): it mediates between the highest-level descriptions of fully symbolic Optimality Theory and the lowest-level descriptions purely in terms of connectionist networks. What does OT add to grammatical theory, beyond what HG provides? And how exactly are the two connected in a consistent overall theory? The first question is addressed via several general subissues concerning the similarities and differences, real and apparent, between OT and HG. The second question is addressed by revisiting the problem at the syntax-semantics interface studied with HG in Chapter 11, split intransitivity; a new OT analysis of this phenomenon is developed and compared with the HG account (contributing to ② of Figure 6 in Chapter 2's ICS map). Finally, how exactly does HG make possible a link between an OT grammar and a connectionist network? (See ⑤ and ⑦ of Figure 5, and (27c), Chapter 2.) To illustrate this, we explicitly reduce an OT grammar (for syllabification) to a harmonic grammar, in turn reducing that to a local connectionist network. Simulations show that the dynamics of this network allows it to build correct syllabifications, sometimes by quite indirect routes. Reducing local connectionist networks to still lower-level distributed networks is discussed in general in Chapter 11.

Contents

The Integrated Connectionist/Symbolic Cognitive Architecture (ICS) incorporates two optimization-based grammatical frameworks, Harmonic Grammar (Chapters 6, 10, and 11) and Optimality Theory (Chapters 4, 12, and 13–19). HG provides a level of description intermediate between the highest, fully symbolic level of OT and the lowest, fully connectionist level. Like those in OT, the representations employed in HG are symbolic. As in connectionist computation, constraints interact in HG via numerical weighting. In this chapter, we explore the HG bridge between the connectionist and the symbolic. Primarily, we do this through two extensive case studies. The first considers how an HG account changes when it is pulled up to the level of OT; the second examines how an OT account can be pushed down to an HG account, which can then be pushed down to a connectionist network. The first study concerns syntax, the second, phonology.

The first study (Section 2) starts with the HG account of split intransitivity in Chapter 11 and recasts the analysis in OT. This highlights how OT provides a theory of universal typology: while the HG account is fully language particular, the OT analysis focuses on crosslinguistic variation. The contrast with OT's rigidly restrictive constraint interaction by strict domination also throws into relief how HG's numerical interaction allows it to describe more complex language-internal patterns. The new theory of split intransitivity developed in this section uses OT to bring into sharp focus the phenomenon's highly challenging mix of strong universal tendencies and dramatic crosslinguistic differences.

The second case study (Section 3) proceeds in the other direction. It starts with an OT analysis of the unusual syllabification system of Berber (from Prince and Smolensky 1993/2004). This is then recast in HG terms. A harmonic grammar for Berber syllabification can be readily realized as a local connectionist network—BrbrNet.[1] The computational properties of this network are, like the linguistic data it models, quite remarkable. While the connectionist level of ICS is assumed to involve distributed representations, Chapter 11 shows how a local network can itself be regarded as a kind of higher-level description—of a still lower-level, distributed network. Thus, BrbrNet has a place in the overall ICS picture linking high-level OT grammars to low-level distributed connectionist networks.

Before launching into these two case studies, we begin in Section 1 by considering general conceptual issues concerning the OT-HG relationship. OT and HG are both relatively new frameworks, and most of the questions we will address concerning their relationship are still open; much of the discussion will therefore be somewhat speculative.

---

[1] Chapter 10 shows how harmonic grammars for formal languages can be realized in local connectionist networks.

1 THE OPTIMALITY THEORY–HARMONIC GRAMMAR CONNECTION: GENERAL REMARKS

The fundamental similarities between Optimality Theory and Harmonic Grammar are fairly evident: the output of the mappings specified by the grammar—the structures declared grammatical—are those that optimally satisfy a set of constraints that apply in parallel to evaluate alternatives. The constraints are simple—that is, general—and therefore typically in conflict. Conflicts are adjudicated by the differential strength the grammar assigns to constraints. Intricate grammatical patterns emerge from the complex interaction of fundamentally simple constraints.

But there are also differences between the two formalisms. In some ways, OT imposes further restrictions on a harmonic grammar. In other ways, the two theories appear to be in fundamental conflict. In certain respects, the kinds of grammatical questions the two theories have focused on differ. And the levels of description the theories adopt differ in their distance from a lower connectionist level. (For a direct comparison of the fundamental principles of OT with those of connectionism, see Chapter 22 (6).)

1.1 Universality

A principle central to OT is the universality of grammatical structures and constraints. This is one respect in which OT is more restricted than HG. The constraints employed in the HG analysis of split intransitivity discussed in Chapter 11 were intended to embody universal tendencies, but the emphasis was on capturing difficult interactions within a single language. While language-particular analysis plays an important role in OT as in all grammatical theory, OT places a strong emphasis on explaining crosslinguistic patterns via the reranking of a fixed set of hypothesized universal constraints.

1.2 Numerically weighted constraints versus strict domination

The most obvious difference between HG and OT is also one that underlies many of the other differences: both theories resolve constraint conflict by differentiating the strengths (or 'weights') of constraints, but in HG this is formalized with numerical strengths and in OT with a strict priority ranking. We consider two facets of this issue: empirical and computational.

1.2.1 Empirical considerations

The empirical question at issue is whether in fact grammatical constraints interact in accord with the principle of strict domination. The body of empirical work in OT to date seems to say yes—with qualification. Though we don't attempt to justify it here, our judgment is that, with respect to those constraints that seem implicated in broad crosslinguistic patterns, much empirical evidence supports the hypothesis that strict domination captures the core of grammatical constraint interaction, in at least most of phonology and much of syntax.

1.2.1.1 Grammars can't count

A central component of the empirical basis for strict domination is synopsized in the oft-repeated adage, *Grammars can't count*. A concrete and simple illustration is provided by the interaction between two constraints from stress theory. The constraint STRESSHEAVY (more properly, WSP, the 'weight-to-stress principle' — Prince 1990; Prince and Smolensky 1993/2004) requires that heavy syllables be stressed. (Essentially, a syllable is heavy if it has a long vowel or, in many languages, if it ends in a consonant.) The other constraint, MAINSTRESSRIGHT, requires a word's primary stress to fall on the rightmost syllable; it is **gradiently violable**, violated once for each syllable that separates the main stress from the right edge of the word. Let's compare the possible patterns arising from the interaction of these two constraints under OT and HG.

In OT, there are only two possibilities: either STRESSHEAVY dominates MAINSTRESSRIGHT or the opposite ranking holds. These two situations are considered in tableaux (1)–(2). A light syllable is denoted by σ, a heavy syllable by σ_H. The acute accent marks the syllable bearing main stress: $\acute{\sigma}$. The input is a word with a heavy syllable σ_H followed by n light syllables σ (such as hypothetical *beetata$\cdots$ta*). The question is, where is the stress? On the heavy (leftmost) syllable, satisfying STRESSHEAVY, or on the rightmost syllable, satisfying MAINSTRESSRIGHT? As always, this conflict between constraints is resolved in OT by ranking, with the higher-ranked constraint taking priority.

(1)

Candidates		MAINSTRESSRIGHT	STRESSHEAVY
a.	$\underbrace{\acute{\sigma}_H\sigma\sigma\cdots\sigma}_{n}$	$\underbrace{**\cdots*}_{n}$	
b. ☞	$\underbrace{\sigma_H\sigma\cdots\sigma\acute{\sigma}}_{n}$		*

The tableau in (1) illustrates a language where MAINSTRESSRIGHT is dominant. The optimal candidate, (1b), has final stress, satisfying the higher-ranked constraint. For our purposes, the interesting case is the reverse ranking, illustrated in (2).

(2)

Candidates		STRESSHEAVY	MAINSTRESSRIGHT
a. ☞	$\underbrace{\acute{\sigma}_H\sigma\sigma\cdots\sigma}_{n}$		$\underbrace{**\cdots*}_{n}$
b.	$\underbrace{\sigma_H\sigma\cdots\sigma\acute{\sigma}}_{n}$	*	

Tableau (2) depicts a language where STRESSHEAVY dominates; now the optimal candidate has stress on the initial syllable, (2a). The point is this: the force of strict domination is to ensure that initial stress is optimal, *no matter how much this violates* the lower-ranked constraint favoring final stress, that is, no matter how many light syllables σ follow the initial heavy syllable. That is, a single violation of the top-ranked constraint must outweigh *any number* of violations of the lower-ranked constraint.

So under OT, the typology of possible languages, with respect to the interaction of these two constraints and this type of input, contains only two language types. In one type (1), stress will always fall on a heavy syllable (as in Hindi); in the other (2), stress will always be final (as in French).

Under HG, however, the typology implicit in these two constraints exhibits *infinitely many* possibilities. For suppose the numerical strengths of the two constraints are $w_{\text{STRESSHEAVY}}$ and $w_{\text{MAINSTRESSRIGHT}}$: each violation of a constraint lowers the Harmony by a quantity equal to its strength. Then the Harmonies of the two candidates are as shown in (3).

(3)

Candidates		STRESSHEAVY	MAINSTRESSRIGHT	**Harmony**
a.	$\underbrace{\acute{\sigma}_H \sigma\sigma\cdots\sigma}_{n}$		$\underbrace{**\ldots*}_{n}$	$-n(w_{\text{MAINSTRESSRIGHT}})$
b.	$\underbrace{\sigma_H\sigma\cdots\sigma\acute{\sigma}}_{n}$	*		$-w_{\text{STRESSHEAVY}}$

Now suppose STRESSHEAVY is the stronger constraint; under strict domination, this implies that initial stress (3a) is optimal. Under HG, initial stress maximizes Harmony if and only if

$$-n(w_{\text{MAINSTRESSRIGHT}}) > -w_{\text{STRESSHEAVY}},$$

that is, if and only if

(4) $n < w_{\text{STRESSHEAVY}}/w_{\text{MAINSTRESSRIGHT}} \equiv r.$

STRESSHEAVY's being dominant means its weight is greater, so the ratio r in (4) is greater than one. How much greater presumably varies typologically; in HG, r can in principle be any number. So if the word is short enough, if n is less than r, then initial stress maximizes Harmony, as with strict domination. But if the word is long enough, if n exceeds r, then stress flips to the final syllable: many violations of MAINSTRESSRIGHT — the cost of stress falling n syllables from the right edge of the word — **gang up** and overcome the single violation of the higher-ranked constraint STRESSHEAVY that mars the final-stress alternative (3a). The word length at which the stress flips from initial to final, set by the ratio of constraint weights r, can be any number. Thus, the HG typology predicts that in some languages, in words with a single, initial, heavy syllable, stress will be initial for words shorter than four syllables, but final for longer words; in other languages, stress will be initial for words shorter than five syllables, otherwise final; and so on ad infinitum.

It is exactly this sort of typology that is banned as empirically impossible by the high-level generalization *Grammars can't count.*

Moreover, the above example is only the very simplest typological prediction of

HG-style, numerically weighted constraint interaction: even more empirically suspect predictions are readily obtained by simply considering more than two constraints. If the weights of three conflicting constraints are, say, $w_A = 11$, $w_B = 3$, $w_C = 2$, then the strongest constraint A will override the preferences of the two weaker constraints B and C, if each of them is violated at most once; but the weaker constraints can gang up and overrule A if B is violated four or more times, or C is violated six or more times, or B is violated three times and C twice, or … . Once a realistically sized set of conflicting constraints is considered, the counting required of such grammars is staggering, and, it would appear, utterly without empirical basis in the many crosslinguistic studies of the world's grammars. (For a concrete example highlighting strictness of domination in an actual phonological analysis, see Prince and Smolensky 1993/2004, Sec. 7.4n.)

1.2.1.2 Conjunctive constraint interaction

A wide variety of empirical studies employing OT have confirmed strict domination as the basic mode of constraint interaction. However, a number of language-specific analyses, and some typological studies, have observed deviations from this basic mode. Even in this regard, however, strict domination serves two crucial roles: it identifies the basic interactive mode, providing the baseline for identifying these deviations; and it provides a formal device that can be deployed to develop a theory of the new type of interaction.

This theory asserts that in addition to strict domination, universal constraints sometimes interact via **local conjunction** (Chapter 12 (43); Chapter 14). That is, when two constraints are simultaneously violated within the same local domain, their joint effect can be stronger than their linear sum. In particular, if an isolated violation of $\mathbb{C}_1$ is weaker than a violation of $\mathbb{C}_0$, and an isolated violation of $\mathbb{C}_2$ is also weaker than a violation of $\mathbb{C}_0$, it can sometimes happen that simultaneous violations of $\mathbb{C}_1$ and $\mathbb{C}_2$ 'at the same place' are *stronger* than a violation of $\mathbb{C}_0$.

The formalism developed to capture strict domination can actually be called into the service of a theory of such conjunctive interactions. Given two constraints $\mathbb{C}_1$ and $\mathbb{C}_2$, their **local conjunction with respect to a domain** $\mathcal{D}$, written '$\mathbb{C}_1 \,\&_{\mathcal{D}}\, \mathbb{C}_2$', is violated whenever $\mathbb{C}_1$ and $\mathbb{C}_2$ are both violated in a common domain $\mathcal{D}$.[2] This new constraint $\mathbb{C}_1 \,\&_{\mathcal{D}}\, \mathbb{C}_2$ is then ranked with all the other constraints in the hierarchy defining a language's grammar.

Obviously, allowing such conjunctive interactions makes OT considerably less restrictive, and there are currently many open questions about whether the empirical facts require lessening the theory's restrictiveness in this way. Regardless of the ultimate fate of the theory of local conjunction, there seems to be considerable consensus that OT has made a major contribution in identifying simple strict domination as the fundamental mode of grammatical constraint interaction.

---

[2] For example, if $\mathbb{C}_1$ = NoCoda, $\mathbb{C}_2$ = NoVoicedStops, and $\mathcal{D}$ = a segment, then the conjunction is violated by a voiced stop in a syllable coda.

1.2.1.3   Grammaticalization

The HG study of split intransitivity in French discussed in Chapter 11 provides some evidence of numerical constraint interaction. How does this relate to OT's assumption of strict domination? One possibility is this. Knowledge relevant to language processing may combine (i) a system of constraints one might consider more strictly 'grammatical', interacting exclusively or primarily via strict domination, and (ii) a set of more pragmatically based constraints, reflecting more directly, perhaps, statistical characteristics of experience, and interacting in a less restricted manner, via arbitrarily weighted constraints. **Grammaticalization** may be one process in which constraints effectively move from the latter category to the former. It may be that both types of constraints are interacting in the HG analysis and that those focused upon in OT studies are mainly from the grammatical class. Computationally, it is possible to combine both types of constraints into one analysis (as perhaps the HG analysis of Chapter 11 does), because the strict domination interaction required by OT can be implemented by numerical weighting, putting the grammatical constraints into a computational arena where they can interact with more pragmatic constraints bearing arbitrary numerical weights. The OT analysis of split intransitivity in Section 2 explores the implications of strict domination interaction of some types of constraints included in the HG study of French.

1.2.2   Computational considerations

In a sense, strict domination is one respect in which OT adds further restrictions to HG: strict domination can be seen as a special relation among numerical weights (Prince and Smolensky 1993/2004, Chap. 10). Several of the relevant considerations have already made their appearance in Section 1.2.1.1's discussion of counting by grammars.

1.2.2.1   Exponential constraint weighting

Suppose first that each candidate can violate each constraint only once. What strengths will yield the strict domination hierarchy $\mathbb{C}_n \gg \ldots \gg \mathbb{C}_2 \gg \mathbb{C}_1 \gg \mathbb{C}_0$? To set the arbitrary origin of weights, let the strength of $\mathbb{C}_0$ be 1. Then obviously the weight of $\mathbb{C}_1$ must be greater than 1; to set the arbitrary scale of weights, let the weight of $\mathbb{C}_1$ be 2. Now in order that $\mathbb{C}_2$ have strict priority over both lower-ranked constraints, the cost of violating $\mathbb{C}_2$ must be higher than the cost of violating both $\mathbb{C}_1$ and $\mathbb{C}_0$, that is, greater than $2 + 1 = 3$; we can keep integer weights by taking the strength of $\mathbb{C}_2$ to be 4. Continuing this logic, we see that strict domination can be achieved by setting the weight of $\mathbb{C}_k$ to be 2^k. We will refer to this as **exponential weighting**: the strengths of constraints grow exponentially as the hierarchy is mounted (see Chapter 21 (22c)).

Typically, however, constraints can be violated more than once in a candidate linguistic structure (e.g., NoCoda is violated once for each syllable that ends in a consonant; MAINSTRESSRIGHT is violated once for each syllable separating the main-stressed syllable from the word's right edge). Suppose each constraint can be violated anywhere from 0 to 9 times in a single candidate. If $\mathbb{C}_1$ is to strictly dominate $\mathbb{C}_0$, the cost of a single violation of $\mathbb{C}_1$ must exceed that of any number of violations of $\mathbb{C}_0$, so the weight of $\mathbb{C}_1$ must exceed 9—say, 10. Iterating this logic, we see that the strength of $\mathbb{C}_k$ must be 10^k. This is exponential weighting, but the base of exponentiation has grown from 2 to 10.

In one sense, then, OT's strict domination is a special case of HG's numerical weighting: exponential weighting. But in another sense, strict domination is an idealization that no set of numerical weights can actually achieve. For strict domination puts no limit on the number of lower-ranked violations that a higher-ranking constraint overrides; thus, no finite base of exponentiation—whether it be 2, or 10, or 10^6—can *truly* implement strict domination. Thus, it is most accurate to state that, as an idealized competence theory, OT constitutes a certain *limiting* case of HG: exponential weighting, in the limit as the base of exponentiation goes to infinity.[3]

Exponential weighting of constraints poses a number of unanswered questions about an underlying connectionist realization. Even for a small base of exponentiation, such weights quickly become enormous as the number of crucially ordered constraints increases. The challenge this presents to a connectionist realization is the large *dynamic range* required by computation with exponential weighting: no matter how the actual range of weights involved might be compressed by multiplying by a small scale factor, the number of *distinct values* of Harmony that must be accurately compared is large. It is unknown whether there is a way of embedding constraints in a network such that effective weighting of constraints will naturally be exponential.

1.2.2.2 Functional speculations

A quite different question is, *why* should constraint weighting be exponential? From the perspective of familiar connectionist networks, exponential weighting is entirely unexpected; is there some consideration from which it might actually follow? One possible functional motivation may come from the demands that grammar be a *sharable* knowledge system. The optimization involved in, say, planning a reaching movement can produce a different result each time. There's no strong requirement for reproducibility; any trajectory that basically meets the constraints is good enough. But

---

[3] It is worth noting that it is not possible to have strict domination without finite, discrete levels of constraint violation. Thus, continuous constraint penalties typical in phonetics, such as $c([\text{actual value}] - [\text{target value}])^2$, contrast with the discrete penalties of OT phonology (Flemming 2001). Suppose the weights of $\mathbb{C}_2 \gg \mathbb{C}_1$ are nonstandard, infinite real numbers $w_2 > w_1$. For strict domination, any degree of violation ε_2 of $\mathbb{C}_2$ must overpower any finite degree of violation—say, 1—of $\mathbb{C}_1$; that is, it must be the case that $\varepsilon_2 w_2 > w_1$. Thus, ε_2 must not be an infinitesimal with $\varepsilon_2 < w_1/w_2$. So continuous degrees of violation of $\mathbb{C}_2$ are incompatible with $\mathbb{C}_2$'s strictly dominating $\mathbb{C}_1$. (For a less transparent argument, replace the infinite penalties with large finite ones.)

If phonological representations are discrete, it follows that degree of violation will be discrete, as required for strict domination. If, contrary to standard assumptions, phonological representations are continuous (Kirchner 1998), then strict domination requires that each individual constraint discretize its relevant representational continuum, assessing violations in a discrete, discontinuous fashion.

it won't do if each hearer's optimization yields a different structure for a sentence, and each speaker's optimization yields yet another structure. One suggestion, due to David Rumelhart (personal communication), and independently to James McClelland (personal communication), is that exponential weighting of constraints may enable quick-and-dirty optimization algorithms of the sort embodied in connectionist computation to consistently find a single global Harmony optimum, whereas arbitrarily weighted constraints typically lead such algorithms to produce widely varying solutions, each only a local optimum. (See Section 6:2.4 for the relation of the competence/performance distinction to the global/local optimum distinction.) Some experimental evidence favoring this suggestion is discussed in Section 3.

Another possibility is that *learnability* demands exert pressure for strict domination among constraints of unknown strength. Rather strong formal results have been obtained concerning the efficient learnability of strictly ranked constraints (see Section 12:3), but it remains an open problem to formally characterize exactly what is essential about strict domination to guarantee efficient learning.

In either case—whether to meet demands of reliable, rapid optimization, or efficient learnability—the idea is that while arbitrarily weighted constraints may be the typical case in connectionist networks, evolutionary pressures on the language system may have led to the development of a special architecture—as yet unknown—in which strict domination obtains, at least to the degree needed to ensure that an OT-like grammar would provide a good competence-theoretic idealization.

1.2.3 Local conjunction and strict domination

Consider for the sake of argument the following oft-repeated line of reasoning.

(5)   The ganging-up argument: General form

The central premise of OT is strict domination—that is, no number of violations of lower-ranked constraints can overpower a single violation of a higher-ranked constraint. In particular, if $\mathbb{C} \gg \mathbb{A}$ and $\mathbb{C} \gg \mathbb{B}$, then no degree of violation of the lower-ranked constraints $\mathbb{A}$ and $\mathbb{B}$ can overrule a single violation of $\mathbb{C}$. The conjunction $\mathbb{A} \& \mathbb{B}$ is designed specifically so that in this situation, the ranking $\mathbb{A} \& \mathbb{B} \gg \mathbb{C}$ *does* entail that a violation of both $\mathbb{A}$ and $\mathbb{B}$ overrules a violation of $\mathbb{C}$. Thus, admitting local conjunction into OT nullifies its most basic principle.

In fact, the need for local conjunction shows that strict domination is simply empirically incorrect. Strict domination in OT eliminates the potentially much richer possibilities for constraint interaction provided by a theory that is like OT except that constraints have numerical strengths, and each constraint violation incurs a numerical penalty equal to that constraint's strength. Such a theory is in fact exactly HG, developed in Chapters 6, 10, and 11. Strict domination corresponds to a very special property of constraint strengths: stronger constraints are numerically *so much* stronger that it is simply numerically impossible for weaker constraints to gang up on and overpower a stronger constraint; as explained in Section 1.2.2.1, constraint strengths essentially need to grow exponentially as the ranking is mounted. What the need for local conjunction is telling us is that empirically, HG is correct and OT is not — that weaker constraints *can* gang up in the way that HG allows, but OT does not (without local conjunction).

The basic arguments developed in Chapter 14 for introducing local conjunction into OT center on the **BOWOW** pattern: inventories that ban only the worst of the worst. In this context, the argument in (5) can be made more concrete.

(6)   The ganging-up argument: BOWOW inventories

An element that violates the markedness constraint $*\alpha$ is acceptable (i.e., allowed in the inventory); an element that violates the markedness constraint $*\beta$ is acceptable; but an element that violates both is unacceptable (banned from the inventory). This BOWOW inventory requires the local conjunction $*\alpha \, \& \, *\beta$ in an OT analysis:

$*\alpha \, \& \, *\beta \gg F \gg *\alpha, *\beta$.

(F is the faithfulness constraint opposing elimination of the marked structures.)

Numerically, the BOWOW inventory requires these constraints to have numerical strengths such that, individually, the weight of the markedness constraint $*\alpha$, $w_{*\alpha}$, is less than that of F, w_F; similarly, individually, $w_{*\beta}$ is less than w_F; but together, the sum $w_{*\alpha} + w_{*\beta}$ is greater than w_F, so the markedness constraints gang up and overpower F when violated together. This sort of ganging up is exactly what is barred by strict domination, which requires that $w_{*\alpha} + w_{*\beta}$ never be greater than w_F; under strict domination, w_F would be so large that no summation of weights of lower constraints could be larger. Thus, BOWOW inventories show that strict domination is fundamentally incorrect, that weights for constraints must be allowed to gang up. Using local conjunction amounts to admitting this failure of strict domination.

To understand the implications of local conjunction for OT, it is important to see that *this argument is a fallacy*, in either its more general (5) or more concrete (6) form. Whether the weights satisfy the strict domination condition — whether the weight of the weaker constraints together, $w_{*\alpha} + w_{*\beta}$, exceeds that of the stronger constraint, w_F — *has nothing to do with* generating a BOWOW inventory.

The reason is extremely simple. To ban the worst of the worst, it is not sufficient that $w_{*\alpha} + w_{*\beta}$ exceeds w_F; what is required is that $w_{*\alpha} + w_{*\beta}$ exceed *twice* w_F. This is because in the 'worst of the worst' input, competition pits two markedness violations ($w_{*\alpha} + w_{*\beta}$) against *two* faithfulness violations ($2w_F$). And it is simply impossible for $w_{*\alpha} + w_{*\beta}$ to exceed $2w_F$ if, individually, neither $w_{*\alpha}$ nor $w_{*\beta}$ exceeds w_F — no matter what the numbers, regardless of whether the weights satisfy the strict domination condition $w_F > w_{*\alpha} + w_{*\beta}$. Eliminating strict domination could allow two weaker violations to exceed *one* stronger violation, but *nothing* can allow two weaker violations to exceed *two* stronger violations.

To see why the competition is in general between two lower-ranked markedness violations and *two* higher-ranked faithfulness violations, consider the simple subset of the English obstruent inventory where place markedness and manner markedness interact: {*t, k, s, *x*}; *x*, the velar fricative, is banned from the English inventory.

(7)   BOWOW subset of English obstruent inventory

	Place	*[vel]
Manner	t	k
*[cont]	s	**x**

The unmarked segment *t* is in the inventory; and violating either *[vel(ar)] (place markedness) or *[cont(inuant)] (manner markedness) individually is allowed, admitting *k* and *s* into the inventory. But the segment violating both markedness constraints, *x*, is banned. This is a classic BOWOW inventory. Its analysis under numerically weighted constraint interaction is simple. In order that the input /k/ have as its optimal output [k] (*[velar]) as opposed to [t], faithfulness to place, F[vel], must outweigh place markedness, *[vel].

(8)   *k* admitted $\Rightarrow w_{F[vel]} > w_{*[vel]}$

By identical reasoning, for the segment *s* to be admitted, F[cont] must outweigh *[cont].

(9)   *s* admitted $\Rightarrow w_{F[cont]} > w_{*[cont]}$

Together, (8) and (9) entail that faithfulness to place and manner combined outweigh markedness of place and manner combined—so *x* must be in the inventory (10).

(10) $w_{F[vel]} + w_{F[cont]} > w_{*[vel]} + w_{*[cont]}$ $\Rightarrow$ *x* admitted

This is displayed in the **HG tableaux** of (11), where for concreteness actual numerical weights have been employed. To emphasize the irrelevance of strict domination, the weights chosen for faithfulness constraints exceed those chosen for markedness constraints by less than 3%; the strict domination condition is not even close to being satisfied, as a single stronger violation is much less than the sum of two weaker violations.

In (11), numbers show the Harmony of candidates, the optimal output being the one with highest Harmony; the Harmony is the sum of negative contributions from each violation, weighted by the weight of the constraint violated.

The situation is depicted in another way in (12). For input /k/, the move from faithful [k] to unmarked [t] must be Harmony-decreasing, since *k* is in the inventory; call the Harmony difference $-\varepsilon$ (this is just $-(w_{F[vel]} - w_{*[vel]})$ in the notation above; in the example (11), $-\varepsilon = -0.02$). Similarly, for input /s/, a move to [t] must produce a Harmony decrease, call it $-\delta$. Now consider input /x/. The move from [x] to [s] incurs the same Harmony penalty as that from [k] to [t], $-(w_{F[vel]} - w_{*[vel]})$; this is $-\varepsilon$, so /x/→ [x] has higher Harmony than /x/→[s]. Similarly, /x/→ [x] has higher Harmony than /x/→[k] (by the amount δ). And finally, eliminating both marks via /x/→[t] incurs the Harmony penalty that is the sum of the other two, −ε−δ; this too must be less harmonic than the faithful mapping. Since the faithful mapping /x/→[x] has highest Harmony, *x* must be in the inventory.

(11)   HG tableaux: Impossibility of BOWOW in HG

		F[vel] 5.02	F[cont] 5.01	*[vel] 5.0	*[cont] 4.9	Constraint Weight	
/k/→						**Harmony**	
☞	[k]			* −5.0		− 5.00	✓ *k*
	[t]	* −5.02				− 5.02	
/s/→							
☞	[s]				* −4.9	− 4.90	✓ *s*
	[t]		* −5.01			− 5.01	
/x/→							
☞	[x]			* −5.0	* −4.9	− 9.90	✓ *x*
	[s]	* −5.02			* −4.9	− 9.92	
	[k]		* −5.01	* −5.0		−10.01	
	[t]	* −5.02	* −5.01			−10.03	

(12)   Net Harmony penalties for unfaithful mappings

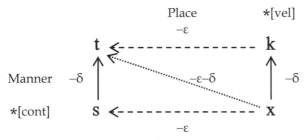

The difficulty of banning only the worst of the worst cannot be overcome by manipulating the strengths of constraints, which is why strict domination is not a relevant issue. The problem resides in the *means of combining* markedness dimensions: simple summation. The above analysis shows that what is needed for a BOWOW inventory is that *the penalty for violating two markedness constraints is more than the sum of their individual penalties.* We could say that markedness combination must be super-additive or **superlinear**.[4] It is the additive or linear character of HG that prevents

---

[4] Alternatively, FAITHFULNESS combination could be *sublinear*, with the Harmony penalty of two faithfulness violations *less* than the sum of the individual penalties. (This would be a version of Burzio's (2002) **gradient attraction**, where the strength of FAITHFULNESS between *A* and *B* diminishes as *A* and *B* become less similar.) Sublinear FAITHFULNESS is instantiated in segmental-MAX: if this replaces the individual-feature faithfulness constraints F[φ] in the text, then deleting the entire segment

BOWOW; as long as markedness combination remains additive, it makes no difference whether strict domination is required of the weights.

What local conjunction centrally achieves is superlinear interaction, not nonstrict domination. For the numerical example in (11), the sum of the penalties for *[vel] and *[cont] is 9.9; if superlinear interaction instead yields a sufficiently higher penalty (e.g., 9.93), then the faithful mapping is no longer the most harmonic (/x/ → [s] is), and x is now banned (13).

(13)   Possibility of BOWOW with superlinear constraint combination

	*[vel]& *[cont] 0.03 [+5.0+4.9=9.93]	F[vel] 5.02	F[cont] 5.01	*[vel] 5.0	*[cont] 4.9	Constraint Weight
/x/ →						**Harmony**
[x]	* −0.03			* −5.0	* −4.9	−9.93
☞ [s]		* −5.02			* −4.9	−9.92
[k]			* −5.01	* −5.0		−10.01
[t]		* −5.02	* −5.01			−10.03

The argument developed above is quite general. Indeed, it applies directly to the general formalization of basic inventories developed in the Appendix of Chapter 14, so the theorems derived there all pertain to a general setting in which it is superlinearity, not nonstrict domination, that is required to achieve the effects that can be achieved with local conjunction.

The above situation is covered by a general theorem formulated by Prince (2002).

(14)   The "Anything Goes" Theorem

Let $\mathcal{H}$ be a strict domination hierarchy and let A be an optimal output for some input, and B a suboptimal output for that input. Suppose the following holds: for every constraint $\mathbb{C}$ in $\mathcal{H}$, the total number of violations by A of the constraints ranked higher than $\mathbb{C}$ is less than the total number of violations by B of the same constraints. Then A has higher numerical Harmony than B when computed by summing weighted constraint violations, for any set of numerical weights that order the constraints in accord with the ranking $\mathcal{H}$.

This theorem gives a sufficient condition for numerical weights to produce the same optimal outputs as OT harmonic evaluation with no restriction on the rate at which

---

avoids *both* marks *[vel] and *[cont] given /x/, while incurring the same *single* mark *MAX that is incurred if either one alone is avoided by whole-segment deletion given /k/ or /s/. In general, however, it is not sublinear FAITHFULNESS but superlinear MARKEDNESS that is the numerical implementation of local conjunction. Given how optimality is computed in OT, making [α, β] more marked than [α] + [β] is straightforwardly achieved by a higher-ranked conjoined constraint, which adds a third mark to *α and *β; but making two FAITHFULNESS violations *less* costly than the two individual violations cannot be achieved by adding an additional mark: it requires *removing* at least one of the individual marks when two violations occur. Thus, a general means of weakening FAITHFULNESS would require considerably more alteration to the basic theory than does strengthening MARKEDNESS.

weights grow as the hierarchy is mounted (exponential growth is *not* required).[5] (Prince shows that this is a necessary condition as well.)

The condition of the "Anything Goes" Theorem is met in the little example just discussed, and in fact, it is met in general for all **basic inventories** as defined in the Appendix of Chapter 14.[6] Thus, the conclusion we have reached is quite general: for *any* numerical weighting of the constraints, the numerically optimal candidate is the same as that in plain OT. Thus, the inability of OT without local conjunction to generate BOWOW inventories applies equally to a theory employing unrestricted numerical weights. Since neither system can derive BOWOW inventories, as discussed at length in Chapter 14, neither is strongly harmonically complete. To achieve strongly harmonically complete typologies, local conjunction is needed in OT, and superlinear constraint combination is needed in HG. Strict domination is irrelevant.

1.3 Relative versus absolute Harmony; graded acceptability

In the HG analysis of split intransitivity, a structure's absolute level of Harmony was taken to model its acceptability. Since multiple Harmony values are possible, this means multiple levels of acceptability can be modeled, and indeed the French data analyzed in that study consisted of a graded acceptability judgment, on a 5-point scale, for each sentence. In OT, however, only relative, not absolute, levels of Harmony matter: the highest-Harmony member of a candidate set is the only grammatical one, all other candidates being equally ungrammatical. Indeed, it is readily seen upon inspecting many OT analyses that use of relative, not absolute, Harmony is crucial: in many cases, the absolute Harmony value of the optimal (and indeed correct) candidate in one candidate set is lower than the absolute Harmony of suboptimal

---

[5] *Proof sketch.* Since $A \succ B$, by the Cancellation/Domination Lemma (Prince and Smolensky 1993/2004), every mark of A is either canceled or dominated by a mark of B. In both OT and the numerical theory, cancellation eliminates irrelevant marks. The highest uncanceled mark of A, call it *W, is dominated by a mark of B, *L. In the numerical theory, this condition is equivalent to $w_W > w_L$, with no restriction on the magnitude of the weights or their difference. Now throw out these two marks, noting that their respective contributions to the Harmonies of A and B favor A (lower penalty), and proceed to the new highest mark of A and repeat. When all marks of A have been discarded in this way, it is proved that the Harmony of A is higher than that of B (there may be remaining marks of B, but these just make it even lower in Harmony). This procedure can be executed whenever the condition of the theorem is met: for every uncanceled mark of A, there is guaranteed to be a higher-ranked remaining mark of B, even after some B-marks have been discarded. Each mark of A is canceled or dominated by *its own distinct* mark of B. Thus, the numerical Harmony of A is greater. But if the conditions of the theorem are not satisfied, all we know from the Cancellation/Domination Lemma is that each uncanceled mark of A is dominated by *some* uncanceled mark of B: but a *single* higher mark of B can dominate any number of lower-ranked marks of A—this is strict domination.

[6] *Proof* (assuming the definitions and notation from the Appendix of Chapter 14). Given an input I specified with feature values φ_i, the optimal output A has features ψ_i, where $\psi_i \equiv \varphi_i$, except $\psi_i \equiv -\varphi_i$ if φ_i is the marked value and $M[\varphi_i] \gg F[\varphi_i]$. That is, for A, for all i, either φ_i is unmarked, generating no mark $M[\varphi_i]$ and no mark $F[\varphi_i]$ as ($\psi_i \equiv \varphi_i$), or φ_i is marked, and A violates the lower-ranked constraint of $\{M[\varphi_i], F[\varphi_i]\}$. Let B be a suboptimal output for I. Then consider any mark of A; it is for some i the lower ranked of $\{M[\varphi_i], F[\varphi_i]\}$. Either this mark is canceled in B because B has the same value for ψ_i, or it is dominated because B is marked by the other, higher-ranked constraint of $\{M[\varphi_i], F[\varphi_i]\}$. Every mark of A has *its own* canceling or dominating mark in B. This ensures the condition of the theorem; indeed, it's just what the condition of the theorem is designed to ensure—see the proof in Footnote 5.

(and indeed incorrect) candidates in a different candidate set. An essential feature of competition-based explanation in OT is that a structure can be grammatical *even though it violates constraints that are fatal in other competitions,* because it is the best option in the candidate set. According to an OT grammar, the best of a bad batch is grammatical, while the second-best of a good batch is not. For this reason, use of absolute Harmony values as a model of graded acceptability, or graded processing accuracy or difficulty, is at odds with the fundamental structure of OT.

And indeed, there is no natural sense in which a connectionist network has access to its own absolute Harmony level: that is just a convenient measure for the analyst looking at the system from outside. Implicitly, a network has access to relative Harmony levels, because its processing algorithm takes it from a state at one moment to a state at the next moment that has higher relative Harmony; and this can be computed entirely locally, by spreading activation. But the absolute Harmony value of the state as a whole is a global quantity that would seem inaccessible to the network itself. It would be surprising, then, if informants reporting acceptability judgments are in effect reporting absolute Harmony levels. Indeed, we suspect it is OT rather than HG that is on the right track here: only relative, not absolute, Harmony levels should be cognitively relevant.

How, then, can HG be reconceived without appealing to absolute Harmony? Simply by making it consistent with OT. To illustrate, we take the relatively clean case of harmonic grammars of formal languages, discussed in Section 6:2.3 and Chapter 10. As it will turn out, our proposal involves the final difference between HG and OT we consider here, that between a theoretical bias toward grammatical mappings in the interpretation direction and one in the production direction.

1.4 Interpretation versus production orientation

Section 6:2.3 and Chapter 10 describe how, given a context-free formal language $\mathcal{L}$, a harmonic grammar can be designed so that a string of terminal symbols μ is in $\mathcal{L}$ if and only if $H(\mu) \geq 0$, that is, if and only if the maximum-Harmony parse tree of μ has nonnegative (in fact, 0) Harmony. There, following what we will now refer to as the **absolute-Harmony interpretation** of HG, we took this criterion to *define* grammaticality. This is essentially an *interpretation-oriented* criterion: what is given is an 'overt' string of symbols μ (idealizing a sequence of words a hearer might receive), and this is mapped onto the parse tree that maximizes Harmony. The absolute Harmony of this tree is then consulted: if it is negative, μ is not in the language $\mathcal{L}$; otherwise, it is.

There is, however, another view of HG, the **relative-Harmony interpretation**, which relies on the same *production-oriented* criterion for grammaticality that is used in OT. To generate, rather than recognize, strings in a formal language $\mathcal{L}$, we start with the grammar's start symbol, **S**, which we think of as denoting the category of grammatical sentence. We then use the grammar to generate all legal trees with **S** at the root and terminal symbols at the leaves of the tree. In the HG context, that means we take **S** as the 'input' and assign it to the maximum-Harmony tree with **S** at the root and terminal symbols at the leaves. What tree is this? There are many such trees — infinitely many, typically. For every grammatical string μ in L, there is a zero-Harmony tree with μ at the leaves and **S** at the root; all other trees have negative Harmony. So the maximum-Harmony trees with **S** at the root are exactly the legal parse trees of grammatical strings in L. Thus, simply by reinterpreting the harmonic grammar using a production- rather than interpretation-oriented definition of grammaticality, we get a relative- rather than absolute-Harmony characterization of the formal language.

How might the HG analysis of split intransitivity (Chapter 11) be recast in a production-oriented, relative-Harmony framework? In such a framework, to determine the grammaticality of a sentence, it does not suffice to simply evaluate the maximum-Harmony parse for that sentence; we must compare this Harmony with alternative parses of the same input, employing other constructions. A given syntactic expression, with a particular verb and set of arguments, is thus ungrammatical if the corresponding input — the proposition it would express — is optimally expressed via another expression.[7] Note that, as with OT, in this revised conception of grammaticality under HG, it is unclear how to model graded judgments of acceptability.[8]

For reasons discussed at some length in Chapter 16, there are some subtle conceptual and technical issues in OT syntax regarding propositions that have *no* grammatical expression in a language. Most of the unaccusativity tests discussed in Chapter 11 are of the form, 'If a verb V is grammatical in construction X, then V is unaccusative'. For a verb that fails the test, there is no grammatical output for the input that corresponds to the construction X. It is most straightforward, then, to consider a different type of unaccusativity test. In this type, unaccusative verbs are grammatically expressed one way, and unergative verbs a different way: in every case, there is a well-formed expression for the grammar to select. An extremely well-known test of this type is **auxiliary selection**: in certain constructions where a main verb requires an auxiliary verb, unaccusative main verbs 'select' (employ) one auxiliary verb ('be'), while unergative main verbs select another ('have'). A detailed analysis of this phenomenon is a primary topic of Section 2, a case study to which we now turn. It shows how a production-oriented, relative-Harmony approach can be developed to study

---

[7] In some cases, the optimal output for a given input may be semantically unfaithful to that input, so that it does not in fact express the input proposition, which is only a semantic *target*. In this case, no grammatical sentence expresses the input semantics. See the discussion of ineffability in Chapter 16.
[8] It is a common misconception that OT is naturally more suitable than previous generative theories for modeling graded judgments because it employs violable rather than inviolable constraints. "The concept of violable constraint has still other potential advantages over derivational approaches that have yet to be explored. A prime example is the way such a model easily lends itself to the task of capturing the graded nature of alternative surface forms so characteristic of many variable processes" (Nagy and Reynolds 1997, 39). Ironically, exactly the opposite is the case. With inviolable constraints, it is simple enough to stipulate that, while the normal consequence of violating a constraint is a '*' (ungrammatical), for certain constraints, a violation only induces a '?' (questionably grammatical). But in OT, for the reasons discussed in the text, the characterization of grammaticality in terms of relative Harmony makes a theory of partial grammaticality more difficult. It may be possible to construct an adequate theory of graded grammaticality by equating 'less grammatical' with 'less frequent' in the theory of variation provided by partial constraint ranking, developed in fact by Nagy and Reynolds (1997) among others (see Chapter 18).

split intransitivity. The analysis is cast in OT, but in principle the same approach could be adopted with numerically weighted constraints in the style of HG.

2 A CASE STUDY AT THE SYNTAX-SEMANTICS INTERFACE: REVISITING SPLIT INTRANSITIVITY

In this section, we inspect the OT-HG relation from the perspective of empirical linguistics, taking an HG account discussed earlier in the book and recasting it in OT terms to compare the views of a single phenomenon that are revealed by the two different theoretical lenses.

2.1 Symbolic approaches to crosslinguistic unaccusativity mismatches

Recall from Section 6:2.5 and Box 11:1 that the Unaccusative Hypothesis formalized in Perlmutter 1978 and Burzio 1986 states that the class of intransitive verbs divides into two subsets—**unaccusatives** and **unergatives**—that have distinct syntactic properties. The **grammatical relation** (GR) of the argument of an unaccusative verb is that of an underlying or **deep direct object**, so this argument displays many of the syntactic properties of the direct object of a transitive verb. In contrast, the single argument of an unergative verb is a **subject** at all levels of representation and thus consistently displays the same syntactic behavior as the subject of a transitive verb. This syntactic difference, discussed at length in Chapter 11, can be represented as in (15).

(15) a. Unergative: NP [$_{VP}$ V]   deep subject   e.g., *he works hard*
     b. Unaccusative: ___ [$_{VP}$ V NP]   deep object   e.g., *he died recently*

The earliest formulations of the Unaccusative Hypothesis noted that the distinction is also systematically related to certain lexicosemantic characteristics of the predicate: agentivity tends to correlate with unergativity and patienthood with unaccusativity (Perlmutter 1978; Dowty 1991). Much subsequent crosslinguistic research has shown, however, that the alignment between syntactic and semantic properties is not as consistent as originally predicted: some verbs with similar lexical semantics exhibit different syntactic behavior across languages (e.g., 'blush' is unaccusative in Italian and unergative in Dutch; Rosen 1984), and some verbs are classified as both unaccusative and unergative by the same diagnostic.[9] For example, Italian *continuare* 'continue' can take both auxiliary *essere* 'be' (like an unaccusative) and auxiliary *avere* 'have' (like an unergative) in the past tense (for the relevance of auxiliary verbs, see Chapter 11 (3)).

Nevertheless, a substantial body of research has shown that these **unaccusative mismatches** are problematic only to the extent that one expects unaccusative and unergative verbs to represent syntactically *and* semantically homogeneous classes.

---

[9] See Rosen 1984 for an early discussion of the absence of complete crosslinguistic overlap between a given semantic class and a given syntactic class. See also Legendre and Rood 1992 for a detailed illustration in the Siouan language Lakhóta.

Most of the syntactic diagnostics of unaccusativity/unergativity reported in the literature tend to identify semantically coherent subsets of verbs (Levin and Rappaport Hovav 1995). French, however, is a particularly challenging case, as summarized in Chapter 11, based on Legendre 1989 and Legendre, Miyata, and Smolensky 1990a, b, 1991. (See Legendre and Sorace 2003b for a detailed discussion of the relevant empirical facts in French.)

The challenge has long been to identify the syntactically relevant components of meaning in different languages and to develop a theory that can account for the reciprocal syntax-semantics interaction. The principle underlying this endeavor is that neither a verb's ability to occur in the unaccusative or unergative syntactic configuration, nor its particular semantic characteristics, are by themselves sufficient conditions to satisfy particular diagnostics, as explored in the HG account discussed in Chapter 11. A syntactic characterization of unaccusativity in terms of deep grammatical relations is necessary to account for phenomena not easily reducible to purely semantic explanations, such as the similarity between unaccusatives and passives, the resultative construction in English, auxiliary selection in Italian,[10] and the complex facts of French (see Chapter 11; Legendre 1989).[11] The identification of syntactic constraints, however, is not sufficient; it is also crucial to explain how semantic characteristics (e.g., agentivity) and aspectual properties (e.g., telicity)[12] of individual verbs map to the binary syntactic representations underlying split intransitivity.[13]

Two main proposals have been made in strictly symbolic terms in the last decade or so. One, known as the 'projectionist' approach (see Levin and Rappaport Hovav, in press, for discussion), maintains that the lexical semantics of a verb *deterministically* specifies the hierarchical classification of its arguments, and that this in turn produces

[10] In Italian, split intransitivity also manifests itself in participial absolute and reduced relative constructions (both illustrated in Table 11:1 for French), as well as use of the pronoun *ne*. *Ne* is a weak pronoun equivalent to *some* in English. Sorace (1995a, b) shows that whether a verb allows *ne* or not systematically varies with whether the verb selects the auxiliary *essere* or *avere*. (Examples from Rosen 1984, 50.)

(i) a. Ne sonno (*essere*) morte tre. b. *Ne hanno (*avere*) risposto tre.
       of-them were   died three   of-them have   replied three
       'Three of them died.'   'Three of them replied.'

The corresponding French pronoun *en* does not distinguish unaccusatives from unergatives (despite claims to the contrary in the literature). See Legendre and Sorace 2003b for thorough discussion.

[11] For example, the resultative construction in English is subject to a 'direct object restriction' (Levin and Rappaport Hovav 1995)—it can be predicated only of a direct object NP governed by the verb.

(i) a. John licked his finger clean. (transitive)
    b. The bottle broke open. (unaccusative)
    c. *John shouted hoarse. (unergative)

[12] Telicity is a temporal property of an event (Box 11:1). A telic event includes achievement of a location, goal, or state as part of its meaning (e.g., *go to the train station*: one hasn't gone there until one is there). An atelic event is unbounded (*draw*, *cry*, etc.). The standard test is to add the temporal phrases *in an hour* and *for an hour*, which are respectively felicitous with telic and atelic verbs only. A given verb may describe both telic and atelic events (e.g., *draw for an hour* vs. *draw a picture in an hour*). See further discussion in section 2.3.

[13] Various recent theories of argument structure (focused on the syntactically relevant properties of verb arguments) and event structure (focused on the temporal and aspectual organization of the event described by a verb) have pursued this goal (e.g., Grimshaw 1990; Pustejovsky and Busa 1995; van Hout 1996; Rappaport Hovav and Levin 1998).

the syntactic behavior associated with unaccusativity or unergativity (e.g., Hale and Keyser 1986, 1993; Levin and Rappaport Hovav 1992, 1994, 1995, in press). The most comprehensive account of this type is Levin and Rappaport Hovav's (1995) model based on English, in which a small number of linking rules map semantic components of verb meaning (such as 'immediate cause', 'directed change', and 'existence') onto positions at argument structure. Under this approach, verbs with variable behavior have multiple meanings and therefore multiple semantic representations, each with its own regular argument structure realization.

Alternatives to the projectionist view that have gained ground in recent years are the 'constructional' approaches (see Borer 1994, 1998; McClure 1995; van Hout 1996, 2000; Arad 1998). These models regard unaccusativity and unergativity not as lexical properties of verbs, but as clusters of properties derived from the syntactic configurations in which verbs appear, which in turn determine their aspectual interpretation. Since the lexical entry of a verb does not specify the grammatical relations of its arguments, any verb is free to enter into more than one syntactic configuration and consequently to receive multiple aspectual interpretations. Unlike the projectionist model, this approach predicts flexibility in the syntactic realization of arguments, but at the price of insufficient restrictiveness. Constraints preventing overgeneration must thus be present at other levels (e.g., Cummins 1996; van Hout 1996).

2.2 Modeling crosslinguistic gradience in auxiliary selection as a lexico-semantic hierarchy

A challenge to both the projectionist and the constructional views has come from two directions. One is the HG account discussed in Chapter 11, as it demonstrates the need for soft constraints to handle the kind of variation displayed by split intransitivity. The other is a series of empirical studies by Sorace and her collaborators (Sorace 1993a, b, 1995a, b; Keller and Sorace 2000; Sorace and Cennamo 2000; Sorace and Shomura 2001); together, these establish variation of a particular type as the norm crosslinguistically. The starting point of the latter studies are facts that characterize split intransitivity in a number of western European languages in two ways: (i) across languages, certain verbs tend to show consistent unaccusative/unergative behavior, whereas others do not; (ii) within languages, certain verbs are invariably unaccusative/unergative regardless of context, whereas others exhibit variation. Sorace and colleagues' studies provide supporting evidence for these generalizations, mostly based on experiments testing native speakers' intuitions about auxiliary selection (perhaps the best-known diagnostic of unaccusativity) in various languages that have a choice of past tense auxiliaries (such as Dutch, German, Standard Italian, and the Paduan dialect of Italian). In all these languages—and even to some extent in French—unaccusative verbs tend to 'select' the counterpart of English *be* (henceforth 'E' for Italian *essere*—*bE*) while unergative verbs select the counterpart of *have* ('A' for *avere*—*hAve*).[14] However, native intuitions on auxiliaries are categorical and consistent

---

[14] Legendre 1989, on which the HG account is based, rejected E selection as a *productive* diagnostic test

for certain types of verb, but much less determinate for other types. For example, native speakers have a very strong preference for auxiliary E with change-of-location verbs (e.g., 'arrive'), but express a weaker preference for the same auxiliary (or have no preference at all) with stative verbs (e.g., 'exist'). We discuss the experimental evidence further below.

Sorace's (2000) account of these systematic differences within the syntactic classes of unaccusative and unergative verbs is that there exist gradient dimensions or hierarchies that distinguish **core** unaccusative and unergative verbs from progressively more **peripheral** verbs. These hierarchies, which are based on (potentially universal) event parameters, identify the aspectual notion of **telic dynamic change** as the core of unaccusativity and the semantic property **agentive nonmotional activity** as the core of unergativity. The extremes of the hierarchies thus consist of maximally distinct core verbs—verbs of change of location (e.g., 'arrive') and verbs of agentive nonmotional activity (e.g., 'work')—that reliably display the greatest degree of consistency in auxiliary selection. In contrast, peripheral verb types between the extremes are susceptible to variation.[15]

The overall hierarchy is represented in (16).

(16)   **Auxiliary Selection Hierarchy (ASH)**

      Change of location   Selects 'be' (least variation)
      Change of state
      Continuation of a preexisting state
      Existence of state
      Uncontrolled process
      Controlled process (motional)
      Controlled process (nonmotional)   Selects 'have' (least variation)

Arranged in order of closeness to the unaccusative core or top of the hierarchy, peripheral unaccusative verb types include verbs denoting indefinite change in a particular direction (e.g., 'rise'), change of condition ('wilt'), appearance ('appear'), continuation of a preexisting condition ('stay'), and states ('exist', 'suffice'). Peripheral unergative verbs away from the unergative core or bottom of the hierarchy include verbs denoting motional processes (e.g.,'swim') and various kinds of uncontrolled processes such as bodily functions ('sweat'), involuntary reactions ('tremble'), and emissions ('rattle').[16] The hierarchy in (16) embodies the claim that noncore verbs

for unaccusativity in French, compared with other tests. Here, we show that the nonproductivity of E selection in some languages is actually predicted by the derived typology.

[15] In the proposed analysis, verbs are arrayed along a single scale extending from 'most unaccusative' to 'most unergative' (16). Thus, verbs that are 'core' unaccusatives and unergatives fall at the *extremes* of the hierarchy, while verbs that are 'peripheral' unaccusatives and unergatives fall in the *center*.

[16] The hierarchy does not include intransitive verbs alternating with transitive causative variants (e.g., *break, increase*), which are weakly unaccusative, and in some languages display unergative behavior (see Legendre 1989; Labelle 1992 on French; Haegeman 1994 on English; Sorace and Shomura, in press). Nor does it include intransitive verbs that appear with reflexive morphology, *se, s'* (e.g., French *s'évanouir* 'to faint', *s'évaporer* 'to evaporate'). See Legendre and Sorace 2003b for an analysis of reflexive unaccusatives that extends the present OT analysis.

may receive multiple argument realizations, depending on how they are conceptualized. Thus, these verb classes do not display stable syntactic behavior across languages: they may be unaccusative in some languages and unergative in others. They may also show variable behavior within individual languages—for example, by displaying syntactic characteristics of both unaccusative and unergative verbs.

The generalization that has emerged from these studies is that as soon as one moves away from a core, one finds substantial but predictable indeterminacy in syntax-semantics mapping with intransitive verbs. This indeterminacy is difficult to accommodate insightfully within a projectionist model of the syntax-semantics interface, since it would require multiple lexicosemantic classifications for a great number of verbs (for discussion, see van Hout 1996; Rappaport Hovav and Levin 1998). It is also challenging for a constructional model, since core verbs display categorical behavior and the other verbs are variable, but to different degrees. For example, several verb classes in Italian allow both auxiliaries, as indicated by E*/A* in Table 1 below, but most indeterminate are the stative verbs in the center of the ASH (including verbs of physical and abstract existence, as well as psychological verbs). Verb classes closer to the unaccusative and unergative cores usually show a preference for E or A that follows the ASH: verbs closer to the unaccusative core allow E and A but prefer E, while verbs closer to the unergative core allow E and A but prefer A.

The hierarchy in (16) makes it possible to advance some specific typological predictions. Note that it does *not* predict that all languages differentiate among all verb classes—only that there should not be complete reversals of the hierarchical order of verb types (e.g., languages in which stative verbs are core unaccusatives, or in which verbs denoting involuntary processes are core unergatives). The data on auxiliary selection suggest that within any given language, there is a cutoff point between the verbs that select auxiliary E and those that select A. The cutoff point cannot be the same in all languages, since if it were, all languages with a choice of auxiliaries would have exactly the same system. Thus, the locus of variation must be in the mapping between the lexicon and the syntax. Mapping must be language specific because the location of the cutoff points along the hierarchy may differ. However, variation in the cutoff point mostly affects the verbs in the middle of the hierarchy—crucially, rarely the core.

As mentioned earlier, evidence for gradient variation has been found in several experimental studies in Italian (Sorace 1993a, b, 1995a, b; Bard, Robertson, and Sorace 1996) and in Germanic languages. Experiments on Dutch (Sorace and Vonk 1998) show orderly gradience in native speakers' judgments on *zijn* 'be' and *hebben* 'have', largely corresponding to the intransitive hierarchies identified for Italian. In addition, they show that the acceptability of impersonal passives (a construction traditionally regarded as a diagnostic of unergativity) is affected by semantic factors, particularly agentivity, which cut across the unaccusative/unergative distinction (Zaenen 1993). For German, Keller and Sorace (2000) provide similar findings for native judgments on *sein* 'be' and *haben* 'have', and show that interdialectal variation in auxiliary usage between northern and southern varieties is mostly found with peripheral (but not with core) verbs. In French, proper experiments are yet to be conducted, but the results of a pilot study of speaker variation in judgments of unaccusative and unergative verbs (collected by Legendre from five speakers in the same geographical region and age group) suggest that gradient variation is the norm in French as well. In acquisition of Italian as a nonnative language, syntactic properties such as auxiliary selection and use of *ne* (see Footnote 10) are acquired earliest with core verbs and then gradually extended to more peripheral verb types (Sorace 1993a, 1995b). Moreover, Italian learners of French find it more difficult to acquire *avoir* 'have' as the auxiliary for verbs closer to the core than for more peripheral verbs (Sorace 1993b, 1995a).

A preliminary look at the early acquisition of French verbs by Grégoire, one of the children studied in Chapter 18, confirms the general findings. In his earliest four files (age 1;9–1;10), the only intransitive verbs Grégoire uses are unaccusative; he first produces past tense forms with the correct auxiliary (E) with verbs of location—specifically *tomber* 'fall', *monter* 'go up', *partir* 'leave', in that order. The first unergative verbs to show up in the past tense with auxiliary A are controlled motional processes *bouger* 'move (for a person)' (age 2;0) and *rouler* 'move (for a car)' (age 2;3).

To sum up, auxiliary selection displays a gradient sensitivity to the aspectual and semantic properties of individual verbs; this gradience is captured by the Auxiliary Selection Hierarchy. While the ASH is a generalization and not a theory, it challenges existing theories of the syntax-semantics interface: it cannot be accommodated within a projectionist account because it would entail too much duplication in the lexicon, and it does not fit a constructional account because the amount of variation is related to specific verb types. At the same time, it has features of both accounts: like the projectionist approach, it assumes a systematic relation between the syntax of auxiliary selection and the semantics of individual verbs; like the constructional approach, it allows some (but not all) verbs to have multiple syntactic projections.

The main idea of the HG account is that the overall acceptability (or Harmony) of a given verb in the syntactic context of a given unaccusativity test results from the complex interaction of mapping constraints (or linking rules) pertaining to semantic and aspectual properties of the verb, the semantic properties of its argument, and properties of the diagnostic test itself. The rules themselves are very similar in content to the rules proposed by Levin and Rappaport Hovav (1995). One important difference, however, is that the mapping constraints in HG are formalized as soft constraints rather than hard ones: they express numerically weighted *preferences* of a given feature (e.g., telicity) for mapping to a given deep grammatical function (e.g., direct object). The numerical values themselves are extracted from the French data by a connectionist learning algorithm in a computational model that encodes the strength of a preference for a particular mapping in the connection between abstract units—some of which represent features like telicity and animacy, others underlying grammatical relations, still others the individual verbs—and the diagnostic test itself. Finally, the model incorporates the binary-deep-grammatical-relation distinction, underlying subject versus direct object, in the form of hidden units that are automatically assigned values by the connectionist processing algorithm. There is explicit competition between unaccusative and unergative syntactic configurations for each individual combination of verb, argument, and construction. (See Chapter 11 for details.)

Another notable difference with Levin and Rappaport Hovav's linking rule approach is that the set of possible mappings is far richer in the HG account, allowing for a very fine-grained analysis. Finally, the HG account establishes the importance of telicity in characterizing unaccusativity (contra Levin and Rappaport Hovav's approach).

However, the main import of the HG account is that it establishes a model of gradience as syntactic competition driven by violable mapping constraints.[17] It also documents the need for a featural semantic and aspectual description of verbs in terms of which the constraints themselves are stated. The constraints do not refer to predefined verb classes per se (unlike, say, Levin and Rappaport Hovav's linking rules for directed-change verbs versus existence verbs); the mapping preferences pertain to individual features for specific syntactic configurations. In other words, classes of similarly behaving verbs are *emergent* properties, not analytic premises.

This suggests that the ASH too should be seen as the outcome of grammatical competition. This is indeed what we establish below by demonstrating that the empirical generalization embodied in the ASH is best explained in terms of an existing construct of OT, **Harmonic Alignment of (prominence) scales** (Prince and Smolensky 1993/2004; Chapter 12 (42) of this book).[18] In fact, the OT account builds on the earlier HG account, specifically, on its featural descriptions. The main difference is that HG exploits numerical optimization (or constraint weighting) while OT exploits nonnumerical optimization (based on a domination hierarchy).

The ASH suggests that there are two types of gradience to capture. One is the gradience across languages whereby a different cutoff point on the hierarchy determines which classes are unaccusative in a given language. This is the focus of the OT analysis presented in Section 2.4. The other is the gradience within a language whereby verb classes in the middle of the ASH are likely to exhibit some variation in auxiliary choice. We sketch an analysis of such variation in terms of **partial constraint ranking**, an OT construct well established in studies of variation, including synchronic (Nagy and Reynolds 1997), dialectal (Anttila 1997), diachronic (Slade 2003), and developmental (Legendre et al. 2002; Davidson and Goldrick 2003; Davidson and Legendre 2003; Legendre et al. 2004; Chapter 18).

---

[17] Sorace and Keller (2005) investigate the notion of gradience in syntax and elaborate on the difference between hard and soft constraints, providing experimental data from several domains.

[18] This was originally proposed in the context of the role of the sonority scale in syllable structure (Chapter 13), formally stating that vowels are less marked syllable peaks than nonvowels, sonorant consonants are less marked peaks than obstruents, and so on. Prominence Alignment has been applied to other phenomena in syntax and semantics: see Artstein 1999; Asudeh 1999; and Chapter 15.

2.3 A featural analysis of auxiliary selection in French and Italian

The lexicosemantic and aspectual properties widely implicated in split intransitivity phenomena are telicity, directed change, change of state, motion, displacement (e.g., Van Valin 1990; Dowty 1991; Zaenen 1993; Levin and Rappaport Hovav 1995; Sorace 2000), and homogeneity (McClure 1995). These properties are reflected in the features in (17)—the smallest set of features necessary to exhaustively characterize auxiliary selection in Romance.

(17)   Event features: INHERENT **DIS**PLACEMENT, INHERENT **HOM**OGENEITY, **TE**LICITY, **DIR**ECTION, **ST**ATE, INHERENT **VO**LITION, INTERNAL **MO**TION

Table 1 provides a featural description of each verb class; (17) shows the abbreviations. (A '+' under '–HOM' indicates the feature value –HOM.)

Table 1. Featural composition of French and Italian intransitive verbs

Fr.	It.	Emergent verb classes	DIS	–HOM	TE	DIR	ST	–VO	MO
E	E	Change of location: 'arrive'	+	+	+	+	+	+	–
		Change of state							
E	E	a. Change of condition: 'die'	–	+	+	+	+	+	–
E*	E	b. Appearance: '(dis)appear'	–	–	+	+	+	+	–
		c. Indefinite change in a particular direction:							
E*	E	'go up'	–	–	+	+	+	+	–
A	E	'rot'	–	–	+	+	+	+	–
A	E*	'worsen'	–	–	–	+	+	+	–
		States							
		a. Continuation of a							
A	E*	preexisting state: 'last'	–	–	–	–	+	+	–
		b. Existence of a state:							
A	E*	'exist'	–	–	–	–	+	+	–
A	E	'be'	–	–	–	–	+	+	–
		Uncontrolled processes							
A	A*	a. Involuntary actions: 'shiver'	–	–	–	–	–	+	–
A	A*	b. Emissions: 'resound'	–	–	–	–	–	+	–
A	A	c. Bodily functions: 'sweat'	–	–	–	–	–	+	–
		Controlled processes							
A	A*	a. Motional: 'swim'	–	–	–	–	–	–	+
A	A	b. Nonmotional: 'work'	–	–	–	–	–	–	–

* = Both auxiliaries are possible (see Section 2.4.5 for further discussion).

With the understanding that the relevance of most features in (17) has a solid basis in the literature cited in this chapter, we briefly discuss this choice of features. Among these is TELICITY, determined from diagnostic tests like occurrence with *for* versus *in* adverbials and structures like *spend an hour V-ing* versus *take an hour to V* (e.g., Dowty 1979). On the basis of such tests adapted to French, change-of-location verbs like *arriver* 'arrive' are telic (18) while verbs denoting controlled processes like *travailler* 'work' are atelic (19).

(18) Telicity

    a.   Pierre est arrivé chez lui en une heure.
           'Peter arrived home in one hour.'

    b.   Pierre a pris/mis une heure pour arriver chez lui.
           'Peter took one hour to arrive home.'

    c.   *Pierre est arrivé pendant une heure.
           'Peter arrived for one hour.'

(19) Atelicity

    a.   *Pierre a travaillé en trois heures.
           'Peter worked in three hours.'

    b.   *Pierre a pris/mis trois heures pour travailler.
           'Peter took three hours to work.'

    c.   Pierre a travaillé pendant trois heures.
           'Peter worked for three hours.'

The fact that change-of-state verbs are fundamentally telic does not entail identical choice of auxiliary: *mourir* 'die' selects E, *pourrir* 'rot' selects A. Both processes denote events reaching an endpoint and both are gradual (even if they differ in degree), as shown by their compatibility with modifiers like *petit à petit* 'little by little' (*il est mort/ le fruit a pourri petit à petit* 'he died/the piece of fruit rotted little by little'). Rather, the difference lies in their internal structure event: *pourrir* is incrementally homogeneous while *mourir* is not.

Event HOMOGENEITY denotes the extent to which each subinterval of an event is identical. Events as different as controlled activities (*travailler* 'work') and changes of state (*pourrir* 'rot') are homogeneous in the following way. Each subevent of an ongoing event of working or rotting entails that the referent has worked or rotted at least a bit. In contrast, an ongoing event of dying (since it canonically takes time to die) is not made up of homogeneous subevents: at any point of getting closer to the endpoint, one cannot say that the referent has died (even a bit).

(20) Event homogeneity

    a.   *travailler* 'work'
           Jean est en train de travailler.   ⇒ Il a travaillé.
           'John is (in the process of) working.'   ⇒ 'He has worked.'

Table 1

    b. *pourrir* 'rot'

       Ta pomme est en train de pourrir   ⇒   Elle a pourri (un peu).

       'Your apple is (in the process of) rotting.' ⇒ 'It has rotted (a bit).'

    c. *mourir* 'die'

       Jean est en train de mourir.   ⇏   Il est mort (un peu).

       'John is (in the process of) dying.'   ⇏   'He has died (a bit).'

Another important distinction is between verbs that connote INHERENT DIS-PLACEMENT from point A to point B (e.g., *aller à* 'go to' and more generally change-of-location verbs) and verbs that connote internal motion (e.g., *nager* 'swim', *courir* 'run'). Note that the latter type of motion can occur without displacement, as revealed in the common expression *nager/courir sur place* 'swim/run in place'. In Table 1, the feature INTERNAL MOTION distinguishes among controlled (volitional) processes (e.g., 'swim' vs. 'yell').

Finally, INHERENT VOLITION distinguishes uncontrolled from controlled processes at the bottom of the hierarchy. Change-of-location and change-of-state verbs (e.g., *venir* 'come', *mourir* 'die') are not inherently volitional. Volition, when present, is a property of their argument.

The remaining features in Table 1 are DIRECTION and STATE. The former distinguishes change-of-location and states from the rest because an important component of meaning is 'directed change', and the latter characterizes verbs whose meaning includes being in or reaching a state (or location).

Using these features and their appropriate values, we obtain a set-inclusion hierarchy, as represented in Table 1. What is crucial here is that verb classes that select a different auxiliary be distinguished by at least one feature value and that these feature values express implicational relations (+DIS implies –HOM; –HOM implies +TE; +TE implies +DIR, etc.). This is true of the first six features, counting from the left. This distribution enables us to propose next an OT analysis grounded in a power hierarchy (Section 2.4.2) whose universal scope does not rely on any further stipulation.

2.4 Optimality Theory analysis of auxiliary selection

2.4.1 Harmonic Alignment

One important outcome of much typological-functional research is the discovery of markedness relations (e.g., Jakobson 1965/1995; Croft 1990) that express favored associations in languages of the world.

Scales including 'animacy' (local person > pronoun 3rd > human 3rd >...) and thematic properties (agent > patient) have been associated with the well-known grammatical relation hierarchy in (21)[19] to express markedness relations (e.g., Silverstein 1976; Keenan and Comrie 1977; Perlmutter 1983; Aissen 2001). In a similar

---

[19] For example, languages that allow relativization of a direct object and languages that allow null objects are a subset of the languages that respectively allow relativization of a subject and null subjects (Keenan and Comrie 1977).

vein, we formulate event scales as in (22) for the features relevant to the A/E auxiliary distinction. (The telicity scale, atelic > telic (22c), is adopted in Grimshaw 1990.)

(21)   Grammatical relation scale: 1 (subject) > 2 (object)

(22)   Event feature scales

      a.   Displacement: −DIS > +DIS

      b.   Homogeneity: +HOM > −HOM

      c.   Telicity: −TE > +TE

      d.   Directed change: −DIR > +DIR

      e.   State: −ST > +ST

      f.   Inherent volition: +VO > −VO

      g.   Internal motion: −MO > +MO

By aligning two scales, we come up with relations that express the markedness of the mapping of a certain feature—say, TELIC—to a certain grammatical relation—say, 1. Such **harmonic alignments**, as they are defined in OT, formalize markedness relations for mappings between certain properties *across* scales (Chapter 12 (42)).[20] Note the change of symbol from '>' (higher on a scale) to '≻' (more harmonic—less marked) in the sample harmonic alignments in (23).

(23)   Harmonic alignments

      a.   2/telic ≻ 1/telic   The mapping of +TE onto an unaccusative configuration (underlying 2) is less marked than the mapping of +TE onto an unergative configuration (underlying 1).

      b.   1/atelic ≻ 2/atelic

      c.   2/telic ≻ 2/atelic

      d.   1/atelic ≻ 1/telic

      e.   etc.

Such alignments correspond to a hierarchy of constraints with polarity reversed (note again the change in symbol from '≻' (more harmonic) to '≫' (more dominant)).

(24)   Constraint alignments

      a.   *1/telic ≫ *2/telic   'Don't map +TE onto an unergative configuration' outranks 'Don't map +TE onto an unaccusative configuration'.

      b.   *2/atelic ≫ *1/atelic

      c.   *2/atelic ≫ *2/telic

      d.   *1/telic ≫ *1/atelic

      e.   etc.

[20] Alignment in OT in fact formalizes the concept of 'mirroring' in statements like "The deep syntactic encoding mirrors the thematic hierarchy in markedness." See the Universal Alignment Hypothesis (UAH—Perlmutter 1978; Rosen 1984), also known as the Uniformity of Theta Assignment Hypothesis (UTAH—Baker 1988)—a well-known principle governing the mapping between thematic roles and their (underlying) syntactic instantiation.

Table 1

For the present, we drop the lower-ranked constraints in each of these alignments, which target the unmarked mappings (see Footnote 12:28). Focusing first on those remaining constraints pertaining to GR1, we have {*1/telic ≡ *1/+TE, *1/+DIR, *1/−VO, …}. We now encapsulate all these constraints.

2.4.2 Formulating a *1 power hierarchy

Consider again Table 1. Down to feature −VO, Table 1 expresses implicational relations among feature values. We can thus define a set $\mathscr{C}$ of '2-preferring' feature values (25a) and state an encapsulated constraint *1/$\mathscr{C}$ that is violated each time a constraint in {*1/f | f ∈ $\mathscr{C}$} is violated.

(25) a. $\mathscr{C}$ ≡ {+DIS, −HOM, +TE, +DIR, +ST, −VO}   ('2-preferring' feature values)

  b.   F ≡ *1/$\mathscr{C}$ An event with a $\mathscr{C}$-feature is not mapped to an unergative configuration.

The fact that a candidate violating F = *1/$\mathscr{C}$ six times is more marked than one violating it twice is implemented via a standard OT **power hierarchy** (Smolensky 1995; Legendre, Smolensky, and Wilson 1998). (See Section 12:1.8.3; the analysis here is formally identical to the phonological analysis in Section 14:6.) The power hierarchy is given in (26a); the constraint F^k is violated whenever F is violated k (or more) times.

(26)   Universal Mapping Constraint Hierarchy

  a. $F^6 \gg \cdots \gg F^2 \gg F^1$ (GR/event semantics mapping)

  b.   *1/+DIS $\gg$ *1/−HOM $\gg$ *1/+TE $\gg$ *1/+DIR $\gg$ *1/+ST $\gg$ *1/−VO

Given the implicational relations among features in Table 1, the power hierarchy can be written in the equivalent form (26b). For example, any candidate violating F at least three times must violate the constraints {*1/+DIR, *1/+ST, *1/−VO}: the feature sets yielding at least three violations are exactly {±DIS, ±HOM, ±TE; +DIR, +ST, −VO}. Indeed, any feature set violating *1/+DIR will necessarily also violate {*1/+ST, *1/−VO}, so it will violate F at least three times. F^3 can thus be equated with *1/+DIR.[21]

As shown in Table 2, it is more marked for *arriver* 'arrive' to be assigned an unergative configuration than for *suer* 'sweat' because *arriver* violates constraint F six times while *suer* violates it only once.

Recall that an additional feature is needed to distinguish motional from nonmotional controlled processes: *nager* 'swim' versus *travailler* 'work'. The feature proposed is INTERNAL MOTION. Because all verb classes above controlled motional processes have the value −MO, as does the lowest class on the ASH that includes *travailler*, the feature MO does not stand in an implicational relation with all other features. The constraint *1/+MO is therefore not part of the power hierarchy proper. In fact, Legen-

---

[21] It is worth entertaining the idea that the constraint hierarchy in (26b) derives in fact from the alignment of the scale −VO > +ST > +DIR > +TE > −HOM > +DIS with the grammatical relation scale 1 > 2, yielding two harmonic alignments: (i) 1/−VO ≻ 1/+ST ≻ 1/+DIR ≻ 1/+TE ≻ 1/−HOM ≻ 1/+DIS and (ii) 2/+DIS ≻ 2/−HOM ≻ 2/+TE ≻ 2/+DIR ≻ 2/+ST ≻ 2/−VO. In (26b), we are referring to only one of the two constraint hierarchies this alignment yields, namely, the *1/*feature* hierarchy.

dre (to appear) demonstrates that German auxiliary selection provides independent empirical evidence for placing MO outside the power hierarchy proper.

Table 2. Markedness as determined by the *1 power hierarchy

Power hierarchy Constraint ranking	$(*1/\mathscr{C})^6$ *1/+DIS	$(*1/\mathscr{C})^5$ *1/−HOM	$(*1/\mathscr{C})^4$ *1/+TE	$(*1/\mathscr{C})^3$ *1/+DIR	$(*1/\mathscr{C})^2$ *1/+ST	$(*1/\mathscr{C})$ *1/−VO
1/ *arriver* 'arrive' +DIS, −HOM, +TE, +DIR, +ST, −VO	*	*	*	*	*	*
1/ *suer* 'sweat' −DIS, +HOM, −TE, −DIR, −ST, −VO						*
1/ *nager* 'swim' −DIS, +HOM, −TE, −DIR, −ST, +VO						

In Romance, the constraint *1/+MO must be ranked below the lowest constraint in the power hierarchy to express the relative markedness of assigning GR2 to the *nager* versus *travailler* classes. Diachronic evidence of auxiliary change in Spanish discussed by Legendre (to appear) supports the conclusion that 'work' is "more unergative" than 'swim'; moreover, native speakers do not completely reject selecting auxiliary E in the case of 'swim'. With GR1, 'swim' violates *1/+MO, while 'work' violates no *1 constraint. Combining the *1 power hierarchy and *1/MO gives the *1 constraint hierarchy.

(27) *1 constraint hierarchy

     *1/+DIS ≫ *1/−HOM ≫ *1/+TE ≫ *1/+DIR ≫ *1/+ST ≫ *1/−VO ≫ *1/+MO

Obviously, if no constraint against mapping onto GR2 ever entered the picture, selection of 2 (auxiliary E) would always be optimal, and we would have no crosslinguistic mismatches and no unergative verbs. While the harmonic alignments stated in (24b) result in a hierarchy of *2 constraints antiparallel to that of *1 constraints (24a), for the purposes of this discussion and the formal results we seek, it suffices to state the *2 constraint in the encapsulated version given in (28).[22] Further refinements may be called for in future work.[23]

---

[22] This formulation is independent of which specific structural terms this configuration might be stated in: Agr$_O$P, and so on.

[23] A fuller analysis would consider whether the constraint in (28)—*2—should be replaced with a Harmonic Alignment constraint *2/E, derived from the alignment of the (underlying) grammatical relation prominence scale 1 > 2 (21) with A > E (*have* > *be*). Harmonic Alignment would entail that 1/A is more harmonic than (≻) 1/E and 2/E ≻ 2/A. In turn, the following constraint rankings obtain: *2/A ≫ *2/E and *1/E ≫ *1/A. As a result, the optimization would involve four candidate pairings of grammatical relation and auxiliary. The formal result is the same with the simpler constraint in (28).

Table 2

(28)   *2   Don't map onto an unaccusative configuration.

We propose that across languages, this *2 constraint slides along the hierarchy of the Harmonic Alignment constraints in (27), resulting in a cutoff point that is cross-linguistically variable.

2.4.3   Establishing the language-particular ranking of *2

It should be clear by now that the crosslinguistic choice of auxiliary for a given featural profile will be determined by the relative ranking of *2 —just where *2 is interposed into the fixed *1 hierarchy.

We take the input to optimization to be the featural description of individual predicates or predicate subclasses, as specified in Table 1. The candidate set simply consists of two candidates corresponding to the two assigned configurations— underlying 2 and 1—assumed to be directly mapped to E and A, respectively.[24]

Next, we provide sample tableaux that highlight the crucial optimizations responsible for the language-particular rankings of *2 stated to be derived in (33). (For further exemplification, see Legendre and Sorace 2003a.)

(29)   *pourrir* 'rot'

Input: −DIS, +HOM, +TE, +DIR, +ST, −VO, −MO

French	*1/DIS	*1/−HOM	*2	*1/TE	*1/DIR	*1/ST	*1/−VO	*1/MO
a. 2/E			*!					
b. ☞ 1/A				*	*	*	*	

Even though it is telic, the change-of-state verb *pourrir* selects A. This motivates the French subranking *2 ≫ *1/TE, shown in (29). But *mourir* selects E, even though it is also a telic change-of-state verb. This is where the constraint on mapping the feature HOMOGENEITY comes in: *1/−HOM ≫ *2 in French, as shown in (30).

(30)   *mourir* 'die'

Input: −DIS, −HOM, +TE, +DIR, +ST, −VO, −MO

French	*1/DIS	*1/−HOM	*2	*1/TE	*1/DIR	*1/ST	*1/−VO	*1/MO
a. ☞ 2/E			*					
b. 1/A		*!		*	*	*	*	

In Italian, verbs of state (+ST) select E. This entails that *2 must be outranked by *1/ST in Italian; see (31). In contrast, −ST verbs select A. Thus, *2 ≫ *1/−VO; see (32).

---

[24] This is the consequence of assuming that auxiliary selection is one reflex of the larger unaccusative/unergative distinction to be stated in syntactic terms.

(31) *esistere* 'exist'
      Input: −DIS, +HOM, −TE, −DIR, +ST, −VO, −MO

Italian	*1/DIS	*1/−HOM	*1/TE	*1/DIR	*1/ST	*2	*1/−VO	*1/MO
a. ☞ 2/E						*		
b. 1/A					*!		*	

(32) *sudare* 'sweat'
      Input: −DIS, +HOM, −TE, −DIR, −ST, −VO, −MO

Italian	*1/DIS	*1/−HOM	*1/TE	*1/DIR	*1/ST	*2	*1/−VO	*1/MO
a. 2/E						*!		
b. ☞ 1/A							*	

These crucial cases result in the language-particular constraint rankings stated in (33).

(33) a. French: *2
                                ↓

      *1/DIS ≫ *1/−HOM ≫ *1/+TE ≫ *1/+DIR ≫ *1/+ST ≫ *1/−VO ≫ *1/MO

                                                  ↑
      b. Italian: *2

2.4.4 Verifying predictions in French, Italian, and beyond

For Italian, the position of *2 in the *1 hierarchy entails that verbs that have any of the feature values −DIS, −HOM, +TE, +DIR select E. For example, *peggiorare* 'worsen' selects E in Italian, as expected; see (34). Its French counterpart *empirer*, however, is predicted to select A because *2 outranks *1/DIR in French; see (35).

(34) *peggiorare* 'worsen'
      Input: −DIS, +HOM, −TE, +DIR, +ST, −VO, −MO

Italian	*1/DIS	*1/−HOM	*1/TE	*1/DIR	*1/ST	*2	*1/−VO	*1/MO
a. ☞ 2/E						*		
b. 1/A				*!	*		*	

(35) *empirer* 'worsen'
      Input: −DIS, +HOM, −TE, +DIR, +ST, −VO, −MO

French	*1/DIS	*1/−HOM	*2	*1/TE	*1/DIR	*1/ST	*1/−VO	*1/MO
a. 2/E			*!					
b. ☞ 1/A					*	*	*	

In both languages, controlled processes (motional and nonmotional) are predicted to select A. That is because only *2 and *1/MO are activated in the case of motional processes (36) and only *2 in the case of nonmotional processes (e.g., *travailler/lavorare*

Table 2

'work'). Given that *2 ≫ *1/MO in both languages, A is the preferred option.

(36)　*nager* 'swim'
　　　Input: −DIS, +HOM, −TE, −DIR, −ST, +VO, +MO

French	*1/DIS	*1/−HOM	*2	*1/TE	*1/DIR	*1/ST	*1/−VO	*1/MO
a.　　　2/E			*!					
b. ☞ 1/A								*

Let us sum up. Auxiliary selection results from the competition of two mapping hierarchies: power hierarchies of mapping constraints, themselves derived from Harmonic Alignment of simple scales referring to lexicosemantic and aspectual features and syntactic configuration. This entails that mapping rules cannot be stated in terms of verb classes, contra Levin and Rappaport Hovav (1995).

Significantly, the proposed general OT analysis does *not* predict total, unconstrained variation in auxiliary selection. Rather, it predicts a very specific typology of languages including languages in which all verb classes are syntactically unaccusative, languages in which all verb classes are unergative, and languages that each display one of a tightly limited set of splits.

First of all, it predicts that some languages do not show any split effects in auxiliary selection—in other words, that there are languages in which all verb classes select E and languages in which all verb classes select A. The latter formally result from *2 outranking all *1 constraints and the former from *1 constraints outranking *2. Both are found within Romance: Spanish selects only A and the central Italian dialect Terracinese (Tuttle 1986) selects only E.

The OT analysis also correctly predicts the existence of languages with different cutoffs along the universal hierarchy. Besides Standard Italian with its low cutoff point and Standard French with its high cutoff, we find Dutch and German with a threshold somewhere in between. In both these Germanic languages, change-of-location and change-of-state verb classes select E, while the remaining verb classes—continuation of a preexisting state, existence of state, uncontrolled processes, and controlled processes—select A.

Diachronically, the historical development of auxiliaries in Romance shows that core verb types tend to be the last to be affected by the replacement of E-reflexes by A-reflexes, whereas peripheral verb types are the most vulnerable to the change (see e.g., Benzing 1931; Tuttle 1986). Spanish provides a remarkable example (Aranovich 2003). In Modern Spanish, all verb classes select A. In Old Spanish, only core unergative verbs like *trabajar* 'work' and *pecar* 'sin' selected A. Change from E to A started with the peripheral classes as predicted by our analysis. The first to change were verbs of manner of motion like *errar* 'wander' and verbs of existence of state like *rastar* 'remain' (fourteenth century). Next to change were 'dynamic verbs of existence and appearance' (*aparecer* 'appear', *desaparecer* 'disappear', etc.) in the fifteenth century. *Morir* 'die' and *ir* 'go' were the last ones to give up E (seventeenth century).

Our OT analysis also predicts some languages to be impossible. For example, there could not be a language where existence-of-state verbs selected E but change-of-state verbs selected A. As far as we know, this prediction is correct.

2.4.5 Partial constraint ranking

The OT analysis above captures gradience across languages whereby a different cut-off point on the hierarchy determines which classes of verbs are unaccusative in each language. As we noted in Section 2.2, there is another type of gradience whereby verbs in the middle of the ASH are peripherally unaccusative or unergative in the sense that they are likely to fluctuate to some degree in their choice of auxiliary. For example, verbs of state in Italian and verbs of appearance in French may select either E or A (see Table 1). Can this type of gradience be derived from the present model? The answer is yes, provided the analysis is supplemented by **partial ranking**, that is, some indeterminacy in the relative ranking of *2 and the *1/f constraints. By definition, a partial constraint ranking yields a set of rankings (e.g., Anttila 1997; Boersma 1997; Legendre et al. 2002; Slade 2003). This set of rankings yields potentially different optimal outputs, hence variation in outputs. See Chapter 18 for an illustration in the domain of early acquisition of syntax.

   In the interest of space, we do not provide an actual analysis of such gradience in auxiliary selection. Rather, we illustrate the mechanism in question, leaving a full analysis for future work. Consider, for example, the consequences if *2 were to float over four positions at the top of the *1/f hierarchy (27), as in (37). We would obtain a set of four rankings for the class of +DIS, −HOM, +TE verbs, as represented in (38). (For convenience, the lowest portion of the hierarchy, *1/−VO ≫ *1/+MO, is omitted.)

(37)   Partial ranking with floating *2 constraint
         Fixed: *1/DIS ≫ *1/−HOM ≫ *1/TE ≫ *1/DIR ≫ *1/ST
         Floating: ⟵———— *2 ————⟶

(38)   Corresponding total rankings
         a. ***2** ≫ *1/DIS ≫   *1/−HOM ≫   *1/TE ≫   *1/DIR ≫ *1/ST
         b.   *1/DIS ≫ ***2** ≫ *1/−HOM ≫   *1/TE ≫   *1/DIR ≫ *1/ST
         c.   *1/DIS ≫   *1/−HOM ≫ ***2** ≫ *1/TE ≫   *1/DIR ≫ *1/ST
         d.   *1/DIS ≫   *1/−HOM ≫   *1/TE ≫ ***2** ≫ *1/DIR ≫ *1/ST

Different rankings yield different proportions of verbs selecting a particular auxiliary. Specifically, verbs that are +DIS (hence also −HOM, +TE) are unaccusative in rankings (38b,c,d)—that is, 75% of the time, assuming all four total rankings to be equally probable (see Chapter 18). Verbs that are −DIS, −HOM (hence +TE) are unaccusative for rankings (38c,d)—50% of the time; verbs that are −DIS, +HOM, +TE are unaccusative only 25% of the time—ranking (38d) only. Finally, verbs that are −TE (hence −DIS, +HOM) are unergative 100% of the time. So the more extreme features +DIS or −TE are more homogeneously unaccusative or unergative; the middling feature −HOM (hence

Table 2

–DIS, +TE) wavers 50/50 between the two. Put another way, there is more indeterminacy in the middle of the range than at the extremes.

2.5 Concluding remarks: The larger perspective

Summing up, we have proposed that the ASH derives from Harmonic Alignment of simple scales referring to semantic and aspectual features and syntactic configuration. In other words, verb classes like 'change of state' (see the vertical axis in Table 1) have no theoretical status in our OT analysis. They are emergent classes. Yet they serve the important function of making explicit how, given a set of constraints stated on relatively fine-grained semantic and aspectual features, and given a (typically binary) choice between two auxiliaries, verbs alternatively select E or A, albeit differently in the languages forming the focus of this case study, Italian and French.

Another property of the OT analysis worth emphasizing is that the constraints are the same in different languages. What varies is the position of a single constraint (*2) relative to all others in the hierarchy. Thus, variation results from different interactions of the same set of mapping constraints. This stands in contrast with an OT analysis like that of Bentley and Eyrthorsson (2002), which is grounded in the ASH but posits different mapping rules in different languages.

While much more study is needed to further confirm the predictions of the analysis, these initial results provide new evidence from syntax and semantics for the utility of OT as a formal theory of typology; more specifically, we have shown that the typological properties of split intransitivity (e.g., the existence of systematic crosslinguistic mismatches) receive a straightforward and enlightening account in terms of existing explanatory mechanisms in OT.

In Chapter 11, HG was used to analyze the complex French pattern of language-internal unaccusativity mismatches as delicate quantitative interactions of general and crosslinguistically attested constraints. But HG is not and was never intended to be a theory of typology. HG and OT provide deeply related but complementary instruments for characterizing human knowledge at the syntax-semantics interface, at different scales. They both find their place in the overall ICS theory. If — as we believe a half-century of work in generative linguistics has demonstrated — typologies are real and robust, then theories of the mind must, among other things, wrestle with this fundamental reality. OT is the component of ICS grappling with this challenge, and the early results reported here give some significant basis for optimism.

3 A CASE STUDY IN PHONOLOGY: SYLLABIFICATION IN BERBER

In this section, we first analyze a remarkable phonological system within OT; next, we transform this OT account into an account in HG; and finally, we implement the HG account in a local connectionist network. Thus, this case study illustrates the general ICS theoretical reduction leading from OT to neural computation, a reduction in which HG plays a crucial bridging role.

There are several ways in which this demonstration is incomplete or unsatisfactory. The OT account involves only two constraints, although one of them arguably encapsulates an entire hierarchy of eight constraints. The structure imposed by the grammar during parsing is very simple: certain segments are marked as syllable nuclei, and that's it; there is no epenthesis or deletion, nor elaborate structure-building. The connectionist network employs local, not distributed, representations. Its temporal behavior is not (as yet) formally analyzed, so a proof of correctness, and calculation of processing times, are not (currently) available; the network's computational behavior is studied only by computer simulation. Nonetheless, means of partly addressing all these shortcomings have been developed within this book.

3.1 Introduction to Berber

Dell and Elmedlaoui (1985) present a spectacular analysis of syllabification in the Imdlawn Tashlhiyt dialect of the language Berber (spoken in the Atlas mountains of northern Africa; henceforth, 'Berber' will refer to this particular dialect). Just like the *m* and *r* of English *prism* and *Berber*, consonants can function as syllable nuclei in this dialect of Berber. But whereas English allows only the most vowel-like—the most **sonorous**—consonants to be nuclei, in Berber *any* consonant can be a syllable nucleus. Berber contains words like *tftkt* and *txznt* in which all segments have low sonority—yet Berber words are sequences of syllables just like words in any other language, and the syllables are governed by universal principles. Since any segment can be parsed into any syllable position, the number of possible syllabifications of Berber words grows very quickly (exponentially) as the words get longer.[25]

Analysis of syllabification in Berber is the starting point of Prince and Smolensky 1993/2004, and it is used throughout that book to illustrate many central concepts of OT. As we will show here, Berber also provides an excellent case study for illustrating the relationship between OT and HG. For this purpose, we accept the approximation to Berber syllabification adopted in Prince and Smolensky 1993/2004, which abstracts away from certain complications, primarily at phrase edges, that are beside the present point. (See Clements 1997 for a fuller OT analysis of the complexity of Berber syllabification.)

3.1.1 Sonority: Nuclear Harmony, HNUC

The key idea is that the universal ideal for syllables is a certain **sonority profile**: starting at a low level, sonority rises quickly in the onset to a peak in the nucleus and then drops gently in the coda (e.g., Clements 1990; see Section 14:6). Sonority is an abstract grammaticalization of the inherent phonetic prominence of segments: the low vowel

---

[25] Consider 6 segments. They can be fully syllabified in two ways: .CV.CV.CV. or .CVC.CVC. (see text below). So a string of $6k$ segments has at least 2^k syllabifications (roughly, then, a string of n segments has at least $2^{n/6}$ syllabifications). This seriously undercounts, since there are many syllabifications that cross the boundaries of the k substrings of 6 segments each, and we have counted only those that don't. Further, the syllabifications counted all satisfy ONSET and *COMPLEX (or *VV and *CCC), so if these constraints are external to *Gen*, then many more syllabifications are also candidates.

Table 2

a has the greatest sonority, while voiceless stops like *t* and *k* have the lowest sonority. The sonority of a segment ρ will be written '*son*(ρ)'. While many aspects of the sonority scale are clearly universal, there are (at least apparent) minor variations across languages; these will not be dealt with here. Dell and Elmedlaoui argue that the sonority scale in Berber is as indicated in (39).

(39)   Sonority scale

Segment class	Example segment ρ	Sonority *son*(ρ)
voiceless stops	t, k	1
voiced stops	d, b, g	2
voiceless fricatives	s, f, x	3
voiced fricatives	z, ɣ	4
nasals	n, m	5
liquids	l, r	6
high vocoids	i/y, u/w	7
low vowel	a	8

The high vocoids are *i/y* and *u/w*. When syllabified as a nucleus, these segments are pronounced as vowels (*i* or *u*), and when syllabified as a syllable margin — onset or coda — the same segments are pronounced as glides (*y* or *w*). (To aid the reader, in examples, the sonority level of each segment will often be indicated as a subscript.)

The central point is that, despite their oddity, syllables in Berber respect the universal ideal for a sonority profile. While in languages like English only the most sonorous segments can appear in the nucleus, in Berber syllable nuclei contain *the most sonorous segments possible*, given the segments provided by the word. In the word $t_1r_6g_2l_6t_1$ 'you locked', the most sonorous segments — the liquids r_6 and l_6 — are the nuclei: the correct syllabification is $.t_1\acute{r}_6.g_2\acute{l}_6t_1.$, where, as in Chapter 13, periods mark syllable edges and the acute accent marks syllable nuclei. In another convenient notation, the syllable structure of $.t\acute{r}.g\acute{l}t.$ will be written .CV.CVC., using 'V' to denote any segment that has been syllabified into a nucleus (not necessarily a vowel) and 'C' any segment that has been syllabified into a syllable margin. The CV string .CV.CVC. will then be called a **parse** of the segment string *trglt*.

The universal constraint demanding that syllable nuclei be sonorous will be formulated below: it is called **Hnuc** (Harmony of the nucleus). Interacting with Hnuc is the Onset constraint requiring syllables to have onsets, familiar from Chapter 13.

It is evident that Onset has priority over Hnuc in words like $t_1x_3z_4n_5t_1$ 'you (sg.) stored', which is syllabified $.t_1\acute{x}_3.z_4\acute{n}_5t_1.$ Conforming to Hnuc, the most sonorous segment in the word, n_5, is parsed as a nucleus. But the next-most-sonorous segment, z_4 (a voiced coronal fricative), is passed over, and a lower-sonority segment, x_3 (a voiceless velar fricative), is selected as the other nucleus. As Dell and Elmedlaoui explain, this is because the syllable headed by *n* must have an onset; this forces *z* to be parsed as an onset, which takes it out of the running for the second nucleus. Of the remaining segments, *x* is the most sonorous, and it is selected.

3.1.2 Syllable structure

Syllables in Berber consist of an obligatory onset containing a single segment, an obligatory one-segment nucleus, and an optional one-segment coda. (In the notation of Chapter 13, Berber belongs to the typological class $\Sigma^{CV(C)}$.) The requirement that syllables must have a nucleus is suspended for the first syllable of the word (or phrase); because this subtlety has no bearing on the topic of this section — the connection between OT and HG — we will simply pretend that the ONSET constraint includes within it the waiver for initial syllables.

(40) (quasi-)ONSET (*VV)

   A noninitial syllable must have an onset.

If a noninitial V is preceded by a C, that C can be parsed as an onset to satisfy ONSET. So the force of this constraint is to ban a noninitial V (i.e., nucleus) preceded by another V; that is, it bans **hiatus**: two adjacent syllable nuclei. The banned structure is simply VV, so it will sometimes be convenient to call this constraint '*VV'.

   Note that, given the syllable structure requirements of Berber, it is always possible to locate syllable boundaries from a string of Cs and Vs: each noninitial V must be preceded by a single onset C. So before each CV there must be a syllable boundary, '.'. Thus, for example, VCCVCV must denote the syllabification shown in (41).

(41) .VC.C**V**.C**V**.

In this parse, each noninitial V, in boldface, determines the '.' before the preceding C; and of course the parse must also begin and end with a syllable edge '.'. Because the location of syllable boundaries is determined by the CV string, the '.' markings will often be omitted below.

   That onsets and codas in Berber are limited to a single segment can be seen as the effect of a universal constraint introduced in Chapter 13: *COMPLEX, which prohibits syllable positions (onset, nucleus, or coda) that are **complex** in the sense of containing multiple segments. That *COMPLEX is unviolated in Berber entails that a legal parse will never contain a sequence CCC: the middle C is not syllabifiable.

(42) *COMPLEX (*CCC)

   No more than one segment may occupy a single syllable position.

Note that any string of Cs and Vs satisfying both the constraints *VV and *CCC is a legal syllabification in Berber. Such a CV string will be called a **legal parse**; for any given input string of segments, the optimal syllabification will be a legal parse. Any string of Cs and Vs at all — not necessarily satisfying *VV or *CCC — will be called a **potential parse**.

3.2 The Dell-Elmedlaoui syllabification algorithm

Given an input like $t_1x_3z_4n_5t_1$, how can a syllabification be found that meets HNUC's demand for maximally sonorous nuclei, while respecting the overriding demand of

Table 2

ONSET? Dell and Elmedlaoui (1985) propose a syllabification algorithm we will call **DE**. It works as follows.

Start with the highest sonority level: 8, the sonority of *a*. Scan the string from left to right, looking for unsyllabified segments with this sonority level. Suppose one is found: call the segment ρ. Then look to see if there is an unsyllabified segment to its left (this is waived for the initial segment). If so, ρ is a **trigger**. Then, parse the trigger ρ as a syllable nucleus V and parse the preceding segment as a syllable onset C. Continue to the end of the string.

Now drop down one level in the sonority hierarchy: 7, the sonority of the high vocoids *i/y* and *u/w*. Follow the same procedure, scanning from left to right for an unsyllabified segment with sonority 7, parsing it as a nucleus if there is an unsyllabified segment to its left to parse as an onset.

Then continue down the sonority hierarchy until the lowest level has been scanned: 1, the sonority of voiceless stops like *t* and *k*.

At this point, unsyllabified segments may remain; parse each as a coda. The result is a complete parse, the output of the parsing algorithm DE.

To illustrate, we parse $t_1x_3z_4n_5t_1$ as in (43). At step (43e), parsing the most sonorous segment in the word, *n*, as a nucleus commits the parser to syllabify the preceding segment *z* as an onset, even though it is more sonorous than the segment to its left, *x*, which is then syllabified as a nucleus in step (43f).

(43)   Dell-Elmedlaoui algorithm (DE) parsing $t_1x_3z_4n_5t_1$

    a. $t_1\ x_3\ z_4\ n_5\ t_1$ (input)

    b. $t_1\ x_3\ z_4\ n_5\ t_1$ *no segments at sonority level 8*

    c. $t_1\ x_3\ z_4\ n_5\ t_1$ *no segments at sonority level 7*

    d. $t_1\ x_3\ z_4\ n_5\ t_1$ *no segments at sonority level 6*

    e. $t_1\ x_3\ .z_4\ \acute{n}_5\ t_1$ on scan at sonority level 5
             .C V   *current syllabification*

    f. $.t_1\ \acute{x}_3\ .z_4\ \acute{n}_5\ t_1$ on scan at sonority level 3
             .C V .C V   *current syllabification*

    g. $.t_1\ \acute{x}_3\ .z_4\ \acute{n}_5\ t_1.$ on final step: parse codas
             .C V .C V C.   (output)

The left-to-right scanning employed in DE is used to disambiguate parsing when two adjacent segments have the same sonority (e.g., *mn*). When that level of sonority is scanned, both segments are triggers: both are potentially available to become syllable nuclei—but both cannot be, since that would create a VV configuration, violating ONSET = *VV. The left-to-right scan disambiguates the situation by selecting the leftmost segment, *m*, for the nucleus. If the rightmost segment *n* were instead selected, the preceding *m* would serve as the onset of a syllable *.mń*. This has a poor sonority profile, as there is no sonority rise at all between onset and nucleus. Dell and Elmedlaoui themselves describe the left-to-right scanning as an indirect means of achieving a goal that is not actually concerned with directionality: maximizing the sonority difference between onset and nucleus (Dell and Elmedlaoui 1985, 127n22). Since, again, this complication is beside the present point, we will restrict attention to inputs that *have no sonority plateaus,* that is, where the sonority values of adjacent segments are never identical. For such inputs, there are no ambiguities of the sort the left-to-right scanning of DE was designed to resolve, and directional scanning is unnecessary. When the algorithm reaches a given sonority level *s,* all unparsed segments meeting the criterion (sonority = *s* with an unparsed preceding segment) can be parsed as nuclei, without conflict.

It will prove useful below to modify DE slightly. Consider the point in DE when a segment α is parsed as a V, and the one preceding it as a C. Now consider the segment β following this new nucleus V. Had β previously been parsed as a V, the segment preceding it—α—would necessarily have been parsed as a C at the same time, which is impossible because α is now being parsed as a V. So if β has already been parsed, it has been parsed as a C. If β has not yet been parsed, we can say with confidence that it will later be parsed as a C: for to be parsed as a V, the segment preceding it, α, would have to be available to serve as an onset, but it is not since it has just been parsed as a nucleus. So in any event, β will end up parsed as a C.

In the modified algorithm, when α is parsed as a V, the segment β following it is also parsed as a C. Instead of inserting CV into the parse, the algorithm now inserts CVC, the final C perhaps already having been parsed. (The second C is of course omitted if α happens to be the final segment and no following segment β exists.) Henceforth, 'DE' will refer to this modified algorithm, which necessarily produces the same output as the original Dell-Elmedlaoui algorithm. The advantage is that in the modified algorithm, to qualify as a trigger at sonority level *s,* it suffices that a segment of that sonority simply be unparsed; there is no need to check its left neighbor to see if it too is unparsed and therefore free to serve as an onset. For if each step of parsing enters a sequence CVC into the parse, any unparsed segment γ must have to its left either a C or an unparsed segment; either way, γ qualifies as a trigger.

Since DE constructs its output by inserting CVC strings, it follows that at most two Cs can end up adjacent to one another. And of course, by construction, DE never generates two adjacent Vs. Thus:

(44)   The output of DE satisfies *CCC = *COMPLEX (42) and *VV = ONSET (40).

3.3 Positive OT

Several OT analyses of Berber syllabification were developed in Prince and Smolensky 1993/2004. The one most intuitively close to DE will be called the **positive** analysis, OT₊. In this formulation, HNUC₊ *rewards* good syllable *nuclei;* in the negative analysis discussed below (OT₋), HNUC₊ is replaced by constraints that *penalize* bad syllable *margins.*

(45)   **HNUC₊** (Nuclear Harmony, positive formulation)
        If $son(\nu) > son(\tau)$, the nucleus v́ has higher Harmony than the nucleus t́.

Table 2

When comparing two parses, compare first the highest-Harmony nucleus of each. If they have equal Harmony, discard them and continue to compare the highest-Harmony remaining nucleus. Continue until a nucleus in one parse has higher Harmony than its counterpart in the other parse; then declare the parse with the higher-Harmony nucleus to be the one best satisfying HNUC+. If all nuclei of one parse are completely exhausted before those of another parse, declare the latter to better satisfy HNUC+.

The positive OT analysis is now simply this:

(46)   OT+: ONSET ≫ HNUC+

We posit that PARSE, FILL, IDENT are undominated, and so consider only candidates that satisfy these constraints.

As an illustration of this analysis, (47) shows a constraint tableau for *txznt*. This tableau will be discussed in the context of theorem (48), one of the earliest results derived in OT.

(47)   OT+ tableau for *txznt*

$/t_1x_3z_4n_5t_1/$		ONSET	HNUC+	Comment
a. ☞	$.t_1\acute{x}_3.z_4\acute{n}_5t_1.$		$\acute{n}_5\ \acute{x}_3$	*DE output*
b.	$.\hat{t}_1.x_3\acute{z}_4.\acute{n}_5t_1.$	*!	$\acute{n}_5\ \acute{z}_4\ \hat{t}_1$	$\acute{z}_4 \succ \acute{x}_3$ *but too late*
c.	$.\hat{t}_1.x_3\acute{z}_4.n_5\hat{t}_1.$		$\acute{z}_4!\ \hat{t}_1\ \hat{t}_1$	$\acute{n}_5 \succ \acute{z}_4$
d.	$.\hat{t}_1x_3.z_4\acute{n}_5t_1.$		$\acute{n}_5\ \hat{t}_1!$	$\acute{x}_3 \succ \hat{t}_1$

(48)   *Theorem.* $opt(\text{OT}_+) = out(\text{DE})$ (Prince and Smolensky 1993/2004)

The optimal parse as defined by OT+ equals the output of DE, for any input with no sonority plateaus.

Note: Subsequent theorems of this type—(49), (58), (59), (60), (63), (66)—all pertain, like (48), to any input with no sonority plateaus.

In the HNUC+ column of tableau (47), $\acute{z}_4$ denotes the violation of HNUC+ by the syllable nucleus containing z; this is a less serious violation of HNUC+ than $\acute{x}_3$ because $son(z) = 4 > son(x) = 3$; that is, $\acute{z}$ is a more harmonic nucleus than $\acute{x}$: $\acute{z}_4 \succ \acute{x}_3$.

> *Proof.* Consider an input (say, $t_1x_3z_4n_5t_1$) and let P be the corresponding output of DE. Is there any competing parse Q that has higher Harmony, on the OT analysis? Since P satisfies ONSET, any competitor Q that does not satisfy ONSET will lose to P when the higher constraint, ONSET, is evaluated (47b). So we need only consider competitors that satisfy ONSET, and consider evaluation by HNUC+. Now suppose s is the highest sonority level present in the input ($s = 5$ for $t_1x_3z_4n_5t_1$). Segments of sonority s (n_5) will be parsed as nuclei in P (on the first scanning step of DE that finds any triggers). Consider a competing parse Q that does not have these segments parsed as nuclei. Then Q will lose to P when the highest-Harmony nuclei of P and Q are compared, because the highest-Harmony nuclei of P have higher sonority, hence higher Harmony, than any

> alternative nuclei (47c). So we need only consider competitors that have the same highest-sonority nuclei as P. Continuing the same logic, consider the next sonority level at which DE finds triggers (3: x_3). Any competitor Q that does not, like P, parse these triggers as nuclei will lose when the second-highest-Harmony nuclei in P and Q are compared by HNUC$_+$ (47d). So we need consider only competitors with the same second-highest-sonority nuclei as P. And so on to the bottom of the sonority hierarchy. When the lowest-sonority nuclei of P are reached, the logic entails that the only parse Q that does not have lower Harmony than P is a parse in which all nuclei are located at the same segments as the nuclei of P—that is, Q = P itself.

Note that the method employed within the HNUC$_+$ constraint for handling multiple syllables itself employs the strict domination characteristic of OT: if the highest-sonority nuclei of two parses differ, this difference will determine which is more harmonic, preempting all consideration of lower-sonority segments. The general strict domination mechanism of OT will be explicitly employed to achieve this in the second OT analysis presented below (Section 3.6).

(49) *Corollary.* OT$_+$ outputs satisfy *CCC (*COMPLEX) (42) and *VV (ONSET) (40).

> *Proof.* By (49), the maximum-Harmony parse with respect to OT$_+$ is the output of DE; such outputs always satisfy *CCC and *VV by (44).

Note that the ranking ONSET ≫ HNUC$_+$ already achieves the effects of *COMPLEX, without requiring an explicit *COMPLEX constraint: maximal satisfaction of HNUC$_+$ is achieved by having as many nuclei as possible, and ONSET restricts those possibilities to those satisfying *VV. This means the subparse CCC can never appear in an optimal parse, because HNUC$_+$ would be better satisfied by replacing CCC with CVC, and such a move cannot run afoul of ONSET. This has the convenient consequence that the harmonic grammar developed next need not explicitly incorporate rules implementing *COMPLEX; it is sufficient to implement ONSET ≫ HNUC$_+$.

3.4 Positive HG

We are finally ready to develop a harmonic grammar—HG$_+$—comparable to the OT$_+$ analysis. It is easy enough to state ONSET and HNUC$_+$ in HG terms.

(50) **HG$_+$:** Harmonic grammar for Berber syllabification

    a. ONSET A noninitial syllable must have an onset. (Negative)
           Strength: $W_{ONS} = 2^M$

    b. HNUC$_+$ Segment ρ must be a syllable nucleus. (Positive)
           Strength: $W_\rho = 2^{son(\rho)} - 1$

ONSET *penalizes* a parse for each V that is preceded by another V; the Harmony penalty equals the strength W_{ONS}. HNUC$_+$ *rewards* a parse for each nucleus; the quantity of Harmony added for each nucleus depends on the sonority of the nuclear segment: higher sonority yields higher Harmony contribution.

Table 2

The remaining question is, what should the strengths be? The answer is given in (50): the HNUC+ contribution from a nuclear segment ρ is $2^{son(\rho)} - 1 \equiv W_\rho$, where $son(\rho)$ is the sonority level of ρ on the numerical scale given in (39). Letting M denote the maximum sonority value ($8 = son(a)$), the largest possible contribution from a single nucleus is $2^M - 1 = W_a$. The strength of ONSET is larger, by one: $2^M \equiv W_{ONS}$; the HG strength relation $W_{ONS} > W_a$ corresponds to the OT+ ranking ONSET $\gg$ HNUC+. The task now is to derive these values.

The modified Dell-Elmedlaoui algorithm DE successively finds maximum-sonority unsyllabified segments and parses them as a V flanked by a C on either side: CVC is added into the parse, with the V at the trigger, contributing positive Harmony via HNUC+. The *cost* of this move is that the two flanking segments, being assigned C, are no longer available as potential nuclei and therefore no longer able to add positive nuclear Harmony by being parsed as V. In the worst case, the two flanking segments parsed C are just one level of sonority lower than the trigger. The Harmony contributions must be arranged so that a single positive contribution from parsing the trigger as V must be greater than the highest possible cost for the move, which is twice the Harmony contribution from one level down the sonority scale.

(51)   Exponential growth of strength with sonority condition
$$W_s > 2W_{s-1}$$

Let us arbitrarily set the lowest HNUC+ reward — for sonority level 1 — at 1.

(52) $W_1 \equiv 1$

Then (51) requires

(53) $W_2 > 2W_1 = 2$,

so let us choose

(54) $W_2 = 3$.

Repeating the logic, we get $W_3 = 7$, $W_4 = 15$, and so on. The result is

(55) $W_s = 2^s - 1$.

The Harmony function for HNUC+ defined by HG+ (50) is

(56) $H_{NUC+}(P) = \sum_i nuc(\rho^i, P)[2^{son(\rho^i)} - 1]$,

where $\{\rho^i\}$ are the segments in the parse $P = \rho^1\rho^2\cdots$ and $nuc(\rho^i, P) = 1$ if P's ith segment ρ^i is parsed as a nucleus in P, and 0 otherwise. Because this is a simple sum of contributions from individual segments, H_{NUC} obeys (57).

(57)   If the CV parse $P = LR$ is the concatenation of two subparses L and R, then
$$H_{NUC}(LR) = H_{NUC}(L) + H_{NUC}(R).$$

This is useful in proving the next result.

(58)   *Theorem.* $opt(\mathrm{HG}_+) = out(\mathrm{DE})$

For a given input string I, consisting of N segments with no sonority plateaus, let the candidate set $Gen(I)$ be the set of all potential parses of I by a CV string of length N. Within $Gen(I)$, the maximum-Harmony parse according to HG_+ (50) is the same as the output of DE given the input I.

For the proof of this result, it is useful to first establish (59).

(59)   *Lemma.* A maximum-Harmony parse of HG_+ cannot violate ONSET = *VV.

> *Proof.* Consider any parse Q that violates *VV. Intuitively: reparse the first V as C, getting a competing parse P. Changing V to C eliminates one nucleus but also the ONSET violation; the Harmony increases by the strength of ONSET and decreases by the strength of HNUC for the reparsed segment. But since the former is defined to be greater than the latter (corresponding to OT$_+$'s ONSET ≫ HNUC), there is an overall gain in Harmony; P is more harmonic than Q. Therefore, Q cannot be a Harmony maximum. This is a **harmonic bounding** argument: P harmonically bounds Q (Section 12:1.6).
>
>   More formally: Express Q as Q = $\mathrm{LV}^1\mathrm{V}^2\mathrm{R}$, where L and R are respectively the portions of the string Q to the left and right of VV. Now let P = $\mathrm{LC}^1\mathrm{V}^2\mathrm{R}$; this parse eliminates the violation at V^2 of *VV in Q. It may even eliminate a second violation of *VV in Q, if there is a violation at V^1 as well (i.e., if L ends in V); any other violations of *VV that there may happen to be within L or R are shared by P and Q and do not differentiate their Harmony with respect to ONSET, denoted by H_{ONS}. Thus, P has at least one fewer violation of *VV than Q, so
>
> $$H_{\mathrm{ONS}}(P) - H_{\mathrm{ONS}}(Q) \geq W_{\mathrm{ONS}}.$$
>
> Call the segments corresponding to V^1 and V^2 in the parse Q ρ^1 and ρ^2. Let V/ρ^1 denote the segment ρ^1 parsed as a nucleus (as in parse Q); let C/ρ^1 denote ρ^1 parsed as a margin (as in P). Using (57), evaluate the difference between P and Q with respect to $H_{\mathrm{NUC}+}$, the Harmony arising from HNUC+:
>
> $$\begin{aligned} H_{\mathrm{NUC}+}(P) - H_{\mathrm{NUC}+}(Q) \quad &= [H_{\mathrm{NUC}+}(L) + H_{\mathrm{NUC}+}(C/\rho^1) + H_{\mathrm{NUC}+}(V/\rho^2) + H_{\mathrm{NUC}+}(R)] - \\ &\quad [H_{\mathrm{NUC}+}(L) + H_{\mathrm{NUC}+}(V/\rho^1) + H_{\mathrm{NUC}+}(V/\rho^2) + H_{\mathrm{NUC}+}(R)] \\ &= -H_{\mathrm{NUC}+}(V/\rho^1) = -W_{\rho^1}. \end{aligned}$$
>
> So P has higher Harmony than Q with respect to ONSET, by an amount at least W_{ONS}, while P has lower Harmony than Q with respect to HNUC+, by an amount W_{ρ^1} that depends on the sonority of the segment ρ^1, which is nuclear in Q but not P. Now W_{ONS}, the strength of ONSET in HG_+ (50), is defined to be greater than all HNUC+ strengths W_ρ, even that of the most harmonic nucleus, W_a. Thus, P has higher total Harmony. In sum, for any parse Q of I that violates *VV, there is another parse P of I with higher Harmony that satisfies *VV. Thus, the maximum-Harmony parse cannot violate *VV.

Now we can return to theorem (58).

> *Proof.* Lemma (59) establishes that any maximum-Harmony parse for HG_+ satisfies ONSET, just like any output of DE, so we now only need consider $H_{\mathrm{HNUC}+}$, the Harmony due to HNUC+. Given any input I with no sonority plateaus, let that parse of I that maximizes $H_{\mathrm{HNUC}+}$ be denoted $\mathrm{P}^\dagger$. It is now useful to view DE as successively

Table 2

winnowing a candidate set: the initial set consists of all potential syllabic parses of *I*, and each time the algorithm parses a segment of *I*, the candidate set is reduced by discarding all syllabifications not consistent with the newly assigned structure. With no sonority plateaus, DE is deterministic and terminates on a unique complete parse, all other candidates having been eliminated.

Let us jump into DE anywhere during its operation. DE has just found a trigger ν at some sonority level *s*, and assigns CVC to the substring μνρ consisting of ν and its immediate neighbors μ and ρ. This winnows the candidate set; is it possible that the maximum-$H_{\text{HNUC+}}$ parse $P^{\dagger}$ has been erroneously eliminated? There are a few different cases to consider. Exceptions associated with the left and right edges of the string *I* are obvious and will not be stated explicitly.

Suppose the segment μ in the critical substring μνρ has already been parsed. If so, it must be parsed as C since its neighbor ν is a trigger and hence previously unparsed: no unparsed segment can be adjacent to ν since (modified) DE imposes CVC whenever it parses a segment. If μ is already parsed, then the remaining candidates all agree that μ is parsed as a C and that part of the 'assignment' of CVC on μνρ has no effect at all.

Only if μ has not been previously parsed does imposing C on μ (as part of imposing CVC on μνρ) winnow the candidate set. But if μ has not been previously parsed, its sonority must be lower than the current level *s*; for in our version of DE, having sonority higher than *s* and being unparsed would necessarily have qualified μ as a trigger at an earlier step of the algorithm. Now in the worst case, the sonority of μ is just one level lower than *s*. Imposing C on μ eliminates parses that assign V to μ and thereby earn an $H_{\text{HNUC+}}$ reward of W_{s-1}.

Inverting left and right in the previous argument shows that either the segment ρ on the right of the trigger ν is already parsed C and irrelevant, or it is unparsed, has a lower sonority than *s*, and assigning it C winnows candidates that parse ρ as V and receive an $H_{\text{HNUC+}}$ reward no more than W_{s-1}.

In the worst case, when *both* μ and ρ are unparsed and have sonority *s* − 1, imposing CVC on μνρ eliminates candidates with an $H_{\text{HNUC+}}$ reward from μνρ of at most $2W_{s-1}$. The candidates retained receive a benefit of W_s from μνρ under the parse CVC, since the sonority of ν is *s*. Now the strengths have been specifically designed so that for all *s*, $W_s > 2W_{s-1}$, as demanded by the exponential growth condition (51); thus, the winnowed candidates have lower $H_{\text{HNUC+}}$ values than the retained candidates. Winnowing in this fashion can never exclude the $H_{\text{HNUC+}}$-maximizing parse $P^{\dagger}$. And since the algorithm must terminate on a single output, this parse must be $P^{\dagger}$.

$P^{\dagger}$ maximizes $H_{\text{HNUC+}}$ and satisfies ONSET, so it maximizes total HG+-Harmony *H*.

Combining (48) and (58) gives this corollary:

(60)   *Corollary. opt*(HG$_+$) = *opt*(OT$_+$)

Intuitively, the connection between the HG and OT accounts here is quite transparent. It is notable, however, that the strengths needed to implement the OT account in HG do *not* exhibit the full exponential growth that is expected in the general (or perhaps the worst) case discussed in Section 1.2.2.1. To achieve the effect ONSET ≫ HNUC$_+$, it is not necessary to make W_{ONS} exponentially larger than W_{HNUC}: it suffices for the former to be even slightly greater than the latter. Within HNUC$_+$ itself, the strict domination character of cross-sonority-level interactions *does* lead to exponentially growing constraint strengths W_s. But here again the growth is not as severe as predicted by the general analysis of Section 1.2.2.1. There, the strengths grew as C^k, where k is the rank of the constraint and C is the maximum number of possible violations of a single constraint in a candidate. In HG$_+$, the base of exponentiation is fixed at only 2, even though the number of possible constraint violations grows without bound as the length of the input grows. Thus, if parse P of I has a *single* nucleus v that is more sonorous than all the nuclei in parse Q of I, then Q cannot maximize HNUC$_+$, even if *all* the nuclei in Q have the highest possible sonority value less than v. Since the number of such nuclei can grow without bound as the length of I grows, it might have been expected that the strength W_s for sonority s would have to exceed that of W_{s-1} by an unboundedly large factor.[26]

3.5 Negative OT

The positive OT$_+$ analysis introduced in Section 3.3 is the one first introduced in Prince and Smolensky 1993/2004, Chap. 2, but the central constraint HNUC$_+$ does not fit the mold of standard OT in which constraints *penalize* violation rather than *reward* satisfaction. The following **negative** reformulation of HNUC as a **universal constraint subhierarchy** is developed in Prince and Smolensky 1993/2004, Chap. 8 (this hierarchy is introduced in Box 13:1 and derived in Section 14:6). Switching from positive to negative forces the focus of the constraint to shift from nucleus to margin, as we now show.

(61) **HNUC**: The universal margin subhierarchy

$$*C/v_1 \gg *C/v_2 \gg \cdots \gg *C/v_7 \gg *C/v_8$$

universally, where the constraint $*C/v_s$ is defined by

$*C/v_s$: A segment v_s of sonority s is not parsed as a syllable margin.

This version of HNUC is best understood via an example. Tableau (62) is the OT$_-$ counterpart to the OT$_+$ tableau (47). Here, the strict domination structure that had been buried within the positive formulation of HNUC is made explicit by the hierarchy. As in OT$_-$ (and DE), what must be attended to first are the highest-sonority segments. In the positive formulation, this meant that the demand that high-sonority segments be nuclei had to be evaluated before evaluating lower-sonority segments. In the negative formulation, the dominant consideration—the demand placed on high-sonority segments—is that they *not be margins* (i.e., they must be nuclei). The margin subhierarchy ranks highest the ban against putting sonority-8 segments into the margin; next-highest, sonority-7 segments; and so on down to the lowest-ranked

---

[26] It is not necessarily the case that the relative Harmonies of all *suboptimal* parses are the same in OT$_+$ and HG$_+$. Consider the hypothetical input *imrtrtrt⋯rt* (with n repetitions of *rt*) and the two parses P = *.im.ṛt.ṛt.ṛt.⋯.ṛt.* and Q = *.ymr.tṛ.tṛ.⋯.tṛt.* In OT$_+$, HNUC$_+$ prefers P because its most sonorous nucleus, *ɨ₇*, is more sonorous than Q's most sonorous nucleus *m̥₅*, even though the remainder of P has n miserable nuclei *ɨ₁* while Q has $n-1$ respectable nuclei *ṛ₆*. In OT$_+$, P $\succ$ Q, but in HG$_+$, $H(P) = W_7 + nW_1 < H(Q) = W_5 + (n-1)W_6$ provided $n > 3$. But this does not contradict Theorem (60), because neither P nor Q is optimal; the OT$_+$-optimal parse is $^{\rm w}$P = *.i.mṛ.tṛ.tṛ.⋯.tṛt.* and in HG$_+$, $H(^{\rm w}P) = W_7 + nW_6$, which is greater than both $H(P)$ and $H(Q)$, for any n.

Table 2

constraint, which bans sonority-1 segments from margins. Higher-ranked ONSET will of course prevail in requiring that *some* segments must be parsed into syllable onsets; the ranking in HNUC ensures that these segments will be those of lowest sonority. And because this is the negative formulation, the margin hierarchy is not demanding good margins — it is banning bad ones. All of this depends on the fact that in Berber, there is no epenthesis or deletion; every segment is parsed as either C or V.

(62)   OT₋ tableau for *txznt*

/t₁x₃z₄n₅t₁/	ONSET	…	*C/v₅	*C/v₄	*C/v₃	*C/v₂	*C/v₁
a. ☞ .t₁x̂₃.z₄ń₅t₁.					*		**
b. .t̂₁.x₃ẑ₄.ń₅t₁.	*!					*	*
c. .t̂₁.x₃ẑ₄.n₅t₁.				*!		*	
d. .t̂₁x₃.z₄ń₅t₁.				*	*!		*

(63)   *Theorem.* opt(OT₋) = opt(OT₊)

The relative Harmonies of any two parses of a given input as evaluated by OT₊ and OT₋ are identical. Thus, these grammars define the same optimal outputs.

> *Proof.* (It may be helpful to refer to the corresponding OT₊ and OT₋ tableaux for *txznt*, (47) and (62), while following this argument.) ONSET is identical in the two analyses, so it suffices to consider evaluation by HNUC. Given an input *I*, consider two candidate parses P and Q. Consider the highest-sonority segments in *I*, which have sonority value *s*. Either they are all parsed identically in P and Q, in which case HNUC does not differentiate P and Q with respect to these segments, or at least one such segment μ is parsed differently — say, as a V in P, and as a C in Q. In OT₊, P is then declared more harmonic than Q because there is a best nucleus μ̂ in P that is lacking in Q. In OT₋, P is also declared more harmonic than Q because the highest-ranked constraint in the margin hierarchy that is relevant to this input, *C/vₛ, rejects Q for having at least one more violation (at μ) than P. This establishes the equivalence of OT₊ and OT₋ unless all segments in *I* of maximum sonority (level *s*) are parsed identically in P and Q. In this case, proceed to consider the next-most-sonorous segments in ψ. By repeating exactly the same argument, OT₊ and OT₋ will declare the same candidate to be more harmonic unless all these segments too are parsed identically. Continuing this reasoning as long as necessary, the conclusion is that the relative Harmony of P and Q will be decided identically by OT₊ and OT₋ unless *all* segments are parsed identically in P and Q, in which case P = Q and both OT₊ and OT₋ declare their Harmonies equal.

3.6 Negative HG

In the positive HG account, positive Harmony is awarded for satisfying HNUC₊. In the negative account, negative Harmony is assessed for violating HNUC₋. The following harmonic grammar implements the negative OT analysis OT₋ (61). Here, all constraints are negative: they punish violation but do not reward satisfaction.

(64)   **HG$_-$**: Negative harmonic grammar for Berber syllabification

    a.   Onset: A noninitial syllable must have an onset.

                     Strength: $s_{\mathrm{Ons}} = 2^M$

    b.   HNuc$_-$:   Segment ρ must not be a syllable margin.

                     Strength: $s_\rho = 2^{son(\rho)} - 1$

The Harmony function evaluating Onset is as before. But now the Harmony function evaluating HNuc is

(65) $H_{\mathrm{NUC-}}(\mathrm{P}) = -\sum_i mar(\rho^i, \mathrm{P})[2^{son(\rho^i)} - 1],$

where $mar(\rho_i, \mathrm{P})$ is 1 if the ith segment, ρ_i, is parsed as a margin in P, and 0 otherwise.

(66)   *Theorem.* $H_{\mathrm{HG-}} = H_{\mathrm{HG+}} + k$

    For any given input I, the Harmony assigned by HG$_-$ is equal to the Harmony assigned by HG$_+$ up to a constant k (which depends on I). Thus, for any given input, the two grammars declare the same parse to be optimal.

> *Proof.* It suffices to consider only HNuc, since HG$_+$ and HG$_-$ have the same other constraint, Onset, with the same strength. Now every segment ρ^i is parsed either V or C in a parse P, so $mar(\rho^i, \mathrm{P}) = 1 - nuc(\rho^i, \mathrm{P})$. Thus, recalling (56), we have
>
> $$\begin{aligned} H_{\mathrm{NUC-}}(\mathrm{P}) &= -\sum_i mar(\rho^i, \mathrm{P})[2^{son(\rho^i)} - 1] \\ &= -\sum_i [1 - nuc(\rho^i, \mathrm{P})][2^{son(\rho^i)} - 1] \\ &= -\sum_i [2^{son(\rho^i)} - 1] + \sum_i nuc(\rho^i, \mathrm{P})[2^{son(\rho^i)} - 1] \\ &= k + H_{\mathrm{NUC+}}(\mathrm{P}), \end{aligned}$$
>
> where $k \equiv -\sum_i [2^{son(\rho^i)} - 1]$; this is a constant for any given input.

3.7 Connectionist implementation

3.7.1 BrbrNet

The HG$_-$ analysis can readily be translated into a local connectionist network: **BrbrNet** is shown in Figure 1. In this network, each input segment is encoded in the activation of one input unit. The leftmost stack of input units—the lower, smaller circles—represents the first segment of the input. Since Berber syllabification depends only on sonority level, we can simplify the picture by having only one unit for each sonority level. For the example input /tbia/ shown in Figure 1, in the first stack of small circles the lowest unit, labeled t, is active while the remaining units in the stack are inactive. 'Active' and 'inactive' refer to activation values of 1 (indicated by black circles) and 0 (white circles), respectively. This same input unit would be active if the

Table 2

first segment of the input were *p* or any other segment with the same sonority level as that of its label *t*. Thus, in the second stack of input units, the active unit is labeled *d* although the input segment is *b*. The network is given an input by clamping on the input units the pattern of activity representing the input string.

Figure 1. BrbrNet: Syllabifier for Imdlawn Tashlhiyt Berber

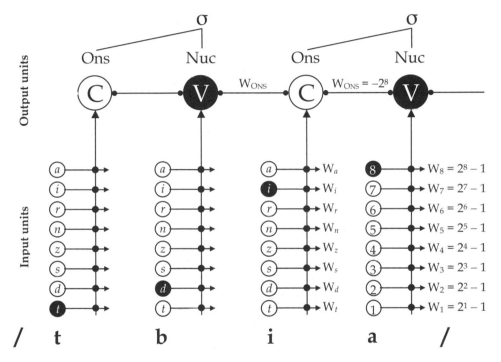

The network computes a syllabification that is represented by a pattern of activity across the output units—the higher, larger circles. The first output unit encodes the syllabic role of the first segment: it is active (1) if the segment is parsed as a syllable peak (nucleus, 'V'), inactive (0) otherwise (margin, 'C'). Each output unit represents the syllabic position assigned to the corresponding input segment (which is represented in the stack of input units directly below the given output unit).

Among the segments parsed as syllable margins, the onset/coda distinction is not explicitly represented in the output: both types of margins are encoded by activation 0. The output representation could be enriched to explicitly make this distinction, but there is no point in doing so here. As pointed out in Section 3.1.2, given the positions of the peaks in a legal Berber syllabification, it is trivial to deduce the onset/coda status of each nonnuclear segment *X*: if *X* immediately precedes a peak, it is an onset; otherwise, it is a coda. It would be trivial to add a second layer of output units encoding the onset/coda distinction, with activity 1 encoding onset and 0 coda; a negative bias on each unit would ensure that a unit is inactive unless it receives positive activation from the following peak unit. Berber is a language in which to study decisions not between onset and coda, but between peak and margin, because of its unique characteristic that any segment can, in the appropriate context, be a peak.

Ultimately, a version of BrbrNet employing distributed rather than local representations is needed to instantiate the principles of ICS, but that requires further progress, as noted in Section 2:8.

The following analysis will address Berber inputs with no sonority plateaus: no two adjacent input segments have the same sonority. This is because for such inputs, there is a uniquely defined correct syllabification. With sonority plateaus, ambiguities arise about which of two equally sonorous segments should be parsed as a nucleus, and the resulting complexities will not be taken up here. (So, with n segments, instead of all 8^n possible input sonority sequences, this analysis addresses only $8 \cdot 7^{n-1}$ inputs — for example, for $n = 5$, only 19,208.)

3.7.2   HG$_+$ $\leftrightarrow$ Net architecture

The connections in BrbrNet realize the harmonic grammar for Berber called HG$_+$ (Section 3.4). This grammar is repeated in (67).

(67)   HG$_+$: Harmonic grammar for Berber syllabification

      a.   ONSET   A noninitial syllable must have an onset. (Negative)
                        Strength: $W_{ONS} = 2^M$

      b.   HNUC$_+$ Segment v must be a syllable nucleus. (Positive)
                        Strength: $W_v = 2^{son(v)} - 1$

The ONSET constraint is implemented by inhibitory connections of strength 2^M between adjacent output units. When two adjacent output units α and β are active, there are two adjacent syllable peaks, a situation that incurs an ONSET violation, changing the Harmony by $\Delta H = a_\alpha W_{\alpha\beta} a_\beta = (1)(-2^M)(1) = -2^M$, just as required by (1a). (Recall that the Harmony contribution made by a connection is the weight of the connection times the activation values of the two units it connects: Section 6:1.)

The HNUC$_+$ constraint is realized by excitatory connections from input to output units. An input unit labeled with a segment v has a connection only to its corresponding output unit (directly above it). The strength of this connection is $W_v = 2^{son(v)} - 1$, $son(v)$ being the sonority level of v, on a scale 1, 2, ..., 8. In Figure 1, the rightmost stack of units is labeled by sonority values, and the corresponding weight values are shown explicitly. The weight pattern is the same for each stack of input units.

When an output unit α is active, a peak has been placed at that segment. In conformity with (1b), the resulting Harmony contributed by the input-output connections is $\Delta H = \Sigma_\beta a_\alpha W_{\alpha\beta} a_\beta = (1)(W_v)(1) = 2^{son(v)} - 1$, where v is the input segment in

Figure 1   *Table 2*

the position of α. That is, all input connections to α come from the input stack beneath it; no other segments are relevant. Suppose the input segment at the position of α is v. Then in the input stack below α, every unit β is inactive except β = v. The inactive units are all connected to α, but they contribute zero Harmony since their activation level is 0. When α is active, the only nonzero Harmony from the input units is $a_\alpha W_{\alpha v} a_v = (1)(W_v)(1)$, which is $2^{son(v)} - 1$ by the design of the connection weights.

In short, the output-output inhibitory connections implement the negative constraint ONSET while the input-output excitatory connections implement the positive constraint HNUC₊: the connection weights are the strengths of these constraints. The Harmony of a pattern of activity **a** as computed by the usual connectionist formula $\Sigma_{\alpha\beta} a_\alpha W_{\alpha\beta} a_\beta$ is the same as the Harmony of the syllabification represented by **a**, as computed by the harmonic grammar (67). At least, when **a** is a pattern of activity that *does* represent a syllabification, this equality holds. These are the activity patterns in which at most one input unit per stack has nonzero activation, and all network units have activation either 0 or 1. These are special network states, the ones with a symbolic semantic interpretation as a string of segments, each parsed as a syllable nucleus or margin. For all other activity patterns, the connectionist formula $\Sigma_{\alpha\beta} a_\alpha W_{\alpha\beta} a_\beta$ gives the correct Harmony value, but since this pattern corresponds to no symbolic structure, it makes no sense to ask for the Harmony assigned by the harmonic grammar.

BrbrNet bears a strong resemblance to the syllabification networks of Goldsmith 1992, an important precursor to this work. But there are critical differences with major implications for general theoretical properties and the correctness of the network's performance. Following the terminology of Prince 1993, where the behavior of these networks is solved analytically, Goldsmith's proposal will be called the **Dynamical Linear Model (DLM)**. DLM's output units represent basically the same information as BrbrNet's, and in both networks each output unit is connected only to its neighbors. But unlike in DLM, in BrbrNet these connections are necessarily symmetric: as strong from right to left as the reverse. This is necessary for the network to perform Harmony optimization (Chapter 9). The input units of DLM also correspond to those of BrbrNet, after a simple transformation that turns BrbrNet into BrbrNet', shown in Figure 2. In BrbrNet, the first input segment v is represented by a unit of activation 1, connected to its corresponding output unit with weight $2^{son(v)} - 1$. From the point of view of Harmony computation, a completely equivalent arrangement would have a single input unit for the first segment, connected to its corresponding output unit with weight 1, and activation value $2^{son(v)} - 1$; since the activation value gets multiplied by the weight in determining the Harmony value, the results are just the same. This new scheme is used in BrbrNet'. In BrbrNet', there is a single input unit for the first segment, and we encode the sonority of this segment in the activation level of this input unit: the higher the sonority, the higher the activation. This is the way the input sonority values are provided to DLM, with an important difference. In DLM, the activation value for sonority level *s* is simply *s*, whereas in BrbrNet', it is $2^s - 1$. The sonority-activation relation in DLM is linear, with sonority values 1, 2, 3, …, 8 be-

ing encoded in activation levels 1, 2, 3, ..., 8. In BrbrNet', the sonority-activation relation is exponential: sonority values 1, 2, 3, ..., 8 are encoded as activation levels 1, 3, 7,
..., 255. This exponential growth is essential for capturing the strict domination structure of the OT Berber analysis OT_+, which is realized in HG_+, which is realized in
BrbrNet'. And this exponential growth is indeed necessary for this sort of network—
with the architecture common to DLM and BrbrNet'—to compute the correct syllabifications.

Figure 2. BrbrNet': Equivalent syllabifier for Berber

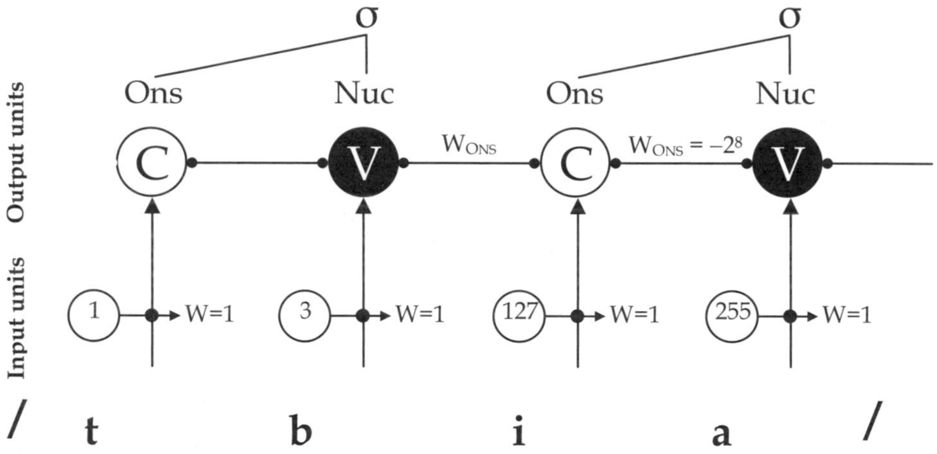

3.7.3 BrbrNet dynamics

To maximize Harmony, BrbrNet uses brain-state-in-a-box (BSB) dynamics (Section
9:3.2.3.4). As usual, the **input** to output unit β is ι_β, the sum of the activations of units
connected to it, weighted by the connection strengths. An output unit in BrbrNet has
two inhibitory connections, one each from its left and right neighbors (end units have
only one neighbor). If we call the left neighbor $\beta - 1$ and the right neighbor $\beta + 1$, the
input from these neighbors to β is $-W_{ONS}(a_{\beta-1} + a_{\beta+1})$, since the weight of these inhibitory connections is $-W_{ONS}$. The input from the input units is just W_v where v is the
input segment at the position of β: the activation value of this input unit is 1, and the
activations of all other input units connected to β—all the other input units in the
stack beneath it—are 0. Thus,

(68) $\iota_\beta = -W_{ONS}(a_{\beta-1} + a_{\beta+1}) + W_v$.   —$v$ = input segment corresponding to β

If the current activation of unit β is a_β, then Δt units of time later—one tick of the
simulated clock—its activation is $a_\beta + \Delta a_\beta$, where the activation change Δa_β is simply
proportional to the input to β, ι_β. If this change would raise a_β higher than 1, then the

Figure 2   *Table 2*

activation is simply set to 1; if the change would lower a_β beneath 0, the activation is set to 0. Thus, the activations are always in the interval from 0 to 1: the space of activation states is the N-dimensional 'box' in which every coordinate — every activation value — lies in this interval. (N is the number of output units.) The activation rule just described is stated formally in (69).

(69)   Brain-state-in-a-box dynamics

$$a_\beta + \Delta a_\beta = \begin{cases} a_\beta + k\Delta t\, \iota_\beta & \text{if this result } r \text{ is in the interval } [0,1] \\ 1 & \text{if } r > 1 \\ 0 & \text{if } r < 0 \end{cases}$$

3.7.4 Competence/performance divergence

From the formal analysis of HG_+ above, we know that the Harmony maxima with respect to that grammar are the correct Berber syllabifications. From the preceding analysis, we know that, among the representations of syllabification as activity patterns in BrbrNet, the maximum-Harmony states are the same as the Harmony maxima defined by HG_+, hence correct syllabifications. From the formal analysis of the BSB dynamics in Chapter 9, we know BrbrNet will maximize Harmony. So it follows that BrbrNet will compute correct Berber syllabifications.

Well, not quite. There are two gaps in the logic. First, we know the Harmony function of BrbrNet is equivalent to the Harmony function defined by HG_+, but only as concerns activation patterns that are symbolically interpretable as syllabifications. It could be that among the network states that are *not* so interpretable, higher Harmony can be achieved. If so, maximizing Harmony in the network should lead to uninterpretable states, not realizations of correct syllabifications.

As concerns a BSB net, however, it turns out that this possibility cannot actually occur. Essentially, the reason is this. If a unit is receiving positive input, it increases Harmony to raise its activation: its Harmony contribution is the product of its input and its activation. So it's always possible to increase Harmony by increasing activation on this unit. Except when that activation level reaches 1, at which point no further increase is allowed by the dynamics: the state cannot leave the box of legal states in which all activations are between 0 and 1 (inclusive). If a unit is receiving negative input, the corresponding reasoning leads to the conclusion that unless the unit's activation is 0, Harmony can be raised by decreasing the unit's activation. If a unit is receiving input exactly equal to 0, its activation level does not affect the Harmony, so any value between 0 and 1 yields the same Harmony, and there is no true maximum. So a real maximum must be one of the 'corners of the box' where all output units' activations are either 0 or 1, and nowhere in between. All such states are symbolically interpretable as syllabifications, or more correctly, as parses of the string into syllable peaks and margins.

The second potential problem is that the BSB dynamics finds a *local* Harmony maximum, and the correct syllabifications are *global* maxima. If there are local Harmony maxima that are not global maxima (necessarily a symbolically interpretable activation pattern), then BrbrNet may produce a suboptimal output, albeit one that has higher Harmony than any 'nearby' states—any states that can be achieved by changing the activation values by an arbitrarily small amount. Are there in fact nonglobal local maxima, and does BrbrNet erroneously produce them as output?

It is easy to show that there are indeed many nonglobal local Harmony maxima. First, since every local maximum is a string of 0s and 1s, interpretable as margin/peak assignments, we can notate any local maximum by a more linguistically evocative string of Cs and Vs, where C denotes 0 and V denotes 1. (Recall that in Berber any segment can be a peak, and any except the most sonorous vowel, *a*, can be a margin. For syllabification, then, it's not useful to attempt to divide the segments into consonants and vowels. So 'C' represents 'syllable margin', not 'consonant' per se.)

Now if a syllabification has three consecutive Cs, $C_1C_2C_3$, it cannot be a local Harmony maximum. (Recall (49).) Raising the middle activation C_2 must increase Harmony. This is because the C_2 unit receives no inhibition from its neighbors, both of which have 0 activation. But this output unit does get excitation from the input units—more excitation the greater the sonority of the corresponding input segment. Hence, increasing this output unit's activation will raise Harmony.

It is also true that a syllabification with two consecutive Vs, V_1V_2, cannot be a local maximum. (Recall (59).) Lowering the activation of either of these two output units from 1 must raise Harmony. Consider V_1; exactly the same reasoning applies to V_2. Since V_1 has a V-neighbor, it receives inhibition equal to $(1)W_{ONS}$ from this neighbor; it may also receive even more inhibition from its other neighbor, but that doesn't matter. The excitation V_1 receives depends on the sonority level of the corresponding input segment: the maximum excitation possible is that for the most sonorous segment, W_a. But by design W_{ONS} is greater than all excitation weights, even the largest one, W_a. Thus, the inhibition V_1 receives must exceed the excitation it receives; its input must be negative, so lowering its activation from 1 will increase Harmony.

So any local maximum must satisfy both *CCC and *VV: *CCC is violated by every C that has no V neighbor, and *VV is violated by every V that has, say, a V to its right. Violating *VV means violating ONSET and violating *CCC means gratuitously violating HNUC$_+$. And any CV string satisfying both *CCC and *VV is a string of legal Berber syllables. Every V must be preceded by a C (except an initial V); thus, every V can be the nucleus of a syllable that has an onset (except initially, where onsets are not required in Berber). Any remaining C (not already serving as an onset) can be syllabified as the coda of the syllable to its left. This C must have a V to its left, since it must have at least one V neighbor to satisfy *CCC, and if its right neighbor were V, it would already be an onset. Thus, a local Harmony maximum must be a candidate that is a string of syllables of shape CV, CVC, #V, or #VC, where # marks the edge of the word. These are exactly the legal syllable structures of Berber.

Figure 2   *Table 2*

It is remarkable that every local maximum is a sequence of legal syllables. Even more remarkable is that the converse is also true. Every string of legal syllables — every CV string satisfying *CCC and *VV — is a local Harmony maximum! Consider any V in the output. It cannot have a V to its left or right, so its neighbors must be either a C unit (activation 0) or an edge of the word. Either way, it receives no inhibition from neighbors. But it necessarily receives some excitation from the input units, so its input is positive, and therefore lowering its activation will lower Harmony. As for an output C, it must have a V either to its left or to its right (or both) to satisfy *CCC. That V unit will send inhibition of strength W_{ONS}, and the excitatory input C receives cannot exceed this inhibition, as observed previously. So this input to this output C unit must be negative, and hence raising its activation from 0 will lower Harmony. In other words, if an output satisfies *CCC and *VV, every C unit is receiving negative input and every V is receiving positive input, so changing the activations can only lower Harmony. Since every small activation change lowers Harmony, the state is a local Harmony maximum. The network is pinned into its corner of the box.

(70) BrbrNet local Harmony maxima

An output pattern in BrbrNet is a local Harmony maximum if and only if it realizes a sequence of legal Berber syllables. That is, every activation value is 0 or 1, and the sequence of values is that given by a sequence of substrings taken from the inventory {CV, CVC, #V, #VC}, where C denotes 0, V denotes 1, and # denotes a word edge.

Thus, the problem of local Harmony maxima in BrbrNet is far from hypothetical. The output space is rife with local maxima, only one of which is the global Harmony maximum, the *correct* output syllabification.

3.7.5 Simulations

Whether BrbrNet will succeed in finding the one global Harmony maximum among the multitude of local maxima cannot, as far as we know, be determined analytically. We therefore performed computer simulations, giving the network 10,000 randomly generated inputs, with length up to 10 segments. The initial value of all output units was 0.[27]

Of these 10,000 inputs, all but 103 were correctly parsed. Of the errors, all but 1 contained a substring of sonority values meeting the template (71).

(71) Problematic input pattern (sonority values)

[Z] Y X 7 8   with [Z <] < Y < X

or the same sequence with left and right reversed. Instead of the correct parse [V].CV.CV, the erroneous output is [C]VC.CV. The bracketed segment may be present or absent.

---

[27] We are extremely grateful to Yoshiro Miyata, who performed these simulations with the PlaNet neural network simulation environment (Miyata 1991).

The one remaining error instantiated the same pattern, with 8 and 7 replaced by 7 and 6, respectively.

Subsequent simulation employed a very small Δt — time interval between 'clock ticks' or steps of the simulation. With this more accurate simulation, every one of the 103 previously problematic inputs was parsed correctly.

Figure 3 shows a trace of the activation trajectory for a rather simple case, our example /txznt/ 'you (sg.) stored', with sonority profile 13451. The correct syllabification is *.tx́.znt́.* or .CV.CVC. With the time step set so that the activation rate coefficient in equation (69) is $k\Delta t = .00008$, after 500 simulation steps, the activation values are 0, 0.27, 0, 1, 0. At this point, the network is guaranteed to ultimately converge to the correct sequence 0, 1, 0, 1, 0 because, while the first peak $\acute{x}$ has only reached activation value 0.27, its neighbors are both 0 so it receives no inhibition, only excitation. The nonpeak segments initially increase in activation because no units receive inhibition until their neighbors have reached a significant activation level. The margin segments *t z t* respectively reach their maximum activation levels of .00034, 0.013, .00011 at time steps 11, 24, 4 and have become completely deactivated by time steps 21, 47, 7. As the lower graph shows, the Harmony monotonically rises throughout the entire computation. The Harmony of the correct parse is $(1)(W_x)(1) + (1)(W_n)(1) = (2^3 - 1) + (2^5 - 1) = 7 + 31 = 38$. After 500 steps, it reaches $32.89 = (1)(7)(.27) + (1)(31)(1)$: because the x unit has only reached activation level 0.27, it is not yet contributing the 7 units of Harmony it will provide when it ultimately reaches activation 1.

Figure 3. Parsing /txznt/ → tx́znt́

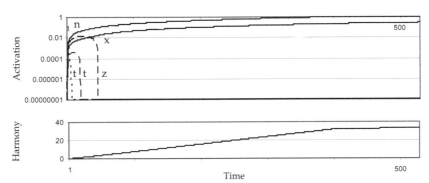

As might be expected, the highest-sonority segment *n* quickly drives its output unit to 1, inhibiting its neighbors (enforcing *VV); the next-most-sonorous segment not thereby inhibited, *x*, drives its output unit up to 1 somewhat less quickly, inhibiting its neighbors in the process. And for longer inputs, this continues, with successively lower-sonority peaks being assigned. The process 'works down the sonority hierarchy' just like the Dell-Elmedlaoui algorithm does, but not because this sequence has been stipulated: the emergent seriality of processing arises from the widely dis-

Figure 3   *Table 2*

parate weights corresponding to different sonority levels.

One might say that stipulating the exponentially growing weights is just a connectionist means of programming seriality into the network's search algorithm. While this is certainly true to a large extent, the story is not so simple. The Dell-Elmedlaoui algorithm *must* monotonically descend the sonority scale, for this is hard-coded in the algorithm. BrbrNet, on the other hand, exhibits much more complex decision-making in cases that are not so clear-cut as the one shown in Figure 3.

In fact, the time course is quite tricky exactly in the cases that were problematic for the less accurate simulation. And observing the network processing these challenging inputs explains why the difficult pattern (71) has the particular shape it does.

Figure 4 shows the activation state trajectory of BrbrNet parsing one of the challenging inputs not correctly parsed in the first, insufficiently fine-grained simulation. The input sonority sequence is 8 1 2 1 3 4 5 7 8 7 as in hypothetical /apbtxznuai/ → *.á.pb.tx̌.zn̩.wáy.* Note that this instantiates the problematic pattern (71) (underlined). While some of the segments exhibit the simple behavior shown in the previous example, others do not. The fifth and seventh segments—hypothetical *x n*, with sonority values 3 5—must be syllabified as peaks in the correct parse (as in actual *txznt* above). Their activation values rise initially, as all do, but are then inhibited to 0. Later, these units rise phoenix-like out of activational oblivion to ultimately assume their proper places atop their respective syllables.

Figure 4. Parsing sonority profile 8 1 2 1 3 4 5 7 8 7

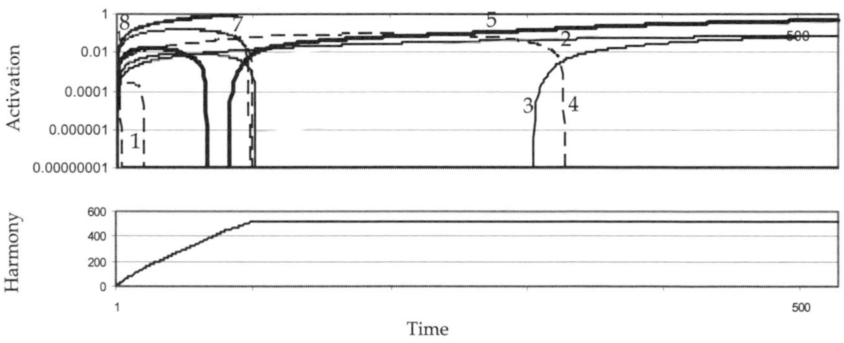

To understand the complex behavior arising in the problematic cases, it is helpful to consider a simpler input also incorrectly parsed in the coarser simulation: 1 2 7 8 as in /txia/ → *.tx̌.yá.*; the relevant incorrect parse is **.tx̌.yá.* The trajectory of BrbrNet while parsing this input is shown in Figure 5.

Examination of this plot reveals why the problematic input pattern is difficult. The sonority-8 final segment quickly rises to its correct value 1: this is the final peak *á*. At the same time, the sonority-7 segment to its left rises to a considerable activation level before it becomes inhibited sufficiently by final *á* to overcome its strong excitatory input $2^7 - 1 = 127$. While the unit for the sonority-7 segment /i/ is active, it inhibits its left neighbor, which, with a mere sonority of 2, receives only excitatory input $2^2 - 1 = 3$ and is easily intimidated by its potent neighbor. It is driven to 0 activation very quickly, and pinned there as long as 7 remains active, which is a considerable amount of time. During that time, when 2 is pinned at 0, it fails to inhibit its left neighbor; with no inhibition, even with its paltry sonority level of 1, /t/ rises appreciably, adding to the inhibition of 2. At this point (around 100 time steps), the net is proceeding directly toward the erroneous parse VCCV, *.*íx.yá*. But the action is not over because it is not yet the case that every active unit has only zero-activation neighbors. In particular, 7 does not. So its impressive rise will soon become a precipitous fall. The critical point is when 7 finally is quashed to activation 0. At this point, 2 is still at 0, but its weaker neighbor 1 has a considerable head start. Released from the inhibition by 7, 2 is now inhibited only by 1. If 1 has such a big head start that it is already highly active, it is possible that its inhibition of 2 can exceed 2's excitation by the input: the weights realizing ONSET $\gg$ HNUC$_+$ ensure that if 1 has reached full activation, its inhibition of 2 is unbeatable. So if 7 takes long enough to give up its ambitions of peakhood, 1 can conceivably have become so close to complete success that 2 cannot even get off the ground. If, however, 1 has not risen sufficiently by the time 2 is released by 7, 2 will receive less inhibition than excitation and it will start to rise. Eventually, it must overtake 1 because of its greater excitation level ($2^2 - 1 = 3$, vs. $2^1 - 1 = 1$ for 1). But eventuality may never arrive. It will take time for 2 to overtake 1, and during that time 1 will continue to rise for a time. If that suffices to get 1 over the finish line of activation 1, the race is over, because (as just observed) the power of ONSET given a fully active peak is dominant and drives 2 back down to 0.

Figure 5. Parsing sonority profile 1 2 7 8

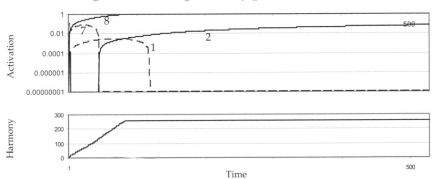

This scenario is responsible for making the difficult inputs difficult. But as Figure 3 shows, in actuality 2 wins the peakness race. Until the dynamics are sufficiently well analyzed to quantify all the timing-dependent interactions played out in this scenario, it is not clear whether the just outcome results from skill or luck. That is, there is as yet no theorem guaranteeing success from BrbrNet. However, it is true

Figure 5   *Table 2*

that in every one of the 103 problematic examples from the first simulation, the correct parse is selected. The network succeeds in avoiding the manifold local Harmony maxima, arriving ultimately at the global maximum.

The case shown in Figure 5 is in some sense the worst of the worst, and success on it is very encouraging. The reason it is the most difficult of the difficult cases is this. To maximize the opportunity for 1 to beat 2, yielding the incorrect parse, we must maximize the time during which 1 is rising and 2 is pinned at 0. And since 2 is pinned by 7, this means maximizing the time required for 7 to be driven to 0 by 8. If the sonority difference between 7 and 8 is increased, the lower-sonority segment will be inhibited more quickly; so to maximize opportunity for error, we need to keep 7 as close in sonority as possible while still less than 8. So if 7 8 is to be modified to make the parsing harder, the replacement must be 6 7 or 5 6 and so on. Of these k $k+1$ pairs, the larger k, the longer the inhibition time of the less sonorous segment, so this time is maximized by the 7 8 pair.

Now to get the most out of the time during which 7 keeps 2 pinned, 1 should be as sonorous as possible: this allows it to rise fastest during that period. But raising 1 to, say, 3 requires raising 2 to 4, which means that after 7 releases its neighbor, now 4, then 4 will overtake 3 more quickly. Since the speed of rise is determined by the weights, which grow exponentially up the sonority scale, the speed difference is much greater for the 3 4 pair than it is for the 1 2 pair. Thus, it appears that with 7 8 maximizing the time for 7 to be inhibited, and 1 2 minimizing the speed at which 2 can overtake 1, the pattern 1 2 7 8 affords the best chance of error.

Figures 6–7 show two more examples of BrbrNet correctly parsing problematic sonority patterns.

Figure 6. Parsing sonority profile 1 2 3 7 8

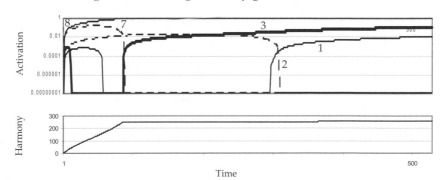

Figure 7. Parsing sonority profile 8 7 2 1 2

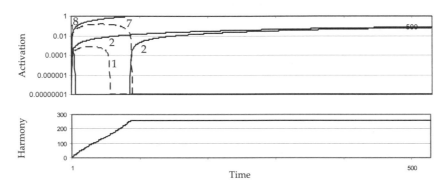

3.8 Summary

In this section, we have examined the core of the complex syllabification system of a dialect of Berber. We have shown how the original Prince and Smolensky 1993/2004 analysis of this system can be directly realized in a harmonic grammar, where exponentially weighted constraints implement strict domination. While exponential weighting is crucial for a core part of the constraint interaction, the need for a large range of weights is not nearly as extreme as expected for the general case. This OT analysis is rather unusual in its use of a positive constraint, so we next examined another OT Berber analysis from Prince and Smolensky 1993/2004 that uses only the standard, negative type of constraint—penalizing violation rather than rewarding satisfaction. This too is readily transformed to a harmonic grammar. The positive OT analysis was then realized in a local connectionist network, BrbrNet, which appears to correctly find the global Harmony maximum—the correct syllabification—amid myriad local maxima, despite using a simple, local Harmony-maximizing activation dynamics that is guaranteed only to find local maxima. For easy inputs, the resulting temporal trajectory implements the sequential parsing algorithm from Dell and Elmedlaoui 1985. But for difficult inputs, the road to the correct parse includes major detours directed toward incorrect competitors.

Figure 7   *Table 2*

References

ROA = Rutgers Optimality Archive, http://roa.rutgers.edu

Aissen, J. 2001. Markedness and subject choice in Optimality Theory. In *Optimality-theoretic syntax*, eds. G. Legendre, S. Vikner, and J. Grimshaw. MIT Press.

Anttila, A. 1997. Variation in Finnish phonology and morphology. Ph.D. diss., Stanford University.

Arad, M. 1998. VP-structure and the syntax-lexicon interface. MIT Occasional Papers in Linguistics 16. MIT, MIT Working Papers in Linguistics.

Aranovich, R. 2003. The semantics of auxiliary selection in Old Spanish. *Studies in Language* 27, 1–37.

Artstein, R. 1999. Person, animacy and null subjects. Ms., Rutgers University.

Asudeh, A. 1999. Linking, optionality, and ambiguity in Marathi: An Optimality Theory analysis. Ms., Stanford University.

Baker, M. C. 1988. *Incorporation: A theory of grammatical function changing*. University of Chicago Press.

Bard, E. G., D. Robertson, and A. Sorace. 1996. Magnitude estimation of linguistic acceptability. *Language* 71, 32–68.

Bentley, D., and T. Eyrthorsson. 2002. Auxiliary selection and the semantics of unaccusatives. Ms., University of Manchester.

Benzing, J. 1931. Zur Geschichte von *ser* als Hilfszeitwort bei den intransitiven Verben im Spanischen. *Zeitschrift für romanische Philologie* 51, 385–460.

Boersma, P. 1997. How we learn variation, optionality, and probability. In *Proceedings of the Institute of Phonetic Sciences of the University of Amsterdam 21*.

Borer, H. 1994. The projection of arguments. In *University of Massachusetts occasional papers in linguistics 17: Functional projections*, eds. E. Benedicto and J. Runner. Graduate Linguistic Student Association, University of Massachusetts at Amherst.

Borer, H. 1998. Deriving passive without theta roles. In *Morphology and its relation to phonology and syntax*, eds. S. Lapointe, D. Brentari, and P. Farrell. CSLI Publications.

Burzio, L. 1986. *Italian syntax: A government-binding approach*. Reidel.

Burzio, L. 2002. Surface-to-surface morphology: When your representations turn into constraints. In *Many morphologies*, ed. P. Boucher. Cascadilla Press. ROA 341.

Clements, G. N. 1990. The role of the sonority cycle in core syllabification. In *Papers in laboratory phonology I: Between the grammar and the physics of speech*, eds. J. Kingston and M. Beckman. Cambridge University Press.

Clements, G. N. 1997. Berber syllabification: Derivations or constraints? In *Derivations and constraints in phonology*, ed. I. Roca. Oxford University Press.

Croft, W. 1990. *Typology and universals*. Cambridge University Press.

Cummins, S. 1996. Meaning and mapping. Ph.D. diss., University of Toronto.

Davidson, L., and M. Goldrick. 2003. Tense, agreement and defaults in child Catalan: An optimality theoretic analysis. In *Linguistic theory and language development in Hispanic languages*, eds. S. Montrul and F. Ordóñez. Cascadilla Press.

Davidson, L., and G. Legendre. 2003. Defaults and competition in the acquisition of functional categories in Catalan and French. In *A Romance perspective on language knowledge and use: Selected papers from the 2001 Linguistic Symposium on Romance Languages (LSRL)*, eds. R. Nuñez-Cedeño, L. López, and R. Cameron. Benjamins.

Dell, F., and M. Elmedlaoui. 1985. Syllabic consonants and syllabification in Imdlawn Tashlhiyt Berber. *Journal of African Languages and Linguistics* 7, 105–30.

Dowty, D. 1979. *Word meaning and Montague Grammar*. Reidel.

Dowty, D. 1991. Thematic proto-roles and argument selection. *Language* 67, 547–619.

Flemming, E. 2001. Scalar and categorical phenomena in a unified model of phonetics and phonology. *Phonology* 18, 7–44.

Goldsmith, J. A. 1992. Local modeling in phonology. In *Connectionism: Theory and practice*, ed. S. Davis. Oxford University Press.

Grimshaw, J. 1990. *Argument structure.* MIT Press.

Haegeman, L. 1994. *Introduction to Government and Binding Theory.* Blackwell.

Hale, K., and S. J. Keyser. 1986. Some transitivity alterations in English. Center for Cognitive Science, MIT.

Hale, K., and S. J. Keyser. 1993. On argument structure and the lexical representation of syntactic relations. In *The view from Building 20*, eds. K. Hale and S. J. Keyser. MIT Press.

Jakobson, R. 1965/1995. Quest for the essence of language. In *On language: Roman Jakobson*, eds. L. R. Waugh and M. Monville-Burston. Harvard University Press.

Keenan, E. L., and B. Comrie. 1977. Noun phrase accessibility and Universal Grammar. *Linguistic Inquiry* 8, 63–100.

Keller, F., and A. Sorace. 2000. Gradient auxiliary selection in German: An experimental investigation. Ms., University of Edinburgh.

Kirchner, R. 1998. An effort-based approach to consonant lenition. Ph.D. diss., UCLA. ROA 276.

Labelle, M. 1992. Change of state and valency. *Journal of Linguistics* 28, 375–414.

Legendre, G. 1989. Unaccusativity in French. *Lingua* 79, 95–164.

Legendre, G. To appear. Optimizing auxiliary selection in Romance. In *Cross-linguistic perspectives on auxiliary selection*, ed. R. Aranovich. Benjamins.

Legendre, G., P. Hagstrom, J. Chen-Main, L. Tao, and P. Smolensky. 2004. Deriving output probabilities in child Mandarin from a dual-optimization grammar. *Lingua* 114, 1147–85.

Legendre, G., P. Hagstrom, A. Vainikka, and M. Todorova. 2002. Partial constraint ordering in child French syntax. *Language Acquisition* 10, 189–227.

Legendre, G., Y. Miyata, and P. Smolensky. 1990a. Can connectionism contribute to syntax? Harmonic Grammar, with an application. In *Proceedings of the Chicago Linguistic Society 26*.

Legendre, G., Y. Miyata, and P. Smolensky. 1990b. Harmonic Grammar—a formal multi-level connectionist theory of linguistic well-formedness: An application. In *Proceedings of the Cognitive Science Society 12*.

Legendre, G., Y. Miyata, and P. Smolensky. 1991. Unifying syntactic and semantic approaches to unaccusativity: A connectionist approach. In *Proceedings of the Berkeley Linguistics Society 7*.

Legendre, G., and D. S. Rood. 1992. On the interaction of grammar components in Lakhóta: Evidence from split intransitivity. In *Proceedings of the Berkeley Linguistics Society 18*.

Legendre, G., P. Smolensky, and C. Wilson. 1998. When is less more? Faithfulness and minimal links in *wh*-chains. In *Is the best good enough? Optimality and competition in syntax*, eds. P. Barbosa, D. Fox, P. Hagstrom, M. McGinnis, and D. Pesetsky. MIT Press and MIT Working Papers in Linguistics. ROA 117.

Legendre, G., and A. Sorace. 2003a. Mapping lexical semantics onto syntactic structure: The problem of unaccusative mismatches in Romance languages. *Journal of Cognitive Science* 4, 43–78.

Legendre, G., and A. Sorace. 2003b. Split intransitivity in French: An optimality-theoretic perspective. In *Les langues romanes: Problèmes de la phrase simple*, ed. D. Godard. CNRS Editions.

Levin, B., and M. Rappaport Hovav. 1992. The lexical semantics of verbs of motion: The perspective from unaccusativity. In *Thematic structure: Its role in grammar*, ed. I. Roca. Foris.

Levin, B., and M. Rappaport Hovav. 1994. A preliminary analysis of causative verbs in English. *Lingua* 92, 35–77.

Levin, B., and M. Rappaport Hovav. 1995. *Unaccusativity: At the syntax–lexical semantics interface.* MIT Press.

Levin, B., and M. Rappaport Hovav. In press. *From lexical semantics to argument realization*. Cambridge University Press.

McClure, W. 1995. *Syntactic projections of the semantics of aspect*. Hitsujishobo.

Miyata, Y. 1991. A user's guide to Planet version 5.6: A tool for constructing, running, and looking into a PDP network. Ms., University of Colorado at Boulder.

Nagy, N., and W. Reynolds. 1997. Optimality Theory and variable word-final deletion in Fætar. *Language Variation and Change* 9, 37–55.

Perlmutter, D. M. 1978. Impersonal passives and the unaccusative hypothesis. In *Proceedings of the Berkeley Linguistic Society 4*.

Perlmutter, D. M., ed. 1983. *Studies in Relational Grammar 1*. University of Chicago Press.

Prince, A. 1990. Quantitative consequences of rhythmic organization. In *Proceedings of the Chicago Linguistic Society: Papers from the parasession on the syllable in phonetics and phonology 26*.

Prince, A. 1993. In defense of the number *i*: Anatomy of a linear dynamic model of linguistic generalizations. Technical report RuCCS-TR-1, Rutgers Center for Cognitive Science, Rutgers University.

Prince, A. 2002. Anything goes. Ms., Rutgers University. ROA 536.

Prince, A., and P. Smolensky. 1993/2004. *Optimality Theory: Constraint interaction in generative grammar*. Technical report, Rutgers University and University of Colorado at Boulder, 1993. ROA 537, 2002. Revised version published by Blackwell, 2004.

Pustejovsky, J., and F. Busa. 1995. Unaccusativity and event composition. In *Temporal reference, aspect and actionality*, eds. P. M. Bertinetto, V. Bianchi, J. Higginbotham, and M. Squartini. Rosenberg and Sellier.

Rappaport Hovav, M., and B. Levin. 1998. Building verb meanings. In *The projection of arguments: Lexical and compositional factors*, eds. M. Butt and W. Geuder. CSLI Publications.

Rosen, C. 1984. The interface between semantic roles and initial grammatical relations. In *Studies in Relational Grammar 2*, eds. D. Perlmutter and C. Rosen. University of Chicago Press.

Silverstein, M. 1976. Hierarchy of features and ergativity. In *Grammatical categories in Australian languages*, ed. R. M. W. Dixon. Australian Institute of Aboriginal Studies.

Slade, B. 2003. How to rank constraints: Constraint conflict, grammatical competition, and the rise of periphrastic *do*. In *Optimality Theory and language change*, ed. D. E. Holt. Kluwer.

Smolensky, P. 1995. On the internal structure of the constraint component *Con* of UG. Talk presented at the UCLA Department of Linguistics. ROA 86.

Sorace, A. 1993a. Incomplete vs. divergent representations of unaccusativity in non-native grammars of Italian. *Second Language Research* 9, 22–47.

Sorace, A. 1993b. Unaccusativity and auxiliary choice in non-native grammars of Italian and French: Asymmetries and predictable indeterminacy. *Journal of French Language Studies* 3, 71–93.

Sorace, A. 1995a. Acquiring argument structures in a second language: The unaccusative/unergative distinction. In *The current state of interlanguage*, eds. L. Eubank, L. Selinker, and M. Sharwood Smith. Benjamins.

Sorace, A. 1995b. Contraintes sémantiques sur la syntaxe: L'acquisition de l'inaccusativité en Italien L2. *Acquisition et Intéraction en Langue Etrangère* 5, 79–113.

Sorace, A. 2000. Gradients in auxiliary selection with intransitive verbs. *Language* 76, 859–90.

Sorace, A., and M. Cennamo. 2000. Aspectual constraints on auxiliary choice in Paduan. Ms., University of Naples and University of Edinburgh.

Sorace, A., and F. Keller. 2005. Gradience in linguistic data. *Lingua* 115, 1497–524.

Sorace, A., and Y. Shomura. 2001. Lexical constraints on the acquisition of split intransitivity: Evidence from L2 Japanese. *Studies in Second Language Acquisition* 23, 247–78.

Sorace, A., and W. Vonk. 1998. Gradient effects of unaccusativity in Dutch. Ms., University of Edinburgh and Max Planck Institute for Psycholinguistics at Nijmegen.

Tuttle, E. 1986. The spread of *esse* as a universal auxiliary in central Italo-Romance. *Medioevo Romanzo* 11, 229–87.

van Hout, A. 1996. *Event semantics of verb frame alteration: A case study of Dutch and its acquisition.* University of Tilburg.

van Hout, A. 2000. Event semantics in the lexicon-syntax interface: Verb frame alterations in Dutch and their acquisition. In *Events as grammatical objects*, eds. C. Tenny and J. Pustejovsky. CSLI Publications.

Van Valin, R. D. 1990. Semantic parameters of split intransitivity. *Language* 66, 221–60.

Zaenen, A. 1993. Unaccusativity in Dutch: Integrating syntax and lexical semantics. In *Semantics and the lexicon*, ed. J. Pustejovsky. Kluwer.

21

Abstract Genomic Encoding of Universal Grammar in Optimality Theory

Melanie Soderstrom, Donald W. Mathis,
and Paul Smolensky

A key feature of Optimality Theory—which distinguishes it from Harmonic Grammar and other facets of the Integrated Connectionist/Symbolic Cognitive Architecture (ICS) more closely tied to the connectionist substrate—is that the knowledge of linguistic well-formedness it ascribes to speakers is *universal*. The origin of this universality is a wide-open question, but of course one influential hypothesis, long associated with Noam Chomsky, is that this universal knowledge is encoded in the human genome. In this chapter, we attempt to couch this hypothesis in more concrete terms, via a case study of a core OT system, the Basic CV Syllable Theory (Prince and Smolensky 1993/2004, Chap. 6; Chapter 13). We reduce the grammatical computation specified by this OT theory to a local connectionist network and then explore what kind of information would need to be genomically encoded for such a network to serve as a Chomskyan Language Acquisition Device embodying innate knowledge of substantive universal principles of grammar. We begin to develop a notion of abstract genome to provide ICS with a bridge between biological genetics and computational cognitive theory, analogous to the bridge that connectionist computation forms between biological neural networks and symbolic cognitive theory.

Contents

Got to be good lookin' 'cause he's so hard to see.
— *John Lennon and Paul McCartney, "Come Together"*

1 AN ICS APPROACH TO THE INNATENESS QUESTION

Perhaps it is not overly optimistic to hope that *this* millennium will see a resolution of the age-old "nature versus nurture" debate concerning the origin of human knowledge. This debate has both stimulated and polarized the field of cognitive science, especially the cognitive science of language, where extreme viewpoints continue to be advocated by leading researchers.[1] In particular, Chomsky's strongly nativist position (e.g., Chomsky 1965) has, since the birth of modern cognitive science, served several generations of researchers as a rallying point attracting fervent defenders and attackers alike.[2]

There seem to be two conceptual difficulties with the nativist hypothesis concerning the type of complex, abstract grammatical knowledge Chomsky presumes in his 'poverty of the stimulus' argument. First, it's hard to see how the nativist story could possibly *work*. Second, it's hard to see how it could possibly *fail*.

For on the one hand, it's very difficult to imagine how genes regulating the manufacture of proteins could program the brain with X′ principles of phrase structure (Box 12:1) and the Minimal Link Condition on *wh*-movement (Box 16:3). On the other hand, it's very difficult to imagine how genes do most of the things we know they must do, so … why not X′ Theory?[3]

This kind of stalemate does not exactly impel cognitive science forward.

A similar impasse might be said to characterize the symbolic theory of cognitive processing, according to which knowledge consists of elaborate rule systems for manipulating complex symbol structures (Chapter 1). On the one hand, it's hard to conceive how this story could actually work: how could the tangled mess of neurons hosting our knowledge provide us with a mental Lisp machine (Box 23:1) performing elaborate symbol manipulation? On the other hand, it's hard to conceive how the brain does most of the things we know it does, so … why not a Lisp machine?

The Integrated Connectionist/Symbolic Cognitive Architecture (ICS) strategy for confronting the latter impasse is to carve out a level of description intermediate between biological neural networks and the symbol-manipulating computer (see Chapter 23) — to seek new organizational principles for abstract neural networks that could

---

[1] Ongoing lively debate on this question can be found in the journal *Trends in Cognitive Science*.

[2] "Doubting that there are language-specific, innate computational capacities today is a bit like being still dubious about the very existence of molecules, in spite of the awesome progress of molecular biology" (Piattelli-Palmarini 1994, 335).

[3] "Although it is quite true that we have no idea how or why random mutations have endowed humans with the specific capacity to learn a human language, it is also true that we have no better idea how or why random mutations have led to the development of the particular structures of the mammalian eye or the cerebral cortex" (Chomsky 1980, 36).

possibly give rise to some sort of symbolic computation, and new sorts of symbolic computation that could possibly arise from an abstract neural network substrate.

In this chapter, we apply this same ICS strategy to the nativism stalemate. We seek a new level of description intermediate between biological genes and abstract grammars—some sort of 'abstract genomic' level that, on the one (upper) hand, is capable of encoding appropriately chosen systems of universal grammatical principles and, on the other (lower) hand, is plausible as a simplified model of the biological system (Figure 1).[4]

Our goal here is not to demonstrate either the success or the failure of nativism. Rather, we hope that progress in conceiving how grammatical knowledge *could possibly be* genetically encoded will help break the stalemate and make it possible to see more clearly how nativist theory could actually succeed or fail. Such progress seems a valuable step toward making nativist theories explicit enough that they can in turn make empirically testable predictions and explain how genes actually influence language acquisition.

Figure 1. Explanatory architecture

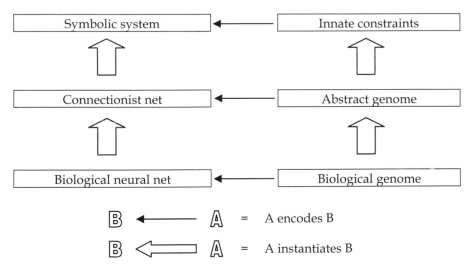

The familiar ICS relationship between biological neural networks, connectionist networks, and symbolic systems is presented on the left. On the right is the complementary relationship between biological genomes, abstract genomes, and innate constraints. In each case, the genomic element encodes (provides the "blueprints" for) its ICS counterpart.

[4] Mitchell (1996, 4) compares the relationship between biological evolution and genetic algorithms to that between biological networks and connectionist networks as described in Smolensky 1988. Here, we take a similar position with respect to the relationship between biological and abstract genomes.

Figure 1

Optimality Theory (OT; Prince and Smolensky 1993/2004) provides a framework conducive to relatively explicit formulations of the nativist hypothesis concerning grammatical knowledge. Indeed, OT versions of the nativist hypothesis in phonology and syntax were respectively the subject of experimental tests in Chapters 17 and 18. We hasten to endorse the position taken in Chapter 2 that the validity of the nativist hypothesis is an empirical question that is currently wide open, and likely to remain so for a long time—we see no sufficiently compelling reason to take a position either way at present.

In this chapter, we explore, not the validity of the nativist hypothesis, but the theoretical commitments it entails. To begin to address this issue, we do not ask, "Is the nativist hypothesis true?"—rather, we ask, "How could it possibly be made to work, given current understanding (admittedly incomplete)[5] of the function and structure of the brain, the genome, and grammar?"

Our strategy is familiar: hypothesize computational primitives that, although extremely simplified, nonetheless capture important biological principles, and that, despite their simplicity, can support cognitive computation with a relevant degree of complexity. The computational primitives we hypothesize here constitute a first attempt to formalize an **abstract genome** that relates to the biological genome roughly as abstract neural networks relate to biological neural networks.

In this chapter, we attempt to develop an abstract genome sufficient to genetically encode a simplified but still relevantly complex component of universal grammar under OT: the Basic CV Syllable Theory of Prince and Smolensky 1993/2004, Chap. 6 (see Chapter 13 of this book). While this first-pass attempt has significant shortcomings, we nonetheless believe it has progressed sufficiently to warrant presentation as one important current boundary of ICS research—the deepest frontier of the ICS attempt to vertically integrate the theory of mind and brain.

1.1 The nativist hypothesis

The version of the nativist hypothesis concerning grammatical knowledge that we target here is formulated in general terms in (1).

(1)   The nativist hypothesis (general formulation)

      a.   *Language.* A language $\mathcal{L}$ is a rich combinatorial system governed by complex structural well-formedness conditions, $G_\mathcal{L}$.

      b.   *Typology.* The well-formedness conditions $G_\mathcal{L}$ for all human languages $\mathcal{L}$ share a great deal of common ('universal') structure, $\mathcal{U}$. The typological

---

[5] It might be objected that current understanding of genetics is so meager as to make the present enterprise extremely premature. It seems to us that current understanding of genetics is not clearly much more incomplete than current understanding of the brain. It has proved worthwhile for cognitive science to explore abstract characterizations of neural computation, so it is not unreasonable to ask whether the same might be true of genetic encoding. It might be objected that abstracting neural computation is also premature and that current connectionist research therefore cannot contribute to cognitive science. This position, however, leads to the conclusion that the entire project of this book—not just the nascent genetic component—is not worth pursuing.

space of possible human languages, $\mathcal{T}$, is intricately structured, the boundary separating possible from impossible languages being subtly determined by the universals of well-formedness $\mathcal{U}$.

    c.   *LAD*. The genome equips the learner with a Language Acquisition Device (LAD) that encodes knowledge of $\mathcal{U}$ in the following sense: the LAD is incapable of learning an impossible human language—one that violates $\mathcal{U}$—but it is capable of effectively and efficiently homing in on any target possible human language $\mathcal{L}$ in $\mathcal{T}$, given examples of well-formed items in $\mathcal{L}$.

Within the framework of ICS, and OT (Chapters 4 and 12) in particular, this hypothesis takes the form (2). A constraint hierarchy is implemented numerically (Section 20:1.2) via a set of numerical weights for the constraints—via a **harmonic grammar** (**HG**; Chapters 2 and 6).

(2)   The nativist hypothesis (ICS/OT/HG formulation)

    a.   *Language*. A language $\mathcal{L}$ is a subset of a combinatorially structured candidate set of linguistic forms S. $\mathcal{L}$ consists of those forms that best satisfy a set of violable well-formedness constraints Con_L, as ranked in a strict domination hierarchy, $\mathcal{G}_L$.

    b.   *Typology*. The set of candidate forms S, the set of well-formedness conditions Con, and the formal definition of 'best satisfying a hierarchy of violable constraints' are exactly the same for all possible human languages: they define $\mathcal{U}$. The typological space of possible human languages $\mathcal{T}$ is the space of all languages $\mathcal{L}$ consisting of the optimal forms relative to some ranking $\mathcal{G}_L$ of the constraints Con.

    c.   *LAD*. The genome g equips the learner with a Language Acquisition Device (LAD) encoding knowledge of $\mathcal{U}$ in the following sense.

        i.   During development, g drives the construction of a neural network $\mathcal{N}$ that maximizes Harmony.

       ii.   The activation patterns in $\mathcal{N}$ can realize any candidate linguistic structure in S.

      iii.   The connections in $\mathcal{N}$ encode the constraints Con: maximizing Harmony constructs the realization of the structure that best satisfies the constraints Con, with each constraint $\mathbb{C}_i$ in Con having a numerical strength s_i.

      iv.   During language acquisition, $\mathcal{N}$ adjusts the constraint strengths s_i while processing example linguistic forms in S. The learning algorithm finds a set of strengths s_i such that each constraint in Con strictly dominates all weaker constraints—that is, it finds the grammar of a possible language in $\mathcal{T}$.

       v.   If the learning data derive from a language $\mathcal{L}$ in $\mathcal{T}$, the learning algorithm efficiently converges to a set of strengths s_i realizing a ranking of Con that correctly generates $\mathcal{L}$.

Figure 1

Recall that we will not address whether this hypothesis *is* true; rather, we will explore how, in principle, it *could* be true. The OT literature provides numerous examples of how the theoretical linguistics hypotheses (2a) and (2b) could be true. (See Chapters 12–16 and the references therein, especially the Rutgers Optimality Archive, http://roa.rutgers.edu/. The particular example we will examine is the Basic CV Syllable Theory of Prince and Smolensky 1993/2004, Chap. 6, reprinted here as Chapter 13; this theory is briefly reviewed below.)

The question, then, is how (2c) could be true, with respect to the universals $\mathcal{U}$ of the Basic CV Syllable Theory. In this chapter, we attempt a proof-in-principle of the possibility of such a LAD, presenting the design for a demonstration system we call 'CV$_{net}$'. This design has not yet been subject to extensive computer simulation; as discussed below, prior theoretical work remains to be done. One significant theoretical gap concerns (2c.iv): under some conditions, CV$_{net}$ may learn a set of constraint strengths that violates strict domination. Our network $\mathcal{N}$ does, however, strongly reflect a genomic encoding of the universal constraints *Con*: its knowledge always consists exactly of a weighted sum of these constraints, even though the weights need not necessarily realize strict domination. For the particular case of the Basic CV Syllable Theory, problematic situations appear to be rare, but addressing the general case would seem to require further theoretical insights.

In the following sections, we will describe the development of a biologically inspired abstract genome to encode a network architecture and constraint system that together determine a particular symbolic linguistic typology. In Sections 1.2–1.3, we motivate this new facet of the ICS research program from a biological perspective, discussing the theoretical role of the abstract genome and reviewing a few relevant basic findings on genetic encoding. Then in Section 2, we quickly lay out the Basic CV Syllable Theory, working at the symbolic level (top right of Figure 1): this provides the presumptive innate constraints. A given language's grammar is a particular ranking of these constraints (top left of Figure 1). In Section 3, we descend to a lower level, presenting the structure of a connectionist network—CV$_{net}$—that realizes the symbolic grammar (middle left of Figure 1). The network design exploits a general mathematical analysis of the realization of strict domination in connectionist networks; this analysis is presented in the chapter's Appendix. In Section 4, we derive an abstract genome—called **CV$_{gene}$**—that encodes the development of the CV$_{net}$ network (middle right of Figure 1). In Section 5, we note a few of the many unanswered questions, particularly with regard to unresolved issues of biological and computational significance. Since this research program is still in its preliminary stages, we do not present this work as a direct contribution toward a conclusive answer to any of the larger issues of innateness in language acquisition. Instead, it demonstrates how the ICS perspective allows such issues to be addressed, and how it raises new questions (and recasts old ones).

1.2 The role of an abstract genome

The past 50 years have seen enormous advances in understanding of genes and gene transmission and expression. Given the sometimes direct relationships that have been established between a particular gene and a particular malady or biological function in general, one might expect that understanding of the genetics of cognition has progressed as well. In fact, very little can be said with certainty about this issue.

Considerable biological evidence suggests that there is hardly ever a one-to-one mapping between a gene and a mechanism. Even the simplest mechanisms in human biology can encompass long, complicated cascades of enzyme activity or other protein interaction, even within a single cell—all ultimately under genetic control. Diseases can have as a source an anomaly of a single gene, but of course this does not mean that a single gene is responsible for the functions disrupted by that gene: if the fuel line is removed from a car's gas tank, the car won't run, but this hardly means that the fuel line is solely (or even primarily) responsible for getting the car from point A to point B. Even extremely simple functions can require complex mechanisms, and interrupting any one subcomponent can render the whole system inoperative or cause it to malfunction. And our linguistic capabilities can hardly be considered extremely simple. We must assume, therefore, that the relationship between our linguistic capabilities and our genetic endowment is extraordinarily complex.

Yet many linguists insist, drawing on arguments about universality and learnability, that certain very abstract yet very specific characteristics of our linguistic knowledge are innate—they do not need to be learned from experience by the infant acquiring a first language (e.g., Chomsky 1965; Wexler and Culicover 1980; Pinker 1984). The Chomskyan perspective views this innateness in terms of a LAD, which is part of the innate (and hence ultimately genetic) endowment of each infant. As articulated in (1), this LAD can be viewed as the infant's knowledge of the nature of universal grammar (UG), the set of grammatical properties, $\mathcal{U}$, that characterizes all and only the possible human languages.

But if the relationship between genes and language is as complex as biology suggests it must be, what exactly could it mean to say that children possess such a LAD? Is there a way to reconcile the linguistically motivated hypothesis that genes encode very specific grammatical knowledge with the biological fact that the means by which genes actually regulate function are highly complex and indirect?

There are several different ways in which genetics might influence linguistic knowledge. Elman et al. (1996) argue that some of these possibilities are more likely than others, given current knowledge of genetics and development. In particular, representational nativism, which posits direct genetic control of structural representations of knowledge, is viewed as unlikely; architectural and chronotopic nativism—which appeal to a host of other possibilities, including higher-order structural constraints and constraints on the timing of maturation—are considered to be the most likely source of genetic influence on knowledge representation. In our view, such analysis constitutes definite progress—defining the problem this way allows one to

Figure 1

ask more fruitful questions than "Nature or nurture?" Elman et al. are also right to stress the importance of development, which is a primary point of contact between genes and the environment. Yet at present not much is known about how higher-order symbolic knowledge, such as linguistic knowledge, is realized in the brain. Until progress is made on this hard problem, we think it premature to flatly eliminate major classes of hypotheses about how genes might encode knowledge.

Within the ICS framework, symbolic theory benefits from insights at lower levels of analysis. OT owes its major innovation (violable constraints) to an understanding of the fundamental nature of harmonic connectionist networks: that such systems can settle into a stable state through the interaction of a number of local, conflicting forces. This insight about connectionist networks is in turn based on understanding of the state of affairs at the neural level: that neurons speak to each other locally through synapses in a primarily additive manner, and in parallel.

Similarly, we suggest that what is needed to advance research on innate knowledge is some understanding of how (indeed, whether) a nativist LAD could possibly exist within an ultimately biological system. To address this, we need to go back to the underlying biology and look at what *kinds* of structures and processes are available. We need to formally connect the symbolic linguistic concept 'innate' with the biological concept 'genetic': this we propose to do by building an abstract encoding of a connectionist network realizing innate symbolic knowledge—an abstract genome. This abstract genome ought then to help us address the innateness question, just as connectionist models provide insight into the problem of symbolic processing in a neural system.

Connectionist computation provides a valuable intermediate level between biological neural computation and symbolic computation (Smolensky 1988; see also Chapter 23). While many questions remain open, some of the basic facts about the biology of neural networks, and their relationship to abstract networks, are well established. Regardless of whether the 'units' in a given connectionist network model individual neurons, or collections of neurons, or some mathematical conception of a pattern of neural activation, it is generally accepted that the computational notion of a connectionist 'unit' is intimately tied to the biological notion of 'neuron'. Similarly, whether loosely or tightly, computational 'connections' pair with biological synapses, and 'Hebbian learning' in the algorithmic sense with 'Hebbian learning' in the neuroscience sense. Some concepts, like the back-propagation learning algorithm (Rumelhart, Hinton, and Williams 1986), are important tools at one level of analysis, but lack compelling correlates at the other. Clearly, reliance on such single-level concepts should ultimately be minimized in a research program like ICS that seeks a vertically integrated theory of the mind/brain. This is true of the relationships among neuroscience, abstract connectionist network theory, and symbolic knowledge, and also of the relations among biological genetics, abstract genetics, and innateness.

We suggest that biological grounding is important to a good model of innately driven language acquisition, but that some kind of intermediate level of analysis is a crucial step in relating symbolic innateness to the biology of genetics—just as we believe the intermediate level provided by connectionist networks is crucial to linking symbolic theories of cognition to their neurobiological embodiment. The intermediate level is the *abstract genome* we seek to develop in the research reported here. And our proposal is that the intermediate *genetic* level, the abstract genome, is in fact a specification of the intermediate *processing* level, the connectionist network. We limit ourselves here to those aspects of the genetic endowment that in some way directly specify aspects of the network in question. We expect that more indirect genetic influences on cognition, and specifically on language, play an important role in the acquisition process (e.g., Jusczyk and Bertoncini 1988). But these indirect influences are largely irrelevant to the question of Chomskyan innateness.

Two general approaches to building an abstract genome for a connectionist network can be distinguished. In the first approach, the genome directly specifies the relevant components of the network itself. This might include the number of layers of units and their organization, the number of units in each layer and their connectivity, the type of learning rule, the learning rate, and other numerical parameters. Crucially, in this approach there need be no account of how the bits of information in the abstract genome bring about their interpreted manifestation in the network. Thus, in this approach, we could build a genome for any arbitrary neural network. Such a genome specifies a network precisely enough that a computer can simulate an evolutionary process by altering the genomic parameters systematically to optimize the success of the encoded network. This seems to be the current method of choice among evolutionary modelers of neural networks (see the sources in Whitley and Schaffer 1992; Batali 1994; Nakisa and Plunkett 1998; Kvasnicka and Pospichal 1999; for examples of more constrained specifications, see Gruau 1992; Kitano 1994).

An alternative approach is considerably more biologically constrained. The bits of information in the abstract genome are not only given an interpretation in terms of the connectionist network that they specify; they are also given an explicit biological interpretation, albeit an abstract one. This parallels the sense in which the activity of connectionist units in cognitive models can simultaneously carry an interpretation at the level above (say, as a letter sequence) and at the level below (say, as the average firing rate of groups of neurons). In this second approach, the modeler attempts to provide a biologically plausible account of how, given the biological interpretation of the information in the abstract genome, it follows that the network has the properties it ought to, according to the network interpretation of the genomic information.

For the task of relating innateness and genetics, the second approach is likely to be more fruitful in the long run, probably for the same reason that the first approach is currently preferred in many circumstances. While the first approach makes it easy to build a genome for any type of network we want, the second approach is limited to those networks that can be given a biologically plausible genomic encoding. Our working hypothesis is that, in the same way that linguistic theory itself profited from a union with biologically plausible ideas about the nature of neural computation, innateness theory can profit from a union with biologically plausible ideas about genomic encoding.

Figure 1

At the same time, the second approach is currently untenable if taken to the extreme, in part because we do not have complete understanding of the capabilities of a biological genome, and in part because we do not completely understand the relationship between an abstract genome and a biological one. As with connectionist network models, we may be forced to make some back-propagation-like assumptions in our genome—assumptions that are less than ideally biologically plausible—in order to account for what is known about linguistic typologies. These difficulties must be viewed as an overall challenge for the integration of knowledge at the different levels. Rather than invalidating the abstract genome approach, they underscore its importance in identifying crucial inconsistencies between current biological theory and current cognitive theory, and in exploring hypotheses for how these inconsistencies may one day be resolved.

1.3 Biological genomes

A biological genome is a set of blueprints for making proteins. These proteins can interact with each other and with other chemicals (including the DNA that specifies the genome) to build structures, send signals, modulate the production of more proteins, and carry out the basic maintenance of a biological system, as well as controlling the growth and development of a complex organism. Any limitations on what can be an innately driven system are limitations on what can be specified ultimately (directly or indirectly) by the actions and interactions of these proteins. Fortunately, many things can be accomplished this way—but not just anything. What is needed is an understanding of what such mechanisms would look like.

One important respect in which a biological genome differs from most kinds of abstract neural network genomes that have been used so far is that much of the specification of a biological system occurs, not directly, but via a gradual course of development. The wiring of a complex network in the nervous system takes place through the interplay of peptide signals acting on individual neurons' axons as they wind their way toward the ultimate synapse destination (see, e.g., Nichols, Martin, and Wallace 1992, Chap. 11, for an introductory review of neural development). These signals might originate from preferences for substrate molecules (Letourneau 1975), from guidepost cells along the way (Kuwada 1986), or from the target cell itself (Lumsden and Davies 1986), or via a chemical gradient that provides an axis for orienting the direction of travel (Tessier-Lavigne et al. 1988; Tessier-Lavigne and Placzek 1991; Tosney 1991). Although the cited studies have focused on the signals needed to specify long-distance sensory connections, we can use this paradigm to think about the shorter-distance but highly specific connections necessary for a network specifying our UG.

All of these different kinds of signals and signal receptors originate from a single genome. The trick is then to ensure that various peptide signals are sent by, and heeded by, some cells and not others. This might happen because the cells are of different types from "birth," or because their environments are different. Both of these sources of differentiation have been found in the development of simple nervous systems, where cell lineage can be easily traced (Horvitz 1982; Stent and Weisblat 1982; Rubin 1989).

Yet another source of influence on the wiring of a neural system is activity-dependent axonal growth and pruning, which is well studied within the primate and cat visual systems (e.g., Hubel, Wiesel, and Levay 1977; see Nichols, Martin, and Wallace 1992, Chap. 18, for an introductory review) and more generally (e.g., Dantzker and Callaway 1998; see Cowan et al. 1984; Van Ooyen 1994, for reviews).

In the demonstration system developed below, we will show that the nature of the signal needed to specify the connectivity of the network is related to the type of wiring that is being specified. In other words, the nature of the genomic specification of a particular wiring pattern, and its simplicity or complexity, is related to the type of *computation* being performed, and ultimately to the nature of the symbolic typology. This is very different from an abstract neural network genome in which connectivity is simply specified by a matrix pattern of 1s and 0s, where a 1 means there is a connection, and a 0 means there is not. The difference is not simply a matter of the detail of representation. Certain patterns of connectivity might be impossible to set up in the biological system, and others very easy, whereas any such insights would be masked in the simple matrix representation, where all patterns are equal. The nature of genomic encoding is intimately tied to the facts of development.

2   BASIC CV SYLLABLE THEORY: SYMBOLIC DESCRIPTION

Essential to Chomsky's arguments for the innateness of grammatical knowledge is the abstractness and combinatorial intricacy of this knowledge. Thus, for a case study to be relevant to the debate concerning innate linguistic knowledge, it is important to address a formal model of 'language' that, extremely simplified though it must surely be, nonetheless contains essential elements of grammatical systems. Because it incorporates many of these elements (3), albeit in simple form, for the present exercise we study the Basic CV Syllable Theory (CVT) of Prince and Smolensky 1993/2004, Chap. 6. (For an introduction to CVT, see Chapter 12 or 13.)

(3)   Essential linguistic properties of Basic CV Syllable Theory

    a.   The cognitive function—simplified syllabification—maps underlying linguistic forms to surface forms, an essential aspect of the generative perspective on all grammar.

    b.   While the forms are extremely simple—mere strings of Cs and Vs, denoting sequences of unspecified consonants and vowels—they have unbounded combinatorial structure, another essential linguistic property. (Thus, the functions in question display the hallmark of the symbolic cognitive architecture: productivity, explained through the combinatorial strategy introduced in Chapter 1.)

Figure 1

   c.   The CV-syllabification functions of different languages possess universal properties, yet vary crosslinguistically. They constitute a known typology with prototypical linguistic structure (see Chapter 13).

   d.   CVT is not just a simplification of natural language; it is a minicomponent of real natural language grammar that, in combination with other components, plays a crucial role in many actual accounts proposed in the current phonology literature (e.g., Prince and Smolensky 1993/2004, Chap. 7).

   e.   It is a (perhaps *the*) canonical model of UG in OT.

2.1 Input-output function of Basic CV Syllable Theory

In CVT, the grammar of a language defines a mapping of strings of Cs and Vs from an underlying form to a surface form, in a manner that optimally satisfies a set of ranked and violable well-formedness constraints, *Con*, as well as a set of inviolable and unranked constraints (encoded in *Gen*). For example, a string of Cs and Vs like

(4) $C^1V^2C^3V^4C^5C^6$

enters the grammar as input (an underlying form, such as /fɪnɪš+s/ *finish* + *s*, third person singular of *finish*). The system produces an output, such as

(5) $.C^1V^2.C^3V^4.C^5\boxed{V}C^6.$

(the surface form, in the present case [.fɪ.nɪ.šə̌z.] *finishes*). In this example, to improve the sound sequence, the grammar has inserted a vowel between the two final Cs; this **epenthetic** vowel is written here as $\boxed{V}$. The output (5) is a CV sequence; for each output segment C or V, the output indicates which (if any) C or V in the input it **corresponds** to. This correspondence relation is indicated here by superscripts: the output segment written C^3 corresponds to the input segment that is also designated C^3. Correspondences between input and output segments play a central role in CV_{net}. By definition, a segment like $\boxed{V}$ is epenthetic if it has no input correspondent: it has been inserted by the grammar. The grammar is also capable of *deleting* an input segment, in which case there is no output segment corresponding to the deleted input segment. The function from underlying to surface string can potentially introduce many alterations and is by no means trivial computationally (see Chapter 13).

    The segments of the output (5) are grouped into a sequence of **syllables**; '.' marks a syllable boundary. In CVT, however, these boundary marks are redundant in outputs: their location can be computed from the CV string. This is because in CVT, a syllable consists of a **nucleus** containing a single V, optionally preceded by an **onset** consisting of a single C, and followed optionally by a **coda** consisting of a single C. Thus, every V in the output string constitutes a syllable nucleus, and every nucleus consists of a single V. The output of our demonstration network CV_{net} will be a CV string in which a distinction is made between C_{onset} and C_{coda}. Each V comprises the nucleus of a separate syllable; if the segment preceding V is C_{onset}, then the syllable has an onset; if the segment following V is C_{coda}, then the syllable has a coda.

2.2 The constraints of Basic CV Syllable Theory

The function from underlying CV string to surface CV string is determined by the grammar: a language-particular ranking of the universal constraints in *Con*. For CVT, *Con* consists of the following five universal constraints:

(6)   *Con* constraints

    a. PARSE   For every element in the input there is a corresponding element in the output.

    b. FILL^V Every syllable nucleus in the output has a corresponding V in the input. (This V *fills* the syllable nucleus.)

    c. FILL^C Every syllable onset or coda in the output has a corresponding C in the input.

    d. ONSET   Every syllable nucleus has a preceding onset.

    e. NOCODA   There are no codas.

These definitions of ONSET and NOCODA are the same as those in Chapters 12 and 13, except they employ the Correspondence Theory of faithfulness, a central component of contemporary OT developed in McCarthy and Prince 1995 (where the general versions of the PARSE and FILL constraints of (6) are respectively called 'MAX' and 'DEP').

In addition, the generator of candidate outputs for CVT, *Gen*, imposes the inviolable constraints in (7). (Unlike in this simplified theory, in real natural language typologies, these are violable constraints in *Con* rather than inviolable constraints in *Gen*. These constraints were introduced in McCarthy and Prince 1995.)

(7)   *Gen* constraints

    a. IDENTITY   Each correspondence index i may label at most one pairing: either $C^i \leftrightarrow C^i$ or $V^i \leftrightarrow V^i$, but not both.

    b. LINEARITY   Output segments maintain the order of their corresponding input segments.

    c. INTEGRITY   Each segment in the input corresponds to at most one segment in the output.

    d. UNIFORMITY   Each segment in the output corresponds to at most one segment in the input.

Finally, we present four inviolable constraints that are enforced by the very data structure of outputs: strings of onset, coda, and nucleus segments. We will refer to these as **structural** constraints. The necessity of these constraints (and their descriptions) will be clearer within the context of the connectionist realization, where the symbol-string data structure is not directly available.

(8)   Structural constraints

    a. OUTPUTIDENTITY   Every output segment is either an onset, a coda, or a nucleus, but not more than one of these.

    b. NOOUTPUTGAPS   There are no gaps between consecutive segments in

Figure 1

		an output string.
c.	CORRESPONDENCE	No correspondence relation exists without both an input and an output element.
d.	NUCLEUS	There must be a nucleus following every onset and preceding every coda.

One final property of CVT: as in any substantive theory in OT, constraint interaction is governed by strict domination hierarchies. In general, realizing strict domination with numerical constraint weighting requires weights with a special property: they grow exponentially as the hierarchy is mounted, so that the cost of violating any constraint $\mathbb{C}$ will dominate the maximal cost possible from all constraints ranked lower than $\mathbb{C}$, combined (see Section 20:1.2.2.1; also (22) and the Appendix below). This is a general problem for which no solution has yet been found: limiting the strengths of the constraints in a connectionist network to those meeting the special exponential growth condition. Reconciling a numerical learning algorithm with necessarily exponential weighting is probably the single most pressing open problem in this line of research.[6]

Within OT, the nativist hypothesis (2) posits that knowledge of the universal violable constraints in *Con* (6), the universal inviolable constraints in *Gen* (7), and the universal inviolable structural constraints in (8) are all innate. Constraints are not created de novo or altered by the learning process; they are simply ranked relative to one another. To understand what it might mean for these constraints to be innate, it is first necessary to have a picture of what it would mean for the constraints to be explicitly realized in a network.

3 BASIC CV SYLLABLE THEORY AT THE NETWORK LEVEL: $\mathrm{CV_{NET}}$

According to ICS, a grammar is a system of violable well-formedness constraints that apply in parallel to evaluate the "goodness" or **Harmony** of mental representations. The conflicting demands of the constraints are resolved in favor of stronger constraints, the relative strengths being language particular while the constraints themselves are universal. Learning a particular language requires learning the relative strengths of the constraints. According to the nativist hypothesis (2), the constraints

---

[6] To a surprisingly large extent, exponential weighting is *not* actually needed to get correct syllabification in CVT. This is because most of the constraint interaction is local to either the onset or the coda, and the relevant decisions there (e.g., "Should an onset be epenthesized, or should ONSET be violated?") are determined solely by the relative weights of two constraints (e.g., FILL$^\mathrm{Ons}$ vs. ONSET). As long as the numerical strengths of the constraints match an OT ranking, the same optima will result even without exponentially growing weights. This is not entirely true, however. An example of an exception is the input /CC/, where decisions about the onset and coda interact with one another: epenthesizing *one* medial V allows *two* Cs to be parsed, simultaneously creating an onset and a coda. Here, to implement the ranking FILL$^\mathrm{Ons}$ ≫ PARSE, the weight of FILL$^\mathrm{Ons}$ must exceed *twice* the weight of PARSE; it is not good enough that the weight of FILL$^\mathrm{Ons}$ simply exceed the weight of PARSE. The key to understanding this issue is Prince's (2002) "Anything Goes" Theorem (Chapter 20 (14)). We are extremely grateful to Alan Prince for his proof that, because of such exceptions, CVT as a whole does require exponential weights.

themselves, along with all other universal elements of grammar, do not need to be learned: they are innate.

In the symbolic, high-level description, the relative constraint strengths are encoded in a strict domination hierarchy, forming an OT grammar G. At a subsymbolic level, the constraints are encoded in patterns of connection weights in a network $\mathcal{N}$. The relative strength of constraints is manifest numerically, along the lines of HG (Chapters 6, 10, 11, and 20). $\mathcal{N}$ is a harmonic network (Chapters 6 and 9): its activation-spreading algorithm maximizes Harmony. $\mathcal{N}$ will (ideally) compute the input-output function of the grammar G provided the network's Harmony function correctly realizes the constraint hierarchy of G.

The formal relationship between an OT grammar as a symbolic system and a harmonic network as a subsymbolic system is discussed in general terms in Chapter 20; indeed, it constitutes a core result of ICS. Yet no harmonic network that realizes CVT has previously been *explicitly* specified, nor has there been an explicit specification of the learning algorithm that handles the reranking of innate constraints within the network system. (But see the purely symbolic learning algorithm of Tesar and Smolensky 1993, discussed in Section 12:3, and the numerical/symbolic algorithm of Boersma 1998.) For an abstract genomic encoding of a network to be developed, there must first be a network to encode. Therefore, this section is devoted to specifying the LAD at the network level.

The demonstration LAD we develop—CV_{net}—consists of the four components given in (9).

(9)   Network-level description of CV_{net}

    a. *Architecture.* CV_{net} is a connectionist network architecture supporting representations of an underlying and a surface CV string, along with the correspondence relations linking them.

    b. *Constraints.* The connections in CV_{net} encode a set of linguistic constraints $\{\mathbb{C}_i\}$, those of CVT defined in Section 2.1. Each constraint $\mathbb{C}_i$ is realized by a set of unchanging **connection coefficients** $c^i_{\Phi\Psi}$ that determine the relative weights of connections between units of type Φ and units of type Ψ. Each constraint $\mathbb{C}_i$ has an overall strength s_i that will change during learning; this is the numerical HG counterpart of the OT rank of $\mathbb{C}_i$.

    c. *Activation dynamics.* The activation algorithm describes how activation spreads in CV_{net}, given the connection coefficients and the overall strengths of the constraints.

    d. *Learning dynamics.* CV_{net}'s learning algorithm governs how the strengths of constraints s_i change in response to data from the target language.

Network-level descriptions of these four components are described next, first generally (Section 3.1), then in detail (Sections 3.2–3.4). Section 3.5 shows formally that CV_{net} possesses the competence necessary to realize CVT. Descriptions pertaining to CV_{net}'s abstract genomic encoding—CV_{gene}—will be presented in Section 4.

Figure 1

3.1 CV$_{net}$ in a nutshell

From a structural standpoint, the CV$_{net}$ network must be capable of representing input strings, output strings, and the correspondence relationships between them, since each of these are the basic elements of the symbolic description to which the OT constraints apply (9a). The overall structure of the CV$_{net}$ network is a variant of the Sequence-Mapping Network of Touretzky 1989; Touretzky and Wheeler 1990, 1991.

One crucial innovation relative to Touretzky and Wheeler's network—and indeed relative to standard connectionist networks in general—is that the weight of any connection is not a primitive, atomic quantity, but a composite of finer-grained elements we can call **subconnections**, for the moment; their relative strengths are given by the connection coefficients (9b). This innovation results from the network implications of several general properties of the constraints of an OT grammar. First, a single constraint is realized by a set of subconnections that is distributed throughout the network: the ONSET constraint applies to all onsets, everywhere. Second, these subconnections are essentially a local pattern repeated over and over throughout the network; thus, the units of the network can be divided into various *types*, and the subconnections realizing a particular constraint are simply determined by the types of units connected, thus repeating themselves throughout the network, everywhere units of these types are found. And finally, several constraints may involve subconnections between the same types of units; the subconnections associated with one constraint simply add their contribution to those of the other constraints, all contributions being weighted by the strength of the corresponding constraint. The weighted sum of the contributions of all the subconnections between two units is the total connection weight between those units. As the strength of a constraint changes during learning, all the subconnections throughout the network that realize this constraint must adjust their contributions in concert, to maintain the pattern of subconnections defining that particular constraint.

More formally, consider the connection to a unit φ of type Φ from a unit ψ of type Ψ. The weight of this connection, $W_{\varphi\psi}$, is a sum of contributions from all the constraints (their 'subconnections'). Each constraint $\mathbb{C}_i$ contributes a quantity $s_i c^i_{\Phi\psi}$: the constraint's connection coefficient to units of type Φ from units of type Ψ, $c^i_{\Phi\psi}$, multiplied by the strength s_i of the constraint.

(10)   Connection weights in CV$_{net}$

   The weight of the connection to a unit φ of type Φ from a unit ψ of type Ψ is the sum of contributions from the N_{con} constraints $\mathbb{C}_i$:

$$W_{\varphi\psi} = \sum_{i=1}^{N_{con}} s_i c^i_{\Phi\psi} \,.$$

   The ranking of constraints is realized via the multiplicative factor, the strength s_i of each constraint $\mathbb{C}_i$, where higher rank is realized by larger s_i.

With regard to activation dynamics (discussed in Section 3.5), CV$_{net}$ is a stochastic Boolean harmonic network (Section 9:4), like those of Boltzmann machines (Ackley, Hinton, and Sejnowski 1985; Hinton and Sejnowski 1986) or Harmony Theory (Smolensky 1984, 1986).

Under the nativist hypothesis, learning an OT grammar in the symbolic description consists of ranking constraints with respect to one another. At the network level, learning occurs by altering the strengths of individual connection weights; nonetheless, each constraint must maintain its integrity throughout the learning process. The learning dynamics of CV_{net} is therefore given by a learning algorithm in which each constraint $\mathbb{C}_i$'s strength s_i is altered, thereby raising or lowering in concert the contributions of all subconnections realizing a constraint $\mathbb{C}_i$, rather than separately altering the weights of individual connections. This procedure is a generalized version of the Boltzmann machine learning algorithm, discussed in Section 3.6.1.

This feature of the network structure, in which constraints are described as subcomponents of the network, appears to be crucial to implementing an OT grammar in this kind of system. Such a system has to our knowledge not been explored previously within the connectionist framework. Therefore, it should be considered both a novel hypothesis regarding the possible nature of some connectionist systems in cognition and an essential (and falsifiable) prediction made by OT grammatical theory concerning these same systems.

The CVT constraints realized in CV_{net} (Section 2.1) are of several kinds. The violable constraints of *Con* (PARSE, FILL^V, FILL^C, ONSET, and NOCODA) are subject to 'reranking' (strength adjustment) in the learning process and to domination by other constraints. Inviolable constraints, both *Gen* constraints (IDENTITY, LINEARITY, INTEGRITY, and UNIFORMITY) and structural constraints (OUTPUTIDENTITY, NOOUTPUTGAPS, CORRESPONDENCE, and NUCLEUS), are not subject to reranking and are never dominated.

3.2 Overall network architecture of CV_{net}

As shown in Figure 2, the CV_{net} network consists of three layers: an input string layer, an output string layer, and a correspondence layer. The input and output segments are represented in a strictly local fashion. The set of input units consists of pairs of adjacent nodes, one for C and one for V. The C-V pairs of input units each designate the segment in a given position relative to the left edge of the string; we draw the pair designating the leftmost segment in the leftmost position on the page, and so on. Thus, the string always begins at the leftmost position in the input layer.

The output string is represented in a similar fashion. The initial segment of the output string is always represented by the uppermost triple of $C_{onset}/C_{coda}/V$ units in the output string layer. The initial output segment is determined by the activation of these three units: it is a C parsed as a syllable onset if the C_{onset} unit is active; it is a C parsed as a syllable coda if the C_{coda} unit is active; and it is a V (parsed, as always, as a syllable nucleus). In an interpretable output, at most one unit can be active per triple. Units designating V are triangular; those designating C_{onset} are circular; those

Figure 1

Figure 2. The basic network: Input, output, and correspondence layers

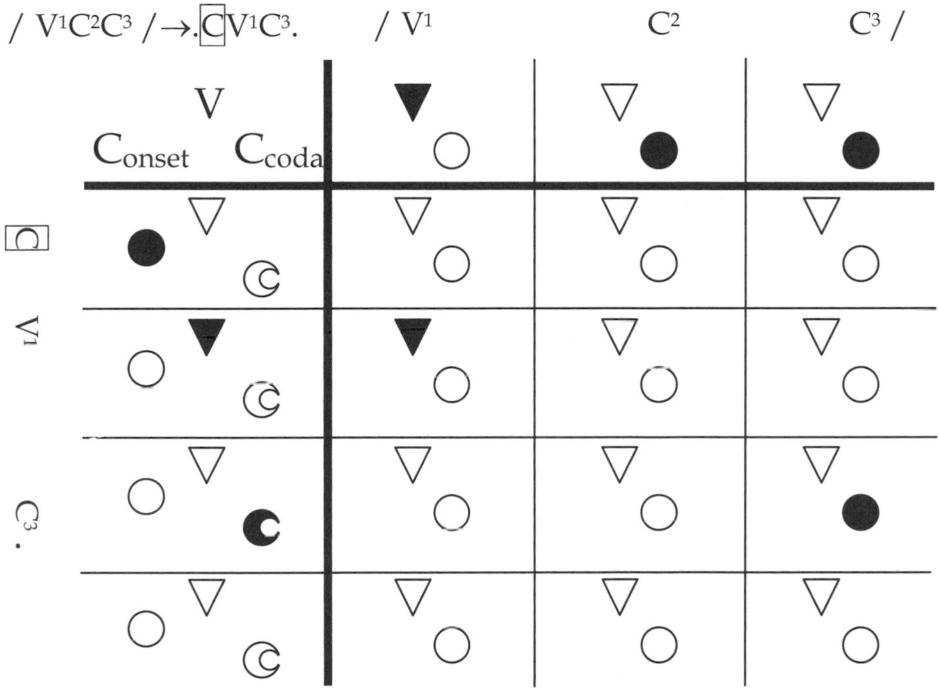

designating C_{coda} are crescent-shaped.

The architectural relationship between the input and output string layers and the correspondence layer is best understood by considering the correspondence layer as a two-dimensional grid (see Figure 2; the gridlines are added only for ease of viewing). This technique for representing string-to-string mappings was proposed by Touretzky and Wheeler (1991).[7] The activity pattern shown is interpreted as an input string $/V^1C^2C^3/$ mapped to an output string $.\fbox{C}V^1C^3$. The appropriate input and output units are active, shown as shading (black = 1, white = 0). The activation in the correspondence layer is interpreted as follows. The first segment of the input (V^1) is in correspondence with the second segment of the output: there is an active correspondence unit that is both directly below this input unit and directly to the right of this output unit. Beneath the input V^1 unit, exactly one correspondence unit is active; it indicates the output position into which V^1 is parsed. The first segment of the output is an epenthetic onset C ($\fbox{C}$): it is in correspondence with no input segment; there is no active correspondence unit directly to the right of the topmost output C_{onset}

---

[7] Interestingly, this connectionist innovation anticipated by several years the closely related, independently developed OT proposal by McCarthy and Prince (1995), Correspondence Theory.

Figure 3. Microstructure of a connection

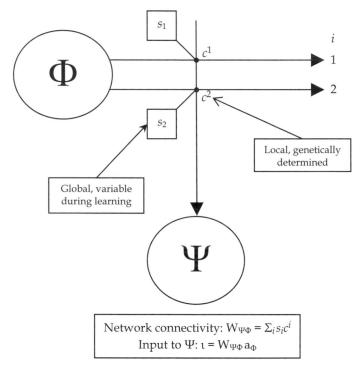

Network connectivity: $W_{\Psi\Phi} = \Sigma_i s_i c^i$

Input to Ψ: $\iota = W_{\Psi\Phi} a_\Phi$

unit. The second input segment (C^2) is not parsed into the output (it is deleted); there is no active correspondence unit directly below the second input C unit.

Each C-V input pair is connected to each $C_{onset}/C_{coda}/V$ output triple via a pair of correspondence units: each V correspondence unit connects to the V input unit directly above it and the V output unit directly to its left; each C correspondence unit connects to the input C unit above it and both output C units to its left (C_{onset} and C_{coda}). Additionally, there are connections between the correspondence units themselves (described in detail below) and between the output units. All connections are symmetric, as usual for harmonic constraint-satisfaction networks (Chapter 9).

3.3 Constraints and connections in CV$_{net}$

Section 3.4 describes the connections realizing each constraint. The numbers given for any constraint $\mathbb{C}_i$ are its connection coefficients $c^i_{\Phi\Psi}$, which ultimately contribute to connection weights $W_{\Phi\Psi}$ in proportion to the constraint's strength, s_i (10) (see Figure 3). Thus, a constraint's fixed connection coefficients determine the sign and relative magnitude of the weights realizing that constraint's contribution to the grammar; the

Figure 3

absolute magnitude of this contribution is determined by the varying constraint strength. Thus, the *relationship* between different connection weights is the innate knowledge provided by a constraint. This relationship is maintained over the course of learning, although the absolute magnitude of the weights changes as a particular grammar is learned.

Because the numbers specifying each constraint given below are merely connection coefficients, comparison of these numbers between *different* constraints is not meaningful (independent of the constraint strengths).

The inviolable constraints in CV_{net} can be thought of as one large constraint, since their strengths relative to one another are unchanging, and their strengths must simply be sufficiently large relative to the strengths of all violable constraints. The distinct inviolable constraints are discussed separately below for the sake of comprehensibility. In discussions of CV_{net} at the network level (and later at the genome level), 'Gen' will denote the collection of all inviolable constraints (7) and (8), including those called 'structural' in the symbolic description.

The particular nature of the inviolable constraints is intimately tied to the nature of the representation chosen for the network. There are two ways that an inviolable constraint can be encoded. The first, and simplest, is for there not to be a state of the network that corresponds to a violation of the constraint. For instance, there is no explicit constraint preventing the network from outputting some symbol other than C or V, such as P or Q; but since there is no unit in the local representation corresponding to any other symbols, there is an implicit constraint on the network that the output symbols are C_{onset}, C_{coda}, V, or nothing.

The second, more complicated way to realize an inviolable constraint in the network is the same way the violable constraints are realized: explicitly, through a set of connection weights.[8] Only those inviolable constraints for which it is necessary to have an explicit realization are described below: these constitute what we here call *Gen*. At the network level, the constraints in *Gen* have the potential to be ranked among the constraints of *Con*; yet they must not be, if the network is truly to contain innate knowledge of UG. This is an issue that must be addressed in CV_{net}'s learning algorithm (Section 3.6).

Finally, CV_{net} units have biases (or thresholds) as well as connections. As explained in Section 9:1.5, a unit's bias can always be replaced by a 'bias connection' to that unit from a special 'bias unit' B that is always ON ($a_b \equiv 1$).[9] In our diagrams of the network realization of a constraint $\mathbb{C}$, this unit B will not be shown explicitly. Instead,

---

[8] This distinction may be similar to Elman et al.'s (1996) distinction between representational and architectural nativism. To the extent that the right representation could generate the appropriate implicit constraints to account for the linguistic data, architectural nativism has much to offer. The main difference between such an account and the current one seems to be the role of learning in the system. At first glance, architectural nativism does not seem to allow for constraints of the type linguistic theory suggests remain intact during the learning process. However, implicit constraints are set aside here not for theoretical reasons, but because on a practical level they are more difficult to study.

[9] A 'bias unit' is a construct of expository and computational convenience and does not have any conceptual significance of a biological nature. Its connection w to a unit a is computationally equivalent to a threshold $-w$ for a, which is a feature of biological neurons.

Figure 4. IDENTITY. All connection coefficients are –1.

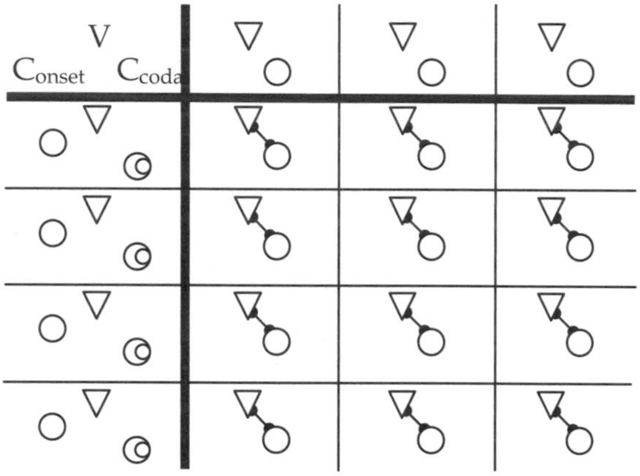

the connection coefficient from B to a given unit will be shown as a number placed within that unit; this **bias coefficient**, when multiplied by the strength s_i of $\mathbb{C}_i$, gives $\mathbb{C}_i$'s contribution to the unit's absolute bias (or **bias weight**). Bias connections are implicitly included in all our general references to the network's 'connection coefficients' or 'connection weights'—in particular, the equations defining the activation-spreading and learning processes also govern bias connections. Thus, for example, among the connection coefficients $c^i_{\Phi\psi}$ of (9b) are the bias coefficients $c^i_{\Phi B}$; among the connection weights described by equation (10) are the bias weights. For a unit of type Φ, the bias weight is as follows:

$$(11) \quad W_{\varphi B} = \sum_{i=1}^{N_{con}} s_i c^i_{\Phi B}$$

3.4 Constraints realized in CV_{net}

We now describe the connection coefficient pattern, including bias coefficients, that realizes each individual constraint. These patterns are illustrated in Figures 4–15, which should be consulted while reading the verbal explanations to follow.

Constraints in *Gen*: (7)–(8)

3.4.1 IDENTITY

A –1 connection coefficient between paired C and V correspondence units prevents both from being active at the same time; this coefficient pattern, illustrated in Figure 4, realizes IDENTITY.[10] (That is, a candidate activation pattern in which both paired

[10] This constraint may not be strictly necessary, since the combination of OUTPUTIDENTITY and

Figure 4

Figure 5. LINEARITY

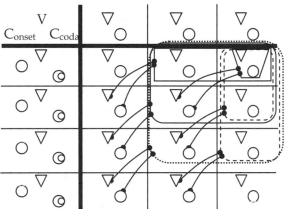

units are active has Harmony value –1, while the pattern resulting from deactivating any one, or both, of these units has higher Harmony: 0. Here we consider only the Harmony contributions from connections realizing the single constraint in question, in this case, IDENTITY.)

3.4.2 LINEARITY

Although visually complex (see Figure 5), LINEARITY is conceptually simple. Linear order is preserved from input to output by inhibitory (–1) connection coefficients between correspondence units. Each correspondence unit (φ) has mutually inhibitory connections with every other correspondence unit (ψ) for which the following is true: the input unit connected to φ linearly precedes the input unit connected to ψ, but the output unit connected to φ linearly follows the output unit connected to ψ. Connections are formed between C and V units as well as from C to C and from V to V. (As in the case of IDENTITY, these inhibitory connections entail that a maximum-Harmony state will not have active two correspondence units that would instantiate a violation of LINEARITY.)

3.4.3 INTEGRITY

The connection coefficient pattern for INTEGRITY is shown in Figure 6. Mutual inhibition (–1 connection coefficients) between correspondence units in the same *column* penalizes multiple output correspondents of a single active *input* unit. (Such multiple

CORRESPONDENCE indirectly guarantees that the simultaneous activity of paired C and V correspondence units is harmonically dispreferred. However, there is some benefit to conceptual compartmentalization of the different constraints, particularly for the sake of generalizability to future analyses (if, for instance, a constraint is eliminated or becomes violable), so it is separately specified. Note also that IDENTITY bears only partial resemblance to the IDENT constraint of Correspondence Theory.

Figure 6. INTEGRITY. All connection coefficients are –1.

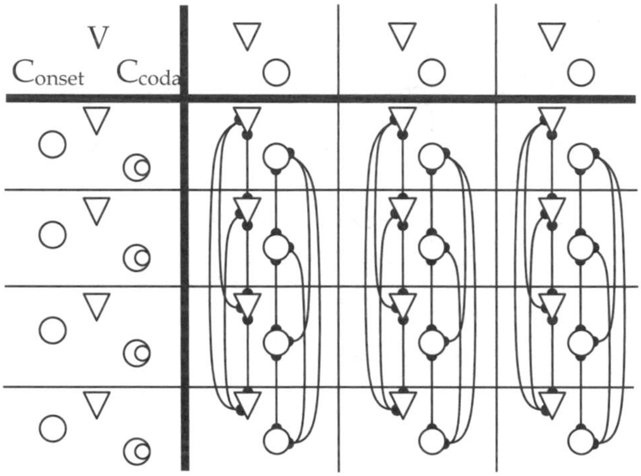

correspondents will in fact be explicitly encouraged by the realization of the PARSE constraint below.)

3.4.4 UNIFORMITY

Analogously to INTEGRITY, for UNIFORMITY mutual inhibition between correspondence units in the same *row* penalizes multiple correspondents of a single active *out-*

Figure 7. UNIFORMITY. All connection coefficients are –1.

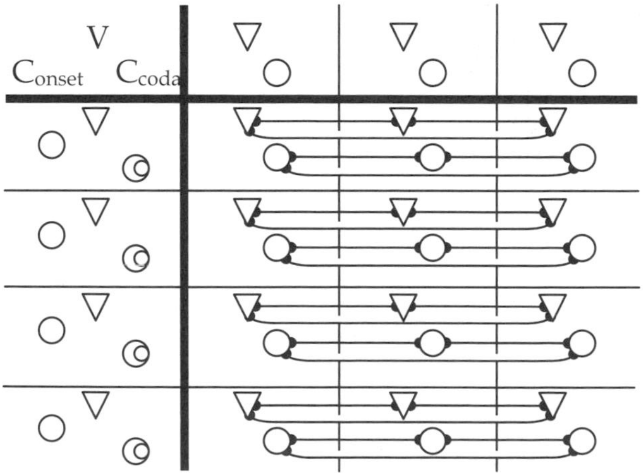

Figure 7

Figure 8. OUTPUTIDENTITY. All connection coefficients are –1.

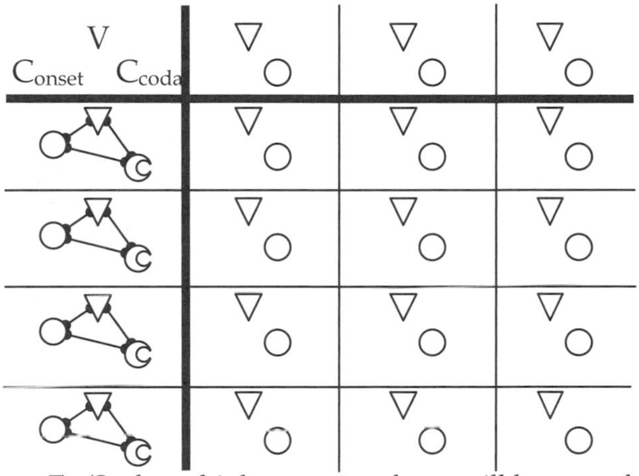

put unit (see Figure 7). (Such multiple correspondence will be rewarded by the realizations of the FILL constraints below.)

3.4.5 OUTPUTIDENTITY

OUTPUTIDENTITY is realized by –1 connection coefficients between the elements in each output $C_{onset}/C_{coda}/V$ triple (see Figure 8). These inhibitory connections have the effect of penalizing states in which more than one unit in each triple is active. In preliminary simulations, we have found that this constraint must be "ranked" significantly higher than some other *Gen* constraints (e.g., CORRESPONDENCE), that is, the –1 connection coefficients listed here must be multiplied by a factor greater than 1 when the *Gen* constraints are combined. Otherwise, some other *Gen* constraints will force multiple units to be active within the same triple.

3.4.6 NOOUTPUTGAPS

In the connection coefficient pattern for NOOUTPUTGAPS, all output units (except the first set) have a –1 bias (see Figure 9). Positive (+1) connections between each unit in an output triple and each unit in the following triple repay this Harmony deficit when one of the units immediately preceding an output unit is also active.

3.4.7 CORRESPONDENCE

CORRESPONDENCE (Figure 10) makes use of the same wiring pattern as PARSE and FILL, but it is a purely structural constraint. The –2 bias on each correspondence unit creates a Harmony deficit when the unit is active; this is repaid only when *both* the input unit and one of the output units it is connected to are active. If only one of its

Figure 9. NOOUTPUTGAPS. All connection coefficients are +1,
biases −1.

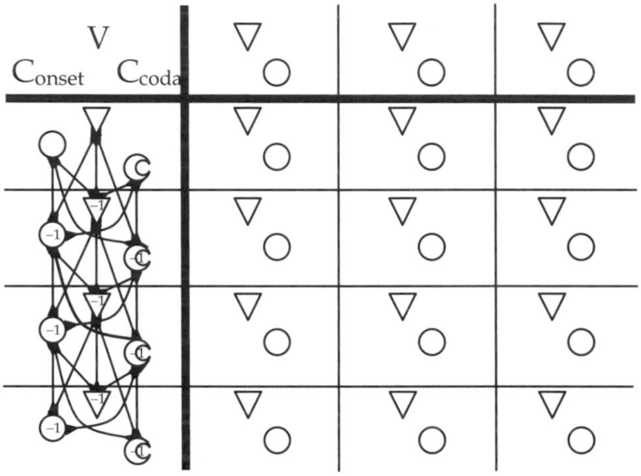

corresponding input and output string units is active, the Harmony of an inactive
correspondence unit ($H = 0$) exceeds that of an active unit ($H = -1$).

3.4.8 NUCLEUS

The connection coefficient pattern for NUCLEUS is shown in Figure 11. Each C_{coda} and
C_{onset} unit (except the first C_{coda} unit) has a –1 bias. A +1 connection to the preceding

Figure 10. CORRESPONDENCE. All connection coefficients are +1.

Figure 10

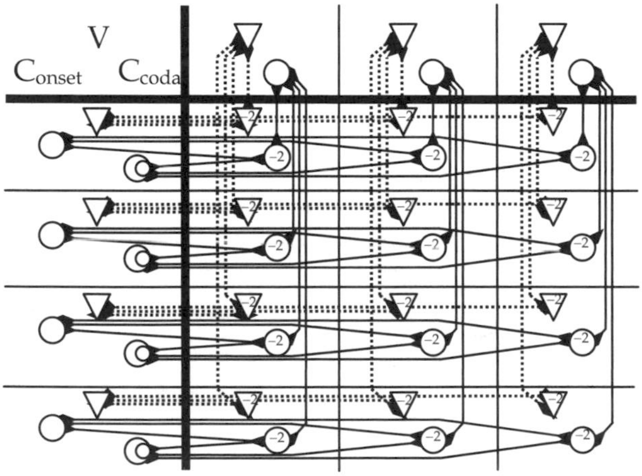

Figure 11. NUCLEUS. All connection coefficients are +1.

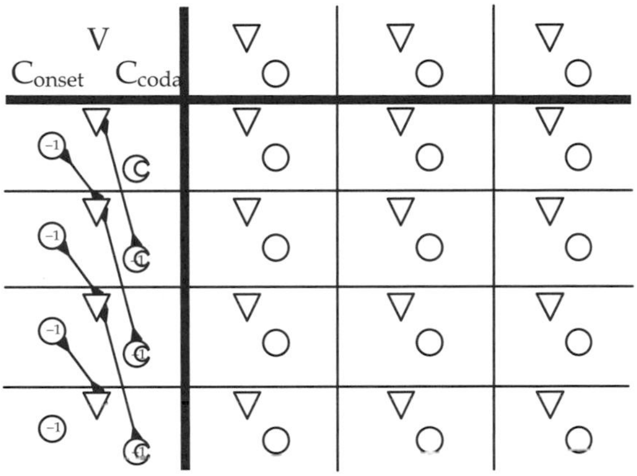

V (for C_{coda}) or following V (for C_{onset}) allows this Harmony deficit to be resolved if this V is also active.

Constraints in *Con*: (6)

We now assume that the *Gen* constraints have sufficiently high strength that they must be satisfied by any optimal activation pattern. The realizations of the violable constraints in *Con* can be designed under the assumption that all relevant activation patterns obey *Gen*.

3.4.9 PARSE

PARSE is realized through connections between each input unit (both C and V) and its associated column of correspondence units, as well as connections between each $C_{onset}/C_{coda}/V$ output unit and its associated row of correspondence units (see Figure 12). PARSE has the same connectivity pattern as CORRESPONDENCE. The two constraints must be handled separately nonetheless, because PARSE is a rerankable violable constraint while CORRESPONDENCE is an inviolable *Gen* constraint.

For PARSE, a bias coefficient of −1 is associated with each input node, and a coefficient of −3 with each correspondence node. All connection coefficients are +2. This has the effect that for any active input unit, a Harmony deficit of −1 is created (from the bias); this deficit can be made up for by the activation of any output unit *as well as* the correspondence unit that is associated with both the active input unit and the active output unit. The Harmony of this configuration is (−1) + (−3) = −4 from the biases, plus (+2) + (+2) = +4 from the connections, for a total of zero net Harmony.[11]

---

[11] The biases on the input units are solely for convenience; they are not necessary. For formal and conceptual purposes, it is often convenient if maximum-Harmony subpatterns have $H = 0$ (e.g., see

Figure 12. PARSE. All connection coefficients are +2.

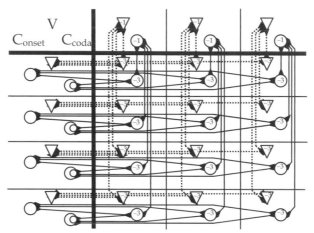

Note that this analysis applies to any output–correspondence unit pair connected to the input unit in question, regardless of the activity of other units in the column. This version of PARSE thus rewards expression of the input signal in the output layer, as much expression as possible. Once is enough for zero Harmony; activating $n > 1$ output correspondents of a single input creates a positive Harmony value of $n - 1$. While PARSE itself exhibits this preference for multiple output correspondents for a given input, two *Gen* constraints discussed above — INTEGRITY and OUTPUTIDENTITY — ensure that no more than one correspondent can appear in an optimal representation.

3.4.10 FILL^V and FILL^C

The FILL constraints function equivalently to PARSE, with the roles of input and output exchanged. The negative bias is associated with any active output unit, and this Harmony deficit is made up for by the activation of input–correspondence unit pairs associated with the output unit in question. Analogously to PARSE, these versions of FILL prefer representations with multiple input correspondents of a single output; these are rendered suboptimal by a *Gen* constraint, UNIFORMITY.

In Figure 13, the constraints FILL^C and FILL^V are shown together, but they are different constraints and are ranked separately. All C units and the connections between them are part of FILL^C (solid lines); all V units and the connections between them are part of FILL^V (dotted lines). All connection coefficients are +2.

Chapter 10); this is the reason for assigning a bias of –1 to each input unit. Since the input units are clamped, such a bias cannot affect processing in the network, although it does change the absolute level of Harmony achieved by the optimal pattern. Only relative, not absolute, Harmony values are relevant to processing and hence to determining the optimal output.

Figure 12

Figure 13. FILL (C and V). All connection coefficients are +2.

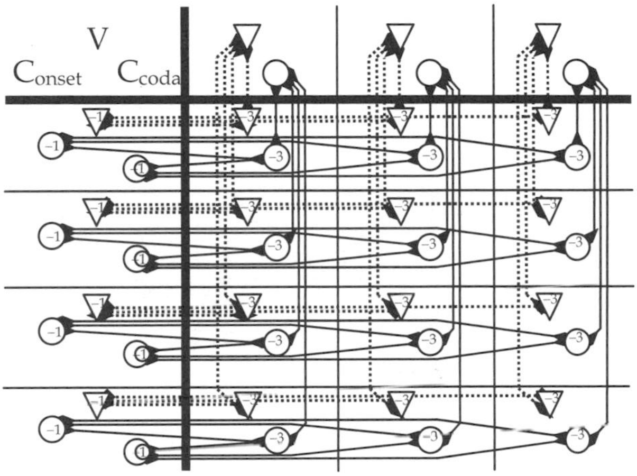

3.4.11 ONSET

ONSET (Figure 14) is realized by a negative bias (–1) on all V output units. This negative Harmony is offset by a +1 connection coefficient between each V unit and the preceding C_{onset} unit.

3.4.12 NOCODA

NOCODA (Figure 15) is implemented by a –1 bias on every C_{coda} unit in the output.

Figure 14. ONSET. All connection coefficients are +1.

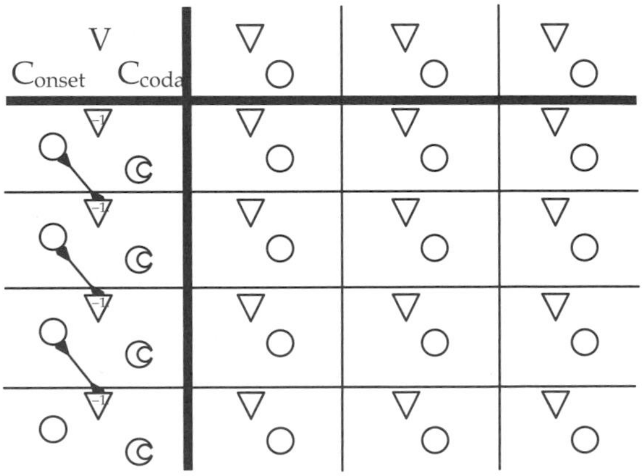

Figure 15. NoCODA. Biases only (–1).

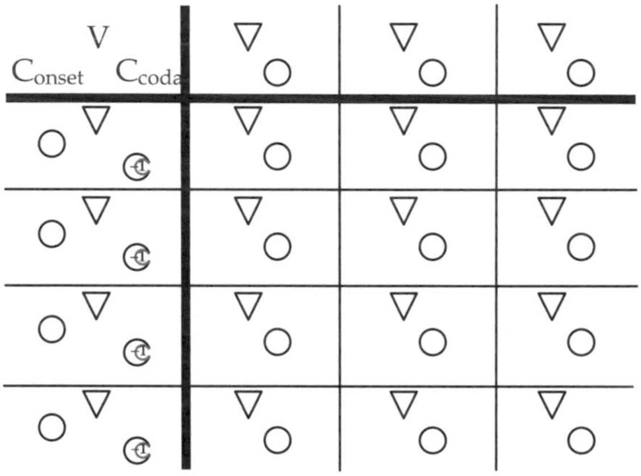

3.5 The activation dynamics of CV$_{net}$

CV$_{net}$ must be a harmonic—Harmony-maximizing—network. Among these networks, we choose the Boltzmann machine architecture, which provides a good environment for learning as well as Harmony maximization (Section 9:4.1). As required for this architecture, the connection matrix of CV$_{net}$ is symmetric (all connections are two-way, with the same weight in each direction).

The units of CV$_{net}$, like standard Boltzmann machine units, have Boolean activation values: 0 and 1. These units are stochastic: the activation-spreading algorithm (12) contains a degree of randomness regulated by the **computational temperature** parameter T. The greater the input to a unit, the higher the probability it will be active (activation 1); the lower the temperature T, the higher the probability the unit will be active if its input is positive, or inactive if its input is negative.

(12)   Boltzmann machine activation dynamics

Upon updating its activation value, a unit φ with input ι_φ stochastically chooses a value 0 or 1 according to

$$pr(a_\varphi = 1) = \frac{1}{1 + e^{-\iota_\varphi/T}} = f^{\log}(\iota_\varphi/T), \qquad \iota_\varphi \equiv \sum_\psi W_{\varphi\psi} a_\psi,$$

where $f^{\log}$ is the logistic sigmoid function $f^{\log}(x) \equiv 1/[1 + e^{-x}]$.

The CV$_{net}$ network operates as follows. An input is provided to the net by clamping the appropriate C/V units in the input layer. An initial high value of T is set. The correspondence and output string units update their activation values asynchronously (one at a time), with a high initial degree of randomness. Updating continues as T is lowered and the randomness is 'cooled' out of the system; this procedure is

Figure 15

called **simulated annealing**. In the idealized limit of a sufficiently gentle cooling schedule, the network state, with probability 1, approaches the state that globally maximizes Harmony. If the constraint strengths s_i are appropriately set for realizing a particular OT ranking of the CVT constraints, the maximal Harmony state will realize the correct (optimal) parse of the input. The remaining question for the network-level description of CV_{net} is thus, how are the correct constraint strengths learned for a target language in the CV typology?

3.6 Learning constraint strengths from examples of optimal forms

Our design for CV_{net} provides a connectionist network and a set of Harmony functions (connection patterns) realizing the constraints in *Gen* and *Con*. What this LAD needs to accomplish is to learn a set of constraint strengths s_i realizing the correct constraint ranking for the language $\mathcal{L}$ to be acquired. We assume, as is the norm in nativist learning theories, that this is to be achieved on the basis of examples of complete, optimal forms from $\mathcal{L}$. The problem is to find a set of constraint strengths s_i such that the composite Harmony function $H_{\mathfrak{H}}$ they define (described below in (22)) realizes the underlying constraint hierarchy $\mathfrak{H}$; that is, every observed form is optimal according to $H_{\mathfrak{H}}$, among all forms that share the observed form's input. As discussed in Section 3.7, such a set of constraint strengths s_i must exist.

We apply a variant of the **Boltzmann Machine Learning Algorithm (BMLA)** to the problem of estimating the s_i parameters from the observed data. The BMLA distinguishes **visible** and **hidden** units: the visible units are the input and output units,[12] whose activation values are given for training examples. Any remaining units — never specified by training data — are hidden units. The version of CV_{net} presented here has no hidden units, but extensions will likely require them, so they will be included in the following general discussion of learning.

3.6.1 Boltzmann learning

The BMLA is an optimization algorithm that realizes gradient descent in the space of network weights, in order to minimize an **error function** that measures the degree to which the network's behavior differs from its desired behavior, in the following sense. When stochastic unit updating is performed in the Boltzmann machine, at a given computational temperature, each point in weight space gives rise to a probability distribution over network activation states, and in particular, over visible-unit activation patterns. The empirical distribution of observed data (patterns on the visible units) is viewed as specifying a **target** distribution. The error function that the BMLA tries to minimize is a measure of the difference between the target distribution and the distribution generated by the network. For networks like CV_{net} in which the visible units are partitioned into input and output sets, the error function measures the

---

[12] In the general computational discussions of this section and the next, the 'input' units are our C/V input string units, and the 'output' units are all the remaining units, including both the $C_{onset}/C_{coda}/V$ output string units and the correspondence units.

difference between the conditional distributions of output patterns given input patterns.

The BMLA updates each individual network weight $W_{\varphi\psi}$ in proportion to $W_{\varphi\psi}$'s potential for decreasing the error function: the weight-change vector is proportional to the (negative) gradient of the error function in weight space. But in our case, we do not wish to allow the network weights to be modified independently. Rather, we would like to modify only the constraint strengths s_i. So the approach we take is to derive a learning rule that modifies the s_i values in (negative) proportion to the gradient of the same BMLA error function in s_i-space. In the normal BMLA, the amount by which a given network weight $W_{\varphi\psi}$ changes when updated is as computed in (13).

(13) $\Delta W_{\varphi\psi} = \varepsilon[E\{a_\varphi a_\psi \mid \text{input \& output clamped}\} - E\{a_\varphi a_\psi \mid \text{input clamped}\}]$

ε is a small positive constant, the learning rate. The quantity $E\{a_\varphi a_\psi \mid \text{input \& output clamped}\}$ is the expected value (E) of the product of the activations of the units φ and ψ—that is, the probability that the units φ and ψ are ON together—when all the visible units are clamped by training data; $E\{a_\varphi a_\psi \mid \text{input clamped}\}$ is that probability when only the input units are clamped. Intuitively, equation (13) says that if the units φ and ψ are ON together more frequently when *observing* the outputs (all visible units are clamped) than when *computing* the outputs (only inputs are clamped: the output is determined by the weights), then the weight connecting φ and ψ should be increased. This has the effect of increasing the conditional probability that one unit will turn ON given that the other one is ON, which will increase the probability that they are ON together. Similarly, the learning equation has the opposite effect if the probabilities fall in the other order.

One common way to apply the BMLA computationally is as follows. For each observed visible pattern p, run two phases: in the (output) **clamped phase** $\mathcal{P}^+$, all visible units are clamped to the observed pattern p, and the hidden units (if any) are allowed to update stochastically using simulated annealing; the computational temperature is lowered to a small value, until (ideally) the unclamped units reach a fixed activation pattern. The expected value $E\{a_\varphi a_\psi \mid \text{input \& output clamped}\}$ is computed for each unit pair (φ, ψ) and saved. Next, the process is repeated in an **unclamped phase** $\mathcal{P}^-$, in which only the input units are clamped and the output and hidden units are allowed to update stochastically; then $E\{a_\varphi a_\psi \mid \text{input clamped}\}$ is computed for all unit pairs (φ, ψ). Finally, the weight $W_{\varphi\psi}$ is changed according to the update equation (13).

3.6.2   Learning in CV_{net}

In the case of CV_{net}, a rederivation of the gradient-descent-in-error learning algorithm in which the s_i values are taken to be the modifiable parameters results in the following learning rule (Mathis, in preparation):

(14)   Learning equation: Strengths for sub-Harmony functions

$$\Delta s_i = \varepsilon[E\{H_i \mid \text{input \& output clamped}\} - E\{H_i \mid \text{input clamped}\}]$$

Figure 15

Here, H_i is the **unscaled** value of the Harmony function H_i. That is, when running the network, we must use the full composite Harmony function $H_{\mathcal{H}}$, in which each of the individual Harmony functions H_i is weighted by the corresponding s_i, but the quantities $E\{H_i\}$ that we compute for learning must be the Harmonies of the H_i *without* the s_i scaling factor. The s_i are changed in proportion to the difference in these unscaled Harmonies.

Equation (14) strongly resembles the original learning algorithm (13), except now we are comparing *Harmonies* in the clamped and unclamped phases. The intuition is rather similar: For a given observed visible pattern, imagine running the network in the unclamped phase $\mathcal{P}^-$ under $H_{\mathcal{H}}$ and obtaining a single final visible pattern. Now consider an individual Harmony function H_i. Suppose that the network's final state in the unclamped phase $\mathcal{P}^-$ has *lower* Harmony according to H_i than does the fully clamped visible pattern (phase $\mathcal{P}^+$). This means that the network found an output pattern that didn't satisfy the ith constraint as well as the target output pattern did. In this case, the learning rule will increase the weighting on H_i. This has the effect of making the term $s_i H_i$ more important in $H_{\mathcal{H}}$, thus increasing the probability that the network will find a state that satisfies H_i better next time. Similarly, if the network's output state satisfies H_i better than the target pattern does, then perhaps H_i is *too important* in the current $H_{\mathcal{H}}$. Decreasing s_i in this case should have the effect that the state the network finds next time will not reflect as strong a priority for satisfying H_i.

This learning algorithm, when viewed as a LAD for OT, does not in general have the important property that it is incapable of learning impossible languages, since it is in theory able to learn languages that correspond to settings of the s_i parameters that do not realize strict domination—they do not meet the 'exponential strength' condition (22c) discussed below. Unlike the symbolic OT learning algorithms of Tesar and Smolensky 1993, 1998, 2000 and Tesar 1998a, b (see Section 12:3 of this book), our CV$_{net}$ learning algorithm is not informed by the a priori knowledge that the target language is generated by a strict domination hierarchy of the *Con* constraints. Indeed, the result of learning in CV$_{net}$ could potentially be any linear combination of these constraints. Hence, the learning algorithm is in general too unconstrained to be a true realization of the LAD we seek.

It is important to note that, while it may not yet be *fully* informed by UG, the learning algorithm for constraint strengths (14) is nonetheless extremely strongly constrained: it is only capable of learning grammars consisting of the universal constraints *Con*, interacting via numerical weighting. This is far more constrained than would be a standard application of Boltzmann learning (13) to the same network architecture, in which all the weights in the network would need to be independently estimated from the observed data. For example, if our example network had N_{in} input units and N_{out} output string units, even with our restricted connectivity and enforced weight symmetry, there would still be at least $\frac{1}{2}(N_{in}N_{out}^2 + N_{out}N_{in}^2 + 20N_{out}N_{in})$ modifiable weights. For $N_{in} = N_{out} = 6$, this would mean at least 1,152 weights. In contrast, regardless of the size of the input and output string layers, our constrained learning algorithm has only as many underlying modifiable parameters to estimate as there are constraints: in this case, 6 (if *Gen* is treated as one constraint; otherwise, 13). Thus, while our system is not constrained to realize and learn only systems of strictly ranked constraints, its limited representational capacity should in principle result in greatly speeded learning as a function of the number of observed examples; accordingly, for a fixed number of examples, it should be expected to generalize better to new examples from the same language than would the unconstrained system.

3.6.3 *Gen*

In the CV_{net} learning algorithm as discussed so far, all of the constraint strengths are modifiable, even the one (or ones) corresponding to the inviolable constraint(s) in *Gen*. To encode the a priori knowledge that the *Gen* constraints must effectively outrank all the constraints of *Con* requires distinguishing the *Gen* constraints in the learning algorithm. The strength of these constraints must be greater than that of the *Con* constraints, in a sense made precise in the exponential strength condition (22c) below.

This condition arises from the requirement that no combination of Harmony differences contributed by the (scaled) violable constraints in *Con* can ever exceed the (scaled) Harmony differences from the *Gen* constraints between a state that satisfies *Gen* and one that does not (see the Appendix). To anticipate (22), let $\mathbb{C}_0$ denote *Gen* (considered as a single constraint), and let $\delta_{min}(H_0)$ be the smallest Harmony difference between a state that satisfies *Gen* and one that does not. Denote the largest Harmony difference contributed by a violable constraint $\mathbb{C}_i$ by $range(H_i)$. Then the sum of Harmony differences due to all the violable constraints $\mathbb{C}_i$ in *Con*—each weighted by its strength s_i—must never exceed $\delta_{min}(H_0)$ weighted by s_0, the strength of $\mathbb{C}_0$ = *Gen*. So the preeminence of *Gen* requires its strength s_0 to satisfy (15).

(15) $s_0 > \Sigma_i \, s_i \, range(H_i)/\delta_{min}(H_0)$

There are many ways a learning algorithm might achieve such a condition. The method we propose for CV_{net} is one for which a relatively straightforward genomic encoding can be provided. The initial value of s_0 is set so that the condition (15) is satisfied in the initial state. Then, each time a *Con* constraint's strength s_i is altered during learning, the *Gen* strength s_0 is also altered to ensure that (15) remains satisfied. This can be achieved by the following learning equation for s_0:

(16)   Each change Δs_i induces an accompanying change $\Delta s_0 = k_i \Delta s_i$,

where $k_i \equiv range(H_i)/\delta_{min}(H_0)$. If the connection coefficients $c^i_{\Phi\psi}$ defining all H_i are appropriately normalized—by multiplying them by $k_r/range(H_i)$—it can be arranged that, after normalization, all values of $range(H_i)$ are the same: k_r. Then all k_i have the same value, as in (17).

(17) $k_i = k_r/\delta_{min}(H_0) \equiv k_G$ for all $i = 1, 2, ..., N_{con}$

Figure 15

3.6.4 Local computation of global parameters

The learning equation in (14) is stated in terms of the expected value of Harmony functions:

(18) $\Delta s_i = \varepsilon[E\{H_i \mid \text{input \& output clamped}\} - E\{H_i \mid \text{input clamped}\}]$

Harmony functions are defined globally, over the entire network. Yet network learning rules must be local. Can (18) be locally computed?

   As discussed above, the two expected values can be computed by running the network in two phases: $\mathcal{P}^+$, during which both input and output units are clamped to training data values, and $\mathcal{P}^-$, during which only input units are clamped. A way to achieve the difference in expected values is to *increase* s_i in proportion to the expected value during $\mathcal{P}^+$, and *decrease* s_i in proportion to the expected value during $\mathcal{P}^-$. What then needs to be locally computed, separately, are the two expected values $E\{H_i \mid \mathcal{P}^+\}$ and $E\{H_i \mid \mathcal{P}^-\}$. The Harmony function is

(19) $H_i(\mathbf{a}) \equiv \sum_{\varphi,\psi=1}^{N} c_{\Phi\Psi}^{i}\, a_\varphi a_\psi ,$

where N is the total number of units in the network. Each expected value (in $\mathcal{P}^+$ and $\mathcal{P}^-$) is an average over the N_p training patterns p:

(20) $\varepsilon E\{H_i \mid \mathcal{P}^\pm\} = \varepsilon E\left\{ \sum_{\varphi,\psi=1}^{N} c_{\Phi\Psi}^{i}\, a_\varphi a_\psi \,\middle|\, \mathcal{P}^\pm \right\}$

$$= \frac{\varepsilon}{N_p} \sum_{p=1}^{N_p} \left\{ \sum_{\varphi\psi} c_{\Phi\Psi}^{i}\, a_\varphi^{(p\pm)} a_\psi^{(p\pm)} \right\}$$

$$= \varepsilon' \sum_{\varphi\psi} \left\{ \sum_{p} c_{\Phi\Psi}^{i}\, a_\varphi^{(p\pm)} a_\psi^{(p\pm)} \right\},$$

where $\varepsilon' \equiv \varepsilon/N_p$; $a_\varphi^{(p\pm)}$ is the activation of unit φ when pattern p is processed in phase $\mathcal{P}^\pm$; and in each term of the sum, Φ and Ψ denote the types of the units φ and ψ. Thus, to increase s_i in $\mathcal{P}^+$ by $\Delta s_i = \varepsilon E\{H_i \mid \mathcal{P}^+\}$, it suffices to increment s_i by an amount $\varepsilon' c_{\Phi\Psi}^{i}$ at every connection between a type-Φ unit φ and a type-Ψ unit ψ, for every pattern p for which φ and ψ are simultaneously active. Decrementing s_i in exactly the same manner during $\mathcal{P}^-$ achieves a change $\Delta s_i = -\varepsilon E\{H_i \mid \mathcal{P}^-\}$. The net result of these two learning phases is exactly the change to s_i required by equation (18).

(21) CV_{net} learning algorithm

   During the processing of training data in phase $\mathcal{P}^\pm$, whenever unit φ (of type Φ) and unit ψ (of type Ψ) are simultaneously active, modify s_i by $\pm\varepsilon' c_{\Phi\Psi}^{i}$.

Included in (21) is a modification of s_i by $\pm\varepsilon' c_{\Phi B}^{i}$ whenever a unit of type Φ is active during $\mathcal{P}^\pm$, where $c_{\Phi B}^{i}$ is the $\mathbb{C}_i$ bias coefficient for unit type Φ (11).

3.7 Is CV$_{net}$ formally a subsymbolic realization of Basic CV Syllable Theory?

To assess whether CV$_{net}$ indeed realizes CVT, we first consider the general case.

The problem of realizing OT constraint interaction in a connectionist network can be formalized along the following lines. Suppose we are given a network $\mathcal{N}$ supporting patterns of activity realizing the candidate linguistic structures S of an OT grammar (perhaps by a tensor product realization: Chapters 5, 7, and 8). Suppose further that each individual symbolic, macrolevel constraint $\mathbb{C}_i$ of the grammar can be realized by a set of microlevel constraints between units in $\mathcal{N}$ encoded in some weight matrix $\mathbb{W}^i$. 'Realize' here means the following. Consider the network $\mathcal{N}^i$ with weight matrix $\mathbb{W}^i$. Consider any two network activation vectors **a** and **a'** that realize two symbolic linguistic structures **S** and **S'** that are candidate parses of a common input **I**. Then the Harmony values of **a** and **a'** in the network $\mathcal{N}^i$ must accord with the relative degrees to which the structures **S** and **S'** satisfy the constraint $\mathbb{C}$: if **S** and **S'** satisfy $\mathbb{C}$ equally well, **a** and **a'** must have equal Harmony, and if **S** satisfies $\mathbb{C}$ better than does **S'**, the Harmony of **a** must be greater than the Harmony of **a'**.

All this is the setup for the problem. Given is a collection of N_{con} Harmony functions H_i (or weight matrices $\mathbb{W}^i$) that respectively realize the OT constraints $\mathbb{C}_i$ in a common connectionist network architecture $\mathcal{N}$. The problem is, what Harmony function (weight matrix) for $\mathcal{N}$, if any, realizes the OT grammar given by the strict domination hierarchy $\mathbb{C}_1 \gg \mathbb{C}_2 \gg \cdots \gg \mathbb{C}_{N_{con}}$?

This problem is formalized and analyzed in the Appendix to this chapter. The resulting theorem (proved in Mathis, in preparation) is given in (22).

(22)   Composite Harmony function for a constraint hierarchy

    a. Suppose G is an OT grammar defined by the strict domination hierarchy

$$\mathcal{H} \equiv \mathbb{C}_1 \gg \mathbb{C}_2 \gg \cdots \gg \mathbb{C}_{N_{con}}$$

        and let $\mathbb{C}_0$ denote *Gen*.

    b. Suppose constraint $\mathbb{C}_i$ is realized in a network $\mathcal{N}$ by a Harmony function H_i encoded in a weight matrix $\mathbb{W}^i$, for $i = 0, 1, \ldots, N_{con}$.

    c. Define a set of constraint strengths $\{s_i\}_{i=0}^{N_i}$ that satisfy the **exponential strength condition**:[13]

$$s_0 = 1,$$

$$s_i < \tfrac{1}{2} s_{i-1}\, \delta_{min}(H_{i-1})\,/\,range(H_i),$$

        where $\delta_{min}(II_i)$ is the minimum, and $range(H_i)$ the maximum, difference in distinct values of H_i for network states realizing candidate symbolic structures.[14]

---

[13] To see transparently why this condition yields weights that exponentially shrink as the hierarchy is descended, rescale each H_i by the factor $1/range(H_i)$, which converts $range(H_i)$ to 1. Then let δ be the largest of the values $\{\delta_{min}(H_i)\}$. Then the condition entails $s_i < \tfrac{1}{2} s_{i-1}\delta$, which in turn implies $s_i < \delta(\tfrac{1}{2})^i$.
[14] H_0 realizes *Gen* by assigning equal Harmony K to all states of $\mathcal{N}$ that satisfy *Gen*, and Harmony less than K to all other states. $\delta_{min}(H_0)$ is the minimum difference in H_0 values between a state that satisfies

Figure 15

d. Then $\mathcal{H}$ is realized in $\mathcal{N}$ by the Harmony function and weight matrix

$$H_{\mathcal{H}} = \sum_{i=0}^{N_{con}} s_i H_i \; ; \quad \mathbb{W}_{\mathcal{H}} = \sum_{i=0}^{N_{con}} s_i \mathbb{W}_i \; .$$

e. Thus, the maximum-Harmony activation vectors of $\mathcal{N}$ realize the optimal structures of $\mathcal{G}$.

This result entails that once we have found a way to realize the individual constraints of CVT in a network $\mathcal{N}$, we are guaranteed that, for each language $\mathcal{L}$ in the CVT typology $\mathcal{T}$, there exists some weight matrix for $\mathcal{N}$ such that the maximum-Harmony states give the correct input-output function for $\mathcal{L}$.

Furthermore, if only the constraint strengths s_i can change as $\mathcal{N}$ learns, the only input-output functions $\mathcal{N}$ is capable of learning are those that derive from a weighted combination of the universal CV constraints. In the general case addressed in (22), for $\mathcal{N}$ to realize a strict domination hierarchy, the connection strengths must obey the special condition (22c), a precise and general version of the exponential growth exhibited in the specific case of Berber syllabification discussed in Section 20:3. Thus, if $\mathcal{N}$ could learn any set of constraint strengths, then it could learn impossible languages — languages outside the typology $\mathcal{T}$ because they correspond to no strict domination hierarchy. And indeed this is, in general, an open problem for our approach at present. (See discussion of numerical constraint weighting in HG in Section 20:1.2.)

Any LAD for CVT consists of four elements: (i) a representation of inputs, outputs, and correspondence relations; (ii) a realization of each individual constraint of CVT; (iii) a way to compute maximum-Harmony forms; (iv) a way to represent and learn the constraint strengths s_i. These four elements correspond, respectively, to the four elements of CV$_{net}$ outlined in (9a–d). Element (i) was addressed in Section 3.2, (ii) in Sections 3.3–3.5, (iii) in Section 3.6, and (iv) in Section 3.6.

4 CV$_{GENE}$: AN ABSTRACT GENOME FOR CV$_{NET}$

Having described CV$_{net}$ at the network level, we now turn to the question posed in Section 1: how, in principle, could the kind of innate knowledge of UG embodied in CV$_{net}$ be encoded in an abstract genome? As outlined in (9) and recapitulated at the end of the previous section, CV$_{net}$ consists of four elements: the architecture, the constraints, the activation dynamics, and the learning dynamics. The complete abstract genomic encoding of CV$_{net}$, CV$_{gene}$, specifies all four of these elements. Sections 4.1 and 4.2 describe the encoding of the architecture. Section 4.3 describes the encoding of constraint-specific weightings in CV$_{gene}$. Section 4.4 addresses briefly the question of activation dynamics. Section 4.5 addresses in detail the question of learning dynamics. Finally, Section 4.6 summarizes CV$_{gene}$.

Gen and one that does not. For CV$_{net}$, $\mathcal{N}$ will be a Boolean network with a finite set of states, so this difference is guaranteed to be nonzero.

As discussed in Section 1.3, a biological genome is a set of blueprints for making proteins. A biological genome specifies a biological neural network via a process of development. Proteins are used as chemical signals to (among a great many other things) direct the growth of an axon toward a target neuron, modulate the strengths of connections, and regulate the learning process. Yet the relationship between chemical signals and a biological neural network is extremely complex. While the task of describing this system at the most explicit level is important and ultimately necessary for a complete understanding of the brain, not all of the details of this mechanism will be relevant to our innateness question. Indeed, considering only the most explicit description of the system serves to mask important insights and generalizations at higher levels. The purpose of developing an abstract genome like CV_{gene} is to find those insights and generalizations. The "genes" of the abstract genome CV_{gene} do not specify the proteins that are relevant at the biological neural network level. Instead, they encode and specify higher-order elements relevant to the connectionist network level at which CV_{net} is described. Still, these elements must be informed and constrained not only by the connectionist network they encode, but also by the biological genome of which they are an abstraction. To remain focused on the question of Chomskyan innateness, as discussed in Section 1.2, the specification of CV_{gene} is limited to those elements directly responsible for building and maintaining the network that instantiates the OT symbolic system.

A biologically inspired genomic representation of the connectivity of the demonstration network CV_{net} must be conceived within the context of developmental processes. The developmental picture will provide a basis for making inferences about the nature of the abstract genome—what kind of machinery is necessary, and what information is explicitly or implicitly represented. Questions related to the development of a system like CV_{net} are of the following nature: How many different kinds of units are there? What information is necessary (from the source unit's point of view) to identify the location of a target unit, and the strength of the connection with it? How are constraints initially specified? How are they maintained through the learning process?

4.1 Unit types

In terms of the symbolic interpretation of the network, there are basically three different kinds of units in our network: input units, correspondence units, and output units. Additionally, there is a distinction between C and V units for input and correspondence units, and between C_{onset}, C_{coda}, and V for output units. This yields a total of seven types of units. This differentiation along two representational dimensions ($C_{onset/coda}$/V vs. input/correspondence/output) is a consequence of the local representation employed in CV_{net}. In a more distributed representation, the binary C/V distinction might well disappear.

The question of how unit types are differentiated has a direct parallel with biological cells. Cell differentiation is an interesting biological process (consider that *all*

Figure 15

of the different cell types in the human body, from hair cells to liver cells to neurons to white blood cells, originate from one original cell, the fusion of a sperm and an egg—a zygote). But the details of how it is accomplished are outside the scope of the current project. Suffice it to say that there is evidence that several different types of neurons exist in the human brain. How many is still a matter of research. It is possible that further study of cell differentiation might yield insight into the representation of different unit types in the abstract genome. For the moment, CV_{gene} simply represents different unit types by having a separate section in the genome for each unit type.

4.2 Connectivity information

We now consider the information that must be specified in order to account for the connectivity of each constraint. In the descriptions (23)–(32), it is assumed that the physical organization of the network corresponds roughly to that of Figures 4–15, with the added provision that adjacent C and V units are aligned linearly in a third dimension; see Figure 16. The axis running from the top to the bottom of the figure will be referred to as the **north-south axis**; that from left to right, as the **east-west axis**. The third C/V axis is the **front-back axis**. The information in (23)–(32) is summarized in Table 1, page 451.

(23)   PARSE/FILL/CORRESPONDENCE

Input units grow south and connect, output units grow east and connect. Correspondence units grow north and west and connect with input and output units.

(24)   ONSET

Short connections grow north-south between C_{onset} units and the following V units in the output.

(25)   NOCODA

No external connections necessary (bias only).

(26)   OUTPUTIDENTITY

Within a single output position, V, C units connect with short-distance front/back growth; C_o, C_c units connect with short-distance east/west growth.

(27)   INTEGRITY

Each correspondence unit (C and V) grows long connections, and connects with all other correspondence units for the same segment type (either C or V) along the north-south axis.

(28)   UNIFORMITY

Each correspondence unit (C and V) grows long connections and connects with all other correspondence units for the same segment type (either C or V) in the east-west axis.

Figure 16. CV$_{net}$ from CV$_{gene}$

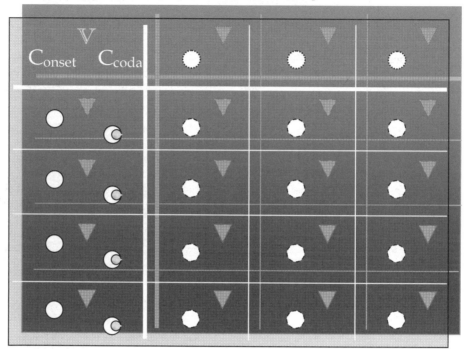

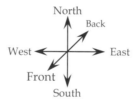

(29)   LINEARITY

Each correspondence unit (C and V) grows long connections toward all correspondence units (C and V) to its north-east (not including due north and due east) and to its south-west (not including due south and due west).

(30)   NoOUTPUTGAPS

Each unit in the output layer grows short connections north-south.

(31)   IDENTITY

Similarly to OUTPUTIDENTITY, short-distance connections grow along the front-back axis between adjacent C and V units in the correspondence layer.

Figure 16

(32) NUCLEUS

V units grow short-distance connections north to the preceding C_{onset} and south to the preceding C_{coda}. C_{onset} units grow south, and C_{coda} units north, to the adjacent V units.

The necessary kinds of information for this connectivity in CV_{gene} can be categorized as **direction**, **extent**, and **target unit type**.

4.2.1 Direction

Using direction in CV_{gene} to specify network connectivity stems from some assumptions about the physical organization of the units, particularly the three-dimensional topography, where each axis constitutes a symbolically meaningful distinction. Topographic organizations are widely attested throughout the known neural structures, including the visual system (orientation: Hubel and Wiesel 1963), the auditory system (pitch: Merzenich and Brugge 1973), and the somatosensory system (anatomical proximity: Mountcastle 1957). The layout of these structures reflects the organization of the sensory modalities from which they take input; the topographic organization of the CV_{net} network, however, is clearly less obvious. Furthermore, the layers in our network are organized two-dimensionally, with output units perpendicular to input units. The use of directionality relies on this two-dimensionality to achieve the right connections. Directionality is used here because it is the most straightforward source of connectivity information, but other sources, such as patterning of unit activity, may prove important, or better, in more complex future models.

The orientation information needed to specify the axes in the present network might stem from sources either external or internal to the network. Axes in biological nervous systems determined by chemical gradients exist from very early on in development (Nusselein-Volhard 1991). Information of this sort regarding an external axis could be used by the units in a network to orient the placement of units and the growth of connections. Alternatively, we hypothesize that a network-internal axis might be created simply by the relationship between an ordered growth pattern and the age of individual cells in the system, although we are not aware of neuroscientific data either for or against such an idea.

CV_{gene} abstracts away from the details of how chemical signals specify the growth of connections. As described in Section 1.3, controlling this growth can be accomplished in multiple ways. Since the effect is ultimately the same regardless of the signal type, directions of growth are simply specified explicitly in CV_{gene} for each combination of unit types and constraint. For example, a gene involved in the INTEGRITY constraint specifies that V correspondence units grow north. Another gene specifies that V correspondence units grow south. Yet another gene specifies that C correspondence units grow north; and so on. Note that more than one constraint may direct the growth of the same connection. This redundancy is not explicitly utilized — it is assumed that a connection is either made or not (connection *strength* is determined through other means), and one directive is enough to cause a connection to be formed. Note also that the symmetric connections must be specified separately. This will be discussed further in Section 5.

4.2.2 Extent

The need for information about extent of connectivity stems from the idea that some projections may grow farther from the source in search of a target than others. Some constraints, such as NoOutputGaps and Onset, require connections that are specifically targeted at adjacent units, while others, such as Correspondence, Parse, and Fill, require connections over a long distance and to multiple targets of the same unit type. So a genomic distinction must be drawn between *local* (short-distance, single-target) and *nonlocal* (long-distance, multiple-target) projections. As with direction, this information is encoded explicitly for each connection. These 'genes' may be thought of as stemming from the type and locality of the growth signal used in each case. For example, if the source of the growth signal is the target itself, and the target is contacted, growth may cease.

4.2.3 Target unit type

The other source of information necessary for specifying connectivity is the unit type of the target. Although the first two sources go a long way toward specifying the target (particularly in the network in question, which is relatively simple), they cannot handle all of the necessary parameters. The connections necessary for Parse, Fill, and Correspondence are a good example. The connections from the input and output units to the correspondence units can be specified simply by the directive to the input and output units 'Grow south' and 'Grow east', respectively, with connections being formed along the way. However, the reverse connections, from the correspondence units to the input and output units, cannot be specified this way, because each correspondence unit does not connect (at least for these constraints) with every unit it encounters along the way as it grows 'north' and 'west'; it targets only units in the input and output layers. Like direction and extent, target unit type is specified explicitly in the genome. It is not difficult to imagine systems of chemical signals that specify whether or not a connection is made; but again, a detailed representation of this system is not relevant.

4.3 Constraint-specific connection weights

We now pass from the genomic encoding of connection formation to the genomic specification of connection weights. At the network level, the weight of a connection to unit φ (of type Φ) from unit ψ (of type Ψ) is the sum of contributions from each constraint $\mathbb{C}_i$, each contributing $s_i c^i_{\Phi\Psi}$, where s_i is the constraint strength (variable during learning) and $c^i_{\Phi\Psi}$ is $\mathbb{C}_i$'s connection coefficient between units of type Φ and Ψ (constant during learning) (10). This constraint-specific connection weighting is an

Figure 16

important difference between this model of connection strength and other neural network models, and it is a crucial component of CV_{net}. Somehow, in such a system, the constraint-specific contributions to the strength of a connection must be specified during the initial development of the network, and also remain constant during the learning process. Since no biological models exist of this kind of system, we must descend briefly to the level of a biological network and consider how such a system could possibly be implemented there, before considering how it might be encoded in CV_{gene}. Additionally, the theoretical strength of the connectivity component of CV_{net} rests at least partly on the biological plausibility of its implementation, so it is important to address this issue explicitly. However, it is equally important to keep in mind that this "biological" model is only a best-guess attempt to describe this aspect of the network in a biologically plausible manner. We do not pretend to be neuroscientists, nor do we present this model as a finished product; rather, it is an exploration of what the theoretical implications of our learning algorithm might be at the biological level.

There are likely other formally equivalent ways to achieve the desired end besides the one we propose. These alternative hypotheses may entail different degrees of abstraction of the relationship between the computational and biological entities, akin to the differing ways that a connectionist unit may be thought to relate to a neuron. We present one relatively straightforward version, in which units are transparently cells (or at least, groups of cells), to see whether it is possible to conceive of how this relationship between connection weights might hold. To the best of our knowledge, the system sketched below is in basic accord with, although not directly supported by, current neuroscientific knowledge. Whether such a system (or some reasonable variant) exists in the human brain is, of course, an open empirical question.

We need two biological quantities: physical embodiments of the strength s_i and of the connection coefficient $c^i_{\Phi\Psi}$. The product of these quantities must be a contribution to "synaptic efficacy." The mechanism we hypothesize to serve this function is spelled out in (33) (see Figure 17).

(33)   Mechanism of constraint-specific connection weights

    a.   For each constraint $\mathbb{C}_i$, $i = 1, 2, \ldots, N_{con}$, there is a distinct chemical messenger (a peptide) P_i circulating in the intercellular space. Define s_i to be the concentration of P_i divided by some constant k_0 (which will be set for convenience below). This concentration will change during learning.

    b.   For each peptide P_i there are two distinct types of *receptors*, R^+_i and R^-_i; R^+_i receptors are found at excitatory synapses, R^-_i receptors at inhibitory synapses. Consider the connection coefficient $c^i_{\Phi\Psi}$, which governs the synapses between type-Φ and type-Ψ units. If the connection coefficient $c^i_{\Phi\Psi}$ is positive (excitatory), then there are $k_1 c^i_{\Phi\Psi}$ receptors of type R^+_i at excitatory synapses between units of type Φ and Ψ. If the connection coefficient $c^i_{\Phi\Psi}$ is negative (inhibitory), then there are $k_1|c^i_{\Phi\Psi}|$ receptors of type R^-_i at inhibitory synapses between units of type Φ and Ψ. The number of receptors

Figure 17. Hypothetical synaptic mechanisms

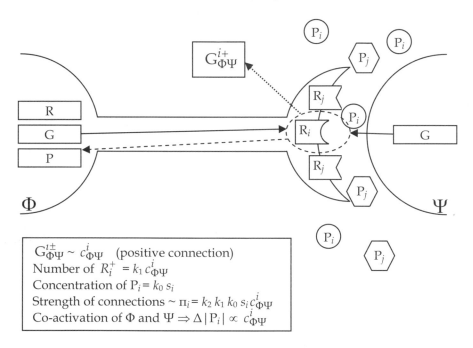

$G_{\Phi\Psi}^{i\pm} \sim c_{\Phi\Psi}^{i}$ (positive connection)

Number of $R_i^+ = k_1 c_{\Phi\Psi}^i$

Concentration of $P_i = k_0 s_i$

Strength of connections $\sim \pi_i = k_2\, k_1\, k_0\, s_i c_{\Phi\Psi}^i$

Co-activation of Φ and $\Psi \Rightarrow \Delta|P_i| \propto c_{\Phi\Psi}^i$

is set during development and does not change thereafter. (Alternatively, the efficacy of the receptors, rather than the absolute number, is proportional to $c_{\Phi\Psi}^i$, and the number of receptors is relatively constant.)

c.   The efficacy of a synapse is maintained by an active process involving the receptors $R_i^\pm$. When a receptor $R_i^\pm$ in a synapse binds peptide P_i, a process π_i is initiated that contributes k to the efficacy of the synapse.

d.   The rate at which π_i occurs is therefore proportional to both the number of receptors $(k_1|c_{\Phi\Psi}^i|)$ and the concentration of P_i $(k_0 s_i)$; call the (positive) constant of proportionality k_2. Then

rate of $\pi_i = k_2\,(k_1|c_{\Phi\Psi}^i|)\,(k_0\, s_i) = k_2 k_1 k_0\,(s_i|c_{\Phi\Psi}^i|)$.

e.   Therefore, combining (33c) and (33d), the magnitude of the contribution of π_i to the efficacy of the synapse to a type-Φ unit φ from a type-Ψ unit ψ is

$|\delta W_{\varphi\psi}| = k k_2 k_1 k_0\,(s_i|c_{\Phi\Psi}^i|)$.

If $c_{\Phi\Psi}^i$ is positive, this contribution is excitatory; if negative, inhibitory. Thus,

Figure 17

$$\delta W_{\varphi\psi} = k k_2 k_1 k_0 \, (s_i c^i_{\Phi\Psi}).$$

f. The efficacy of a synapse is the sum of the contributions of the receptors of all types i at the synapse. Thus, the total connection weight to φ from ψ is

$$W_{\varphi\psi} = k_3 \sum_{i=1}^{N_{con}} s_i c^i_{\Phi\Psi},$$

where $k_3 \equiv k k_2 k_1 k_0$ is a positive constant. Now choose the constant k_0 in the definition of s_i (33a) to be $1/k k_2 k_1$; then $k_3 = 1$.

(Included in this account is the bias weight $W_{\varphi B} = \Sigma_i s_i c^i_{\Phi\Psi}$; this provides a constant input $W_{\varphi B}$ to unit φ. This is the consequence of receptors $R^{\pm}_i$ not in synapses but, say, on the soma; these receptors, when binding P_i, contribute a steady current 'leak', independent of the activation of φ's neighbors.)

The proposal (33) achieves the connection weights demanded by the network-level specification of CV_{net} (10). To generate the correct connection weights, what the genome needs to encode are the coefficients $c^i_{\Phi\Psi}$: the number of receptors of type $R^{\pm}_i$ at synapses between cells of type Φ and Ψ. This number is determined by three things: the identity of the presynaptic cell, the identity of the postsynaptic cell, and the constraint. One possible approach to this encoding is sketched in (34).

(34)   Development of connection coefficients

a. Each cell type produces a chemical identifier, G. During neural development, when two units of types Φ and Ψ come in contact, a certain number of receptors of each type of constraint ($R^{\pm}_i$) are produced at the synapse. This number is modulated by the two chemical signals, $G(\Phi)$ and $G(\Psi)$; their particular chemical structures determine the strength of this modulation on production of $R^{\pm}_i$ receptors. The nature of the interaction of Gs with each other and with the process of each type of receptor production would be fully, but implicitly, specified by the chemical structures, which in turn would be explicitly encoded in the *biological* genome.

b. At the *abstract* genome level, by contrast, the details of the chemical structures of the Gs are not relevant. What is relevant at the abstract level is simply that for each connection type (defined by three things: the two unit types involved in the connection and the constraint), a connection weight is specified. The abstract genome therefore contains '$G^{i\pm}_{\Phi\Psi}$ genes', which regulate the relative *strengths* of connections; the *existence* of a connection is determined by other genes, those encoding the connectivity information discussed in Section 4.2.

c. The relationship between the signals $G(\Phi)$ and the $G^{i\pm}_{\Phi\Psi}$ values is as follows: each $G^{i\pm}_{\Phi\Psi}$ represents the strength of a chemical interaction between $G(\Phi)$ and $G(\Psi)$, and the subsequent effect on the production of a given $R^{\pm}_i$. Since the number of receptors of type $R^{\pm}_i$ is proportional to $c^i_{\Phi\Psi}$, as stated in (33b), $G^{i\pm}_{\Phi\Psi}$ is proportional to $c^i_{\Phi\Psi}$.

The values of the various $G^{i\pm}_{\Phi\Psi}$s are listed in Table 2.

An assumption here is that for each pair of unit types Φ and Ψ, there is one signal, $G^{i+}_{\Phi\Psi}$, for each receptor type R^+_i. Since each cell type produces only one identifier $G(\Phi)$, there are not two different signals, $G^{i+}_{\Phi\Psi}$ and $G^{i+}_{\Phi\Psi}$. (And similarly for $G^{i-}_{\Phi\Psi}$ and R^-_i.) This has the consequence that the result of development will be a *symmetric connection matrix*. For example, for the IDENTITY constraint, symmetric inhibitory connections are formed between adjacent C and V units in the correspondence layer. Suppose the types of the C and V correspondence units are numbered 3 and 4, and the IDENTITY constraint is numbered 5. Then the strength of expression of the G^{5-}_{34} gene determines the strength of type 5 inhibitory connections that form between units of type 3 and type 4—both those to 3 from 4 and those to 4 from 3. At the biological level, the density of R^-_5 receptors at these synapses will be the same; and this density determines the contribution of R^-_5 receptors to the efficacy of both the 3←4 and the 4←3 inhibitory synapses at a later time t: the contribution is proportional to the number of R^-_5 receptors times the concentration of peptide P_5 in the intercellular space at time t. These contributions must therefore always be the same for 3←4 and 4←3. Since this is true for all receptor types $R^\pm_i$, not just $i = 5$, it follows that the total connection weight between type 3 and type 4 units must be the same in both directions.

If such a system of chemical signals turns out to be a realistic biological model, there will be significant implications for the plausibility of symmetric connection weights. Symmetry of connection weights, and preservation of the relative strengths of different connection weights as these weights change during learning, are computational constraints that seem biologically implausible under the usual conceptions of how connectionist processing and learning might be biologically realized. It seems to us an important aspect of the abstract genome approach that the plausibility of these computational constraints can change significantly as a result of the shift in plausible computational primitives that accompanies the conceptualization defining the abstract genomic level of description.

In this section and the last, we have discussed the genomic encoding of the connectivity and the connection weights needed for CV$_{net}$. We now turn briefly to the activation dynamics.

4.4 Activation dynamics

We will assume that the activation of the units in CV$_{net}$ can be described, at least approximately, by the Boltzmann machine activation dynamics. This amounts to assuming some mechanism by which activations are clamped on input units, and a mechanism by which the activations of output units are stochastically determined by the input they receive through their weighted connections, subject to a noise level modeled by the computational temperature T, which starts high when an input is first presented and then lowers as the network settles on an output. This is, of course, a huge and controversial assumption. We make it here because the current exercise addresses the problem of how innate knowledge of UG could conceivably be en-

Figure 17

coded genetically, not the problem of how standard connectionist activation-spreading algorithms might be biologically realized. We do not presume the latter problem to be solved, or uninteresting, or unimportant—just orthogonal to the point of our demonstration here.

4.5 Learning

Like the initial constraint specification, the learning algorithm developed at the network level (21) must be viewed at a more biological level before we look at the consequences for an abstract genome.

(35)   Learning at the biological level

  a. The $R_i^{\pm}$ receptors are involved in controlling the production of P_i. This assumption is crucial in linking the relative rates of synaptic modification to the relative strengths of those synapses. This will allow the different types of synapses realizing a constraint to maintain constant ratios as their overall strengths are modified during learning.

  b. When two cells of type Φ and Ψ are simultaneously active, they each alter the intercellular concentration of P_i via their respective $R_i^{\pm}$ receptors.

  c. In learning phase $\mathcal{P}^+$, the R_i^+ receptors cause an increase in the production of P_i and the R_i^- receptors cause a decrease in the concentration of P_i. The reverse holds in learning phase $\mathcal{P}^-$ (the 'second phase'): the R_i^+ receptors *decrease*, and the R_i^- receptors *increase*, the concentration of P_i.

  d. During each learning phase, a set of N_p patterns is presented to the network, each pattern clamped on the appropriate cells for a time Δt. Consider $\mathcal{P}^+$. Suppose cells φ and ψ are simultaneously active. The φ-ψ synapse changes the concentration of P_i by $\Delta t\, k_4 \big| c_{\varphi\psi}^i \big|$, where k_4 is a constant representing the strength of the effect of $R_i^{\pm}$ receptors on the production of P_i. If $c_{\varphi\psi}^i$ is positive, there are R_i^+ receptors, so the concentration of P_i increases. If $c_{\varphi\psi}^i$ is negative, there are R_i^- receptors, so the concentration of P_i decreases. Thus, the change in P_i concentration is $\Delta t k_4 c_{\varphi\psi}^i$. Since s_i is the concentration of P_i (33a) divided by k_0, it follows that the contribution of the synapse to changing s_i is

$$\Delta s_i = k_0^{-1}\, \Delta t\, k_4\, c_{\varphi\psi}^i = \varepsilon'c_{\varphi\psi}^i,$$

where $\varepsilon' \equiv k_0^{-1}\Delta t\, k_4$. In phase $\mathcal{P}^-$, simultaneous activation of φ and ψ produces exactly the negative of this change to s_i.

Thus, we have realized exactly the CV_{net} learning rule for rerankable constraints (21). The *Gen* constraints are subject to a somewhat different learning rule (16)–(17), one in which they accrue strength along with the *Con* constraints, to ensure that *Gen* remains stronger than *Con*.

(36)   Each change Δs_i induces an accompanying change $\Delta s_0 = k_G \Delta s_i$.

There are several ways to realize this at the biological level. Let $\mathbb{C}_i$ be any constraint in *Con*. Then it might be that the receptors $R_i^{\pm}$ affect the concentration not only of P_i, but also of P_{Gen}, the peptide(s) regulating the strength of the *Gen* constraint(s). Or a different mechanism altogether might regulate the concentration of P_{Gen}, a mechanism sensitive to the concentration of P_i, in such a way that any change in P_i also causes a proportional change in P_{Gen}. Or it might even be possible to eliminate P_{Gen} altogether and assume that *Gen* receptors R_{Gen} can bind all the peptides P_i corresponding to any constraint $\mathbb{C}_i$ in *Con*.

Since the $G(\Phi)$ genes indirectly control learning as well as initial constraint development in this model, the $G_{\Phi\psi}^{i\pm}$ genes already encode the information necessary for constraint-specific learning (see Table 2).

4.6 The abstract genome — summing up

An abstract genomic representation of the model network requires assumptions about the general developmental machinery of the system and abstract 'genes' that specify the particular network in question.

4.6.1 Developmental machinery

The genomic representation assumes a system that will handle the differentiation of the various unit types of CV_{net} (C/V, and input-output/correspondence), as well as their organization into its general topographic layout. It also assumes that directional information is available during connection formation via some kind of gradient or other orienting signal (as discussed above). The hypothetical mechanisms of (33)–(35) also assume processes through which (i) receptors bind peptides to maintain a level of synaptic efficacy, (ii) synapses increase or reduce concentrations of peptides during simultaneous activation of the connected units, (iii) two learning 'phases' are executed during which some signal regulates whether peptide production increases or decreases, and (iv) genes regulate the construction of such 'receptors' and the rate of peptide production. There are also presumed to be genes for specifying the internal structure of the peptides and the receptors, which are constraint specific in that there is hypothesized to be one type of each per constraint.

Legend for Tables 1–2, Figure 18

C_I	C input	C_c	C_{coda} (output)	W	West	D	Direction
V_I	V input	V_O	V output	F	Front	E	Extent
C_C	C correspondence	S	South	B	Back	T	Target
V_C	V correspondence	N	North	L	Long	B	Bias
C_o	C_{onset} (output)	E	East	Š	Short		

Figure 17

Table 1. Connectivity encoding

	C_I			V_I			C_C			V_C			C_o			C_c			V_O		
	D	E	T	D	E	T	D	E	T	D	E	T	D	E	T	D	E	T	D	E	T
IDENTITY							F	Š	V_C	B	Š	C_C									
LINEARITY							NE	L	C_C V_C	NE	L	C_C V_C									
							SW	L	C_C V_C	SW	L	C_C V_C									
INTEGRITY							S	L	C_C	S	L	V_C									
							N	L	C_C	N	L	V_C									
UNIFORMITY							E	L	C_C	E	L	V_C									
							W	L	C_C	W	L	V_C									
OUTPUT-IDENTITY													B	Š	V_O	B	Š	V_O	F	Š	C_o
													E	Š	C_c	W	Š	C_o	F	Š	C_c
NOOUTPUTGAPS													N S	Š	C_o C_c V_O	N S	Š	C_o C_c V_O	N S	Š	C_o C_c V_O
NUCLEUS													S	Š	V_O	N	Š	V_O	N	Š	C_o
																			S	Š	C_c
CORRESPONDENCE	S	L	C_C	S	L	V_C	N	L	C_I	N	L	V_I	E	L	C_C	E	L	C_C	E	L	V_C
							W	L	C_o C_c	W	L	V_O									
PARSE	S	L	C_C	S	L	V_C	N	L	C_I	N	L	V_I	E	L	C_C	E	L	C_C	E	L	V_C
							W	L	C_o C_c	W	L	V_O									
FILL^V				S	L	V_C				N	L	V_I									
										W	L	V_O							E	L	V_C
FILL^C	S	L	C_C				N	L	C_I				E	L	C_C	E	L	C_C			
							W	L	C_o C_c												
ONSET													S	Š	V_O				N	Š	C_o
NOCODA																					

Table 2. Strength encoding

Constraint	From	To	Strength
IDENTITY	C_C	V_C	−1
LINEARITY	$C_C \& V_C$	$C_C \& V_C$	−1
INTEGRITY	C_C	C_C	−1
	V_C	V_C	−1
UNIFORMITY	C_C	C_C	−1
	V_C	V_C	−1
OUTPUTIDENTITY	$C_o \& C_c \& V_O$	$C_o \& C_c \& V_O$	−1
NOOUTPUTGAPS	$C_o \& C_c \& V_O$	$C_o \& C_c \& V_O$	+1
	$C_o \& C_c \& V_O$	B (except first)	−1
NUCLEUS	$C_o \& C_c \& V_O$	$C_o \& C_c \& V_O$	+1
	$C_o \& C_c$	B (except first C_c)	−1
CORRESPONDENCE	$C_C \& V_C$	B	−2
	C_C	$C_I \& C_o \& C_c$	+1
	V_C	$V_I \& V_O$	+1
PARSE	$C_C \& V_C$	B	−3
	$C_I \& V_I$	B	−1
	$C_I \& C_o \& C_c$	C_C	+2
	$V_I \& V_O$	V_C	+2
FILL^V	V_C	B	−3
	V_O	B	−1
	$V_I \& V_O$	V_C	+2
FILL^C	C_C	B	−3
	C_O	B	−1
	$C_I \& C_o \& C_c$	C_C	+2
ONSET	V_O	C_o	+1
	V_O	B	−1
NOCODA	C_c	B	−1

4.6.2 Network-specific genes

A specific set of genes is expressed by each unit type of CV_{net}. These genes encode all of the information necessary to specify all connections made by each unit (direction, extent, and target unit identity). They also encode the constraint-specific information for each connection, the $G^{i\pm}_{\phi\psi}$ values. All the information specified within these sets of genes is provided in Tables 1 and 2. For a schematic map of the network-specific abstract genome we have developed, see Figure 18.

Figure 18. Abstract genome map

Large-scale view

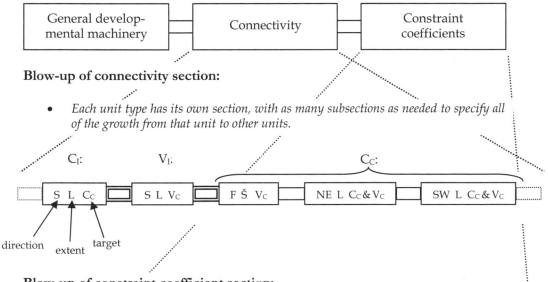

Blow-up of connectivity section:

- *Each unit type has its own section, with as many subsections as needed to specify all of the growth from that unit to other units.*

Blow-up of constraint coefficient section:

- *Each constraint type has its own section, with as many subsections as needed to specify all of the connectivity types.*

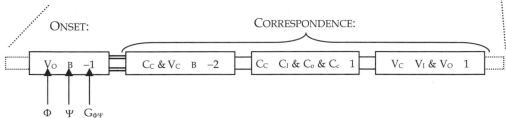

5 FURTHER ISSUES OF COMPUTATIONAL AND BIOLOGICAL SIGNIFICANCE, AND FUTURE DIRECTIONS

The task of creating an abstract genome for a simple language typology provides, we believe, some useful insights into the computational and biological significance of claims about the innateness of linguistic constraints. Just as connectionist modeling helps in bridging the gap between understanding of symbolic knowledge and understanding of neuroscience, so too can a model using an abstract genome bridge the gap between genes and innate constraints. As with connectionist models, in the long term it will be important to separate the model-specific conclusions from those that are generally true across systems. For the time being, the current exercise has generated some points to consider.

5.1 Network issues

A number of issues remain to be resolved that are obviously particular to the current network, CV_{net}. We single out two for discussion because they are of a type likely to arise in other attempts of this kind.

5.1.1 Edges are strange

The linear, local nature of the representation in the CV_{net} network causes some odd behavior at the edges of the network. This was particularly true of a previous version of the network, but it has been resolved somewhat by the division between C_{onset} and C_{coda} units in the output layer. That some edge-related oddness remains is particularly clear in the genomic description of the NoOutputGaps constraint, in which the first set of output units have a unique bias. This edge-related difficulty is likely a general fact about architecturally linear models such as the one used in the demonstration. More time-sensitive models, such as recurrent networks, which can represent a given output across time as well as space, might be less subject to these kinds of problems.

5.1.2 Local representation

The static, local representation was chosen to conceptually simplify the hand-design of particular constraints and their genomic description. So far, it is unclear how well this conceptual simplicity from the human designer's point of view maps onto the representational simplicity from the genomic perspective. After all, as discussed in Chapters 5, 8, and 11, there are certain computational equivalences between local and distributed representations in connectionist networks. In a similar vein, would an abstract genomic encoding of a time-dependent, distributed constraint representation actually be more complex from an informational standpoint (or from an evolutionary perspective), or just more difficult to understand and analyze?

5.2 Biological issues

In Section 1.2, we argued that apparent inconsistencies between symbolic and biological plausibility highlight important areas for future work. Given the incompleteness of the current project, there are evidently several such inconsistencies; other issues are raised by the abstract genome perspective, CV_{gene}, and the network, CV_{net}.

Figure 18　　　　　　　　　　　　　　　　　　　　　　　　　　　　　　　*Table 2*

We discuss some of these issues here.

5.2.1 Symmetry of connection growth

The connections in CV_{net} (and any comparable harmonic network) all grow symmetrically. (This is not to be confused with symmetry of connection *strength*, as discussed in Section 4.3—although the two properties are related.) In known biological systems, axons grow in particular directions in response to a signal such as a chemical gradient. By its very nature, a chemical gradient is an asymmetric signal: if it encourages growth in one direction, then it discourages growth in the opposite direction. By contrast, symmetric connections require growth in *opposing* directions along a particular axis. It is not unreasonable to suppose that different units might respond to a particular gradient in opposite fashion. For example, in the case of IDENTITY, C units might respond to a gradient along the in-out axis by growing toward a signal, and V units by growing away from the same signal. It is even reasonable to consider that the same unit might grow some connections toward, and some away from, the same signal, as would be necessary for INTEGRITY and UNIFORMITY. This is perhaps less plausible in a case like LINEARITY, in which connections grow broadly in the south-west and north-east directions, but not in south-east and north-west directions, nor in the due north/east/south/west directions. Still, it might be possible to generate a scenario in which this kind of growth might occur (possibly by having two different stages of growth, one to the north-east, and a separate one to the south-west). But more importantly, the unidirectionality of the chemical gradient concept (and indeed, any of the directional growth signals discussed) fails to capture the fundamental bidirectionality of symmetric connection growth within the entire system. It is unreasonable to suggest that such a situation might arise from the haphazard design of evolutionary change.

5.2.2 Biological plausibility is model dependent

Some aspects of innate constraints for a given network type are more biologically troubling than others. In the demonstration network, the quantitative symmetry of connections from a learning perspective turns out to have a potentially reasonable justification in the context of the proposed "biological" system, while the qualitative symmetry of the growth of those connections is more difficult to explain. The ability of connection strengths to change between positive and negative sign during learning in many connectionist models (which is improbable at the neural level) may not be a significant factor in this model, because the 'ranking' of different constraints will never require a negative constraint strength s_i. This is a direct consequence of the nature of the learning algorithm, in which relationships between different connections are preserved (the innate part of the model), while learning alters only the ratios between different groupings of connections. Put differently, a constraint might be strong or weak, but will never reverse itself. Other kinds of networks would represent innate constraints differently, and thus presumably would generate different conclusions about biological plausibility.

5.2.3 Scalability

A main argument from biology against the idea of innate linguistic constraints stems from the relatively "small" number of genes. Current estimates place the number of genes in the human genome at roughy 35,000, about 98% of which are shared with our closest primate neighbors. Given that there are around 10^{11} neurons, and 10^{15} synaptic connections, there are of course not remotely enough genes to individually encode each synaptic connection. Nor is this a particularly reasonable way to think about how genes might encode information about the connectivity of the brain. Aside from the counting argument, it is implausible that there are structures in the human brain that diverge radically from those of other primates. Evolution is conservative, tending to alter existing structures rather than generate new ones. While the view of the abstract genome sketched above does not suggest a one-to-one relationship between connections and genes, it does generate a large number of genes for a very simple symbolic constraint satisfaction system. It is important to consider how well this relationship will scale to more reasonably complex linguistic systems, and to multiple cognitive systems. One point in favor of the scalability of CV_{gene} is that it is not the case that a 'gene' in the abstract genome must correspond precisely to one gene coding for one protein at the neural level—illustrated by the difference between the biological and abstract genomes in (34). A 'gene' in the abstract genome might be thought of as a bit of information that can be modified by evolutionary pressures, and might correspond, for example, to a small section of an actual protein, which might radically change the protein's behavior in a certain context, but leave that behavior unchanged in a different context. Another point to consider is that individual genes are likely to be involved in specifying multiple distinct systems. This sidesteps the number game, to a certain extent, yet is radically different from the kinds of abstract genomes envisioned to date. Ultimately, the types of mechanisms at the connectionist network level hypothesized to underlie any symbolic constraint system, and the directness or indirectness of the relationship between elements at the connectionist and neural levels, will have consequences for the claims that can be made about the scalability of a particular model. The challenge for any conception of an abstract genome lies in making specific, ultimately testable hypotheses about the nature of the encoding of symbolic constraints within the biological system.

5.2.4 Development

The developmental picture in this model is evidently quite simple, mostly a matter of straightforward growth patterns of connectivity. More complex developmental interactions, such as activity-dependent pruning of connectivity, exist at the biological level. Incorporating abstractions of these interactions would likely allow us to derive further insights from the abstract genome concept and enrich its biological ground-

Figure 18   *Table 2*

ing. A more complex developmental model might generate very different conclusions about which aspects of the genomic instantiation of a connectionist network are the most troublesome, and which the most biologically realistic.

5.2.5 Robustness

An important question for future study is, how robust is the developmental picture? For instance, if a small number of wrong connections are made, or some other parameter is slightly off, will the constraint specification degrade gracefully?

5.3 Computational issues

Among the many computational issues left open in this work, three seem particularly significant.

5.3.1 Optimization

The demonstration LAD, like all of ICS theory, depends upon Harmony maximization in a harmonic connectionist network (CV_{net}) to compute optimal linguistic representations. The effectiveness of Harmony maximization in practice depends on the detailed properties of the Harmony function in question, and it is important to determine whether the particular type of Harmony function embodied in CV_{net} enables effective Harmony maximization algorithms.

5.3.2 Structured representations

The symbolic representations realized in CV_{net} are symbol strings. This is a nontrivial data structure, with full-blown combinatorial structure. Actual linguistic representations, however, employ more complex symbol structures. This is obviously true of syntax, where recursive embedding is a defining characteristic, but it is also true of phonology, which relies on a rich set of structural devices. One of the simplest is grouping of segments into syllables, the essence of syllabification; this has only been approximated in CV_{net}, which lacks explicit syllables and as a result could not extend to syllabification beyond the simplifications employed in CVT. It remains for future work to determine whether the ideas developed for CV_{net} can be upgraded for connectionist networks realizing symbol structures more complex than strings—perhaps via vectorial realizations in the tensor product family (Chapters 5, 7, and 8).

5.3.3 Restriction to strict domination hierarchies

The open problem most directly connected to ICS linguistic theory is finding a natural means of limiting the outcome of numerical connectionist learning to the special constraint strengths that realize OT's strict domination hierarchies. Whatever strict domination may have to say about the proper connectionist realization of grammar, it remains a mystery. While this obviously constitutes an important gap in the current state of our approach, it should not obscure the degree of success that has been achieved: the realization of highly specific, substantive linguistic principles admitting intricate crosslinguistic variation in a connectionist network specified by a biologically constrained abstract genome. This squarely addresses the primary general challenge facing the design of a Chomskyan LAD; the further challenge posed by strict domination is one entirely internal to the particular linguistic theory under study, OT.

5.4 Conclusion

Although a main objective of this project is to incorporate biological plausibility into the debate surrounding innateness, it is not our goal to develop a biologically explicit model of linguistic knowledge acquisition at the genetic level. Instead, we seek to create a level for conceptualizing the innateness question that is intermediate between the symbolic and the biological, but informed by both. Inspired by the successes of connectionist modeling in an analogous role, we suspect that this is the right level at which to analyze innateness and, in future work, the best level at which to run evolutionary simulations and test hypotheses concerning knowledge representation, which will in turn inform both the symbolic and biological levels. What we have achieved thus far is an explicit design for an abstract genomic encoding of the type of innate substantive knowledge of linguistic principles required by a Chomskyan LAD. The preceding discussion highlights some of the insights generated from this work to date, both positive and negative. We anticipate that future formal simulations at the connectionist network level will promote further progress. It is our hope that the abstract genome concept will eventually become biologically and linguistically well motivated enough, and formally explicit enough, so that evolutionary simulation can be attempted. Of course, it remains to be seen whether the general ideas developed for this demonstration abstract genome can be applied to the design of more powerful connectionist networks encoding more linguistically sophisticated knowledge, and whether the attempts to describe this system within a biologically motivated framework hold up to further scrutiny. Ultimately, the success of this research program will depend on the capacity of interlevel channels carrying scientific information down from symbolic cognitive theory and up from biology. Success would also mean sending new insight through these same channels, down to biology, and up to symbolic cognitive theory.[15]

[15] This material is based on work supported in part by a National Science Foundation Graduate Research Fellowship awarded to the first author. Any opinions, findings, conclusions, or recommendations expressed in this publication are those of the authors and do not necessarily reflect the views of the National Science Foundation. Thanks to Karen Arnold for valuable feedback on a previous draft of this chapter, and to Géraldine Legendre for very helpful discussions of the innateness question.

Figure 18   *Table 2*

APPENDIX. CONNECTIONIST REALIZATION OF CONSTRAINT HIERARCHIES WITH HARMONY FUNCTIONS

Our general approach to realizing a system of OT constraints in a connectionist network is to use a harmonic (or constraint satisfaction) network, which is a recurrent network in which all connections between units are symmetric; see Chapters 6 and 9, which we now quickly review. We will assume here that the units take on binary values: either 0 ('OFF') or 1 ('ON'). Networks with the symmetric weight property allow the definition of a Harmony function, which assigns a numerical value to each activation pattern over the units of the network and can be viewed as a measure of the degree to which the activation pattern satisfies the constraints defined by *individual* weights and biases in the network. In this simple sense of 'constraint', a positive weight on a connection between two units embodies the constraint that if one of the two units is ON, then the other unit should also be ON. A negative weight embodies the constraint that the two units should not be ON together. A positive bias on a unit says that unit should be ON, and a negative bias says it should be OFF. The standard form of the Harmony function is $H = \Sigma_{\varphi\psi} a_\varphi W_{\varphi\psi} a_\psi$.

When constraints are defined in this simple way, it is rather easy to see how one could configure the weights in a network to realize strict domination. Consider, for example, a network with N input units and one output unit, with all zero biases, and imagine that the inputs represent the presence or absence of N binary features of an input (underlying) form and the output unit represents a binary feature of an output (surface) form. Presentation of an input consists of setting (**clamping**) the input units to fixed values (0 or 1) and letting the output unit compute its activation in order to maximize the Harmony function. The constraint embodied by a (say) positive weight between a particular input unit and the output unit says that the output feature should be present whenever that input feature is present; a negative weight means the output feature should *not* be present when that input feature is present. One can verify from the Harmony function that Harmony is maximized if the output unit turns OFF except when the sum of the weights connecting the output to inputs that are ON is positive, in which case it turns ON. Then, for a particular constraint to dominate all others, the weights must be set such that whenever that input unit is ON, the sum of the weights from *all* ON units is the *same sign* as that unit's weight. A sufficient condition for achieving this is that the weight from the unit in question to the output unit is larger in absolute value than the sum of the absolute values of all other weights. For example, suppose we have four input units, the first input unit's weight is –8, and the other weights are 4, 1, and 2. Then if input 1 is ON, the total Harmony will be negative if the output unit turns ON, no matter what the values of the other three inputs are. Therefore, the output unit will turn OFF to maximize Harmony (with the value 0), and constraint 1 will thus always be satisfied.

In contrast, if the weights are (–8, 4, 3, 2), constraint 1 does not dominate the others. For example, if the input pattern is (1, 1, 1, 1), the optimal state would have the output unit ON; but this violates constraint 1. Constraints 2–4 have outweighed con-

straint 1, which therefore does not dominate them. Repeating this construction iteratively from lower-ranked constraints, we can define a strict domination hierarchy by
setting each weight to be larger than the sum of the absolute values of all those
weights that we want it to dominate. If the lowest-ranked constraint is assigned a
weight of ±1, this process results in an exponentially increasing set of weights (in absolute value), for example, $\pm 1, \pm 2, \pm 4, \ldots, \pm 2^N$ (see Prince and Smolensky 1993/2004,
Chap. 10, and Section 20:1.2.2.1 of this book).

This construction suffices for single-connection constraints; but for nontrivial
problems, we should expect that constraints will need to be defined over larger units
than pairs of single features. In general, a constraint may need to be defined over the
entire representation of the form, and in our example, this includes all three layers of
the network CV_{net}: input, output, and correspondence layers. Our approach is to define each constraint as a distinct Harmony function on the network, and then to find
a way to combine the Harmony functions so that they realize a strict domination hierarchy. It turns out that, given a set of appropriately defined Harmony functions
(the requirements for which will be described below), and given any desired ranking,
it is always possible to find a set of coefficients multiplying the Harmony functions
such that the resulting composite Harmony function, a linear combination of the
component functions, realizes the desired domination hierarchy. This appendix details a procedure for constructing this composite Harmony function. We will proceed
as follows. First we will define our symbolic domain and what it means to have constraints on forms in that domain, independent of any network representation. Then
we will define the kind of network we will use, the Harmony functions, and certain
assumptions about network computation. Next we will define the representation
mapping that allows us to represent domain forms in the network, describe how
Harmony functions can realize individual constraints, and finally give sufficient conditions under which Harmony functions can be made to realize strict domination.

A.1 Domain entities

Let $\mathcal{T}$ denote a symbolic domain space of "forms" (e.g., all strings of **C**s and **V**s); not
all forms in $\mathcal{T}$ need be considered valid candidate linguistic representations. A function *Gen* is assumed to exist that in some way distinguishes a subset $\mathcal{D}$ of $\mathcal{T}$ as the set
of valid candidate forms in the domain (e.g., the set of strings of **C**s and **V**s that have
'valid syllabifications'). We will not make any more specific assumptions about $\mathcal{T}$ and
Gen than this, and will focus on the set $\mathcal{D}$ of candidate forms. A form is assumed to
be a *complete* form, consisting of an (input, output) pair. In our example domain, the
input consists of the underlying form, and the output consists of the surface form together with the correspondence relation, since the latter must be computed along
with the surface output, given the input.

A **constraint** $\mathbb{C}$ over the domain $\mathcal{D}$ can be formalized as a **penalty function** p that
maps a form **d** in $\mathcal{D}$ to a nonnegative integer, the number of violations (or 'marks' in
the terminology of Chapter 12) that $\mathbb{C}$ assesses to **d**. Each constraint's penalty func-

Figure 18   *Table 2*

tion thus induces the binary preference relation on $\mathcal{D}$ called '$\succ$': $\mathbf{a} \succ \mathbf{b}$ if and only if $p(\mathbf{a}) < p(\mathbf{b})$. It also induces an equivalence relation '$\sim$': $\mathbf{a} \sim \mathbf{b}$ if and only if $p(\mathbf{a}) = p(\mathbf{b})$. Thus, for every $\mathbf{a}, \mathbf{b}$ in $\mathcal{D}$, either $\mathbf{a} \sim \mathbf{b}$, $\mathbf{a} \succ \mathbf{b}$, or $\mathbf{b} \succ \mathbf{a}$. This stratifies all forms in $\mathcal{D}$ into a set of equivalence classes: within a class all forms are $\sim$, and if two forms are in different classes, one is preferred to the other.

We define a **constraint domination hierarchy** $\mathcal{H}$ to be an ordered sequence of constraints that together act as a composite constraint, in the sense that $\mathcal{H}$ defines a relation that stratifies $\mathcal{D}$ in the same way as an individual constraint, although there need be no explicit penalty function specified for $\mathcal{H}$. Let $\mathcal{H}$ be the hierarchy $\mathbb{C}_1 \gg \mathbb{C}_2 \gg \cdots \gg \mathbb{C}_{N_{con}}$ (note that constraint numbering is top to bottom). Given any two forms $\mathbf{a}, \mathbf{b}$ in $\mathcal{D}$, $\mathbf{a} \succ \mathbf{b}$ with respect to $\mathcal{H}$ if and only if there exists some constraint $\mathbb{C}_i$ such that $\mathbf{a} \succ \mathbf{b}$ with respect to $\mathbb{C}_i$ and for all $j < i$, $\mathbf{a} \sim \mathbf{b}$ with respect to $\mathbb{C}_j$ (see Chapter 12). That is, $\mathbf{a} \succ \mathbf{b}$ with respect to $\mathcal{H}$ if some constraint prefers $\mathbf{a}$ to $\mathbf{b}$, and all higher-ranked constraints consider $\mathbf{a}$ and $\mathbf{b}$ equivalent. $\mathbb{C}_i$ is thus the highest-ranked constraint that has a preference between $\mathbf{a}$ and $\mathbf{b}$, and the fact that this constraint's preference prevails in $\mathcal{H}$ means that this constraint **dominates** all lower-ranked constraints. Similarly, say that $\mathbf{a} \sim \mathbf{b}$ with respect to $\mathcal{H}$ if and only if for all $\mathbb{C}_i$, $\mathbf{a} \sim \mathbf{b}$ with respect to $\mathbb{C}_i$: $\mathbf{a}$ and $\mathbf{b}$ are equivalent with respect to $\mathcal{H}$ if and only if no constraint has a preference between them.

A.2 Network entities

Define a Harmony network to be a set of N units, a symmetric matrix of real-valued weights connecting the units, and a vector of real-valued unit biases. The units are partitioned into three disjoint sets: input, output, and hidden. The input and output units will be used to represent domain forms, and the hidden units are used to increase the computational capacity of the network; they allow the network to realize a larger class of Harmony functions. The input and output units collectively will sometimes be called the **visible** units. The units are assumed to take on only binary activation values ($a_\psi \in \{0, 1\}$), and we denote the activation space $\Omega = \{0, 1\}^N$. A single activation pattern will be denoted $\omega \in \Omega$. Define a Harmony function on the network to be the usual function $H = \Sigma_{\varphi\psi} a_\varphi W_{\varphi\psi} a_\psi$.

To run the network, an input pattern is clamped on the input units, and an activation-updating rule is used to iteratively update the units' activation values. The goal of network computation is to find an activation state in Ω that is the global maximum of a given Harmony function, given that the input units are clamped as they are. The simulated annealing algorithm (see Sections 3.5, 9:4.1) is a good candidate for this purpose, and we will assume that it does an adequate job of maximizing Harmony. In particular, we will assume that, for any given binary input pattern clamped on the input units, the algorithm will succeed with acceptably high probability in finding a binary network state that maximizes Harmony. We will therefore focus on the Harmony function and set as our goal to design the Harmony function whose global optima represent the optimal domain forms. If we can do this, then maximizing Harmony in the network will deliver an optimal domain form consistent with the input. (This will be made more precise below.)

A.3 Representing domain entities with network entities

To represent domain forms in the network, we define a mapping from the domain space to network activation space (as in the general theory of Chapter 8). Because we must be able to represent input forms by themselves, as well as paired with arbitrary output forms, we will define two mappings, r_I and r. r_I maps an input form to a network input pattern. r maps a complete form (input, output) to a network visible-unit pattern. (Recall that correspondence information is part of the output.) These mappings are assumed to be 1-to-1 and invertible, which means that, for any network state whose visible units represent a domain form, we can recover the form that they represent (in the terminology of Chapter 8, the representation mappings are **faithful**). Because these mappings do not specify hidden unit activations, all network activation patterns with $r(\mathbf{d})$ on their visible units have the same domain interpretation: $\mathbf{d}$. It is useful to define extensions of the representation functions r_I and r to the full network activation space, Ω, as follows: $R(\mathbf{d}) \equiv r(\mathbf{d}) \times \mathcal{H}$, where $\mathcal{H}$ is the N_h-dimensional activation space of the hidden units. Thus, $R(\mathbf{d})$ is the set of all $\omega \in \Omega$ that have $r(\mathbf{d})$ on their visible units. Similarly, $R_I(\mathbf{I}) \equiv r_I(\mathbf{I}) \times O \times \mathcal{H}$; that is, all ω that have $r_I(\mathbf{I})$ on their input units, where O is the N_o-dimensional space of all states of the output layer.

For a given domain form, $\mathbf{d}$, the members of $R(\mathbf{d})$ differ only in their hidden unit activations. Since, in general, hidden units will have nonzero weights and biases in a Harmony function, not all members of $R(\mathbf{d})$ will have equal Harmony. Given a Harmony function H and a domain form $\mathbf{d}$, denote by $H^\dagger(\mathbf{d})$ the highest Harmony value achieved by any member of $R(\mathbf{d})$. Denote by $R^\dagger(\mathbf{d})$ the set of all Ω in $R(\mathbf{d})$ that have this maximum Harmony.

(37)   A Harmony function H **realizes a domain constraint** $\mathbb{C}$ if and only if the following is true for each input, $\mathbf{I}$, separately:

   For every pair of domain forms $\mathbf{a}$ and $\mathbf{b}$ in $Gen(\mathbf{I})$ (where $Gen(\mathbf{I})$ is the set of valid candidate forms that include $\mathbf{I}$ as input),

   $\mathbf{a} \succ \mathbf{b} \Leftrightarrow H^\dagger(\mathbf{a}) > H^\dagger(\mathbf{b})$ and

   $\mathbf{a} \sim \mathbf{b} \Leftrightarrow H^\dagger(\mathbf{a}) = H^\dagger(\mathbf{b})$.

That is, for any fixed input, the *highest-Harmony representations* of $\mathbf{a}$ and $\mathbf{b}$ must stand in the same relation according to H as they do according to $\mathbb{C}$. It doesn't matter what the relationship is between lower-Harmony representations of $\mathbf{a}$ and $\mathbf{b}$. And it also doesn't matter what Harmony values H assigns to members of Ω that do not represent domain states (i.e., are not in $R(\mathcal{D})$). Also note that the condition that the above be true for each input $\mathbf{I}$ separately makes this condition easier to satisfy than if it were required to hold across all inputs. That is, we are not requiring that the Harmony function agree with the constraint's preference relationships between forms with different inputs. For example, we could imagine a case in which some form $\mathbf{x}$

Figure 18   *Table 2*

with input $\mathbf{I}_1$ incurs a single violation of the constraint $\mathbb{C}$, while a different form $\mathbf{y}$ with different input $\mathbf{I}_2$ incurs two violations, and therefore the domain constraint would prefer state $\mathbf{x}$ to $\mathbf{y}$, given its definition as a penalty function. But in this case we put no restriction whatsoever on the Harmonies of $R(\mathbf{x})$ and $R(\mathbf{y})$. We only require that the Harmony relationships between forms that could potentially compete be correct, and in the present context those are only forms that share the same input.

We will need to define a Harmony function H_{Gen} that realizes *Gen*; however, it will realize *Gen* in a slightly different way than the other constraints are realized, because the *Gen* function is defined on all of $\mathcal{T}$, while constraints are defined only on $\mathcal{D}$. The role of the *Gen* Harmony function will be similar to *Gen*'s role in distinguishing $\mathcal{D}$ within the domain $\mathcal{T}$, except it will serve to distinguish network states that lie in $R(\mathcal{D})$ from those that do not. Roughly speaking, we will require that for each input $\mathbf{I}$, separately, H_{Gen} must assign *equal and maximal* Harmony K to all network states that represent domain states that include the input $r_I(\mathbf{I})$, and it must assign lower (but not necessarily equal) Harmony to all other network states. To make this exact, we must account for the effects of hidden units on Harmony values, and so we will require only that the *maximum-Harmony* pattern representing each domain state have this maximum Harmony K. The exact definition is given in (38).

(38)   A Harmony function H_{Gen} **realizes *Gen*** if and only if, for each input $\mathbf{I}$ separately,

$$H_{Gen}(\omega) \begin{cases} = K & \text{if } \omega \in R^{\dagger}(\mathcal{D}) \\ < K & \text{otherwise} \end{cases},$$

where the constant K may depend on $\mathbf{I}$.

Again, this is easier to satisfy than a condition in which all members of $R^{\dagger}(\mathcal{D})$ are required to have a single Harmony value K; for example, one could imagine a case in which the maximum Harmony assigned to a form by H_{Gen} depends on the length of the symbolic input string. In this case, $K(\mathbf{I})$ would grow as the length of $\mathbf{I}$ grows. As before, we are requiring H_{gen} to agree with *Gen* only for states that could potentially compete — in other works, states that share the same input.

A few facts will be useful later. First, note that there is a positive difference between the maximum H_{gen} Harmony value K and the largest H_{gen} Harmony value less than K. This follows from the fact that Ω is a discrete (and finite) space. Second, if a Harmony function H realizes a constraint $\mathbb{C}$, then if we multiply H by any positive constant c, we get another Harmony function cH that also realizes $\mathbb{C}$. And third, if we add two Harmony functions defined on the same network, we get a Harmony function whose weights are just the sum of the weights of the component functions. Thus, any linear combination of Harmony functions is a ("composite") Harmony function.

A.4 Realizing strict domination with Harmony functions

If we assume we have obtained a set of Harmony functions realizing each of our constraints and *Gen*, we can ask by what factors these functions should be multiplied to achieve strict domination for a ranking we specify. To approach this question, the following definition will be useful: Given two functions H and G (e.g., Harmony functions) defined on a space X, we say that

(39)   **H ε-dominates G with ε equal to Δ** if and only if for any x_1, x_2 in X,

$$H(x_1) - H(x_2) \geq \Delta \;\Rightarrow\; [H(x_1) + G(x_1)] - [H(x_2) + G(x_2)] > 0.$$

This says that if the value of H at x_1 exceeds the value at x_2 by at least Δ, then the value of the composite function $(H+G)$ at x_1 exceeds that at x_2 (by more than zero). If we take H and G to be Harmony functions, we might paraphrase this as follows: H ε-dominates G with ε equal to Δ if and only if 'all preferences by H of size at least Δ are preserved when H and G are added' (preserved in the sense that they are still preferences).

Now, suppose we have two Harmony functions H and G realizing constraints $\mathbb{C}_H$ and $\mathbb{C}_G$, and also suppose (for technical reasons) that if these Harmony functions make use of hidden units, they make use of *disjoint* sets of the hidden units; that is, each function assigns all zero weights to the hidden units used by the other function. The fact that H realizes $\mathbb{C}_H$ implies that the optimal Harmony values that H assigns to representations of domain states (i.e., the $H^\dagger(\mathbf{d})$ values) are stratified in the same way that domain states are stratified into equivalence classes by $\mathbb{C}_H$. Since the network activation space, Ω, is discrete and finite, it is guaranteed that the difference between any two unequal Harmony values in H will be at least a certain finite positive amount. Call the minimum difference in Harmony between any two optimal $\mathcal{D}$-representations $\delta_{min}(H)$. This is the minimum Harmony gap between any two strata defined by H. Now, suppose it happened to be the case that H ε-dominated G with ε equal to $\delta_{min}(H)$. This would imply, by definition, that all preferences by H of size at least $\delta_{min}(H)$ are preserved when H and G are added. Since the Harmony difference between any two optimal $\mathcal{D}$-representations is at least $\delta_{min}(H)$, every ordering that H imposes on elements of $\mathcal{D}$ would be preserved if H and G were added. That is, in the composite constraint $H + G$, H would strictly dominate G. (Clearly, any preference between two states that G imposed would only apply if H had no preference between those states.)

The foregoing assumed that H happened to ε-dominate G. But what if it doesn't? It turns out that we can *make* H ε-dominate G with ε equal to $\delta_{min}(H)$ by "shrinking" G (multiplying it by a small positive factor) so that its entire Harmony range falls within $\delta_{min}(H)$. That is, we make a given preference in H survive the addition of G by making sure that G can't possibly change the relative Harmony of two states by more than their H-difference. Since $\delta_{min}(H)$ is the minimum size of all such differences, all preferences will survive, and H will dominate G. Take for example two states $\mathbf{d}$ and $\mathbf{d}'$ in $\mathcal{D}$, and let $H^\dagger(\mathbf{d}) - H^\dagger(\mathbf{d}') = \delta$ (positive). Now, in the worst case (for H), G disagrees with H and assigns $\mathbf{d}'$ higher Harmony than $\mathbf{d}$, by assigning its maximum possible Harmony to $\mathbf{d}'$ and its minimum possible Harmony to $\mathbf{d}$. If we denote the range of G by $range(G) = max(G) - min(G)$, then the difference in Harmony between $\mathbf{d}$ and $\mathbf{d}'$

Figure 18   *Table 2*

when H and G are added will equal $\delta - range(G)$. So as long as $range(G) < \delta$, all preferences on H will survive and H will dominate G. We can therefore define the composite Harmony function F as in (40).

(40)   Composing two Harmony functions to realize strict domination

$F = H + sG$,   where s is chosen such that

$s < \delta_{min}(H)/range(G)$.

This works when we have just two constraints. To build a domination hierarchy from a longer sequence of Harmony functions, it is not enough for each Harmony function H_i to ε-dominate its immediately following neighbor. It must be the case that each H_i dominates the *sum* of all Harmony functions that follow it in the sequence. It turns out that this can be achieved if the s values are defined recursively as in (41) (going from the highest-ranked constraint to the lowest). Again, it must also be true that the Harmony functions use disjoint sets of hidden units.

(41)   Scaling multiple Harmony functions to realize a hierarchy

$s_0 = 1$,   then s_i is chosen to satisfy

$s_i < \frac{1}{2} s_{i-1} \delta_{min}(H_{i-1})/range(H_i)$.

H_{Gen} must be treated slightly differently. For H_{Gen}, the only preferences we care about are those in which a **feasible** state ω—a state in $R^\dagger(\mathcal{D})$, a maximum-Harmony representation of a valid candidate form—is preferred to an **infeasible** state ω'—a state not in $R^\dagger(\mathcal{D})$ (ω' might be a non-maximum-Harmony representation of a candidate form in $\mathcal{D}$, or a representation of a noncandidate form in $\mathcal{T}$ outside $\mathcal{D}$, or no representation of a form in $\mathcal{T}$ at all). In this case, the size of the gap between the Harmony of any feasible state and the highest-Harmony infeasible state plays the role of $\delta_{min}(H_{Gen})$ in the above formula. Defining $\delta_{min}(H_{Gen})$ this way allows H_{Gen} to be used as H_0 in the above formula, resulting in a complete domination hierarchy with H_{Gen} at the top. The full composite Harmony function is thus defined as in (42).

(42)   Composite Harmony function for a constraint hierarchy

$$H_{\mathcal{H}} = \sum_{i=0}^{N_{con}} s_i H_i$$

The key facts about $H_{\mathcal{H}}$ in (43) can be proved (Mathis, in preparation).

(43)   Suppose given a sequence of constraints $\{\mathbb{C}_i\}$ and the resulting domination hierarchy that they generate, $\mathcal{H}$. Then for any input $\mathbf{I}$,

a. $\mathcal{H}$ prefers a state $\mathbf{d}$ to state $\mathbf{d}'$ (both of which include the input $\mathbf{I}$) if and only if $H_{\mathcal{H}}$ assigns strictly higher Harmony to $R^\dagger(\mathbf{d})$ than to $R^\dagger(\mathbf{d}')$,

b. $\mathcal{H}$ considers states $\mathbf{d}$ and $\mathbf{d}'$ equivalent if and only if $H_{\mathcal{H}}$ assigns equal Harmony to $R^\dagger(\mathbf{d})$ and $R^\dagger(\mathbf{d}')$, and

c.   every network state that maximizes $H_{\mathcal{H}}$ is the representation of an optimal domain state in $Gen(\mathbf{I})$.

The final result (43c) in particular means that, for any domain input, when the representation of that input is clamped onto the network's input units, every maximum-Harmony state in the network's activation space represents a complete, valid candidate domain form that includes the input and that is optimal according to the constraint domination hierarchy $\mathcal{H}$.

A.5 Applying the general technique to our example domain: CV_{net}

We have shown that *if* one can design a network, a representational scheme, and a set of Harmony functions that realize *Gen* and each constraint individually, then for any desired constraint ranking there exists a set of strengths $\{s_i\}$ such that the composite constraint $H_{\mathcal{H}}$ realizes the desired ranking. Next we must show that it is possible to satisfy these requirements in our example domain of Basic CV Syllable Theory.

To apply the general technique to our domain, we must perform the tasks in (44).

(44)   General method
   a.   Define a symbolic domain.
   b.   Define a set of rerankable constraints in the domain.
   c.   Design a binary network and representation function that support the representation of domain forms in the network (both complete forms and inputs alone).
   d.   Define Harmony functions realizing *Gen* and each constraint individually.
   e.   Derive from the Harmony functions and the desired ranking the strength factors *s* to use to construct the final composite Harmony function $H_{\mathcal{H}}$.

Of these tasks, only (44d–e) remain to be done. The Harmony functions have been described above, but we have not yet verified that these functions realize the constraints and *Gen* in the sense required by our general method.

We will start with the *Gen* Harmony function, H_{Gen}. We showed above (38) that to realize *Gen* it must satisfy, for each input separately,

$$(45)\quad H_{Gen}(\omega) \begin{cases} = K & \text{if } \omega \in R^{\dagger}(\mathcal{D}) \\ < K & \text{otherwise} \end{cases}.$$

First note that there are no true hidden units in our network, since the correspondence units are considered part of the output. So $R^{\dagger}(\mathbf{d}) = R(\mathbf{d}) = \{r(\mathbf{d})\}$, that is, each domain state has a single network representation. As described above, H_{Gen} is the sum of nine component Harmony functions each capturing part of *Gen*, and each part was designed to impose a penalty (negative Harmony) whenever *Gen* is violated. Reviewing them, we see that IDENTITY, LINEARITY, INTEGRITY, UNIFORMITY, and OUTPUTIDENTITY consist only of negatively weighted connections; therefore, the maximum Harmony value will be zero for these components, and zero Harmony will be achieved only by states representing valid candidate forms—states in which no pair of units connected by these constraints are both active. For NOOUTPUTGAPS, CORRESPONDENCE, and NUCLEUS, the maximum Harmony value, which is assigned

Figure 18   *Table 2*

only to valid candidate forms, is also zero. Thus, the value of K above, the Harmony value that all valid-candidate-representing patterns share, is zero.

We also need to determine the minimum Harmony difference between K and the best network state in Ω that does not represent a valid candidate. To do this, notice (Table 2) that all nonzero weights have magnitude either 1, 2, or 3. This means that the value 1 is a lower bound on the difference in Harmony between any two binary patterns. A lower bound is sufficient because we just need to choose an s that is less than this number over a constant, so we do not need to verify in general whether the lower bound is achievable. So we can set $\delta(H_{Gen}) = 1$.

Now we turn to the individual constraints. As stated in (37), these must satisfy, separately for each input form $\mathbf{I}$,

(46) $\mathbf{a} \succ \mathbf{b} \Leftrightarrow H^\dagger(\mathbf{a}) > H^\dagger(\mathbf{b})$ and

  $\mathbf{a} \sim \mathbf{b} \Leftrightarrow H^\dagger(\mathbf{a}) = H^\dagger(\mathbf{b})$

for any pair of *valid candidate forms* $\mathbf{a}$ and $\mathbf{b}$ that contain $\mathbf{I}$. Note that, because *Gen* will be realized by a dominating Harmony function, we can restrict our attention to just the network states satisfying *Gen*. This is generally a big help in this task. In (47), we verify that each Harmony function satisfies (46), and we find $\delta_{min}(\mathbb{C})$ and *range*$(\mathbb{C})$ for every constraint (or lower and upper bounds on these, respectively).

(47) Verifying (46) and bounding $\delta_{min}(\mathbb{C})$ and *range*$(\mathbb{C})$

  a. ONSET   The Harmony assigned to a state by H_{Onset} is equal to minus the number of violations of the constraint. So all forms in $\mathcal{D}$ that have equal numbers of violations, and are therefore $\sim$ according to the constraint, have equal Harmony. If state $\mathbf{d}$ has fewer violations than state $\mathbf{d}'$, and thus $\mathbf{d} \succ \mathbf{d}'$, $H(\mathbf{d})$ will be greater than $H(\mathbf{d}')$. Finally, $\delta_{min} = 1$, and *range* $= N_{rows}$.

  b. NOCODA   As with ONSET, the Harmony is minus the number of violations and the result follows. $\delta_{min} = 1$, and *range* $= N_{rows}$.

  c. PARSE   Again, the Harmony is minus the number of violations. For every violation, there must be an input ON and no correspondence unit ON in its column. This produces Harmony of -1. At first glance, it might seem possible to have a PARSE violation in which the input is ON, one correspondence unit is ON, and the corresponding output unit is OFF, but this would violate *Gen*'s correspondence component. Indeed, the design of PARSE crucially relies on that fact. Finally, $\delta_{min} \geq 1$ (lower bound), and *range* $= N_{cols}$.

  d. FILL^V This is nearly identical to PARSE, including the reliance on *Gen*. $\delta_{min} \geq 1$ (lower bound), and *range* $= N_{rows}$.

  e. FILL^C This is exactly the same as FILL^V.

The values for the δ_{min} and *range* of each constraint found above result in a fairly simple set of constraint strengths. Each δ_{min} is 1, and each *range* is N_{rows} except for

PARSE, which is N_{cols}. So the ratios of interest ($\delta_{min}(H_{i-1})/range(H_i)$) will be either $1/N_{rows}$ or $1/N_{cols}$. A single constant factor that would be sufficient for every weight would be

(48) $f \equiv 1/max(N_{rows}, N_{cols})$,

and the corresponding strengths would be

$$s_i = f^i = max(N_{rows}, N_{cols})^{-i}, \ i = 0, 1, ..., 5.$$

Figure 18   *Table 2*

References

ROA = Rutgers Optimality Archive, http://roa.rutgers.edu

Ackley, D. H., G. E. Hinton, and T. J. Sejnowski. 1985. A learning algorithm for Boltzmann machines. *Cognitive Science* 9, 147–69.

Batali, J. 1994. Innate biases and critical periods: Combining evolution and learning in the acquisition of syntax. In *Proceedings of the Artificial Life Workshop 4*.

Boersma, P. 1998. *Functional phonology: Formalizing the interactions between articulatory and perceptual drives*. Holland Academic Graphics.

Chomsky, N. 1965. *Aspects of the theory of syntax*. MIT Press.

Chomsky, N. 1980. On cognitive structures and their development: A reply to Piaget. In *Language and learning: The debate between Jean Piaget and Noam Chomsky*, ed. M. Piattelli-Palmarini. Harvard University Press.

Cowan, W., J. Fawcett, D. O'Leary, and B. Stanfield. 1984. Regressive events in neurogenesis. *Science* 225, 1258–65.

Dantzker, J. L., and E. M. Callaway. 1998. The development of local, layer-specific visual cortical axons in the absence of extrinsic influences and intrinsic activity. *The Journal of Neuroscience* 18, 4145–54.

Elman, J. L., E. A. Bates, M. H. Johnson, A. Karmiloff-Smith, D. Parisi, and K. Plunkett. 1996. *Rethinking innateness: A connectionist perspective on development*. MIT Press.

Gruau, F. 1992. Genetic synthesis of Boolean neural networks with a cell rewriting developmental process. In *Proceedings of the International Workshop on Combinations of Genetic Algorithms and Neural Networks (COGANN-92)*.

Hinton, G. E., and T. J. Sejnowski. 1986. Learning and relearning in Boltzmann machines. In *Parallel distributed processing: Explorations in the microstructure of cognition*. Vol. 1, *Foundations*, D. E. Rumelhart, J. L. McClelland, and the PDP Research Group. MIT Press.

Horvitz, H. 1982. Factors that influence neural development in nematodes. In *Repair and regeneration of the nervous system*, ed. J. G. Nicholls. Springer-Verlag.

Hubel, D., and T. Wiesel. 1963. Shape and arrangement of columns in cat's striate cortex. *Journal of Physiology* 165, 559–68.

Hubel, D., T. Wiesel, and S. Levay. 1977. Plasticity of ocular dominance columns in monkey striate cortex. *Philosophical Transactions of the Royal Society of London B* 278, 377–409.

Jusczyk, P. W., and J. Bertoncini. 1988. Viewing the development of speech perception as an innately guided learning process. *Language and Speech* 31, 217–38.

Kitano, H. 1994. Neurogenetic learning: An integrated method of designing and training neural networks using genetic algorithms. *Physica D* 75, 225–38.

Kuwada, J. 1986. Cell recognition by neuronal growth cones in a simple vertebrate embryo. *Science* 233, 740–6.

Kvasnicka, V., and J. Pospichal. 1999. An emergence of coordinated communication in populations of agents. *Artificial Life* 5, 319–42.

Letourneau, P. C. 1975. Cell-to-substratum adhesion and guidance of axonal elongation. *Developmental Biology* 44, 92–101.

Lumsden, A., and A. Davies. 1986. Chemotropic effect of specific target epithelium in the developing mammalian nervous system. *Nature* 323, 538–9.

Mathis, D. W. In preparation. On the implementation of optimality-theoretic processing and learning in neural networks.

McCarthy, J. J., and A. Prince. 1995. Faithfulness and reduplicative identity. In *University of Massachusetts occasional papers in linguistics 18: Papers in Optimality Theory*, eds. J. Beckman, L. Walsh Dickey, and S. Urbanczyk. Graduate Linguistic Student Association, University of Massachusetts at Amherst. ROA 60.

Merzenich, M., and J. Brugge. 1973. Representation of the cochlear partition on the superior temporal plane of the macaque monkey. *Brain Research* 50, 275–96.

Mitchell, M. 1996. *An introduction to genetic algorithms.* MIT Press.

Mountcastle, V. 1957. Modality and topographic properties of single neurons of cat's somatic sensory cortex. *Journal of Neurophysiology* 20, 408–34.

Nakisa, R., and K. Plunkett. 1998. Evolution of a rapidly learned representation for speech. *Language and Cognitive Processes* 13, 105–27.

Nichols, J., A. Martin, and B. Wallace. 1992. *From neuron to brain: A cellular and molecular approach to the function of the nervous system.* Sinauer Associates.

Nusselein-Volhard, C. 1991. Determination of the embryonic axes of *Drosophila. Development (Supplement)* 1, 1–10.

Piattelli-Palmarini, M. 1994. Ever since language and learning: Afterthoughts on the Piaget-Chomsky debate. *Cognition* 50, 315–46.

Pinker, S. 1984. *Language learnability and language development.* Harvard University Press.

Prince, A. 2002. Anything goes. Ms., Rutgers University. ROA 536.

Prince, A., and P. Smolensky. 1993/2004. *Optimality Theory: Constraint interaction in generative grammar.* Technical report, Rutgers University and University of Colorado at Boulder, 1993. ROA 537, 2002. Revised version published by Blackwell, 2004.

Rubin, G. 1989. Development of the *Drosophila* retina: Inductive events studied at single cell resolution. *Cell* 57, 519–20.

Rumelhart, D. E., G. E. Hinton, and R. J. Williams. 1986. Learning internal representations by error propagation. In *Parallel distributed processing: Explorations in the microstructure of cognition.* Vol. 1, *Foundations,* D. E. Rumelhart, J. L. McClelland, and the PDP Research Group. MIT Press.

Smolensky, P. 1984. The mathematical role of self-consistency in parallel computation. In *Proceedings of the Cognitive Science Society* 6.

Smolensky, P. 1986. Information processing in dynamical systems: Foundations of Harmony Theory. In *Parallel distributed processing: Explorations in the microstructure of cognition.* Vol. 1, *Foundations,* D. E. Rumelhart, J. L. McClelland, and the PDP Research Group. MIT Press.

Smolensky, P. 1988. On the proper treatment of connectionism. *Behavioral and Brain Sciences* 11, 1–74.

Stent, G., and D. Weisblat. 1982. The development of a simple nervous system. *Scientific American* 246, 136–46.

Tesar, B. B. 1998a. Error-driven learning in Optimality Theory via the efficient computation of optimal forms. In *Is the best good enough? Optimality and competition in syntax,* eds. P. Barbosa, D. Fox, P. Hagstrom, M. McGinnis, and D. Pesetsky. MIT Press and MIT Working Papers in Linguistics.

Tesar, B. B. 1998b. An iterative strategy for language learning. *Lingua* 104, 131–45. ROA 177.

Tesar, B. B., and P. Smolensky. 1993. The learnability of Optimality Theory: An algorithm and some basic complexity results. Technical report CU-CS-678-93, Computer Science Department, University of Colorado at Boulder. ROA 2.

Tesar, B. B., and P. Smolensky. 1998. Learnability in Optimality Theory. *Linguistic Inquiry* 29, 229–68.

Tesar, B. B., and P. Smolensky. 2000. *Learnability in Optimality Theory.* MIT Press.

Tessier-Lavigne, M., and M. Placzek. 1991. Target attraction: Are developing axons guided by chemotropism? *Trends in Neuroscience* 14, 303–10.

Tessier-Lavigne, M., M. Placzek, A. Lumsden, J. Dodd, and T. Jessel. 1988. Chemotropic guidance of developing axons in the mammalian central nervous system. *Nature* 336, 775–8.

Tosney, K. 1991. Cells and cell-interactions that guide motor axons in the developing chick embryo. *Bioessays* 13, 17–23.

Touretzky, D. S. 1989. Towards a connectionist phonology: The "many maps" approach to sequence manipulation. In *Proceedings of the Cognitive Science Society 11*.

Touretzky, D. S., and D. W. Wheeler. 1990. A computational basis for phonology. In *Advances in neural information processing systems 2*, ed. D. S. Touretzky. Morgan Kaufmann.

Touretzky, D. S., and D. W. Wheeler. 1991. Sequence manipulation using parallel mapping networks. *Neural Computation* 3, 98–109.

Van Ooyen, A. 1994. Activity-dependent neural network development. *Network: Computation in Neural Systems* 5, 401–23.

Wexler, K., and P. W. Culicover. 1980. *Formal principles of language acquisition*. MIT Press.

Whitley, L., and J. Schaffer, eds. 1992. *Proceedings of the International Workshop on Combinations of Genetic Algorithms and Neural Networks (COGANN-92)*. IEEE Computer Society Press.

Part IV

Philosophical Foundations of Cognitive Architecture

Parts I–III developed the Integrated Connectionist/Symbolic Cognitive Architecture (ICS), focusing on the challenges and results internal to that theory. In Part IV, we turn attention outward to address the relation between ICS and other general approaches to cognitive architecture. The two chapters of Part IV can be read independently of each other; they contain a number of pointers to relevant material in earlier chapters in the book, but Part I provides minimally sufficient background material.

Chapter 22 argues that the connectionist and generative approaches to language are compatible, contrary to the prevailing assumption. The integration of these two approaches is one of the more striking facets of the ICS research program. But the respective roles of connectionist and symbolic explanation in ICS, for language in particular and cognition in general, are not easy to disentangle. Chapter 23 confronts this issue, developing a general multilevel analysis of computational systems and using it to sort out the contributions of symbolic and connectionist principles in the ICS integrative approach to cognitive explanation.

22

Principle-Centered Connectionist and Generative-Linguistic Theories of Language

Paul Smolensky

The computational unification inherent in the Integrated Connectionist/Symbolic Cognitive Architecture (ICS) often makes it challenging to clearly characterize the roles of connectionist and symbolic principles in ICS explanation. For example, standard connectionist modeling develops concrete network models to simulate concrete data on linguistic behavior (in the laboratory, say). Generative grammar develops universal symbolic principles of grammar to formally derive both concrete language-particular patterns and crosslinguistic generalizations. ICS does not primarily follow the standard connectionist route: see ❹ of Figure 6 in the ICS map of Chapter 2. Rather, ICS explanation develops grammar formalisms whose computational structure is explained by connectionist principles, and uses those grammatical theories to formally derive language-particular and crosslinguistic patterns. This style of explanation illustrates the 'principle-centered' (as opposed to 'model-centered') methodology, characterized in Chapter 3. Such explanation is possible because the fundamental theoretical and methodological commitments of connectionism and generative grammar are in fact mutually consistent, common opinion notwithstanding. This chapter argues the consistency of connectionism and generative grammar, and defends the value of principle-based connectionist research as a complement to model-based connectionist research on language.

This chapter is a slightly expanded and revised version of Smolensky 1999.

Contents

This chapter defends two main claims. The first is that there are two general styles of research that both deserve a central place in connectionist approaches to language: these illustrate the 'model-centered' and 'principle-centered' methods defined in Section 3:2.3. The former style, which will be called **model-based** research, is well established. The latter style, **connectionist grammar-based** research, is less so. Each approach, I will argue, has important strengths lacking in the other. The second main claim is that the time has come to stop regarding generative grammar and connectionist approaches to language as incompatible research paradigms. Each has significant potential for contributing to the other.

In Section 1, I will suggest a view of the core theoretical commitments of the two paradigms, connectionism and generative linguistics, and argue that these commitments combine to support a coherent and fruitful research program in connectionist-grounded generative grammar. It is my belief, although I will not attempt to justify it in detail here, that the core commitments I identify are indeed consensus beliefs of the connectionist and generative linguistics research communities.

Going beyond the core commitments, individual researchers have further commitments that are often not mutually compatible, and these competing scientific hypotheses must of course be adjudicated by the usual types of theoretical and empirical arguments. But at this level, competition between incompatible hypotheses is readily found among generative grammarians themselves, or among connectionists themselves—not just between generative linguists and connectionists. Thus, it seems to me more accurate to regard the current *scientific* debates about language as individual conflicts between individual hypotheses, rather than as a war between two monolithic paradigms, connectionism and generative grammar.

1 COMMITMENTS OF CONNECTIONISM

The parallel distributed processing (PDP) school of connectionism is founded, it seems to me, on the following general principles (Rumelhart, McClelland, and the PDP Research Group 1986; see Section 1:2 of this book):

(1)   Fundamental commitments of connectionism: The PDP principles
   a.   Mental representations are distributed patterns of numerical activity.
   b.   Mental processes are massively parallel transformations of activity patterns by patterns of numerical connections.
   c.   Knowledge acquisition results from the interaction of
         innate learning rules,
         innate architectural features, and
         modification of connection strengths with experience.

Testing the implications of these fundamental principles is a challenge in part because of their great generality: depending on how they are instantiated, they can be used to support a number of contradictory claims even concerning issues as fundamental as modularity and nativism. This diversity of potential implications of the PDP principles was already rather clearly in evidence in the earliest PDP models, as the representative citations in the following paragraphs show.

Consider the first PDP principle: *Mental representations are distributed patterns of numerical activity.* This can easily be seen as entailing that mental representations are crucially graded (nondiscrete). Indeed, this is the default case illustrated by many connectionist models, including the majority of the early ones discussed in Rumelhart, McClelland, and the PDP Research Group 1986 and McClelland, Rumelhart, and the PDP Research Group 1986.

However, this same PDP principle is consistent with the claim that mental representations are discrete, as seen in a number of classes of connectionist model. Most obviously, representations are discrete in networks with discrete-valued units (e.g., the original architectures of the Boltzmann machine—Hinton and Sejnowski 1983—and Harmony Theory—Smolensky 1983). But discreteness also plays a crucial role in the important class of models with continuous units that converge to discrete representations (e.g., Anderson et al. 1977; Rumelhart et al. 1986), including models with 'winner-take-all' subnetworks (e.g., Grossberg 1976; Feldman and Ballard 1982; Rumelhart and Zipser 1985; Mozer 1991). And of course discreteness of representations is also a central property of a number of connectionist techniques for embedding symbolic structures as patterns of activity (e.g., Touretzky 1986; Touretzky and Hinton 1988; Dolan 1989; Pollack 1990; Smolensky 1990).

The conclusion must be that the PDP principle concerning representations, (1a), is consistent with both crucial discreteness and crucial nondiscreteness of mental representations.

In a similar vein, consider the second PDP principle, (1b): *Mental processes are massively parallel transformations of activity patterns by patterns of numerical connections.* This can readily be viewed as entailing that mental processing is highly interactive, nonmodular, nonsequential. Indeed, this is the case for "classic" PDP models (e.g., Sejnowski and Rosenberg 1987) in which one layer of input units, containing information of many types, projects directly to one layer of output units (possibly through a hidden layer), with connectivity unrestricted.

But clearly this PDP principle is also consistent with the claim that mental processing is modular or sequential. Modularity of a certain type is central to connectionist models in which different types of information are represented over different groups of units, and in which restricted connectivity between groups of units allows only certain types of information to interact directly (e.g., Mozer 1991; Plaut and Shallice 1994). Modularity is the heart of networks that learn to specialize different subnetworks for different subtasks (e.g., Jacobs et al. 1991). And sequentiality is crucial for many applications of simple recurrent networks (Elman 1990) and related recurrent architectures, including the early model of Jordan 1986.

Again, the conclusion must be that the PDP principle governing processing, (1b), is consistent with modular or nonmodular processing, and processing with or without essential sequentiality.

Finally, consider the most controversial of the PDP principles, (1c): *Knowledge acquisition results from the interaction of innate learning rules, innate architectural features, and modification of connection strengths with experience.* At first glance, this principle would seem to imply that knowledge acquisition consists entirely in the statistical associations gathered through experience with some task. And this does characterize the early connectionist tabula rasa models with simple Hebbian-like learning rules (e.g., Kohonen 1977; Stone 1986) and input-output representations that have no built-in domain structure (e.g., local representations as in Hinton 1986).

However, much of the most noteworthy progress in connectionist learning is more appropriately characterized by another claim: connectionist knowledge acquisition consists in fitting to data the parameters of task-specific knowledge models. To varying degrees, this describes somewhat more recent networks (e.g., Rumelhart et al. 1996; Smolensky 1996c) in which more sophisticated error functions that embody Occam's razor force closeness-of-fit to data to compete with simplicity of generalizations or knowledge. The principle (1c) also describes networks with specialized activation functions, connectivity patterns, and learning rules that provide task-appropriate biases to the learning process (e.g., McMillan, Mozer, and Smolensky 1992), and models in which input-output representations reflect, even implicitly, task-specific regularities (e.g., see Lachter and Bever 1988, and Pinker and Prince 1988, on Rumelhart and McClelland 1986).

Thus, a commitment to the PDP principles (1) does not per se constitute a commitment regarding the degree to which discreteness, modularity, or innate learning bias applies to human cognition. This conclusion is no surprise to the practicing connectionist, of course, but it seems to deserve considerably more recognition than it tends to get in polemical debates between pro- and anticonnectionists. The reason for bringing it up here, however, is to point out that *the indeterminism of the basic connectionist commitments toward most central issues of cognitive theory forces a major choice of research strategy.* The most popular choice is this:

(2)   Model-based strategy for connectionist research on language

Because the basic connectionist principles (1) are too general to have definitive consequences for key theoretical issues, less vague connectionist proposals are needed. These can be achieved as follows:

a.   Choose a *particular* set of cognitive data on which these issues bear (e.g., a set of specific input-output pairs).

b.   Propose a *specific connectionist model* in which, for the particular data in question, choices are made of a specific input-output representation, specific activation functions and learning algorithms, specific numbers of internal layers of specific sizes and connectivity, and so on.

c.   Evaluate the proposed model based on closeness of fit to the data achieved by a computer simulation of the model, and on the internal structure in the model that allows it to achieve its performance.

As I will discuss in Section 4, there are many advantages to this research strategy, and it has produced many important results (for a fairly recent overview, see Christiansen and Chater 1999). The main point of this chapter is to argue that there is, however, *another* strategy available within PDP connectionism, and while this new approach has significant limitations, it also has certain strengths lacking in the model-based strategy. This alternative strategy has been formulated in Section 3:2.3 at the highest level of generality as 'principle-centered' research; here I specialize to the case of language. (For another cognitive domain, say, reasoning, a description of the analogous strategy results from replacing 'grammar formalism' with 'formal theory of human reasoning,' and so on.)

(3)   Grammar-based strategy for connectionist language research

Because the basic connectionist principles (1) are too general to have definitive consequences for key theoretical issues, less vague connectionist proposals are needed. These can be achieved as follows:

a.   Choose a mathematically precise formulation of the PDP principles (1).

b.   Derive from these principles a precise but general grammar formalism (or grammatical theory).

c.   To evaluate the proposed formalism, choose a particular class of target empirical generalizations concerning human language.

d.   Apply the grammar formalism to language data instantiating the target generalizations, defining a formal 'account' of the target phenomena.

e.   Compare the degree of explanation of the target generalizations that can be achieved under the new account with that achieved under previous grammar formalisms. ('Explanation' here means deduction of generalizations and particular data from the principles defining the account.)

I would not argue that all, or even most, connectionist research on language should pursue this grammar-based strategy; my claim is only that a central place in connectionist language research should be reserved for a certain amount of such work, because the model- and grammar-based strategies complement each other nicely. What the grammar-based strategy seeks to provide is a way of pursuing the explanatory goals of linguistic theory while incorporating computational insights from connectionist theory concerning mental representation, mental processing, and learning.

In the remainder of this chapter, I will briefly illustrate the grammar-based strategy with Harmonic Grammar and Optimality Theory (Section 2); identify some of the central goals and commitments of one approach to linguistic theory, generative grammar, and illustrate how Optimality Theory addresses these goals while introducing certain general connectionist insights (Section 3); and discuss the complementary strengths and weaknesses of the model- and grammar-based strategies for connectionist research on language (Section 4).

2 CONNECTIONIST GRAMMAR ILLUSTRATED

If we believe that a mind is an abstract, higher-level description of a brain—as most cognitive scientists presumably do—and if we believe that connectionist networks provide a useful stand-in for a solid theory of neural computation yet to be constructed—as most connectionists presumably do—then it follows that abstract, higher-level descriptions of connectionist computation should provide the basis for theories of mind (Smolensky 1988). The nature of the abstract, higher-level descriptions of connectionist computation will depend on which types of connectionist networks we adopt: some more discrete than others, some more modular than others, some containing more innate knowledge than others, and so on.

Among many such possibilities, here is one, the **symbolic approximation**:

(4)   The symbolic approximation

In the domain of language, the patterns of activation constituting mental representations admit abstract, higher-level descriptions that are closely approximated by the kinds of discrete, abstract structures posited by symbolic linguistic theory.

That this is indeed *a possibility* is suggested by research over the past 15 years showing how distributed patterns of activity can possess the same abstract properties as symbolic structures like syntactic trees. (One such proposal, tensor product representations (Smolensky 1990), is mentioned below in this section; it is introduced in Chapter 5 and more formally in Chapter 8, and discussed extensively in Part II. For related proposals, see Dolan 1989; Pollack 1990; Plate 1991. See also Tesar and Smolensky 1994, and Chapter 7 for relations to temporal-synchrony schemes such as those proposed in Hummel and Biederman 1992; Shastri and Ajjanagadde 1993; Hummel and Holyoak 2003.) That the symbolic approximation is the *correct* possibility is, of course, a working hypothesis; indeed, it seems to me that it is the hypothesis underlying all symbolic language research that takes linguistic representations to be psychologically real. Evidence for the correctness of this hypothesis comes from the successes of symbolic linguistic theory in explaining the overall structure of human language, successes I take to be most impressive.

To be somewhat more precise, the relevant hypothesis is that *some*—not *all*— aspects of the mental representation of linguistic information are well approximated by the abstract symbolic structures posited by linguistic theory. Everyone agrees that such representations do not capture all that cognitive theory wants to capture. The claim is that what they *do* capture has great explanatory power.[1]

The two approaches to connectionist grammar I will now briefly describe both

---

[1] The situation seems highly parallel to what I see as the relation of connectionism to neuroscience. To the criticism that connectionism ignores a tremendous amount of knowledge about the brain, I would respond, "The hypothesis justifying connectionism is that *some*—not *all*—cognitively relevant aspects of neural structure are well approximated by the abstract computational systems posited by connectionist theory. Everyone agrees that such systems do not capture all that cognitive theory wants to capture. The claim is that what they *do* capture has great explanatory power." (See also Box 1:6.)

assume the symbolic approximation. However, this assumption is not required by the grammar-based strategy for connectionist research outlined in (3); indeed, it would be extremely interesting to develop a connectionist grammar based on an alternative formal higher-level description of linguistic representations (for example, less discrete representations, perhaps along the lines of certain proposals of "cognitive linguistics" — e.g., Fauconnier 1985; Lakoff 1987; Langacker 1987; Talmy 1988).

2.1 Harmonic Grammar

As a first illustration of the connectionist grammar strategy, I indicate explicitly for each step of the strategy (3) how that step is instantiated in **Harmonic Grammar**, first introduced in Section 2:4 (Legendre, Miyata, and Smolensky 1990a, b, c, 1991b).The presentation here is brief and informal; more formal discussions may be found in Chapters 6, 10, 11, and 20.

a. *Choose a mathematically precise formulation of the PDP principles (1).*

The first principle, *Mental representations are distributed patterns of numerical activity* (1a), is made more precise via the symbolic approximation: linguistic representations are assumed to be patterns of activity in a connectionist network, patterns that are well approximated by tensor product realizations of the types of symbolic structures proposed in symbolic linguistic theories. Tensor product representations are a general class of schemes by which structured information is encoded in distributed representations (Legendre, Miyata, and Smolensky 1991a). The distributed pattern realizing a symbolic structure is the sum or superposition of distributed patterns realizing its constituent parts, each of which is a distributed pattern realizing a symbolic filler bound by the tensor (generalized outer) product operation to a distributed pattern realizing its structural role. (See Figure 4:3.)

The second principle, *Mental processes are massively parallel transformations of activity patterns by patterns of numerical connections* (1b), is more precisely rendered as 'Linguistic processing is performed by a connectionist network with a **harmonic** architecture, which entails that network outputs maximize Harmony — that is, optimally satisfy the simultaneous soft constraints encoded in the connections'. (The connectionist principle of Harmony maximization, introduced briefly in Chapter 2, was central to Chapter 4; it is discussed more formally in Chapters 6 and 9.)

The final principle is *Knowledge acquisition results from the interaction of innate learning rules, innate architectural features, and modification of connection strengths with experience* (1c). More precisely, the connections in the language-processing network are adjusted so that the higher the Harmony of a linguistic structure, the more well formed it is in the language; specifically, the Harmony-to-well-formedness function is assumed to be a monotonically increasing logistic function.

b. *Derive from these principles a precise but general grammar formalism (or grammatical theory).*

Given the assumptions just stated in step (a), it can be shown that the language-processing network has the following property. At a higher level of description, the output of the network corresponds to a symbolic structure that optimally satisfies a set of **soft constraints** of the form 'If a structure contains a constituent of type i, then it must (or must not) contain a constituent of type j (strength: H_{ij})'. A particular set of such constraints defines a **harmonic grammar**.

c. *To evaluate the proposed formalism, choose a particular class of target empirical generalizations concerning human language.*

One example: In a wide range of languages, intransitive verbs divide into two classes according to whether their argument noun phrase displays "object-like" or "subject-like" properties (e.g., in *the river froze*, the argument of *froze — the river —* displays object-like syntactic properties relative to the more subject-like argument of *flowed* in *the river flowed*). Which type of behavior a verb's arguments display correlates in systematic ways with various syntactic and semantic properties of the verb and argument, but precisely characterizing these correlations as grammatical principles is often problematic (see Chapter 11).

d. *Apply the grammar formalism to language data instantiating the target generalizations, defining a formal 'account' of the target phenomena.*

A variety of French intransitive verbs and sentence structures illustrate the correlations referred to in step (c). A set of soft constraints defining a harmonic grammar is developed to account for the overall acceptability pattern of the French sentences (Chapter 11). A typical soft constraint is 'If a structure contains a verb describing an event with an inherent endpoint, then it must not contain a subject-like argument'. These constraints, with their strengths, capture the correlations of interest; the Harmonic Grammar formalism defines formally how the conflicting demands of these constraints are combined to make precise predictions of sentence well-formedness.

e. *Compare the degree of explanation of the target generalizations that can be achieved with the new account with that achieved with previous grammar formalisms. ('Explanation' here means deduction of generalizations and particular data from the principles defining the proposed account.)*

The Harmonic Grammar account allows a complexity of interaction between syntactic and semantic constraints that better fits the French data, while elucidating the nature and grammatical role of the general correlations. The proposed soft constraints provide the means for precise prediction of the well-formedness of particular sentences, as well as deductive links to the general correlations to be explained.

2.2 Optimality Theory

The grammar formalism introduced briefly in Chapter 4 and in more detail in Chapter 12, **Optimality Theory** (OT; Prince and Smolensky 1991, 1993/2004, 1997), is conceptually related to Harmonic Grammar (HG) but considerably more restrictive, and, as we will see in the next section, therefore better suited to the explanatory goals of linguistic theory. The relevant principles of the theory are summarized in (5), which uses the traditional generative concept of the 'input' and 'output' of a grammar; for current purposes, we can roughly take the input to be the "intended interpretation" a speaker wishes to convey, and the output to be the actual linguistic structure which expresses that interpretation in the language (for a more accurate characterization, see Legendre, Smolensky, and Wilson 1998, and Chapters 12 and 16).

(5)   Optimality Theory

    a.   Given an input, the grammar produces as output the linguistic structure that maximizes Harmony.

    b.   The Harmony of a potential output is the degree to which it simultaneously satisfies a set of violable constraints on linguistic well-formedness (including constraints requiring the output to faithfully express the input).

    c.   The constraints have different strengths, determining which take priority when they conflict.

    d.   The grammar of a language is a ranking of constraints from strongest to weakest; a higher-ranked constraint has absolute priority over all lower-ranked constraints.

    e.   The set of possible outputs, and the set of constraints, is the same in all languages; grammars of languages differ only in the way constraints are ranked.

The additional restrictiveness of OT over HG comes from limiting the interactions among constraints to those that can be achieved by ranking (as opposed to arbitrary numerical strengths), and from the principle that the grammatical constraints, and the possible outputs, are the same in all languages. These additional restrictions reflect important *empirical* facts about language, some of which are long-standing observations of linguists, others of which were discovered in the process of developing OT; more on this in the next section (see also Chapter 20).

In (6), connectionism is related to the fundamental principles that define OT and differentiate it from other generative theories of grammar (see also Prince and Smolensky 1993/2004, Chap. 10).

(6)   Fundamental principles of OT and their relation to connectionism

Principles deriving from connectionism

    a.   *Optimality.* The correct output representation is the one that maximizes Harmony.

    b.   *Containment.* Competition for optimality is between outputs that include the given input. (Clamping the input units restricts the optimization in a network to those patterns including the input.)

    c.   *Parallelism.* Harmony measures the degree of simultaneous satisfaction of constraints. (Connectionist optimization is parallel: the constraints encoded in the connections all apply simultaneously to a potential output.)

    d.   *Interactionism.* The complexity of patterns of grammaticality comes not from individual constraints, which are relatively simple and general, but from the mutual interaction of multiple constraints. (Each connection in a network is a simple, general constraint on the co-activation of the units it connects; complex behavior emerges only from the interaction of many constraints.)

e. *Conflict.* Constraints conflict: it is typically impossible to simultaneously satisfy them all. (Positive and negative connections typically put conflicting pressures on a unit's activation.)

f. *Domination.* Constraint conflict is resolved via a notion of differential strength: stronger constraints prevail over weaker ones in cases of conflict.

g. *Minimal violability.* Correct outputs typically violate some constraints (because of point (e)), but do so only to the minimal degree needed to satisfy stronger constraints.

h. *Learning requires determination of constraint strengths.* Acquiring the grammar of a particular language requires determining the relative strengths of constraints in the target language.

Principles not deriving from connectionism

i. *Strictness of domination.* Each constraint is stronger than all weaker constraints combined. (Corresponds to a strong restriction on the numerical constraint strengths, and makes it possible to determine optimality without numerical computation.)

j. *Universality.* The constraints are the same in all human grammars. (Corresponds to a strong restriction on the content of the constraints, presumably to be explained eventually by the interaction of certain innate biases and experience.)

The OT conception of grammar embodied in the first eight principles (6a–h) directly reflects basic connectionist computational principles. The last two principles (6i–j), however, are unexpected from a connectionist perspective. These two principles reflect empirical discoveries about the similarities and differences among human grammars, to be discussed in the next section. These surprising principles would appear to have strong implications for the connectionist foundations of OT, but these potentially important implications remain to be explored in future research.

In Section 4, I will briefly consider the relative strengths and weaknesses of the model-based and grammar-based strategies for connectionist language research. But the strengths of the grammar-based connectionist strategy are closely tied to the goals of grammar-based research more generally, so I digress to discuss these in the next section. In the process, I will argue that generative grammar and connectionism are not incompatible research paradigms, the second main claim of this chapter.

3 Optimality Theory and generative grammar

Within generative linguistics, a grammar is taken to specify a mathematical function: given an input—for now, roughly, an intended interpretation—the grammar determines an output—the linguistic structure that expresses that interpretation. The grammar in the mind of an English speaker is the knowledge which determines that *which theory did he trash?* is the English formulation of a particular question in a particular discourse context, a question that would be rendered in other languages (with appropriate substitution of the corresponding words) as *he which theory trashed?, he trashed which theory?, which theory trashed he?,* and so on. A speaker uses her grammar every time she utters or hears a sentence; popular misconceptions notwithstanding, grammars are for producing and comprehending words and sentences—they are not for producing metalinguistic grammaticality judgments (although they can be indirectly pressed into service for that purpose).

Table 1. Some central generalizations shaping the generative approach to grammatical theory

	Generalizations	Role of theory	Optimality Theory
a.	Grammars of widely scattered languages of the world share a tremendous amount of commonality.	Grammatical theories must identify these common principles.	All human grammars share a specified set of well-formedness constraints.
b.	With respect to some particular aspect of linguistic structure, the grammars of languages differ, but in a remarkably limited number of ways.	Grammatical theories must identify exactly the possible modes of variation across languages.	Language-particular grammars are different rankings of the same constraints.
c.	The principles common across languages are connected to the observed data in complex ways.	Grammatical theories must provide formal accounts of the complex connection between general linguistic principles and the data of a particular language.	The structures of a language are those that maximize Harmony (i.e., those that optimally satisfy the constraints as ranked by the language's grammar).
d.	Relative to the astronomical number of generalizations children *could* formulate given the data of their language, they converge remarkably quickly toward a correct grammar.	Grammatical theories must provide formal accounts of how a correct grammar can be efficiently learned.	The space of possible OT grammars is sufficiently restricted and well structured that algorithms for identifying a correct ranking can be formulated, and efficiency results obtained.

Among the most basic generalizations molding the enterprise of generative grammar are those listed in Table 1; shown also are the roles generative grammar assigns to grammatical theory in response to these generalizations (see Archangeli

Table 1

1997, for a pedagogical exposition). The final column of Table 1 indicates schematically how OT meets the demands of a generative theory of grammar. By using optimal satisfaction of simultaneous conflicting violable constraints as the computational mechanism, OT offers novel proposals for solving the basic problems of grammatical theory, and new types of explanations of the central generalizations of linguistics.

The central column of Table 1 constitutes, I believe, the core of the central commitments defining generative grammar. None of these seems to me inconsistent with connectionist principles. Indeed, in addition to OT, other connectionist-based approaches to generative grammar can be identified, for example, the Linear Dynamic Model (Goldsmith and Larson 1990). (See also Touretzky and Wheeler's (1991) connectionist implementation of a proposal by Lakoff (1988).) The Linear Dynamic Model is a framework proposed for syllabification and stress assignment based on a particular connectionist architecture. This framework has been used to argue for the importance of graded linguistic representations and of numerical weights for encoding phonological grammars; yet it has received serious consideration within generative linguistics. (Indeed, Alan Prince—known to most connectionists for his critical evaluation with Steven Pinker of early claims about grammar based on connectionist modeling (Pinker and Prince 1988)—has studied this model in great mathematical detail in order to evaluate its linguistic implications (Prince 1993). The name 'Linear Dynamic Models' derives in fact from Prince's formal analysis of the linear dynamics of these networks. As part of his analysis, Prince proposes an alternative version of the model that is radically *more* continuous.) It should not be surprising that the Linear Dynamic Model was taken seriously by generative linguists, because, despite its major breaks with mainstream phonology concerning the nature of linguistic representations and grammatical knowledge, this work nonetheless attempts to address the central issues identified in Table 1.

The commitments of generative grammar are not inconsistent with graded representations, grammars encoded as numerical weights, or, indeed, probabilistic models, nonmodular architecture, or theories in which all language-specific knowledge is acquired by induction. The commitments of generative grammar are to explain formally the overarching generalizations about human language summarized in Table 1, and if there is in the generative literature a strong preponderance of grammatical formalisms that rely on discrete representations, sequential symbol manipulation, modular nonprobabilistic rule systems, and a highly constrained role for learning from the environment, it is because those working assumptions have enabled substantial progress in addressing the issues listed in the table. Other proposals that do so as well—be they based in numerical representations and knowledge like the Linear Dynamic Model, or parallel satisfaction of soft constraints like OT—will be seriously considered, and evaluated on the quality of the explanations they provide for the key generalizations in Table 1 and their many particular manifestations in the world's languages. At least that is what I believe the recent historical record shows.

In this section, I have argued one of the main claims of this chapter, that generative grammar and connectionism should not be considered incompatible research paradigms. The practice of generative grammar requires addressing a certain body of generalizations and providing precise theories of grammatical knowledge that can to some degree explain these generalizations. Connectionism provides proposals for the computational architecture underlying grammar: proposals concerning representation, processing, and learning. The grammar-based strategy for connectionist research on language provides a way of integrating connectionism with generative grammar. In the next section, I give reasons why such an integrated research program is a valuable complement to model-based connectionism.

4 COMPLEMENTARITY OF MODEL- AND GRAMMAR-BASED STRATEGIES FOR CONNECTIONIST LANGUAGE RESEARCH

Two criteria are useful for bringing out the complementary strengths and weaknesses of the model- and grammar-based strategies for connectionist language research. The first criterion concerns the feasibility of incorporating connectionist computational proposals into language research; the second, the feasibility of providing explanations of empirical generalizations about language.

4.1 Feasibility of incorporating connectionist computational proposals into language research

It will not have escaped anyone's attention that while OT replaces generative grammar's previous computational architecture—sequential rule application and hard constraints—with parallel optimization over soft constraints (5), it fails to incorporate many other central features of connectionism: graded representations, probabilistic processing, and associationist learning, to name a few. That OT lacks these features, on my view, is not per se a virtue—although what I find most striking is the impact on grammatical theory that can result from incorporating even a *single* connectionist conception, parallel optimization over soft constraints. It is my hope that the grammar-based strategy for connectionist language research will develop further grammatical theories that successfully incorporate more features of the connectionist computational architecture—but one has to start somewhere.

The real point here is that incorporating connectionist computational features into grammar-based research is difficult, because what is needed is a precise characterization of the higher-level consequences of these connectionist features, precise enough that these consequences can be used as the fundamental principles of a formal grammatical theory. The connections between OT and connectionist theory arise from two connectionist features whose higher-level consequences can be related to grammar: tensor product representations—connecting the low-level structure of certain distributed patterns of activity to their higher-level structure as symbolic representations—and Harmony maximization—connecting the low-level structure of certain activation-spreading rules to their higher-level structure as parallel optimization over soft constraints. I believe there are many more such connections to be exploited

Table 1

linking lower- and higher-level structure in neural networks (indeed, hopes of furthering this aspect of connectionist theory was a primary motivation for assembling a book: Smolensky, Mozer, and Rumelhart 1996).

The model-based strategy suffers from no such limitation on incorporating features of connectionist computation into language research. Not relying on a mathematical characterization of the higher-level consequences of lower-level network assumptions, the model-based strategy uses computer simulation to explore the consequences of specific computational proposals for specific linguistic data. This has opened up new ways of conceptualizing linguistic representations via distributed representations, suggested new ways of computing linguistically relevant functions using massively parallel processing, and deepened our perspective on language learning, for example, by providing provocative glimpses into the self-organizing capacities of sophisticated inductive systems. It is my view that this work is still in the exploratory stage, and that the central issues remain open: Can connectionist networks capture real linguistic knowledge without, to a considerable extent, implementing symbolic representations and rules? Can connectionist learning provide an account of the acquisition of bona fide linguistic principles without implementing the innate-knowledge-triggered-by-experience theory? While I consider these questions largely unresolved by modeling research to date, I also believe that our understanding of the issues has already been significantly sharpened and deepened by modeling work.

It seems likely to me that model-based research will always play a central role in connectionist approaches to cognition because the computer-simulation-based study of various features of connectionist computation will likely continue to be decades ahead of strong mathematical results concerning those features. (At the same time, it seems clear that mathematical results, for their part, have frequently precipitated the development of powerful new connectionist techniques.)

4.2 Feasibility of providing explanations of empirical generalizations about language

What, then, is the relative advantage of *grammar*-based connectionist research? The principal advantage, I will argue, concerns scientific explanation. Since this is a notoriously controversial topic, I will attempt to ground my argument in a (very!) concrete little example first introduced in Chapter 4.

Consider the French word for 'small (masc.)', *petit*. Oversimplifying slightly, it is pronounced with a final *t* [pətit] only when it is followed by a vowel-initial word; otherwise, it is pronounced [pəti]. How are we to understand this quite typical example of context-sensitive phonological alternation?

It might well prove interesting to build a connectionist model that learned the contextually appropriate pronunciation of this word—and others like it—from examples. Suppose this done. We are now positioned to address some very interesting questions about data-driven acquisition of phonology. What kind of initial structure in the representations and architecture of the network, and what kind of data, allows learning procedures to master this pattern of alternation?

Another kind of question is extremely important, however: putting aside questions about the learning process itself, we pass to questions of *exactly what knowledge* the network has acquired. That is, we now want an explanation of how the word *petit* is represented (in the model's 'lexicon'), and how the network's connections (its 'grammar') manage to produce the right pronunciation for every possible context.

Why is this type of question important? Isn't it enough to show that the trained network generalizes correctly to, say, 96% of unfamiliar words? Do we really need to characterize the 'lexicon' and 'grammar' that the network has learned?

Perhaps not. But in that case, we can't conclude that connectionism has provided an alternative way to explain linguistic knowledge and its acquisition. This is so, I believe, for at least the following three reasons.

First, the network may not provide an 'explanation' in an acceptable sense of the word because the degree of success that it does achieve may be due to aspects of the simulation that are not actually theoretical commitments of the implicit connectionist theory of language being proposed (McCloskey 1992). For example, aspects of the input-output representations may provide important biases, reflecting principles of symbolic linguistic theory, and these biases may be more crucial than any general connectionist principles in allowing the network to perform reasonably well. Thus, it is important to understand what knowledge the network actually has and what the critical sources of that knowledge are.

Second, for all we know, whatever correct performance the network displays, or whatever explanation of the phenomena the account provides, may arise because the network partially implements some symbolic system of linguistic representations and rules. Proponents of symbolic theories believe that symbolic rules and representations are somehow implemented in neural networks—perhaps they're right, and our network has managed to perform just such an implementation. At least, that is, to the limited degree required to achieve a 96% success rate on its limited data. Unless we adequately understand the network's knowledge at the higher, more abstract levels where symbolic rules and representations *could possibly* reside, we have no grounds to argue that the network's success counts as evidence *against* symbolic theory.

Third (and most likely), it is possible that what the network has learned has little or no relevance to any general conclusions about linguistic knowledge. Surely it would be a staggering feat of modeling to develop a network capable of learning the full phonology of any known human language. In the imaginable future, all models will confront an infinitesimal fraction of this mass of data. The important point to note is that, in contrast, theories of linguistic knowledge developed in theoretical linguistics *are* informed by, and responsible to, an *overwhelmingly* larger body of crosslinguistic data than any feasible connectionist model.

When a theoretical linguist analyzes a set of data *D* of the scope that might feasibly be presented to a network for training, the linguist's analysis is shaped by a huge

Table 1

mass of **implicit data** in addition to the particular data D explicitly under scrutiny. This point will be developed further below, but to briefly illustrate with the case of *petit*, the data informing contemporary symbolic linguistic analysis of the pronunciation of *petit* includes other phonological processes in French that bear little superficial relation to the issue of final-consonant pronunciation, the pronunciation of final consonants in Australian languages, the syllabification of word-internal consonants in all known languages, the pronunciation of certain vowels in Slavic languages, and much more. All these are the implicit data that inform the linguist's analysis of *petit*; a proposed analysis is responsible for generalizing, in the relevant respects, to all of them. Thus, the linguist rejects a large number of logically possible analyses of D because they would have no hope of generalizing beyond D to other phonological phenomena, and other languages. Successfully accounting for D in isolation is usually quite easy; what is hard is devising an account of D that employs representations and processes that might conceivably generalize well beyond D.

Now it is imaginable that we have in our heads one network for handling one data set D, a separate network for another data set D', yet another for D'', ... Such an approach to linguistic knowledge is hypermodular, in a sense favored by no proponent of modularity within linguistics; the burden of proof is on the connectionist modeler to show that it could conceivably work and, if so, that it provides the best explanation. Theoretical linguistic methodology, by contrast, imposes the constant methodological constraint that every proposed analysis exploit every means of generalization possible; thus, the burden of generality is borne within each analysis, and not by splicing together a collection of separate analyses, each employing knowledge of highly restricted generality.

So unless we have some understanding of what knowledge a network is using to cope with a very limited body of data D, we have no basis for believing that this knowledge will generalize beyond D, and indeed no reason to believe the network has solved a relevantly difficult problem: accounting for D in a way that generalizes well beyond D. Furthermore, what makes these problems difficult is often a relatively small set of challenging cases; which cases are the challenging ones depends on the analysis. Unless we understand how the network is analyzing D, for all we know, the challenging cases amount to only 4% of the data, and these are just the cases our network gets wrong; that is, the network has simply failed to handle the pattern that makes D difficult in the first place.

Thus, it seems to me that the model-based strategy provides a researcher two options. The first is to be content with a model that accounts for 96% of its data, and with only very fragmentary understanding of what knowledge the network has that allows it to exhibit this performance. In this case, for the reasons outlined in the previous paragraphs, I believe the model cannot be seen as providing strong evidence one way or the other about whether connectionism provides a viable alternative to symbolic linguistic theory.

The second option is to determine what knowledge the network has, and to show (i) that this knowledge derives from genuine principles of a connectionist theory of language, and not from arbitrary implementation details of the simulation; (ii) that it is not the case that this knowledge is (partially) successful only because it (partially) implements a symbolic linguistic theory; and (iii) that this knowledge encodes regularities of considerable (cross)linguistic generality, and correctly explains the patterns in the data that make it interestingly challenging. Armed with such a characterization of the knowledge in the network, we could take its success as evidence that connectionist principles lead to linguistic knowledge that is not an implementation of a symbolic theory and that is general enough to be significant: that is, as evidence that connectionist principles can provide an alternative to symbolic accounts of linguistic knowledge.

But achieving such a strong understanding of the knowledge residing in a network that is sophisticated enough to perform linguistically complex tasks is a very tall order, well beyond the current state of the art. Unfortunately, while some significant progress has been made over the past decade or two, our ability to understand the knowledge in networks of any sophistication remains quite rudimentary. So suppose we have trained a network to pronounce *petit* and related French words, achieving 96% generalization to novel words. It seems reasonable to expect—given the past decades' experience with such experiments—that with a great deal of insight, skill, and persistence (and a bit of luck), a researcher *might* be able to analyze the trained network to the point of being able to explain why, given the connection weights, and the representation of individual words like *petit* in various contexts, the correct pronunciation behavior *mathematically follows*. It does not seem at all likely, however, that a researcher could produce more than highly fragmentary explanations at any greater level of generality about the lexical and grammatical knowledge of the network and its consequent behavior.

Now how does such depth and breadth of explanation of this tiny bit of phonology compare with that provided by basic linguistic theory? To lend some perspective on this question, Table 2 summarizes some aspects of an explanation of *petit*'s behavior that emerge from contemporary generative phonology.

Starting with row (a) of Table 2, 'pətit ~ pəti' means that the two pronunciations of *petit* are alternants; we have already stated a generalization concerning the contexts in which each form appears. With respect to the generative explanation, the first thing to note is that this behavior is not peculiar to French; in as distant a language as Lardil, an Australian aboriginal language, the noun stem for 'story' is pronounced [ŋaluk] when followed by a vowel-initial suffix, but [ŋalu] otherwise: the final *k* behaves like the final *t* of *petit* (row (b)). (Indeed, even English has a tiny vestige of such behavior, in the indefinite article *an ~ a*.) The next observation is that in French, this behavior is not limited to *petit*; the final *t* in many—but not all—French words behaves the same way. In row (c), this observation is written 't ~ ∅]Wd'; that is, *t* alternates with silence before the right word-boundary, denoted ']Wd'. Again, the situation in Lardil is parallel: before a stem-boundary, *k* alternates with silence—this time, for all words.

Table 1

Table 2. A *petit* explanation

	Level of generality	French	Lardil
a.	Word (target language)	pətit ~ pəti	
b.	Word (other language)		ŋaluk ~ ŋalu
c.	Segment (target language)	t ~ ∅]$_{Wd}$ (certain words)	k ~ ∅]$_{Stem}$ (always)
d.	Segment class (target language)	C ~ ∅]$_{Wd}$ (certain words)	C ~ ∅]$_{Stem}$ (certain Cs)
e.	Universal	Patterns of 'defective segments' cross-linguistically; C ~ ∅ in syllable coda crosslinguistically, especially 'worse' Cs	
f.	Markedness	Cs avoided in syllable coda in adult inventories, adult phonology, child language, language change, ...	

The next observation (row (d)) is that in French, this behavior is not limited to *t*: there is a class of final consonants that all behave the same way. Again, in Lardil, *k* is merely one member of a class of consonants that can appear only before a vowel. In Lardil, this class can be loosely characterized as those consonants specifying a place of articulation different from that of a **simple coronal**—a single occlusion created by the tongue tip in the general area of the alveolar ridge (see Prince and Smolensky 1993/2004, Chap. 7, and the literature cited therein).

The next step (row (e)) is to observe that the behavior of the class of French final consonants like *t* in *petit* is part of a much more general pattern of 'defective segments' seen in a number of the world's languages; for example, Slavic languages have *vowels* that come and go. The general pattern is that defective segments provide phonological material that can be present or absent, depending on whether the resulting phonological structure would be 'better' with or without that material. In the case of final consonants, the relevant notion of 'better' is this: a consonant is better placed at the beginning of a syllable (the **onset**), rather than the end of a syllable (the **coda**). French defective final consonants appear when they would start a syllable (extending through the initial vowel of the following word); they disappear when they would fall into a syllable coda. In Lardil, the syllable coda (unlike the onset) can never contain the 'worst' consonants: those specifying a place of articulation different from that of a simple coronal.

The general notion that certain linguistic structures are 'better' than others was developed in the 1930s by Jakobson, Trubetzkoy, and others of the Prague Linguistics Circle under the name **markedness**, the 'worse' structures being called **marked** (as by a scarlet letter; Trubetzkoy 1939/1969; Jakobson 1941/1968). Thus, syllable codas are marked relative to syllable onsets; simple coronal consonants are *un*marked relative to other consonants. The Prague School view is that markedness pervades all aspects of language (row (f)). Marked structures are avoided altogether in certain languages—that is, entirely absent from their inventories of possible structures (e.g., languages in which no syllables have codas; Blevins 1995). In other languages, these same marked structures may appear, but only under strongly restricted conditions (e.g., in Lardil, codas can appear only if they contain unmarked consonants). In such languages, marked structures are avoided 'when possible' through phonological alternations (e.g., the final *t* of *petit*). Furthermore, marked structures are avoided by changes across time to the language itself (in Old French, the final *t* of *petit* was pronounced even in coda position). Moreover, Jakobson believed marked structures to be acquired later by children, lost first in aphasia, and, presumably, harder to process online.

Exploiting the notion of markedness, the explanation suggested in Table 2 weaves the tiny thread of *t*'s behavior in *petit* into a large web of crosslinguistic empirical generalizations. First, *t*'s behavior is explained as the avoidance of syllable codas. This is then woven together with the tendency of children to avoid syllable codas. These in turn are both instances of how avoiding markedness of all sorts—from syllable codas and noncoronal consonants in phonology through plural number in morphology to passive voice in syntax—pervades all of language: intact and disordered, adult and child.

In important respects, the notion of linguistic markedness parallels that of (negative) Harmony (or "energy") in connectionist networks. OT's basic hypothesis—that the output of the grammar is the structure that maximizes Harmony relative to the given input—can be viewed as a formalization of the notion that languages avoid more marked—less harmonic—structures. OT's formal calculus of markedness—a version of parallel soft constraint satisfaction, Harmony maximization—has for the first time enabled markedness to provide the very core of a generative theory of grammar.

It is crucial to my argument that, although such depth and breadth of explanation seems quite out of reach of model-based connectionism, at *all* the levels of explanation identified in Table 2, OT analyses have provided a formal means to deduce from the basic principles of the theory both detailed language-particular patterns and overarching empirical generalizations, many of them concerning markedness. In OT, a marked linguistic structure is formalized as one that violates one or more universal well-formedness constraints. To express the universal markedness of syllable codas, a universal constraint (first introduced in Chapter 4) on the well-formedness of syllables is posited: NoCODA, 'Syllables do not have codas' (Prince and Smolensky 1993/2004, Chap. 6, reprinted here in Chapter 13). Similarly, universal constraints express the universal unmarkedness of simple coronal consonants relative to other consonants (Prince and Smolensky 1993/2004, Chap. 9; see Chapter 14). The possible phonetic basis of such constraints in articulation and perception is one facet of OT re-

Table 2

search, but what concerns us now is not what gives rise to these constraints, but what the constraints themselves give rise to: a precise account of the forms of particular words in particular contexts in particular languages (rows (a–d)), and the universal generalizations of which language-particular facts are instances (rows (e–f)).

Along with other proposed universal constraints, NOCODA enables correct prediction of the different context-dependent phonological forms of *petit* and other French words with final defective consonants (Tranel 1994, 1995). Such analysis formally captures the explanation that such consonants are present or absent depending on which option gives the 'better'—more harmonic, less marked—form, entailing avoidance of Harmony-lowering violations of NOCODA. NOCODA plays a formally parallel role in predicting the context-dependent forms of Lardil words like *ŋaluk* (Prince and Smolensky 1993/2004, Chap. 7), formally capturing the common properties of final consonants in French and Lardil (rows (a–d) of Table 2).

Moving to a still more universal level (row (e) of Table 2), an OT analysis of the property that distinguishes defective French consonants from ordinary consonants makes it possible to formally deduce a universal typology that spells out the crosslinguistic possibilities for the behavior of defective material (Zoll 1996). This typology situates French defective consonants in a universal picture that situates them relative to the defective vowels of Slavic and even to defective material in African languages, consisting only in a pitch tone. The Lardil prohibition against placing the least harmonic consonants in the least harmonic syllable position (coda) is seen as one instance of a formal pattern of Harmony maximization—'banning the worst of the worst'—that is evident in many linguistic contexts, including, for example, requirements in African languages that vowels in the same word have the same tongue-root configuration (Prince and Smolensky 1993/2004, Chap. 9; Smolensky 1993, 1997; and Chapter 14).

At a yet more general level, the overarching generalizations concerning markedness summarized in row (f) of Table 2 can be formally deduced within OT. Once any markedness-defining constraint $\mathbb{C}$ (e.g., NOCODA) is recognized as a universal constraint, the general computational principles of OT take over and many logical consequences follow.

According to the general OT theory of crosslinguistic variation, languages will differ in where $\mathbb{C}$ is ranked in their grammars. There will be some languages in which $\mathbb{C}$ is very highly ranked, with the effect that marked structures violating $\mathbb{C}$ will never be most harmonic; they will never appear in the language. Thus, there will be languages that ban the class of $\mathbb{C}$-violating structures from their inventory of possible structures, but no languages that ban the class of $\mathbb{C}$-satisfying structures. (For the case $\mathbb{C}$ = NOCODA, this derives the typological fact that among the world's languages there are some that prohibit syllable codas but none that require them (Jakobson 1962; Prince and Smolensky 1993/2004; Chap. 6; Chapter 13 of this book).

In other languages, $\mathbb{C}$ will be less dominant; it will be outranked by other conflicting constraints that are relevant in some contexts but not in others. In such languages, violations of ℂ will be possible in some contexts, but avoided in others by phonological alternations: marked, ℂ-violating structures will not be optimal, except in those limited contexts where conflicting constraints outranking ℂ are relevant.

Furthermore, according to a general OT learning theory (Smolensky 1996a, b; Tesar and Smolensky 1996, 1998, 2000; Tesar 1998; see Section 12:3), markedness-defining constraints ℂ are initially high ranked, so children's early grammars allow only unmarked structures to be produced; only after such a constraint has been demoted in rank during learning can children produce marked, ℂ-violating structures. (When ℂ = NoCoda, this derives the tendency of children's initial syllables to lack codas.)

OT analysis of language change as reranking of constraints over time (e.g., Zubritskaya 1997) predicts that when a constraint ℂ assumes higher rank, the language loses ℂ-marked structures. And at the frontier of current OT research, in studies of online sentence processing, an incremental-optimization theory of parsing connects processing difficulty to relative Harmony or markedness of syntactic structures (Stevenson and Smolensky 1997; Chapter 19 of this book).

The range of formal explanation summarized in Table 2 is possible because OT's formalization of markedness computation brings into sharp focus a number of issues previously obscure. Some of the most central of these—several already introduced in Chapter 4—are reviewed briefly in (7); for further discussion, see Chapter 12.

(7) Issues in markedness theory formally resolved in OT

   a. *Competition.* To say that a linguistic structure *S* is grammatical in a language *L* because it optimally satisfies *L*'s constraint hierarchy is to exploit a *comparative* property: even though *S* might not satisfy all the universal constraints, *every alternative* incurs more serious violations of *L*'s hierarchy than does *S*. Specifying an OT grammar includes explicitly specifying the **candidate sets** of linguistic structures that compete for optimality. This must be universal, for in OT, only constraint ranking varies across grammars.

   b. *Aggregation of multiple dimensions of markedness.* What defines optimality when the constraints defining different dimensions of markedness disagree on which candidate is preferred? OT's formal answer is **constraint ranking**. *S* is optimal if and only if it is **more harmonic** than all other members *S'* of its candidate set; this means that, of the constraints differentiating the markedness of *S* and *S'*, *S* is favored by the highest ranked.[2] It is remarkable that within such a simple mechanism, reranking can succeed in accounting for such a diversity of observed grammatical patterns.

   c. *Faithfulness to targets.* If grammaticality requires optimality, why isn't there just one grammatical structure per language—the 'best' one? In OT, each candidate is evaluated relative to a **target**, faithfulness to which is de-

---

[2] This characterization of the **harmonic ordering** of Prince and Smolensky 1993/2004, Chap. 5, is due to Jane Grimshaw.

Table 2

manded by constraints collectively called **FAITHFULNESS**, an innovation in grammatical theory. The multiplicity of grammatical—optimal—structures in a single language arises from the multiplicity of possible targets. In phonology, the target is a collection of lexical forms, such as French /pətit/, the word *petit* 'small (masc.)' in isolation. Optimal for this target is [pəti]; this omits the final consonant (/t/) of the target, so it violates a faithfulness constraint $\mathcal{F}$. This minimally unfaithful candidate is optimal because $\mathcal{F}$ is outranked by NOCODA in the French grammar.[3] Optimal for a different target, /pətit øf/ *petit œuf* 'little egg', is a different output, [pə.ti.tøf], in which the final /t/ of *petit* is pronounced, satisfying both $\mathcal{F}$ and NOCODA. That a lexical item (like /pətit/) receives different (but closely related) pronunciations, depending on its context, follows in OT from a fixed target form for the item, faithfulness to which is (minimally) violated in many optimal forms, forced by higher-ranked well-formedness constraints governing sounds in various contexts.

It will be a long time, surely, before our ability to analyze specific connectionist models trained on specific linguistic data reaches the depth and breadth necessary to deduce from basic principles the range of generalizations summarized in Table 2. But a product of grammar-based connectionist research, OT, is already able to do so. And that is the primary reason why—despite the significant limitations on the aspects of connectionist theory that can today be successfully exploited—it seems to me that the grammar-based strategy is a valuable complement to the model-based strategy in the arsenal of connectionist approaches to language.

5 SUMMARY

Debates about the relation of connectionism to language often seem to take it for granted that it is possible to identify two broad theories of language, connectionism and generative grammar, and that these theories are locked in deep scientific conflict. I believe this to be quite false. It is not difficult to identify a particular connectionist proposal about language that conflicts with a particular generative proposal about the same aspect of language—the classic debate about the acquisition of the English past tense (Rumelhart and McClelland 1986; Lachter and Bever 1988; Pinker and Prince 1988; et seq.) may be such a case. But, equally, it is easy to identify two connectionist proposals that conflict as accounts of a common phenomenon, and even easier to identify pairs of conflicting generative proposals. There are plenty of disagreements about language to go around; the question is, do the theories divide into two camps, connectionism and generative grammar, with fundamentally incompatible commitments?

---

[3] Violability of FAITHFULNESS plays a less obvious role in syntax. In Legendre, Smolensky, and Wilson 1998 and Chapter 16, it is used to explain why some syntactic targets have *no* grammatical expression in a particular language: for such an ineffable target, every faithful candidate violates sufficiently high-ranking constraints that an unfaithful candidate, with a different interpretation, is optimal.

The basic commitments of PDP connectionism are often taken to entail commitments about modularity, nativism, and other Big Issues, but it seems to me that brief inspection reveals that while a *particular* PDP proposal may entail such commitments, the broad class of PDP models has, essentially from the beginning, encompassed proposals that span the spectrum of possible positions on the Issues. Equally, I believe that the basic commitments of generative grammar entail no commitments on the Big Issues, even though prominent generative linguists, speaking for themselves, have expressed such commitments.

The view I have tried to sketch here is that PDP connectionism is a commitment to fundamental computational mechanisms, and generative grammar is a commitment to certain types of explanations of certain types of empirical generalizations. These commitments are not in conflict. As I believe recent research shows, it is possible to deploy the computational mechanisms of PDP connectionism to advance the explanatory goals of generative grammar.

Doing so is not possible using the standard model-based strategy for developing concrete proposals within the broad compass of PDP connectionism—at least for the foreseeable future. This is because the types of explanations demanded by generative grammar are not currently feasible within this strategy.

Of course, the model-based strategy has produced important advances in cognitive science and will, I believe, continue to do so for a long time to come. While it may not advance the goals of generative grammar, model-based research serves other scientific goals that seem to me at least as important.

But the goals of generative grammar can in fact be advanced by a different, grammar-based strategy for developing PDP proposals concerning language. In this strategy, new grammatical theories based upon fundamental PDP computational mechanisms are developed, and replace grammatical theories based upon computational devices such as serial symbol manipulation and hard-constraint satisfaction.

In these early days of exploring the potential of the grammar-based strategy for connectionist linguistics, we have succeeded in developing new grammatical formalisms that incorporate only a small part of the full arsenal of connectionist computational principles. But such is the power of the approach that even a small amount of connectionist input, that embodied in OT, has already had a major impact on the practice of generative grammar.

Looking to the future, two types of prospect can now be discerned for the relation between connectionism and generative grammar. One is the development of new grammatical theories that incorporate additional PDP principles (including theories going beyond the symbolic approximation). The other is the advancement of connectionist theories of higher cognition. For OT has led to empirical discoveries about universal grammar that are surprising from the current PDP perspective (including (6i–j)), and these discoveries seem to be telling us that current PDP computational principles are missing something—something quite important for language, at least. It will be most interesting to see what this "something" turns out to be.

Table 2

References

ROA = Rutgers Optimality Archive, http://roa.rutgers.edu

Anderson, J. A., J. W. Silverstein, S. A. Ritz, and R. S. Jones. 1977. Distinctive features, categorical perception, and probability learning: Some applications of a neural model. *Psychological Review* 84, 413–51.

Archangeli, D. 1997. Optimality Theory: An introduction to linguistics in the 1990's. In *Optimality theory: An overview*, eds. D. Archangeli and D. T. Langendoen. Blackwell.

Blevins, J. 1995. The syllable in phonological theory. In *Handbook of phonological theory*, ed. J. A. Goldsmith. Blackwell.

Christiansen, M. H., and N. Chater. 1999. Connectionist natural language processing: The state of the art. *Cognitive Science* 23, 417–37.

Dolan, C. P. 1989. Tensor manipulation networks: Connectionist and symbolic approaches to comprehension, learning, and planning. Ph.D. diss., UCLA.

Elman, J. L. 1990. Finding structure in time. *Cognitive Science* 14, 179–211.

Fauconnier, G. 1985. *Mental spaces*. MIT Press.

Feldman, J. A., and D. H. Ballard. 1982. Connectionist models and their properties. *Cognitive Science* 6, 205–54.

Goldsmith, J. A., and G. Larson. 1990. Local modeling and syllabification. In *Proceedings of the Chicago Linguistic Society 26*.

Grossberg, S. 1976. Adaptive pattern classification and universal recording. Part I, Parallel development and coding of neural feature detectors. *Biological Cybernetics* 23, 121–34.

Hinton, G. E. 1986. Learning distributed representations of concepts. In *Proceedings of the Cognitive Science Society 8*.

Hinton, G. E., and T. J. Sejnowski. 1983. Optimal perceptual inference. In *Proceedings of the IEEE Computer Society Conference on Computer Vision and Pattern Recognition*.

Hummel, J. E., and I. Biederman. 1992. Dynamic binding in a neural network for shape recognition. *Psychological Review* 99, 480–517.

Hummel, J. E., and K. J. Holyoak. 2003. A symbolic-connectionist theory of relational inference and generalization. *Psychological Review* 110, 220–64.

Jacobs, R. A., M. I. Jordan, S. J. Nowlan, and G. E. Hinton. 1991. Adaptive mixtures of local experts. *Neural Computation* 15, 219–50.

Jakobson, R. 1941/1968. *Child language, aphasia and phonological universals*. Mouton.

Jakobson, R. 1962. *Selected writings I: Phonological studies*. Mouton.

Jordan, M. I. 1986. Attractor dynamics and parallelism in a connectionist sequential machine. In *Proceedings of the Cognitive Science Society 8*.

Kohonen, T. 1977. *Associative memory: A system-theoretical approach*. Springer.

Lachter, J., and T. G. Bever. 1988. The relation between linguistic structure and associative theories of language learning—a constructive critique of some connectionist learning models. *Cognition* 28, 195–247.

Lakoff, G. 1987. *Women, fire, and dangerous things*. University of Chicago Press.

Lakoff, G. 1988. A suggestion for a linguistics with connectionist foundations. In *Proceedings of the Connectionist Models Summer School*, eds. D. S. Touretzky, G. E. Hinton, and T. J. Sejnowski. Morgan Kaufmann.

Langacker, R. W. 1987. *Foundations of cognitive grammar*. Vol. 1, *Theoretical prerequisites*. Stanford University Press.

Legendre, G., Y. Miyata, and P. Smolensky. 1990a. Can connectionism contribute to syntax? Harmonic Grammar, with an application. In *Proceedings of the Chicago Linguistic Society 26*.

Legendre, G., Y. Miyata, and P. Smolensky. 1990b. Harmonic Grammar—a formal multi-level connectionist theory of linguistic well-formedness: An application. In *Proceedings of the Cognitive Science Society 12*.

Legendre, G., Y. Miyata, and P. Smolensky. 1990c. Harmonic Grammar—a formal multi-level connectionist theory of linguistic well-formedness: Theoretical foundations. In *Proceedings of the Cognitive Science Society 12*.

Legendre, G., Y. Miyata, and P. Smolensky. 1991a. Distributed recursive structure processing. In *Advances in neural information processing systems 3*, eds. R. P. Lippman, J. E. Moody, and D. S. Touretzky. Morgan Kaufmann.

Legendre, G., Y. Miyata, and P. Smolensky. 1991b. Unifying syntactic and semantic approaches to unaccusativity: A connectionist approach. In *Proceedings of the Berkeley Linguistics Society 7*.

Legendre, G., P. Smolensky, and C. Wilson. 1998. When is less more? Faithfulness and minimal links in *wh*-chains. In *Is the best good enough? Optimality and competition in syntax*, eds. P. Barbosa, D. Fox, P. Hagstrom, M. McGinnis, and D. Pesetsky. MIT Press and MIT Working Papers in Linguistics. ROA 117.

McClelland, J. L., D. E. Rumelhart, and the PDP Research Group. 1986. *Parallel distributed processing: Explorations in the microstructure of cognition*. Vol. 2, *Psychological and biological models*. MIT Press.

McCloskey, M. 1992. Networks and theories: The place of connectionism in cognitive science. *Psychological Science* 2, 387–95.

McMillan, C., M. C. Mozer, and P. Smolensky. 1992. Rule induction through integrated symbolic and subsymbolic processing. In *Advances in neural information processing systems 4*, eds. J. Moody, S. Hanson, and R. Lippman. Morgan Kaufmann.

Mozer, M. C. 1991. *The perception of multiple objects: A connectionist approach*. MIT Press.

Pinker, S., and A. Prince. 1988. On language and connectionism: Analysis of a parallel distributed processing model of language acquisition. *Cognition* 28, 73–193.

Plate, T. A. 1991. Holographic Reduced Representations: Convolution algebra for compositional distributed representations. In *Proceedings of the International Joint Conference on Artificial Intelligence 12*.

Plaut, D., and T. Shallice. 1994. *Connectionist modeling in cognitive neuropsychology: A case study*. Erlbaum.

Pollack, J. 1990. Recursive distributed representations. *Artificial Intelligence* 46, 77–105.

Prince, A. 1993. In defense of the number *i*: Anatomy of a linear dynamic model of linguistic generalizations. Technical report RuCCS-TR-1, Rutgers Center for Cognitive Science, Rutgers University.

Prince, A., and P. Smolensky. 1991. Notes on connectionism and Harmony Theory in linguistics. Technical report CU-CS-533-91, Computer Science Department, University of Colorado at Boulder.

Prince, A., and P. Smolensky. 1993/2004. *Optimality Theory: Constraint interaction in generative grammar*. Technical report, Rutgers University and University of Colorado at Boulder, 1993. ROA 537, 2002. Revised version published by Blackwell, 2004.

Prince, A., and P. Smolensky. 1997. Optimality: From neural networks to universal grammar. *Science* 275, 1604–10.

Rumelhart, D. E., R. Durbin, R. Golden, and Y. Chauvin. 1996. Backpropagation: The basic theory. In *Mathematical perspectives on neural networks*, eds. P. Smolensky, M. C. Mozer, and D. E. Rumelhart. Erlbaum.

Rumelhart, D. E., and J. L. McClelland. 1986. On learning the past tenses of English verbs. In *Parallel distributed processing: Explorations in the microstructure of cognition*. Vol. 2, *Psychological and biological models*, J. L. McClelland, D. E. Rumelhart, and the PDP Research Group. MIT Press.

Rumelhart, D. E., J. L. McClelland, and the PDP Research Group. 1986. *Parallel distributed processing: Explorations in the microstructure of cognition.* Vol. 1, *Foundations.* MIT Press.

Rumelhart, D. E., P. Smolensky, J. L. McClelland, and G. E. Hinton. 1986. Schemata and sequential thought processes in parallel distributed processing. In *Parallel distributed processing: Explorations in the microstructure of cognition.* Vol. 2, *Psychological and biological models*, J. L. McClelland, D. E. Rumelhart, and the PDP Research Group. MIT Press.

Rumelhart, D. E., and D. Zipser. 1985. Feature discovery by competitive learning. *Cognitive Science* 9, 75–112.

Sejnowski, T. J., and C. R. Rosenberg. 1987. Parallel networks that learn to pronounce English text. *Complex Systems* 1, 145–68.

Shastri, L., and V. Ajjanagadde. 1993. From simple associations to systematic reasoning: A connectionist representation of rules, variables and dynamic bindings using temporal synchrony. *Behavioral and Brain Sciences* 16, 417–94.

Smolensky, P. 1983. Schema selection and stochastic inference in modular environments. In *Proceedings of the National Conference on Artificial Intelligence 3.*

Smolensky, P. 1988. On the proper treatment of connectionism. *Behavioral and Brain Sciences* 11, 1–74.

Smolensky, P. 1990. Tensor product variable binding and the representation of symbolic structures in connectionist networks. *Artificial Intelligence* 46, 159–216.

Smolensky, P. 1993. Harmony, markedness, and phonological activity. Talk presented at the Rutgers Optimality Workshop-1. ROA 87.

Smolensky, P. 1996a. The initial state and 'Richness of the Base' in Optimality Theory. Technical report JHU-CogSci-96-4, Cognitive Science Department, Johns Hopkins University. ROA 154.

Smolensky, P. 1996b. On the comprehension/production dilemma in child language. *Linguistic Inquiry* 27, 720–31. ROA 118.

Smolensky, P. 1996c. Statistical perspectives on neural networks. In *Mathematical perspectives on neural networks*, eds. P. Smolensky, M. C. Mozer, and D. E. Rumelhart. Erlbaum.

Smolensky, P. 1997. Constraint interaction in generative grammar II: Local conjunction (or, random rules in Universal Grammar). Talk presented at the Hopkins Optimality Theory Conference.

Smolensky, P. 1999. Grammar-based connectionist approaches to language. *Cognitive Science* 23, 589–613.

Smolensky, P., M. C. Mozer, and D. E. Rumelhart, eds. 1996. *Mathematical perspectives on neural networks.* Erlbaum.

Stevenson, S., and P. Smolensky. 1997. Extending Optimality Theory to comprehension: Competence and performance. Talk presented at the Conference on Architectures and Mechanisms for Language Processing (AMLaP-97).

Stone, G. O. 1986. An analysis of the delta rule and the learning of statistical associations. In *Parallel distributed processing: Explorations in the microstructure of cognition.* Vol. 1, *Foundations*, D. E. Rumelhart, J. L. McClelland, and the PDP Research Group. MIT Press.

Talmy, L. 1988. Force dynamics in language and cognition. *Cognitive Science* 12, 49–100.

Tesar, B. B. 1998. Error-driven learning in Optimality Theory via the efficient computation of optimal forms. In *Is the best good enough? Optimality and competition in syntax*, eds. P. Barbosa, D. Fox, P. Hagstrom, M. McGinnis, and D. Pesetsky. MIT Press and MIT Working Papers in Linguistics.

Tesar, B. B., and P. Smolensky. 1994. Synchronous-firing variable binding is spatio-temporal tensor product representation. In *Proceedings of the Cognitive Science Society 16.*

Tesar, B. B., and P. Smolensky. 1996. Learnability in Optimality Theory (long version). Technical report JHU-CogSci-96-3, Cognitive Science Department, Johns Hopkins University. ROA 156.

Tesar, B. B., and P. Smolensky. 1998. Learnability in Optimality Theory. *Linguistic Inquiry* 29, 229–68.

Tesar, B. B., and P. Smolensky. 2000. *Learnability in Optimality Theory.* MIT Press.

Touretzky, D. S. 1986. BoltzCONS: Reconciling connectionism with the recursive structure of stacks and trees. In *Proceedings of the Cognitive Science Society 8.*

Touretzky, D. S., and G. E. Hinton. 1988. A distributed connectionist production system. *Cognitive Science* 12, 423–66.

Touretzky, D. S., and D. W. Wheeler. 1991. Sequence manipulation using parallel mapping networks. *Neural Computation* 3, 98–109.

Tranel, B. 1994. French liaison and elision revisited: A unified account within Optimality Theory. ROA 15.

Tranel, B. 1995. Current issues in French phonology liaison and position theories. In *Handbook of phonological theory,* ed. J. Goldsmith. Blackwell.

Trubetzkoy, N. 1939/1969. *Principles of phonology* (translation of *Grundzüge der Phonologie*). University of California Press.

Zoll, C. C. 1996. Parsing below the segment in a constraint-based framework. Ph.D. diss., University of California at Berkeley. ROA 143.

Zubritskaya, K. 1997. Mechanism of sound change in Optimality Theory. *Language Variation and Change* 9, 121–48.

23

Computational Levels and Integrated Connectionist/ Symbolic Explanation

Paul Smolensky

The vertically Integrated Connectionist/Symbolic Cognitive Architecture (ICS) treats symbolic and connectionist theories as valid descriptions, at different levels of organization, of a single system: the mind/brain. How then is the wide range of data in cognitive science to be understood in ICS: via symbolic explanations, or connectionist ones?

Sorting out the subtleties underpinning this question demands a clear understanding of the multilevel structure characteristic of computational systems. These systems are analyzed here into three overall levels of organization. In ICS, the highest, **functional**-level description is a symbolic account of mental structure; the lowest, a **physical**-level description of relevant neural structure. Bridging these is an intermediate **computational** level that formally reduces a description corresponding to symbols to a description corresponding to neurons.

Standard reductions of symbolic computation have symbols 'all the way down': they reduce to a level of elementary symbolic operations that is fundamentally irreconcilable with neural computation. And standard connectionism does not provide a means of organizing elementary connectionist operations to build up symbolic computation.

ICS solves this reduction problem by splitting the computational level into two sublevels, providing two different ways of decomposing a state of the mind/brain. At the higher sublevel, a state is decomposed into superimposed patterns, corresponding to the decomposition of a symbol structure into its constituents. At the lower sublevel, a state is decomposed into individual unit activations, corresponding to the physical decomposition of a brain state at the neural level. These two decompositions are compatible because the reduction from the higher to the lower is not structure-preserving: because of distributed representations, the mapping between symbol-realizing patterns and individual unit activations is many to many. The notion of structure preservation needed here—isomorphism—is investigated, as are the implications of ICS's split-level computational level for explaining a broad range of data that spans multiple cognitive subdisciplines and several levels of analysis. Symbolic explanation in ICS addresses many important types of phenomena, but ICS models of cognitive processes are connectionist, not symbolic (Figures 8.❽ and 9 of Chapter 2's ICS map).

Contents

1 OVERVIEW

1.1 The problem

As in many other sciences, in cognitive science one central approach to explanation is a type of reductionism. The explanatory strategy of computationalism demystifies cognition by characterizing it in terms of abstract functions and then showing how such complex cognitive functions can be reduced to a set of simple, mechanical operations. These primitive operations are not conceptually mysterious; furthermore, they are realizable in physical systems. Computational reductions give us precise ways of understanding not only what makes cognition possible at all, but also what makes cognition possible in a physical system.

A set of primitive operations, and their modes of interaction, define a **computational architecture** upon which a computational reduction is founded. If reduction to primitive operations is to explain how cognition is possible in a *brain*, then the computational architecture employed must consist of operations and interactions that are not merely simple, but simple in a way that puts them within the capabilities of neural computation.

Connectionist theory undertakes to characterize just such an architecture. Connectionist networks are, however, often criticized as naïvely simple, given contemporary knowledge of neuroscience. Such a criticism makes little sense, though, when connectionism is properly treated: it is a target of computational reduction for theories of cognition, not a tool for explaining the function of fine-grained neural structure. The real danger for a target of cognitive reduction is that it will be too computationally *powerful*—not too *simple*. Accusations of *excessive* computational power in connectionist architectures are thus appropriate—and they are recognized as such by connectionist theorists, who often explore architectural modifications motivated entirely by such concerns.

So while an enormous amount of difficult work remains to be done, connectionist theory appears to have given cognitive science, at the very least, an effective vehicle for launching the formal study of neural computation. At the other extreme of the reductive scale, contemporary cognitive science also possesses an effective means of precisely characterizing many important, high-level mental functions: symbolic cognitive theory. This theory is computational in that it provides a means of reduction to a set of simple, mechanical operations.

The conceptual crisis currently facing cognitive science arises from the simple fact that the elementary, mechanical operations to which symbolic theory reduces cognitive functions do not constitute a computational architecture that is consistent with today's conception of neural computation (see Box 1). The neurally plausible architectures provided by connectionist theory do not appear to support the kinds of cognitive functions described by symbolic theory. It is of course exactly this crisis that motivates the search for an architecture that can successfully integrate symbolic and connectionist computation—that is, solve what was called in Chapter 3 (1) the **central paradox** of cognitive architecture.

The tensions forming the central paradox can be analyzed as the result of incompatibilities among the demands placed on a satisfactory computational architecture for human cognition. These are summarized in (1).

(1)   **Architectural requirements** (initial formulation)

A complete cognitive architecture must provide a formal foundation for developing, within a single unified framework, theories that promise to

a.   formally explain central aspects of higher cognition, such as grammatical universals and the productivity of cognition;

b.   provide a formal framework for theories of cognitive processes that

i.   explains actual human behavior and

ii.   shows explicitly how cognition can be reduced to basic computational operations;

c.   reduce mental computation to neural computation, showing how the basic computational operations can be, and are, physically realized in the brain.

Simultaneously meeting all these challenges within a unified theory is the goal of ICS research.

The incompatibility of symbolic and connectionist theory has been formulated as a challenge to connectionism by Fodor and Pylyshyn (1988) (see Box 2). Connectionism, they assert, faces a serious dilemma. On one horn, connectionist computation could be used to *eliminate* symbols from cognitive theory; but then connectionism couldn't explain central aspects of higher cognition, for which symbols seem necessary. On the other horn, connectionist computation could be used to literally *implement* symbolic computation; but then connectionism can teach us nothing new about cognition proper, only (at best) something about the neuroscience underlying the "classical" symbolic theory of cognition that we already have.

Box 1. Reducing symbolic computation to primitives:

Symbols all the way down

Symbolic computation enables highly abstract conceptions of mental representations, processes, and knowledge to be characterized with formal precision. It also shows how to reduce these abstractions to extremely simple and concrete elements that can be physically realized.

How is this reduction carried out? In this box, I will consider a conventional computer running Lisp—a **Lisp machine** (roughly along the lines proposed in Abelson, Sussman, and Sussman 1985; see also Touretzky 1989). This (hypothetical) computer is programmed to generate sentences from a context-free grammar (see

---

Box 1

Box 6:1). The generation program is written in Lisp, as explained below. While the details would vary tremendously for different choices of cognitive theory and symbolic implementation, the overall picture and the ultimate conclusions hold, I believe, quite generally for symbolic cognitive theory. To convey a sense of the big picture, many simplifications are necessary throughout; for further simplicity, nonstandard notations are employed. This box merits a liberal, not a literal, reading.

Functional level

At the highest level of abstraction, the sentence generator can be functionally described via structures like (1a), a local tree generated by context-free rewrite rules such as (1b).

(1)　　Functional level

　　　a.　*Representation:* trees with all nodes labeled. For example:

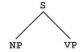

　　　b.　*Grammar:* $G_1 = \{\mathbf{S} \rightarrow \mathbf{NP}\ \mathbf{VP}, \ldots\}$

　　　c.　*Function:* f expands leftmost nonterminal node using G_1.

At this level, descriptions employ abstract mathematical entities defined by the axioms they satisfy. Functions may be defined abstractly, such as the function f (1c). f has an input **I** that is a labeled tree. The corresponding output **O** is the same tree, except at one node. This node is the leftmost unexpanded node, that is, the leftmost node with no children labeled with a nonterminal symbol X. In **O**, this node retains its label X but now has two children A B, where X → A B is a rule of the grammar G_1. For example, if X = **S**, and the selected rule is the one shown in (1b), at the location of childless **S** in the input **I**, the output **O** has the local tree (1a). Starting with **S**, the computer repeatedly applies f to its own output until no further change results; then the output of f is a grammatical parse of a sentence in the language specified by G_1.[1]

Lisp list level

The system under consideration is running a Lisp program built of substructures like those illustrated in (2).

(2)　　Lisp list level

　　　a.　*Representation:* lists (S (NP VP))

　　　b.　*Grammar:* ((S (NP VP)) ⋯)

　　　c.　*Operation:* (substitute node (lhs rule) rule)

The structure being generated is represented as a list of elements each of which is either an atomic symbol, like NP, or another list. A simple example is (2a), the list representation of both the local tree (1a) and its rule counterpart (1b). The grammar is a list

---

[1] It is true, but irrelevant to our purposes, that this depth-first expansion process can fail to terminate if the grammar is left recursive. This exemplifies the level of simplification adopted in this box.

of rules. An operation is a call to a Lisp procedure, such as (2c), which employs the procedure substitute. In Lisp, a procedure call is specified by a list consisting of the procedure name followed by its arguments.[2] This particular procedure call uses a rule of the grammar, rule, to operate on a node in the structure being generated, node, modifying it by substituting for the symbol on the left-hand-side of the rule, (lhs rule), the entire rule itself, which has the effect of inserting the two child nodes. This procedure call uses the access function lhs, which extracts the left-hand side of a rule. The representations and operations at this level match quite closely those of the functional level description (1), operating at essentially the same level of abstraction.

Lisp dotted-pair level

How is a Lisp program using data and operations like those in (2) actually realized in a physical machine? We will work our way down to the machine level in three additional steps. First, in Lisp, lists are actually a special type of data built from more basic elements called **dotted pairs**. Each half of a dotted pair is either an atomic symbol or another dotted pair. The list in (2a) is realized as the dotted-pair structure (3a), shown in both textual and graphical form. In the diagram, a dotted pair is rendered as an unlabeled node; the left and right elements of this pair are drawn as the node's left and right children. The structure is much like a binary tree (except that two nodes with the same label denote the same element). Lists are special dotted-pair structures in that no symbol is ever a right child, except the special symbol nil representing the empty structure.

(3)   Lisp dotted-pair level

      a.   *Representation:* dotted pairs (approximately, binary trees with unlabeled internal nodes); (S . ((NP . (VP . nil)) . nil))

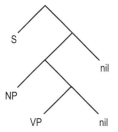

      b.   *Grammar:* ((S . ((NP . (VP . nil)) . nil)) . ⋯)

      c.   *Operation:*   (define substitute (n r)

                          (if (equal? (ex$_0$ n) (ex$_0$ r)) (set (ex$_0$ n) (copy r)) n))

A rule is a dotted-pair structure with the form (3a), and the grammar is just a list of such rules (3b). At this level, all operations such as substitute (2c) are defined in terms of the primitive symbol-manipulating operations of Lisp (3c).[3] These primitives in-

---

[2] Thus, '(f x y)' in Lisp is analogous to '$f(x, y)$' in standard mathematical notation.

[3] For readability, (3c) uses the list notation; the actual procedure definition is the dotted pair imple-

Box 1

clude the operations of extracting the left or right child of a pair (ex₀, ex₁; traditionally 'car' and 'cdr'), attaching a left or right child (set), testing pairs for equality (equal?), assigning definitions to function names (define), and conditional branching of control (if). (In the procedure (if test p q), if test is true, p is performed; otherwise, q.) Procedure definitions can refer to other defined procedures (such as copy, defined from the primitive operation that constructs new dotted pairs, cons); the definition of a procedure can even refer to itself (recursion). This particular procedure takes as input a node n in a tree like (3a), and a rule r like (3b). If the label of n—its left child—equals the 'left-hand side' of the rule r—its left child—then substitute replaces the left child of n with a new copy of r; otherwise, n is unchanged.

Cons-cell level

A dotted pair is in turn realized as a **cons-cell**, each half of which contains a **pointer**— a link to an atomic symbol or another cons-cell. This is graphically depicted in (4). Tags like '⟨p8⟩' are metalanguage labels making it easy for me to refer to particular cells. (The 'p' and 's' in these tags connote 'pair' and 'symbol'.)

(4)   Cons-cell level

    a.   *Representation:* pairs of pointers; symbols

    b.   *Grammar:* same

    c.   *Operations:* insert and follow pointers; create symbols

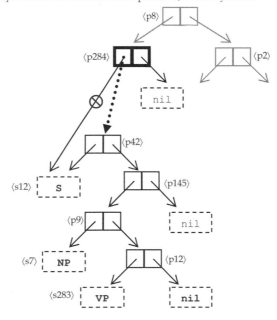

menting this list. Furthermore, as throughout this box, this discussion is oversimplified out of expository necessity.

At this level, operations consist of setting pointers, following pointers, and creating symbols. The actual substitution operation within (3c) (set) is diagrammed in (4); the grammar rule being applied is the one shown in (3b). The targeted cons-cell ⟨p284⟩ (heavy border) is part of a structure that also includes ⟨p8⟩ and ⟨p2⟩ (gray borders); the latter two cells also point to other cells (not drawn). Prior to substitution, the left pointer of ⟨p284⟩ points directly to the symbol named S. The operation changes that pointer so it now points to ⟨p42⟩, the cell heading a structure in which S has two children named NP and VP.

Register-machine level

Finally, the symbols, pointers, and cons-cells are themselves realized as bit patterns, addresses, and bytes of random-access memory within a traditional computer (with a von Neumann architecture). Here I will oversimplify greatly (especially, by pretending a symbol is just a string of letters and by ignoring the stack needed to control the sequencing of procedures and arguments). The situation shown in (4) is depicted schematically in (5a). This is the state of the machine after making the substitution; the discarded pointer is shown as an address (in ⟨L284⟩) that is crossed out.

(5)   Register-machine level

    a. *Representation:* addresses and binary encodings of characters in random-access memory locations

Registers		Pairs				Symbols	
⟨M0⟩	42	⟨L1⟩			⟨R1⟩	⟨S1⟩	
⟨M1⟩	284	⟨L2⟩	...	...	⟨R2⟩	⟨S2⟩	
⟨M2⟩	S12	⋮			⋮	⋮	
⟨M3⟩	S12	⟨L7⟩			⟨R7⟩	⟨S7⟩	N
⟨M4⟩	42	⟨L8⟩	284	2	⟨R8⟩	⟨S8⟩	P
⟨M5⟩		⟨L9⟩	S7	12	⟨R9⟩	⟨S9⟩	•
⟨M6⟩		⋮			⋮	⋮	
⟨M7⟩		⟨L12⟩	S283	0	⟨R12⟩	⟨S12⟩	S
⟨M8⟩		⟨L13⟩			⟨R13⟩	⟨S13⟩	•
⟨M9⟩		⋮			⋮	⋮	
		⟨L42⟩	S12	145	⟨R42⟩	⟨S42⟩	
		⋮			⋮	⋮	
		⟨L145⟩	9	0	⟨R145⟩	⟨S145⟩	
		⋮			⋮	⋮	
		⟨L283⟩			⟨R283⟩	⟨S283⟩	U
		⟨L284⟩	~~S1242~~	0	⟨R284⟩	⟨S284⟩	P
		⟨L285⟩			⟨R285⟩	⟨S285⟩	•
		⋮			⋮	⋮	

The left and right halves of the cons-cell labeled ⟨p42⟩ in (4) are realized by two

Box 1

bytes of memory that I'll refer to with the metalabels '⟨L42⟩' and '⟨R42⟩'. L42 is the address of ⟨L42⟩—a bit string the computer can use to access ⟨L42⟩. 'L42' refers to the content of this register (another bit string). Finally, 'N' designates the bit string that encodes the letter N; the sequence of bit strings in ⟨S7⟩–⟨S9⟩ represents the letter string NP ('•' denotes a special bit string, e.g., all 0s, marking the end of a letter string). '∅' signifies the address of nil.

For example, consider ⟨L42⟩. It contains S12, the address of ⟨S12⟩, which contains the bit string S encoding S. This configuration realizes the left pointer of ⟨p42⟩ in (4), which points at the symbol S. The location of the corresponding right-half pointer is ⟨R42⟩; this contains the (partial) address 145, which realizes a pointer to cons-cell ⟨p145⟩. (Combined with L or R, 145 allows access to ⟨L145⟩ or ⟨R145⟩.)

(5c) shows a program fragment that, for the specific rule **S → NP VP**, achieves the rule application process partially illustrated in (4). The operations at the register-machine level are simple manipulations of memory locations, such as copying the contents of the left half of a cell into a memory register (set-M … L …), storing the location of a symbol in a memory register (set-M … symb-addr …), getting the address of the next available cell for storing new information (M0), and branching conditioned on whether the contents of two memory locations are identical (jump-if-uneq).

(5)   Register-machine level (continued)

   b.   *Grammar:* embedded in operations

   c.   *Operations:*

Instruction	Comment
⋮	
NNode	Landing point for jumps
⋮	[*Operations loading* ⟨M1⟩ *with the address of the leftmost node not yet examined, n:* 284]
set-M M2 L M1	M2 gets the address of the left-child node of *n* (L284): S12
set-M M3 symb-addr S	M3 gets the address of the symbol S: S12
jump-if-uneq M2 M3 *NRule*	If the left child of *n* ≠ S, jump to *NRule* [here, *x* = S, so go to next instruction]
set-M M4 M0	M4 gets M0, the address of the first free pair for constructing a new node: 42
⋮	[*A copy of the rule is constructed, rooted at cell 42; cells 42, 145, 9, and 12 are assigned*]
set-L M1 M4	The left-child cell of *n* is set to M4: 42
jump *NNode*	Jump to instruction initiating selection of the next node *n*
NRule	Landing point for jumps
⋮	[*Proceed to apply the next grammar rule to n*]

The point

The main reason for attempting a five-level description of a symbolic computational system is to explicate the assertion that, in the symbolic computational reduction from abstract to physical, *it's symbols all the way down*. A symbol such as **NP** in the grammar G_1 (1b) remains a localized, unitary entity every step of the way down to its ultimate identity as the memory location $\langle S7 \rangle$. This is strict locality in space. There is a comparable locality in time as well. At each step of the reduction, a higher-level operation is replaced by a group of several simpler operations, which—as a unitary lower-level block—bears a relationship to other such blocks that is the same as the relationship of the original higher-level operation to the other high-level operations. The original atemporal, functional description (1) becomes an inherently serial description and just gets more and more so as the reduction proceeds to lower levels. Ultimately, symbolic computation comes down to a long sequence of steps consisting of following pointers, setting pointers, and checking pointers for equality, and jumping from one stored instruction to another.

What do following, setting, and checking pointers, and jumping to instructions, have to do with neural computation? Does reduction to *those* kinds of simple, mechanical operations shed light on how abstract cognition is realized in the brain? What do we learn about the physical embodiment of *our* minds from a picture in which a mental process consists of a huge number of tiny steps, crucially ordered one after the other in just the right sequence, where at any moment the actual computing activity is localized to only two or three elementary units?

A computational framework, by definition, is one in which complex behaviors are reduced to an organized collection of processes so simple as to be realizable in simple physical systems (Haugeland 1985). It seems uncontroversial to assert that the *reduction* provided by symbolic computation contributes very little to our understanding of how brains realize minds. *Symbolic theory* has a tremendous amount to teach us about the mind, but it is ironic that the property that makes symbolic theory *computational* is itself of little worth for cognitive science.

A primary objective of ICS research is to find new ways of reducing symbolic functional descriptions of cognition to simple, physically realizable processes, well within the power of neural computation. The progress toward this goal within ICS is due to progress in understanding how a computational system that is symbolic at an abstract level *need not be symbolic all the way down*. Reduction of symbolic computation to parallel, distributed, *connectionist* primitive operations holds the promise that the very reduction process that makes such a system computational is also just what makes it highly relevant to understanding how mind is realized in brain.

Box 1

Box 2. The Fodorian challenge to connectionism

In a highly influential paper, Fodor and Pylyshyn (1988) argue that connectionists have two choices: implement the 'classical' symbolic cognitive architecture in their networks, or leave unexplained several fundamental properties of cognition that are explained by the classical architecture. These properties are as follows:

Systematicity. The thoughts a cognitive system is capable of entertaining are not a random collection (like the phrases in a tourist's foreign-language phrasebook) but a systematic set (like the sentences that can be produced by a fluent speaker of a language). For example, if a cognitive system can entertain the thought expressed by *Sandy loves Kim*, then it can entertain the thought expressed by *Kim loves Sandy.*

Productivity. The thoughts a cognitive system is capable of entertaining are unlimited; arbitrarily complex thoughts can be created by composing simpler thoughts.

Compositionality. Thoughts have combinatorial structure, and the semantic content of a thought is determined compositionally by the semantic content of its parts. The thought expressed by *Sandy loves Kim* means what it does because its parts—for instance, those expressed by *Sandy and Kim*—mean what they do.

Inferential coherence. The inferences a cognitive system can draw are not an arbitrary set, but those that arise from the coherent application of certain inference rules. For example, a system able to deduce the proposition P from the proposition $P \& Q \& R$ possesses an inference rule that would enable it also to deduce P from $P \& Q$.

Fodor and Pylyshyn argue that these are *necessary* properties of a cognitive system and that they must be entailed by any adequate theory of cognition. They claim that such entailments follow from the classical symbolic architecture, and presumably would also follow from a connectionist architecture that implemented a classical architecture (although a "mere implementation" of a classical architecture would add nothing to its status as a cognitive architecture). The connectionist's alternative to implementing a classical architecture, on Fodor and Pylyshyn's analysis, would be some neo-Humean associationist architecture that would entail none of their fundamental properties of cognition and would thus fail a fundamental criterion of adequacy.

Fodor and McLaughlin (1990) followed up this argument in a critique of a connectionist architecture based on tensor product representations. A main claim was that these representations do not actually possess constituent structure: the alleged constituent vectors aren't "really there" and so can't have the sort of causal role in mental processing needed to explain Fodor and Pylyshyn's fundamental cognitive properties.[4]

---

[4] Here is a brief synopsis of a main thread of my debate with Fodor and colleagues, with no pretense of objectivity. In Smolensky 1988, I argued that the proper role of connectionism is to explain the successes and repair the failures of symbolic theory by reducing it to a level closer to that of neurons. Fodor and Pylyshyn (1988) asserted that connectionist representations are inadequate for explaining

1.2 The ICS resolution

In this chapter, I argue that ICS furnishes a unified cognitive architecture within which all the challenges of (1) can be faced; among many other things, it resolves the alleged dilemma posed by Fodor and Pylyshyn (1988). The crucial innovation is tensor networks, or **tensorial computation**, the topic of Part II of this book (especially Chapter 5). Tensorial computation furnishes the bridge that allows ICS to cross the chasm separating the high ground of symbolic theories of mind from the low ground of connectionist theories of brain. On the higher side, tensorial computation mirrors — is **isomorphic** to — key aspects of symbolic computation. On the lower side, tensorial computation is simply parallel, distributed connectionist computation, which is plausibly isomorphic to neural computation. Crucially, I will argue, the higher and lower sides of tensorial computation are not isomorphic with one another in the relevant respects. Yet the lower is a formal realization of the higher. The result is a computational theory that reduces symbolic computation to connectionist computation: it provides a formal realization mapping from one to the other. *However*, a crucial transformation occurs within the level of tensorial computation, and this is what enables the symbolic to reduce to the connectionist. This transformation is achieved by distributed representations, which take distinct symbols and realize them in a common set of units, and which enable massively parallel processing. Because of this transformation, in ICS, unlike the purely symbolic architecture, it's *not* 'symbols all the way down' (see Box 1).

An **isomorphism** maps each part of one system to a part of another system in such a way as to preserve the relationships among the parts within each system. Tensorial computation can be isomorphic to both symbolic and neural descriptions because it has two different modes of decomposition into parts. A tensorial representation is a vector with a special structure that enables it to be decomposed into con-

cognition because they are atomic—a compound proposition such as *p & q*, they claimed, is represented by a single unit, connected to a different single unit for *p* and another unit for *q*. In Smolensky 1987, I observed that this is an incorrect characterization of PDP connectionism, in which a composite has a distributed representation that is the *superposition* of the distributed representations of its parts. How this invalidates Fodor and Pylsyhyn's primary argument was spelled out in detail in Smolensky 1991. Fodor and McLaughlin (1990) claimed that it is not sufficient to show that a network *can* have the combinatorial properties needed for an adequate theory of mind; that a network *must* have such properties is necessary. In Smolensky 1995, I pointed out that a viable connectionist theory of mind is not the theory that *any* network is a mind; a viable theory posits a particular set of principles, and it is networks satisfying these principles that realize minds. The principles of ICS were explicitly presented, and shown to logically entail the right combinatorial properties, reducing them to neural computation. The "classical" theory that Fodor and colleagues defend does not *derive* those combinatorial properties at all; it merely stipulates them in its symbolic definition of mind. Against the superpositional representations of ICS, Fodor (1997) claimed that a realization of a symbolic structure must have physically separable realizations of the structure's symbol tokens in order for the symbols to be sufficiently "real" to qualify as a legitimate basis for explaining cognitive generalizations. The falsity of this claim is documented in detail in the present chapter.

The debate through 1995 is reprinted, with enlightening commentary by the editors, in Macdonald and Macdonald 1995. See also van Gelder 1990; Cummins 1991, 1996; Mathews 1997; Phillips 2000; Aizawa 2003; and especially Horgan and Tienson 1996. For learning-oriented conceptions of connectionist systematicity, see, for example, Hadley 1994a, b, 1997a, b; Niklasson and van Gelder 1994; Phillips 1994; Aizawa 1997; Hadley and Hayward 1997; Bodén and Niklasson 2000.

Box 2

stituent vectors; for example, $\mathbf{s} = \mathbf{A} \otimes \mathbf{r}_0 + \mathbf{B} \otimes \mathbf{r}_1$ expresses a decomposition of $\mathbf{s}$ into $\mathbf{A}$- and $\mathbf{B}$-constituents. This decomposition is isomorphic to the decomposition of a symbol structure $\mathbf{s} = [\mathbf{A}\ \mathbf{B}]$ into its $\mathbf{A}$- and $\mathbf{B}$-constituents. This is the sense in which the higher-level description of tensorial computation is 'symbolic'.

At the same time, since a tensorial representation $\mathbf{s}$ is an activation vector, it can be decomposed into a list of numbers $(s_1, s_2, \ldots)$, each the activation value of a single connectionist unit. This lower-level decomposition of $\mathbf{s}$ is isomorphic to the decomposition of a biological pattern of neural activity into a list of numerical activation values of individual neurons.[5]

Tensorial computation thus interfaces isomorphically with symbolic computation at its higher level, and with neural computation at its lower level. *Because of distributed representations, however, the higher and lower levels are not isomorphic with each other*: the two modes of decomposition cannot be put into one-to-one correspondence (see Figure 1).[6] A higher-level part like $\mathbf{A} \otimes \mathbf{r}_0$ corresponds to many lower-level parts: the activation values of the individual units in the pattern of activity $\mathbf{A} \otimes \mathbf{r}_0$. A lower-level part, the activation of unit k, corresponds to many higher-level parts, since it is part of the pattern defining many constituent vectors (e.g., both $\mathbf{A} \otimes \mathbf{r}_0$ and $\mathbf{B} \otimes \mathbf{r}_1$). The higher- and lower-level decompositions crosscut one another.

Figure 1. Interlevel relations in ICS

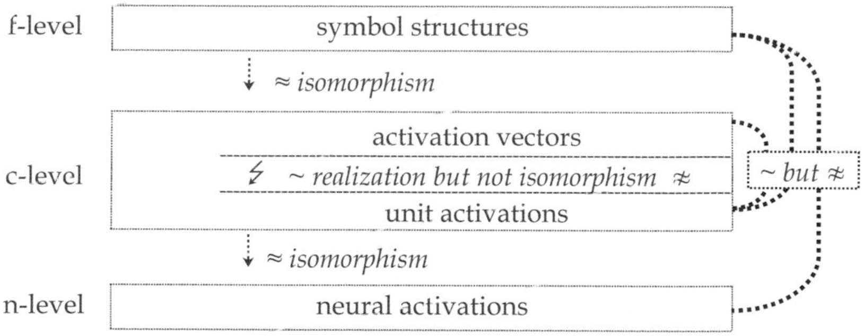

Yet tensorial computation furnishes a fully satisfactory realization mapping from its higher- to its lower-level description. The tensor product operation, for example, has a formal definition that allows exact computation of the unit activations constituting $\mathbf{A} \otimes \mathbf{r}_0$. Likewise, the higher-level tensorial operations such as multiplying representational vectors by weight matrices are fully formally defined with respect to individual unit activations and connection weights. The representational-vector input-output function defined by multiplying an input vector by a matrix corresponds exactly to the input-output function of the connectionist network that realizes it. But the internal causal structure, described by the connectionist network description, has no

---

[5] A one-to-one mapping from connectionist units to neurons is one rather plausible connectionist-neural isomorphism; less obvious mappings may ultimately prove more enlightening, however.
[6] This figure will be elaborated in Figures 7 and 12 below.

corresponding description at the higher, 'symbolic' level. ICS employs symbolic explanation for cognitive *functions*, but connectionist explanation for cognitive *processes*.

1.3 The structure of the argument and the chapter

Integral to the preceding discussion is the notion **level of description of a computational system**. This chapter develops the general analysis of computational levels roughly synopsized in (2). (Section numbers indicate where in the chapter each topic is addressed.)

(2)   **Computational levels** (Sections 2 and 3)

Three levels of descriptive abstraction for physical computational systems (rough)

a.   The f-level: describes the *functions* computed

b.   The c-level: describes the algorithms that *compute* this function

c.   The n-level: describes the *neural* (or other physical) processes that realize the algorithm

The c-level generally consists of multiple sublevels; this is illustrated by the higher- and lower-sublevel descriptions of tensorial nets discussed above (see Figure 1).

Given formal descriptions at two levels, it may be that there is a structure-preserving one-to-one mapping from one description to the other—an isomorphism. Particularly important is isomorphism with the n-level, for that is the level at which the theory makes contact with such observable quantities as reaction times and capacity limitations. For example, in order for the number of steps in an algorithm to necessarily predict the actual time required to perform a computation, the step-by-step structure of the algorithm must be isomorphic to the moment-by-moment structure of the physical system realizing that algorithm. I will argue that the general notion **process-relevance** can be characterized as in (3).

(3)   Process-relevance of a computational description (Section 2.2.1)

In order for a computational description to account for the time, space, or other resource requirements of a process in a physical system, that description must be isomorphic to the n-level description of the system, with respect to the structural decomposition relevant to the given resource.

With this notion, the problem posed by the incompatibility of symbolic and neural computation can be succinctly stated: symbolic theory postulates the process-relevance of its symbolic descriptions of cognitive functions and algorithms, yet the methods of reduction in symbolic theory do not establish a plausible isomorphism with the neural level. (4) states this in the language to be developed in this chapter.

(4)   The central paradox of cognition (Section 5)

f-level $\not\approx$ n-level

The symbolic f-level description is not isomorphic to the n-level.

Figure 1   *Box 2*

(Throughout this chapter, the symbol '≈' will denote the isomorphism relation, and the symbol '~' the weaker relation, realization.)

Exploiting the level distinctions of (2), the argument of this chapter can be summarized with the claims (5)–(9). The comments in square brackets allude to the rationale for individual claims.

The argument begins with a refinement of (1).

(5)   Architectural requirements (interim formulation; final formulation in Section 4)

A complete cognitive architecture must have the following three properties:

   a.   The f-level employs symbolic computation.
   [to explain the combinatorial structure of the representations and functions of higher cognition]

   b.   The c-level
      i.   The c-level provides a realization of the f-level.
      [required for the f- and c-level descriptions to be of the same system]
      ii. The c-level is isomorphic to the physical (n-)level.
      [the c-level of a complete cognitive theory must provide algorithms that are process-relevant—that is, isomorphic to the n-level (3)]

   c.   The physical level is neural computation.
   [this must be the target of reduction in cognitive science]

(6)   Putative incompatibility of the requirements (Section 5)

The three requirements (5), plus (4), are prima facie mutually contradictory.

   a.   They apparently imply that the symbolic f-level must be isomorphic to the neural n-level, in contradiction to the central paradox (4).

   b.   The Purely Symbolic Architecture satisfies only (5a) and (5b.i).

   c.   The Eliminativist Connectionist Architecture satisfies only (5c) and (5b.ii).

(7)   Reconciling the requirements via ICS (Section 6)

Appearances of incompatibility (6) notwithstanding, ICS satisfies all three requirements of (5).

   a.   The f-level is symbolic.

   b.   The c-level is **split** into higher and lower sublevels, the lower realizing the higher.
      i.   The higher sublevel is isomorphic to the f-level.
      ii. The lower sublevel is connectionist, isomorphic to the n-level.

   c.   The physical level is neural.

(8)   ICS explanation (Section 7)

   a.   ICS explanation is symbolic for f-level problems.
   [cognitive functions have symbolic descriptions]

   b.   ICS explanation is connectionist for c-level problems.

[cognitive processes require connectionist descriptions: only the connectionist algorithms of the lower sublevel of the c-level are process-relevant]

(9)   Symbolic explanation in ICS (Section 7.2)

a.   Symbolic explanation in ICS addresses not only "competence data," but important types of "performance data" as well.
[these data actually address f-level problems—explained with functions, not algorithms]

b.   Symbolic explanation in ICS does not address other important types of "performance data."
[these are uniquely c-level problems—explanations require algorithms]

The last point, (9b), identifies a major difference between ICS and the Purely Symbolic Architecture. A defining assumption of the (purely) symbolic theory is the existence of (purely) symbolic algorithms that model cognitive processes. The ICS architecture entails that in general these do not exist.

Points (2)–(9) are taken up in turn in the following sections. The lengthiest section is the next one, which attempts a rather careful and thorough analysis of levels of computational description. This analysis provides the foundation for everything that follows.

In Chapter 1, the problem of explaining the productivity of higher cognition was identified as a central challenge for cognitive science. Readers interested in how ICS explains this productivity will find in Box 3 a relatively simple synopsis of the argument, in question-and-answer format.

Box 3. Is ICS productive?

Q1. How does ICS explain the productivity of cognition?

A1. Symbolic combinatorics. Productivity is an f-level problem, and at the f-level, ICS is symbolic.

Q2. Why is ICS then not just a 'classical architecture' (Fodor and Pylyshyn 1988), that is, a purely symbolic architecture?

A2. The differences lie beneath the f-level. At the c-level, the 'classical' Purely Symbolic Architecture (PSA) assumes process-relevant symbolic algorithms; these do not exist in ICS.

Q3. If there are no such algorithms, how can ICS be a computational theory?

A3. ICS is computational because the symbolic combinatorics of the f-level are reduced, by fully formal realization mappings, to primitive computational operations—connectionist operations. In ICS, the process-relevant algorithms are not symbolic, and the symbolic algorithms are not process-relevant.

Q4. The alleged c-level distinction between ICS and PSA is a mere detail, too low-level to bear on the central issues of cognitive architecture. Who cares about what's beneath the f-level anyway?

Figure 1   *Box 3*

A4. Well, all of 'classical' symbolic cognitive theory must care: this theory *is* the hypothesis that there are process-relevant symbolic algorithms at the c-level. Thus, ICS differs crucially from PSA.

Q5. How can ICS have symbolic f-level accounts of productivity, but no process-relevant symbolic algorithms?

A5. The higher sublevel of the ICS c-level is isomorphic to the symbolic f-level account: symbols are computationally relevant. But only the lower c-sublevel is process-relevant, and at this level there are connectionist but not symbolic algorithms. The reduction from the higher to lower c-sublevel is accomplished by a realization mapping that is *not* an isomorphism; this mapping *does* allow a reduction from symbol structures to connectionist units—but, because representations are distributed, it is a holistic, not a part-by part, reduction. This mapping is formal, as required for a fully computational reduction, but the lack of part-by-part correspondence means symbolic decompositions do not map onto process-relevant decompositions.

2 LEVELS OF DESCRIPTIVE ABSTRACTION IN COMPUTATIONAL THEORIES

This section lays the groundwork for the main argument of the chapter outlined in (5)–(9) by developing a detailed analysis of the level structure of physical computational systems (2).[7]

In the description of a general physical computational system S, three levels of abstraction can be distinguished. These level distinctions derive from those introduced in the seminal work Marr 1982, but are not identical to them. In particular, terminologically, 'computational level' refers to the highest level in Marr 1982 but to the middle level here. I will in fact generally avoid 'computational level' in favor of **c-level**, which emphasizes the technical nature of the level terminology developed here; the label 'computational' for the c-level should be construed as a rough gloss, intended more as a mnemonic than as a meaningful label. The glosses 'functional level' and 'neural level' for **f-level** and **n-level** should be taken in the same spirit.

According to the foundational premise of modern cognitive science—cognition is computation—the ultimate theory of cognition will be a complete, three-level description of a physical computational system, the brain. Available at present are only incomplete theories, which usually specify just one or two levels. Nonetheless, I will argue, these theories typically make implicit but critical assumptions concerning the unspecified levels, so in this chapter it will prove useful to consider every cognitive theory to provide three levels of description—even if, at present, some of these descriptions are rather vague, and the theory largely noncommittal about them.

Figure 2 depicts the three levels, indicating the properties I will now develop.

---

[7] For an explication of the notion of computational level focused on algorithms, see Foster 1992.

Figure 2. Levels of abstraction in the description of a physical computational system $\mathcal{S}$

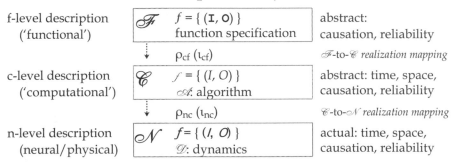

f-level description ('functional')	$\mathcal{F}$	$f = \{ (\mathbf{I}, \mathbf{O}) \}$ function specification	abstract: causation, reliability
		$\rho_{cf}\ (\iota_{cf})$	$\mathcal{F}$-to-$\mathcal{C}$ *realization mapping*
c-level description ('computational')	$\mathcal{C}$	$f = \{ (I, O) \}$ $\mathcal{A}$: algorithm	abstract: time, space, causation, reliability
		$\rho_{nc}\ (\iota_{nc})$	$\mathcal{C}$-to-$\mathcal{N}$ *realization mapping*
n-level description (neural/physical)	$\mathcal{N}$	$f = \{ (I, O) \}$ $\mathcal{D}$: dynamics	actual: time, space, causation, reliability

2.1 The n-level of descriptive abstraction

The lowest-level description is the least abstract, the most detailed and fine-grained. It will be called the **n-level**, in anticipation of the cognitive case in which it is the neural level. At the n-level, our system $\mathcal{S}$ is described like any other physical system. This description, which I will denote $\mathcal{N}$, involves physical states that include the positions of material components in space; it involves a causal dynamics $\mathcal{D}$ that drives change in the state over time, according to physical laws. $\mathcal{N}$ describes how the system $\mathcal{S}$ "lives" in real space, and how its state evolves in real time, according to the indisputably real causal forces of natural science.

Space, time, and causal dynamics are crucial aspects of $\mathcal{N}$ because from a computational perspective these are **resources**. Insufficient space in the memory chips, insufficient size of connectionist networks, will limit what computations can be correctly carried out. The same is true if insufficient time is available, or if operations critical for a computation require certain causal processes that are unavailable.

A fourth resource critical for computation is **precision**. The physical basis of this might be **reliability**. Reliability can be compromised in various ways, but for our purposes we can focus on one: randomness, more randomness of course meaning less reliability. For example, imagine that neurons or semiconductors are damaged or operating under adverse conditions, so that their behavior is, on average, the same as if they were undamaged, but now there is considerable random variance or **noise**. Such damage clearly reduces the degree of computational precision that can be attained.

2.2 The c-level of descriptive abstraction

The intermediate level is the pivotal one for our analysis. At this level, our system $\mathcal{S}$ is given a description that is more abstract than the physical description $\mathcal{N}$. Under this **computational** description, called $\mathcal{C}$, the states of $\mathcal{S}$ involve abstract entities, such as symbols, that are not part of the vocabulary of physical science. These entities "live" in **abstract space**, occupying abstract locations in data structures. They evolve

Figure 2   *Box 3*

in **abstract time**—for example, through the successive discrete "moments" during which they are subjected to step-by-step manipulations. These manipulations are the **abstract causal forces** that together constitute the **algorithm** $\mathscr{A}$ governing the evolution of the system's state through abstract time. Whereas the primitive elements of physical causation include such familiar players as electromagnetic and gravitational forces, the primitive elements of the algorithm's abstract causal powers include "forces" that stick symbols together to form trees, or pry trees apart to extract symbols. These smallest parts of abstract causation—the **primitive operations**—define the **computational architecture** of this description $\mathscr{C}$. The operations of the computational architecture are characterized by a certain level of **abstract reliability** or **precision**; when $\mathscr{S}$ operates under adverse conditions, or is damaged, this level of precision diminishes.

Central to the computational description $\mathscr{C}$ is the notion of **input-output function**. An algorithm $\mathscr{A}$ receives input I (at some point in abstract time) and then (later in abstract time) produces an output O. Viewed as the physical realization of the computation $\mathscr{C}$, the physical system $\mathscr{S}$ is also described in $\mathscr{N}$ as adopting at one point of real time a physical state I corresponding to—or **realizing**—I, and then evolving under the dynamics $\mathscr{D}$ at a later point in real time to a state O realizing O. The **realization mapping** ρ_{nc} associates (or **maps**) a computational state in the description $\mathscr{C}$ to its description in $\mathscr{N}$ as a physical state. The definition of 'realization mapping' requires that the algorithm $\mathscr{A}$ takes an input I to an output O if and only if the dynamics $\mathscr{D}$ takes the realization of I, $\rho_{\text{nc}}(I) = I$, to the realization of O, $\rho_{\text{nc}}(O) = O$. The existence of such a mapping ρ_{nc} defines exactly what it means for $\mathscr{N}$ to realize $\mathscr{C}$; (10) schematizes this relationship, in a form that will recur several times during the course of the chapter.[8] When $\mathscr{A}$ is realized in $\mathscr{D}$, I will write '$\mathscr{A} \sim \mathscr{D}$'.

(10)   Realization of c-level algorithm $\mathscr{A}$ in n-level dynamics $\mathscr{D}$

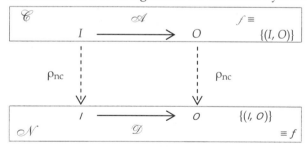

The assignment to I of the output O resulting from the computation $\mathscr{C}$ defines the **function** computed by $\mathscr{A}$, f. The function f consists simply of the set of input-output pairs (I, O) computed by $\mathscr{A}$. Via ρ_{nc}, $\mathscr{N}$ provides a physical realization of f, under the interpretation of $\mathscr{S}$ provided by $\mathscr{C}$. The n-level description of the function computed by $\mathscr{S}$ is f, the set of input-output pairs (I, O).

[8] This is the "Tower Bridge" picture of Cummins and Schwarz 1991, an article that contributed significantly to the development of the analysis presented in this chapter.

2.2.1 The c-level's relation to the n-level

The descriptions $\mathcal{N}$ and $\mathcal{C}$ describe one and the same physical computational system $\mathcal{S}$, and they must therefore be intimately interrelated: $\mathcal{N}$ must be a realization of $\mathcal{C}$ (10). Under the realization mapping ρ_{nc}, the computational description under $\mathcal{C}$ of a state of $\mathcal{S}$ corresponds to a physical description under $\mathcal{N}$ of the same state of $\mathcal{S}$.

Sometimes a stronger relationship holds between $\mathcal{C}$ and $\mathcal{N}$: each *part* of the computational description of a state individually corresponds to a *part* of the state's physical description. In this case, we will say that $\mathcal{C}$ is **isomorphic** to $\mathcal{N}$. This relationship is schematized in (11).

(11)   Isomorphism of c-level algorithm $\mathcal{A}$ with n-level dynamics $\mathcal{D}$: $\Sigma_{cn} \approx \Sigma_n$

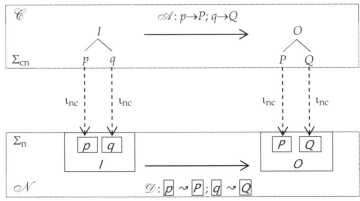

To be somewhat more precise, suppose that under $\mathcal{C}$ a state has internal structure, involving a set of computational 'parts', and that the algorithm $\mathcal{A}$ of $\mathcal{C}$ is defined in terms of these parts. Let Σ_{cn} denote the decomposition of state and algorithm provided by this structure. Analogously, suppose that under $\mathcal{N}$ a state has internal structure Σ_n involving a set of physical 'parts', in terms of which the dynamics $\mathcal{D}$ of $\mathcal{N}$ is defined. Then an **isomorphism** from Σ_{cn} to Σ_n is a realization mapping ι_{nc} that associates to each computational part in Σ_{cn} a part in Σ_n; the latter is a **realization** of the former. To qualify as an isomorphism, ι_{nc} must put the parts into which the algorithm is decomposed by Σ_{cn} into correspondence with the parts into which the dynamics is decomposed by Σ_n. When Σ_{cn} and Σ_n are isomorphic, I will write '$\Sigma_{cn} \approx \Sigma_n$'.

To be able to characterize the isomorphism notion more precisely, we need more precise characterizations of those particular structures within $\mathcal{C}$ and within $\mathcal{N}$ that are 'put into correspondence' by the isomorphism. This will be undertaken in Section 6 for the case of central interest here: the Integrated Symbolic/Connectionist Cognitive Architecture (ICS). The Purely Symbolic Architecture (PSA) will be discussed briefly in Section 5. For the simpler case of serial arithmetic computers, Boxes 4–5 develop and illustrate a notion of isomorphism with respect to temporal structure. Even in this simplest of settings, the concepts are remarkably rich.

Figure 2   *Box 3*

The physical resources required by the processes within S are, at bottom, determined by S's physical description $\mathcal{N}$. Such resources include the actual reliability of operation, the actual time required to produce an output, and the actual size of the machinery required to provide sufficient capacity to process an input. When some computational structure Σ_{cn} within $\mathcal{C}$ is isomorphic to $\mathcal{N}$, that structure can be used to determine the resource demands of the processes required by an input. For example, when Σ_{cn} includes temporal duration structure, isomorphism with $\mathcal{N}$ entails that the *actual* time required to process an n-level input can be determined from the *abstract* time required by the algorithm to process the corresponding c-level input (see Boxes 4–5).

Thus, being isomorphic to $\mathcal{N}$ is an extremely important property; I will use the terminology in (12).

(12)   Process-relevant computational structure Σ_{cn}

Suppose some computational structure Σ_{cn} of $\mathcal{C}$ is isomorphic to some physical structure Σ_n of $\mathcal{N}$: $\Sigma_{cn} \approx \Sigma_n$. Then

a. Σ_{cn} is **process-relevant** (or **physically** or **neurally relevant**), and

b. Σ_n is **computationally relevant**.

A computational description $\mathcal{C}$ may involve several different types of structure, and even when some of these are process-relevant — isomorphic to $\mathcal{N}$ — it may be that other types of $\mathcal{C}$-structure are not. In the case of primary interest here, ICS, this arises from differences in structure at the different sublevels into which $\mathcal{C}$ is stratified (Figure 1) — an important topic that I take up in the next subsection.

Box 4. $\mathcal{C}$-$\mathcal{N}$ isomorphism in arithmetic computers I

The examples developed here and in the following two boxes pertain to serial computation— serial algorithms and (hypothetical) serial machines. At issue is isomorphism between $\mathcal{C}$ and $\mathcal{N}$ with respect to temporal structure: the sequence of states serially traversed during a computation, and the temporal duration of the intervals between them.

Temporal isomorphism defined

First, some basic notation. Let $\mathcal{C}$ be a space of computational states operating under an algorithm $\mathcal{A}$. Let $\mathbf{c}$ denote the sequence of states traversed by an execution of $\mathcal{A}$ from input I to output O: ($I = c_0, c_1, c_2, \ldots, c_k = O$). Let the types of operations over $\mathcal{C}$ that are employed by the algorithm $\mathcal{A}$ be denoted $\{op_\alpha\}$. Then define $\#op_\alpha(\mathbf{c})$ to be the number of times the αth operation op_α executes during $\mathbf{c}$. Define a **duration vector** τ to be a list ($\tau_1, \tau_2, \ldots$) of real numbers, one for each operation op_α; τ_α is interpreted as the (abstract) time, on some relative scale, required for a single execution of op_α. With respect to τ, the abstract processing time T required for the entire computation $\mathbf{c}$ is

(1) $T_{\mathcal{A},\tau}(\mathbf{c}) = \Sigma_\alpha \#op_\alpha(\mathbf{c})\tau_\alpha.$

The function $T_{\mathcal{A},\tau}$ defines the **durational structure** of $\mathscr{C}$, denoted $\Sigma_{\mathscr{C}}^{\mathrm{dur}}$. The **sequential temporal structure** of $\mathscr{C}$—$\Sigma_{\mathscr{C}}^{\mathrm{seq}}$—is defined by the relation *precedes*, where *precedes*(c, c') means that state c precedes state c' as $\mathcal{A}$ operates.

Now let $\mathcal{S}$ be a physical system to be regarded as a serial computer, and let $\mathcal{N}$ be a physical-level description of its states and dynamics $\mathscr{D}$. The sequential structure of $\mathcal{N}$, $\Sigma_{\mathcal{N}}^{\mathrm{seq}}$, is defined by *precedes*(n, n'): the physical state n precedes the state n' under the dynamics $\mathscr{D}$. And the durational structure of $\mathcal{N}$, $\Sigma_{\mathcal{N}}^{\mathrm{dur}}$, is determined by the function $T_{\mathscr{D}}(n, n')$ that gives the duration—in real time—of the interval elapsing between the states n and n' under $\mathscr{D}$.

Now we can define isomorphism between $\mathscr{C}$ and $\mathcal{N}$ as in (2).

(2) $\mathscr{C}$-$\mathcal{N}$ isomorphism with respect to temporal structure

　　a. $\mathcal{A}$ is **isomorphic to** $\mathcal{N}$ **with respect to sequential structure** ($\Sigma_{\mathcal{N}}^{\mathrm{seq}} \approx \Sigma_{\mathscr{C}}^{\mathrm{seq}}$) if and only if there is a general mapping ι_{nc} from computational states of $\mathscr{C}$ to physical states of $\mathcal{N}$ such that when $\mathcal{S}$ is initially in state $I \equiv n_0 \equiv \iota_{\mathrm{nc}}(c_0) \equiv \iota_{\mathrm{nc}}(I)$, its dynamics $\mathscr{D}$ takes it through the states $\{n_i \equiv \iota_{\mathrm{nc}}(c_i)\}$ in the same sequence that $\mathcal{A}$ traverses $\{c_i\}$:

　　　　precedes(n_i, n_j) if and only if *precedes*(c_i, c_j).

　　That is, $\mathscr{D}$ takes $\mathcal{S}$ through $n_0, n_1, \ldots, n_k$ in that order.

　　b. $\mathcal{A}$ is **isomorphic under** ι_{nc} **to** $\mathcal{N}$ **with respect to temporal duration**—$\Sigma_{\mathcal{N}}^{\mathrm{dur}} \approx \Sigma_{\mathscr{C}}^{\mathrm{dur}}$—if and only if there is a duration vector τ such that

　　　　$T_{\mathscr{D}}(I, O) \propto T_{\mathcal{A},\tau}(\mathbf{c})$.

　　That is, the actual time required by $\mathcal{S}$ to go from input $I \equiv \iota_{\mathrm{nc}}(I)$ to output O is proportional to the abstract time (with respect to τ) required by $\mathcal{A}$ to compute O from I via the computation $\mathbf{c}$.

If $\mathcal{A}$ is isomorphic to $\mathcal{N}$ with respect to an aspect of temporal structure (sequence or duration), then $\mathcal{A}$ is **process-relevant** in this respect: the process characteristics of $\mathcal{A}$ model the physical processes at work in $\mathcal{S}$.

2.2.2 Sublevels of c-level description

A computational architecture must be founded upon a set of primitive operations that meet an important criterion: they must require no intelligence and must be so mechanical that they can be materially realized, to a considerable degree of accuracy. (This criterion is motivated quite clearly in Haugeland 1985, an elegant development of the notion of computation in the context of cognitive science.) A complete theory of our system $\mathcal{S}$ will specify exactly how the primitive operations of the computational level are physically realized—how the primitive vocabulary of the computational description $\mathscr{C}$ is related to that of the physical description $\mathcal{N}$.

A set of mechanical primitive operations can be combined in different ways to produce a stock of more complex operations, which can then be taken to be the

Figure 2　　　　　　　　　　*Box 4*

primitive operations of a *higher-level* computational architecture or **virtual machine**. These new primitive operations can in turn be combined to generate a set of primitives for a yet higher-level architecture. This creates a sequence of **sublevels** within the overall c-level. For simple examples see Box 5, which explains Figures 3–4. (For a more complex case, directly relevant to cognitive science, see Box 1.)

Figure 3. S_1 realization mappings

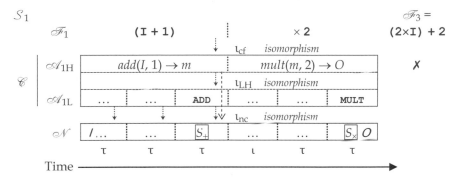

Figure 4. S_2 realization mappings

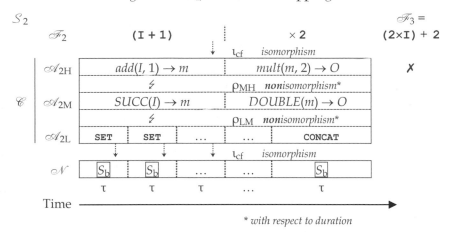

* with respect to duration

   For $\mathscr{C}$ to qualify as computational, it is crucial that the relationships between its sublevels be *completely formal*. The primitives at one sublevel must be precisely defined in terms of the primitives at the sublevel directly below. Thus, descriptions at the highest sublevel of $\mathscr{C}$ are every bit as precise as those at the lowest sublevel of $\mathscr{C}$. The description $\mathscr{C}_k$ at sublevel k is **realized** in the description $\mathscr{C}_{k-1}$ at sublevel $k-1$ via a realization mapping ρ_{ck}. (In actual digital computers, the mapping ρ_{ck} is itself specified precisely by a program: a compiler or interpreter.) The sequence of sublevels $\mathscr{C}_k$

and the chain of realization mappings ρ_k form a completely precise scaffolding stretching from descriptions of $\mathcal{S}$ using the lowest-level primitives of $\mathcal{C}$ potentially up to very high-level, abstract descriptions of $\mathcal{S}$. The highest level is often composed of large modules — the topic of the next subsection.

Box 5. $\mathcal{C}$-$\mathcal{N}$ isomorphism in arithmetic computers II

(Consulting Figures 3 and 4 throughout this discussion is recommended. This box builds upon Box 4.)

First arithmetic computer: $\mathcal{S}_1$

Consider a (hypothetical) physical serial computer $\mathcal{S}_1$ that has dedicated circuitry for each of the arithmetic operations {ADD (+), SUB (−), MULT (×), DIV (÷)}. The circuit for ADD is denoted S_+, that for MULT is denoted $S_\times$, and so on. Each operation takes one tick of the computer's clock, τ seconds. Numbers are represented in this computer via binary numerals. There are two data registers r_1 and r_2; the operations apply to the contents of these registers with the result going into a third register r_0 (r_1 and r_2 being reset to 0). The input-output operations INPUT and OUTPUT respectively put data into and read data out of register r_0. All registers begin with contents 0.

The processes in $\mathcal{S}_1$ can be described by the following algorithm:

(1)   Algorithm $\mathcal{A}_{1L}$

         INPUT; $r_0 \to r_1$; $1 \to r_2$; ADD; $r_0 \to r_1$; $2 \to r_2$; MULT; OUTPUT

This algorithm reads a number x into r_0; copies it to r_1; places the number 1 into r_2; adds r_1 and r_2, placing the result ($x+1$) into r_0; copies this to r_1; places 2 into r_2; multiplies r_1 by r_2, placing the result ($x+1$)×2 into r_0; and outputs this result: $2(x+1)$. Here, x is a metalanguage variable standing in for some particular number given as input to the machine.

This algorithm $\mathcal{A}_{1L}$ is a low-level ('L') algorithm, using primitive operations like ADD and MULT that are directly implemented physically in the device $\mathcal{S}_1$ by the circuits S_+ and $S_\times$. The next algorithm is a higher-level ('H') algorithm.

(2)   Algorithm $\mathcal{A}_{1H}$

         input(n); *add*($n, 1$) $\to$ m; *mult*($m, 2$) $\to$ k; *output*(k)

This algorithm operates over a virtual machine composed of variables like n, m, k, and operations like *add* and *mult* that each take two arguments, each a variable or a constant number. The result of the operation is assigned as the value of a variable. This algorithm takes in a number x as the value of a variable n; adds 1 to it, assigning the result ($x+1$) as the value of a variable m; multiplies m by 2, assigning the result ($x+1$)×2 as the value of a variable k; and outputs k: $2(x+1)$.

The states of $\mathcal{A}_{1L}$ can be described by the contents of the registers $\langle r_0, r_1, r_2 \rangle$: $(\langle x, 0, 0 \rangle; \langle x, x, 0 \rangle; \langle x, x, 1 \rangle; \langle x+1, 0, 0 \rangle; \langle x+1, x+1, 0 \rangle; \langle x+1, x+1, 2 \rangle; \langle 2(x+1), 0, 0 \rangle)$. Ignoring the input and output operations, present in every computation, this particular computation requires six steps. If the time required by each operation is τ, then the

Figure 4   *Box 5*

total time is $T_{\mathscr{A}_{1L},\tau} = 6\tau$.

The states of $\mathscr{A}_{1H}$ can be described with the variables' values: $\langle \boldsymbol{n} = x \rangle$; $\langle \boldsymbol{n} = x, \boldsymbol{m} = x+1 \rangle$; $\langle \boldsymbol{n} = x, \boldsymbol{m} = x+1, \boldsymbol{k} = 2(x+1) \rangle$; $\langle \boldsymbol{n} = x, \boldsymbol{m} = x+1, \boldsymbol{k} = 2(x+1), \boldsymbol{OUT} = 2(x+1) \rangle$. Again ignoring the input and output steps, there are only two operations here (adding 1; multiplying by 2). Each single high-level operation in $\mathscr{A}_{1H}$ does the work of *three* low-level operations in $\mathscr{A}_{1L}$ (in the latter, it takes two additional steps to load r_1 and r_2 before each arithmetic operation). These three steps of $\mathscr{A}_{1L}$ collapse to a single higher-level operation in $\mathscr{A}_{1H}$. So if we define $\tau' \equiv 3\tau$, we have a total computation time of $T_{\mathscr{A}_{1H},\tau'} = 2\tau' = 6\tau$.

The isomorphism from $\mathscr{A}_{1L}$ to $\mathscr{N}_1'$, the $\mathscr{N}$-level description of the machine $\mathcal{S}_1$, is very direct: the physical description $\mathscr{N}_1'$ is of a sequence of states $n_0, n_1, \ldots$, one for each clock-tick; each machine state is a collection of substates, the states of the individual hardware devices that make up the machine. In particular, each register device has its own internal state, which can be described via a binary numeral that is its 'contents'. The isomorphism ι_{nc} maps the $\mathscr{A}_{1L}$-state described above as a sequence of three numbers $\langle r_0, r_1, r_2 \rangle$ into a physical state in which each register device has the internal state described by the binary numeral representing the corresponding number r_i. The transition from one $\mathscr{A}_{1L}$-state to the next corresponds to the transition from one $\mathscr{N}$-state to the state one clock-tick later—hence the isomorphism of sequential and durational structure between $\mathscr{A}_{1L}$ and $\mathscr{N}$.

There is also an isomorphism between $\mathscr{A}_{1H}$ and $\mathscr{N}$, although it is not as complete. The isomorphism mapping ι_{nc} maps the state of $\mathscr{A}_{1H}$ after the operation *add* to the state of $\mathscr{N}$ after the operation of the adding-circuit S_+, and likewise the state of $\mathscr{A}_{1H}$ after *mult* to the state of $\mathscr{N}$ after $S_\times$. The step from one state to the next in $\mathscr{A}_{1H}$ corresponds under ι_{nc} to the transition from one $\mathscr{N}$-state to the $\mathscr{N}$-state *three* clock-ticks later. ι_{nc} is an isomorphism of temporal structure: the sequences of $\mathscr{A}_{1H}$- and $\mathscr{N}$-states correspond in their ordering, and the durations of the steps are proportional to one another (with the actual temporal duration that corresponds to one algorithmic step being three times greater for $\mathscr{A}_{1H}$ than for $\mathscr{A}_{1L}$).

But the $\mathscr{A}_{1H}$ algorithm is not isomorphic to $\mathscr{N}$ with respect to *spatial* structure: there is no general part-by-part mapping from the variables constituting the $\mathscr{A}_{1H}$-states to the register devices constituting the $\mathscr{N}$-states. In this respect, the higher-level algorithm is not as completely isomorphic to the physical description $\mathscr{N}$ as is the lower-level algorithm: the parts making up the $\mathscr{A}_{1L}$-states—data registers—*are* in one-to-one correspondence with the parts comprising the $\mathscr{N}$-states—register devices. Thus, while both $\mathscr{A}_{1L}$ and $\mathscr{A}_{1H}$ are process-relevant with respect to temporal structure, only $\mathscr{A}_{1L}$ is process-relevant with respect to spatial structure. That is, both algorithms can be used to model the temporal resources required by $\mathcal{S}_1$ for its computations, but the spatial resource requirements are accurately modeled only by $\mathscr{A}_{1L}$. Thus, it would *not* be correct to reason that processing one input I would require more memory in $\mathcal{S}_1$ than processing another input I' just because a *higher*-level algorithm might employ more variables in the latter case than in the former; it *would* be correct to reason this way on the basis of *lower*-level algorithms in which the data registers required by a computation map one to one with the register devices required.

For comparison with the next example, let us note finally that the input-output function computed by $\mathcal{S}_1$ is

(3) $f_1: x \mapsto 2(x + 1)$.

Second arithmetic computer: $\mathcal{S}_2$

Now we will consider another (hypothetical) serial computer $\mathcal{S}_2$ with simpler hardware. Instead of circuits like $\mathcal{S}_1$'s that allow any two numbers to be added or multiplied in a fixed time, $\mathcal{S}_2$ only has circuits S_b that manipulate one bit at a time, changing 0 to 1 or 1 to 0, or concatenating (affixing) a 1 or 0 to one end of a string of bits. Each bit operation takes one clock-tick, of duration τ seconds. That is, to add 1 and 3, this computer must perform a sequence of operations of this sort: take the binary representations of each, 1 and 11, and first change the second bit of 11 to 0, getting 10; then change the first bit of 10 to 0, getting 00; and finally concatenate a 1 at the beginning, getting 100, the binary representation of 4.

Our computer $\mathcal{S}_2$ performs the following bit-manipulating algorithm:

(4)   Algorithm $\mathscr{A}_{2L}$
        INPUT($b_k \cdots b_0$)
        zero(β)
        startloop
            if $b_\beta = 0$ then
                SET $b_\beta = 1$
                go to endloop
            else
                SET $b_\beta = 0$
                increment(β)
                go to startloop
        endloop
        CONCAT($b_k \cdots b_0, 0$)
        OUTPUT($b_n \cdots b_0$)

The algorithm inputs a bit string $b_k \cdots b_0$, the binary numeral for a nonnegative whole number x, with each b_i a bit: 0 or 1. (For convenience, the binary numeral has a 0 at its left edge.) β identifies the bit that is the one currently available for examination; zero(β) sets it to 0, so that the rightmost bit is targeted. A loop of instructions starts by examining the bit b_β. If it is 0, it is changed to 1 and the loop is exited; otherwise, it is changed to 0, β is incremented so the next bit to the left is now to be examined, and the loop begins again. After the loop ends, a 0 is concatenated (appended) to the end of the bit string, which is then output.

It is not hard to see that the loop (from 'startloop' to 'endloop') just adds 1; that is, it takes the binary numeral for x and changes it to the binary numeral for $x + 1 \equiv y$. And then the final step of concatenating a 0 to the right of the binary numeral for y produces the binary numeral for $2y$. So in fact, working with binary representations,

Figure 4   Box 5

this algorithm simply computes $2(x + 1)$.

The loop in $\mathscr{A}_{2L}$ computes $x + 1$, so let's abbreviate it by '$SUCC$' for 'successor'. If we take the loop and exchange 0 and 1 everywhere, the resulting algorithm computes $x - 1$, the predecessor of x; we can abbreviate it by '$PRED$'. And since the operation of concatenating a final 0 doubles the number, let's abbreviate it by '$DOUBLE$'. Using variables, the algorithm can be written as in (5).

(5)   Algorithm $\mathscr{A}_{2M}$
$$INPUT(n); \ SUCC(n) \to m; \ DOUBLE(m) \to k; \ OUTPUT(k)$$

Note that the operations $SUCC$, $DOUBLE$, and so on, are completely formally well defined: they are merely abbreviations for sets of bit operations. A realization mapping ϱ_{LM} precisely maps the 'M'-level operators like $SUCC$ and $DOUBLE$ to the combinations of 'L'-level operators like SET and CONCAT that realize them.

Surely $\mathscr{A}_{2M}$ is much preferable to $\mathscr{A}_{2L}$ for understanding the function of S_2. But unlike $\mathscr{A}_{2L}$, $\mathscr{A}_{2M}$ is *not* process-relevant with respect to temporal duration. Each bit manipulation operation in S_2 takes time τ, and since the primitive operations of the algorithm $\mathscr{A}_{2L}$ are just these bit operations, the actual time taken by S_2 to process an input is τ times the number of operations required by $\mathscr{A}_{2L}$ to process the corresponding input. But the primitives employed by $\mathscr{A}_{2M}$ operate at a level higher than bit operations. In particular, $SUCC$ encapsulates numerous bit operations, and most importantly, *different numbers* of bit operations for different inputs. Indeed, the number of bit operations—hence, the actual time—required by $SUCC$ is a highly variable function of its input; see Figure 5.[9] Thus, the number of operations of $\mathscr{A}_{2M}$ *cannot* be used to model the duration of the process within S_2 by which the output is computed. Indeed, $\mathscr{A}_{2M}$ always requires exactly two operations, while the actual processing time varies with the input in the oscillatory manner shown in Figure 5.

At a still higher level, the numerical operations *add* and *mult* can be defined recursively from $SUCC$ and $PRED$:[10]

$add(n, m) \equiv$ if $[m = 0]$ then n else $add(SUCC(n), PRED(m))$;
$mult(n, m) \equiv$ if $[m = 0]$ then 0 else $add(n, mult(n, PRED(m)))$.

Again there is a formal realization mapping ϱ_{MH} translating the H-level operations *add*, *mult* to the combinations of M-level operations $SUCC$, $PRED$ that realize them.

The new operations enable another algorithm for describing S_2:

(6)   Algorithm $\mathscr{A}_{2H}$
$$input(n); \ add(n, 1) \to m; \ mult(m, 2) \to k; \ output(k)$$

---

[9] The number of bit operations required to add 1 to a binary numeral N is determined by the number of 1s at the end of N: each requires a 'carry' operation entailing another iteration through the loop. As soon as a 0 is encountered, it is simply changed to 1 and the process stops: no further 'carrying' is needed. And the number of 1s at the end of N oscillates as shown in Figure 5.
[10] The first of these definitions employs the identities (*a*) $n + 0 = n$, (*b*) $n + m = (n + 1) + (m - 1)$; the second, the identities (*a'*) $n \cdot 0 = 0$, (*b'*) $n \cdot m = n + n \cdot (m - 1)$. The identities (*b*) and (*b'*) have the effect of reducing m by 1, so that if they are repeated, m is eventually reduced to 0 (since m and n are nonnegative whole numbers); then (*a*) and (*a'*) directly give the result.

Like the function *SUCC* from which they are defined, *add* and *mult* encapsulate varying numbers of bit operations, depending on their inputs. So again, while $\mathscr{A}_{2H}$ requires exactly two operations for every input (ignoring input-output as always), the corresponding processes in S_2 consume varying amounts of time for different inputs.

For both $\mathscr{A}_{2M}$ and $\mathscr{A}_{2H}$, there is a realization mapping relating algorithmic states to physical states in S_2, a mapping that preserves temporal sequence but not duration. These algorithms thus provide descriptions of S_2 that are isomorphic to $\mathscr{N}$ with respect to sequential structure but not durational structure.

Note that $\mathscr{A}_{2H}$ exactly equals $\mathscr{A}_{1H}$ (2). So S_2 computes the same function (3).

(7) $f_2 : x \mapsto 2(x + 1)$

A final algorithm

Finally, for contrast with the previous algorithms, consider the algorithm in (8)).

(8)   Algorithm $\mathscr{A}_{3H}$
       input(n); mult(n, 2) → m; add(m, 2) → k; output(k)

This algorithm computes the function in (9).

(9) $f_3 : x \mapsto 2x + 2$

Obviously, $f_3 = f_2 = f_1$; only the input-output mapping individuates a function.

Summary

The two physical systems S_1 and S_2 compute the same function, $f_1 = f_2$, but have very different processing-time behavior. The high-level algorithm $\mathscr{A}_{1H}$ is the same as its counterpart $\mathscr{A}_{2H}$, but with respect to duration, this algorithm is isomorphic to the $\mathscr{N}$-level description—and hence process-relevant—for S_1 but not for S_2. In both systems, the lower-level algorithms $\mathscr{A}_{1L} \neq \mathscr{A}_{2L}$ are isomorphic to their respective $\mathscr{N}$-level descriptions and can (in the case of S_2, must) be used to model processing times. $\mathscr{A}_{2L}$ but not $\mathscr{A}_{2H}$ is process-relevant to S_2 with respect to duration, yet $\mathscr{A}_{2H}$ is clearly more informative for interpreting or understanding or analyzing *what* S_2 computes. $\mathscr{A}_{2H}$ (or $\mathscr{A}_{2M}$) is even somewhat helpful in understanding *how* S_2 computes, since it is process-relevant with respect to temporal sequence, if not duration; for example, $\mathscr{A}_{2H}$ correctly asserts that the output of the process computing *add(n, 1)* is the input to the process computing *mult(m, 2)*. This contrasts with the algorithm $\mathscr{A}_{3H}$, which computes the same function but is not process-relevant at all to S_2: $\mathscr{A}_{3H}$ posits an intermediate state at which the output of *mult* becomes the input to *add*, but just the reverse is true of the actual processes at work inside S_2.

2.2.3   Data-dependency descriptions

In complex computational systems, including the human mind/brain, the global structure of the computation is typically described at the highest level in terms of large *modules* that each perform complex subtasks of their own, and interact in a

Figure 4   *Box 5*

Figure 5. Processing time for the operation *SUCC*

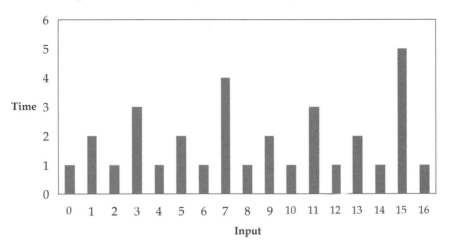

specified way to collectively perform the overall task.

Such descriptions are often depicted with flowchart-like diagrams such as Figure 6, which shows a simple example of what I will call a **data-dependency** description. The overall task in this example is silent word-by-word reading. The upper part of Figure 6 shows the modules, each of which performs a major cognitive task in its own right: recognition that the currently presented visual form is an instance of a particular word; generation of the pronunciation of that word; retrieval of the meaning associated with that pronunciation; integration of that meaning into the conceptual model of the situation described by the passage being read.

An important aspect of each module (box) in such a description is the type(s) of information it receives as input and the type(s) of information it produces as output: this is shown explicitly in the version of the diagram shown in the left-hand part of Figure 6. The input to the pronunciation module, for example, is information identifying a particular lexical item; the information carried by this module's output is a phonological structure, the pronunciation of that lexical item. It is as though the module has converted information of one type into information of a different type — better than 'converted' would be 'extracted' or 'retrieved' or 'made explicit'; but this fascinating and important issue is not our topic here.

The arrows in Figure 6 encode the interaction or interdependencies of the modules. In this case, the arrows specify, for example, that the data serving as input to the meaning retrieval module are the data produced as output by the lexical-item-recognition module together with the output of the lexical-item-pronunciation module.

Figure 6. A simple data-dependency description

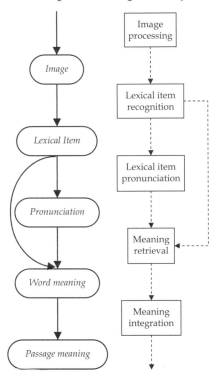

For a programmed computer, something like a data-dependency diagram might provide the overall structure of a large piece of software. In this case, each module (box) is a higher-level description of a chunk of code which performs that module's subtask. This code would typically be written in a high-level programming language, with primitive operations that might include such abstract, complex operations as 'object' creation, 'message' passing among objects, 'inheritance' of message-processing procedures between classes of objects, user-dialogue-management, data-base retrieval, list and tree manipulation, matrix and vector arithmetic, and so forth. These primitive operations of the high-level programming language would each be themselves formally defined as programs stated in a lower-level programming language, which has simpler primitive operations, perhaps ones that involve drawing lines on the screen, arithmetic with simple numbers, and so forth. This scaffolding of sublevels within the c-level would then ultimately extend from extremely complex operations like 'pronounce lexical item' all the way down to the lowest level where very simple operations change a 0 in a memory location to a 1. Despite the increasing complexity and abstractness of information processing that is revealed as the sublevels are mounted, every description is just as precisely defined as the lowest-level

Figure 6   *Box 5*

one. (See Box 1 for an extended example.)

Thus, in the world of software engineering, it would be possible to construct a computational architecture with primitive operations as complex as 'pronounce' (drawn in the right-hand part of Figure 6 as boxes), and with primitive interactions among them (drawn as dashed arrows). In a **serial** version of such an architecture, the 'pronounce lexical item' operation does not begin until the 'recognize lexical item' operation has concluded. In a **cascaded** version of the architecture (McClelland 1979), the 'recognize' operation gives continual output, incomplete or incorrect at first, but converging to the correct output after sufficient processing time; the 'pronounce' operation begins execution immediately, processing the continuously arriving and continuously improving input it receives from 'recognize', in turn continuously producing ever-improving output that is immediately processed by the 'meaning retrieval' operation.

In the world of cognitive science, theories are necessarily incomplete; in particular, theories often propose a data-dependency description of a cognitive process without specifying how each module encapsulated by a box is constructed from lower-level operations, how these are in turn constructed from still lower-level operations, and so on down the formal scaffolding to operations so simple as to clearly require no intelligence, and to be clearly physically instantiable. Such an incomplete theory does not strictly qualify as *computational*, in that it provides no purely mechanical description: there is no substitute for the theorist's knowledge and intelligence in specifying the modules' behavior. Nonetheless, it will be convenient to include such data-dependency descriptions in our discussion, putting them under the rubric of 'computational' descriptions. For despite their incompleteness, these theories play an important role in cognitive science, and a partial explication of that role can be subsumed under the analysis developed here for fully complete, and therefore genuinely computational, descriptions.

2.3 The f-level of descriptive abstraction

The highest-level description of our physical computational system S is the **functional-** or **f-level** description $\mathscr{F}$. (Building on Box 5, Box 6 provides simple illustrations of many of the points made in this section.)

As we have seen, characteristic of the computational description $\mathscr{C}$ is the input-output perspective: an algorithm $\mathscr{A}$ receives input I and then produces an output O; the set of such pairs (I, O) constitutes the function f computed by $\mathscr{A}$. This is the c-level description of the physical dynamics $\mathscr{D}$ of $\mathscr{N}$ that takes a state I of S at some time to another state O at a later time. An f-level description $\mathscr{F}$ also describes this function, but still more abstractly than does the c-level description $\mathscr{C}$.

In cognitive theory, it is often useful to characterize a cognitive function independently of the algorithm $\mathscr{A}$—perhaps because $\mathscr{A}$ is unknown, or because the function can be described more simply and insightfully if some of the nitty-gritty detail present at the c-level is omitted or 'abstracted away'.

In general computation theory, it is necessary to distinguish the f-level from the c-level if we are to study such fundamental questions as whether every function can be computed by an algorithm. Obviously, 'uncomputable function' is simply an oxymoron unless functions can exist independently of algorithms that compute them.

An f-level description is a specification of a function f. f is a set of input-output pairs that will each be denoted ($\mathbf{I}$, $\mathbf{O}$). The function f is **realized by** the c-level function f in the following sense (see the schematic in (13), which parallels (10)). There is a realization mapping ρ_{cf} between the inputs to f and the inputs to f, and between their respective outputs, such that f maps an input $\mathbf{I}$ to an output $\mathbf{O}$ just in case f maps the input realizing $\mathbf{I} - \rho_{cf}(\mathbf{I}) \equiv I -$ to the output realizing $\mathbf{O} - \rho_{cf}(\mathbf{O}) \equiv O$. Since in general the f-level description $\mathscr{F}$ abstracts away from computational details of the c-level description $\mathscr{C}$, the inputs $\mathbf{I}$ and outputs $\mathbf{O}$ of f will typically be simpler entities than their f-counterparts I and O.

(13)   Realization of f-level function f in c-level function f

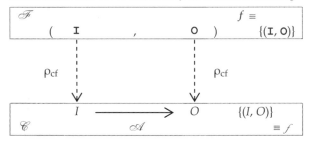

While it makes sense at the c-level to talk of abstract time, this notion has no meaning at the f-level. Functions are ($\mathbf{I}$, $\mathbf{O}$) pairs inhabiting a timeless world.

In recognition of their major contributions to cognitive science, in Section 2.2.3 we granted data-dependency descriptions honorary membership in the c-level by relaxing the requirement that bona fide algorithms be provided for the modules. The same can be done at the f-level, relaxing the requirement that functions be formally specified. The boxes in data-dependency descriptions then represent functions whose behavior is determined intuitively by the analyst interpreting them. The arrows show how representations output by some functions are inputs to others. As we will see in Section 3.4, the arrows can be interpreted as specifying whether one representation is **dependent on** another, in an abstract causal sense.

A data-dependency description takes a large-scale cognitive function f, with unknown formal specification, and reduces it to a system of somewhat smaller-scale functions $\{f_i\}$ with unknown formal specifications. This constitutes a partial specification of f from which cognitively relevant predictions can in fact be made; an example is presented in Section 3.4.

The f-level description $\mathscr{F}$ specifies the function f in some precise, formal language. Specification languages come in qualitatively different types, and the differ-

Figure 6   *Box 5*

ences have important implications for computational architecture, as we begin to see in the next subsection.

2.3.1 Species of function specification

An f-level description is a function specification. The concept of function specification is not highly familiar in much of cognitive science, and it is worth exploring before we proceed because certain aspects of explanation in ICS and in PSA depend crucially on properties of their respective specifications of cognitive functions.

To examine the concept of function specification, I will consider a series of progressively more complex examples. To minimize distraction, I will discuss functions with inputs and outputs that are simply numbers (say, real numbers). At the c-level, it might well be necessary to consider algorithms that manipulate *numerals*, in a given base, with a given precision; but at the f-level, I will abstract away from details of representation with numerals and work simply with numbers.

First, suppose f_1 is a function mapping a number I to the number $2(I + 1)$. This kind of function specification is familiar from algebra; we write $f_1(I) = 2(I + 1)$. The formal language used in this description is that of algebra, which provides as its primitives, say, the arithmetic operations $+$, $-$, $\times$, and $\div$. This specification is $\mathscr{F}_1$.

Next, consider the function specified by $\mathscr{F}_2$: $f_2(I) = 2I + 2$. Clearly, for any input I, f_2 produces the same output as does f_1; that is, for every I, $f_2(I) = f_1(I)$. This means that f_2 is the same function as f_1: $f_2 = f_1$. We have one function, with two different descriptions, $\mathscr{F}_1$: $2(I + 1)$ and $\mathscr{F}_2$: $2I + 2$.

Because the f-level description of a system $\mathcal{S}$ is a function *specification*, different specifications constitute different f-level descriptions even if they specify the same function.

Next consider the function $f_3(I) = \sqrt{I}$. With respect to a description language providing only the primitives of arithmetic, "$\sqrt{I}$" is not a statable description. Yet there is a completely precise way of specifying f_3 using only arithmetic primitives: f_3 pairs I with O if and only if $O^2 = I$, where 'O^2' is simply an abbreviation for $O \times O$. This provides a specification of f_3 by a **constraint**: '$O^2 = I$' is a constraint — a requirement — that a pair (I, O) must satisfy in order to belong to the set of pairs constituting the function f_3. This is a perfectly precise means of specifying f_3, and indeed it is exactly the standard way the square-root function is formally defined in mathematics. The constraint specifying f_3 makes it possible to reason about the function — to prove theorems about it.

As just defined, f_3 includes both the pair $(4, 2)$ and the pair $(4, -2)$. Strictly speaking, a set of pairs constitutes a function only if for each I, there is one and only one O paired with it. For a deterministic physical system, starting in an initial state I — which realizes I — should lead, by the end of the computation, to one and only one state O — which realizes O; so this 'unique output' requirement for f is appropriate. On the other hand, nothing in our analysis will depend on this; it is useful to entertain nondeterministic systems as well, where a single I will lead to several possible outputs O, or even to an infinite number of possible outputs, each with an associated probability. (For example, this is a useful way of describing an unreliable system, where random noise characterizes the unreliability.) For our purposes, then, it is convenient to use the term 'function' to refer to any well-defined set of (I, O) pairs, potentially with an associated probability for each pair.[11]

We can restrict f_3 to exclude pairs like (4, −2) in which O is negative; this gives our next function, f_4 (the 'positive square root'). f_4 is precisely specified by combining the constraint $O^2 = I$ with a second constraint, $O \geq 0$. Now we have a function specified as a set of pairs (I, O) that *simultaneously satisfy* a *set* of constraints (albeit a set of only two).

Our specification of f_3 via the constraint $O^2 = I$ leads to another important mode of function specification. For f_3, a number O will be a possible output for a given input I only if O^2 *exactly* equals I. But what if a constraint can only be *approximately* satisfied?

Imagine, for instance, that we are analyzing a (human or electronic) calculator that uses numerals only to two decimal places, and suppose this is an aspect of the c-level that we don't want to abstract away from now, because, say, we are trying to analyze the consequences of round-off error. Thus, we want to restrict the numbers available at the f-level to those that require only two decimal places—call this set G. Now consider I = 2. The square root of 2 is irrational, so there's certainly no numeral O with two decimal places that will denote a number with a square O^2 that *exactly* equals 2. The obvious move is to do the best we can to approximate f_3, specifying a function f_5 as follows: given an input I, f_5 produces that output O, among the 'candidate set' of possible outputs G, which *minimizes* $|O^2 - I|$, the magnitude of the difference between O^2 and I. This is function specification via **optimization**. Here, '$O^2 = I$' is a **soft** or **violable constraint**; the output of the function f_5 is the number that *minimally* violates it.

It is clear why function specification by optimization would be useful for fields like economics, where theories describe agents actively seeking to optimize a utility function. It is less clear why optimization would be a desirable means of function specification in, say, the natural sciences. Yet it is a remarkable metatheoretic discovery of both classical and quantum physics that, for many important functions describ-

---

[11] The term 'relation' standardly refers to a set of pairs (I, O) for which it is not necessarily the case that a unique O pairs with any given I. I have avoided 'relation' in favor of 'function' because the word 'relation' is so general as to convey almost nothing, whereas at least 'function' makes contact with the relevant notion of functionality. If a set of pairs (I, O) is indeed restricted so that a unique O pairs with any given I, this provides an asymmetry that is consistent with the conception that in a deterministic system I is physically realized at an *earlier* time than O, but not the reverse. This would be an unwelcome residue of the causal connections at the n- and c-levels, where inputs cause outputs (physically and abstractly, respectively). The term 'relation' would in fact more accurately reflect the intended neutrality of directionality in the pairs (I, O) at the f-level. In the cognitive case, the f-level description relates the mental representations that arise during cognitive processing, but does not itself describe the processes themselves. A prototypical case is a grammar, which precisely relates the phonological, syntactic, and semantic mental representations involved in processing a sentence, but does not describe the temporal processes themselves. At the f-level, it does not make sense to ask whether the phonological representation 'precedes' the syntactic one.

Figure 6   *Box 5*

ing physical phenomena, considerable insight is gained by specifying those functions through optimization, rather than through the more direct means of causal dynamical equations. (One of the simplest examples, from the seventeenth century, is Fermat's Principle of Least Time, which asserts that the path taken by a light ray from A to B—say, by bouncing off a mirror or bending through glass—is a path that locally minimizes the travel time required: any small perturbation increases travel time.)

Of course, it has been argued at length in this book, especially in Part III, that in cognitive science too—at least, in the theory of language—function specification by optimization affords significant insight and theoretical power.

2.3.2 The f-c relation

We began with a specification $f_1(\mathbf{I}) = \mathbf{2(I + 1)}$ that provides a ready means of *directly computing* $\mathbf{O}$ from $\mathbf{I}$: assuming we have primitive arithmetic operations available, we just add 1 to $\mathbf{I}$ and then multiply the result by 2. It is important to be clear that *a function specification is not itself an algorithm specification*, although, as here, a function specification may immediately *suggest* an algorithm. But it equally well may not. We have a perfectly precise function specification for the square-root function f_3, via the constraint $\mathbf{O}^2 = \mathbf{I}$. But this specification gives us no clue whatever to a sequence of arithmetic operations that would allow us to directly compute O given I. The constraint may perhaps *suggest* another type of algorithm altogether, one that *guesses* an O value, checks to see whether the constraint is satisfied, and if not, tries again with a new guess (ideally, one informed by the way the previous guess failed). This is a **search algorithm**, and just as the specification for f_1, $f_1(\mathbf{I}) = \mathbf{2(I + 1)}$, may *suggest* but does not *specify* a direct arithmetic algorithm, so too the specification for f_3, $\mathbf{O}^2 = \mathbf{I}$, may suggest but does not specify a search algorithm.

It is the job of the *f*-level description to specify a *function*; it is the job of the *c*-level description to specify an *algorithm*. This will be a critical distinction here because the algorithms of symbolic cognitive theory typically *follow the suggestions* offered by their function specifications, whereas those of the proposed ICS theory do not. Both theories agree on the role of symbols in f-level accounts of cognition, but they disagree on their role in c-level accounts.

In order for the function f specified by the f-level description $\mathscr{F}$ to be a correct description of $\mathcal{S}$, its input-output behavior must be realized by the c-level function f, as shown in (13): the function f contains a pair $(\mathbf{I}, \mathbf{O})$—say, numbers—if and only if the function f contains the corresponding pair (I, O)—say, decimal numerals—where the correspondence is defined by the realization mapping ρ_{cf}. Now such a function f could be described in multiple ways (like $f_1 = f_2$ above, where $f_1(\mathbf{I}) = \mathbf{2(I + 1)}$; $f_2(\mathbf{I}) = \mathbf{2I + 2}$). The most informative descriptions are those with a special property: the *internal structure* of the function specification $\mathscr{F}$ matches the *internal structure* of corresponding aspects of the c-level description $\mathscr{C}$. That is, the realization mapping ρ_{cf} from $\mathscr{F}$ to $\mathscr{C}$ is an **isomorphism**, written ι_{cf}. This notion, illustrated in (14), is parallel to its lower-level counterpart, an isomorphism mapping ι_{nc} from $\mathscr{C}$ to $\mathscr{N}$ (11).

(14)   Isomorphism of f-level function f with c-level algorithm $\mathscr{A}$: $\Sigma_f \approx \Sigma_{cf}$

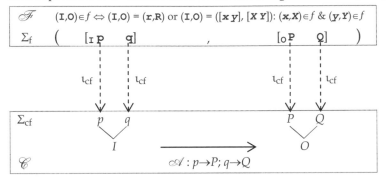

To spell this out a bit more precisely, suppose the function specification $\mathscr{F}$ provides a structural decomposition of f into parts (e.g., a list of symbols); denote this decomposition 'Σ_f'. Suppose further that under $\mathscr{C}$, computational states and the algorithm governing them can be internally decomposed according to some structure Σ_{cf}. Then an isomorphism from Σ_f to Σ_{cf} is a mapping ι_{cf} that associates to each functional part in Σ_f a corresponding part in Σ_{cf}; the latter is a **realization** of the former. To qualify as an isomorphism, ι_{cf} must put the parts into which the function is decomposed by Σ_f into correspondence with the parts into which the algorithm is decomposed by Σ_{cf}. When Σ_f and Σ_{cf} are isomorphic, we write '$\Sigma_f \approx \Sigma_{cf}$'. More precise definition of 'put into correspondence' is possible only with respect to more precise characterizations of the internal structures of $\mathscr{F}$ and $\mathscr{C}$; this is discussed in Sections 5 and 6 for the cases of PSA and ICS. (See Box 6 for simple examples with arithmetic computation.) When an isomorphism ι_{cf} exists, I will use the terminology in (15).

(15)   Functionally relevant computational structure Σ_{cf}

Suppose an isomorphism ι_{cf} exists from $\mathscr{F}$ to $\mathscr{C}$. Then

a.   the decomposition Σ_{cf} provided by $\mathscr{C}$ is **functionally relevant**, and

b.   the decomposition Σ_f provided by the function specification $\mathscr{F}$ is **computationally relevant**.

In any valid, complete three-level theory of a physical computational system $\mathcal{S}$, the *function f* of the f-level description must be computationally relevant, in the sense that its input-output pairs correspond to those of the c-level algorithm, that is, the function f. What is at issue in the isomorphism question is the internal structure of the function *specification* of $\mathscr{F}$, which may or may not be computationally relevant.

Figure 6   Box 5

Box 6. $\mathscr{F}\text{-}\mathscr{C}$ isomorphism in arithmetic computers

(This box continues Box 5. Figures 3 and 4 also illustrate the discussion here.)

Consider the computer S_1 of Box 5. One f-level description of S_1 is clearly that shown in (1).

(1) $\mathscr{F}_1\text{:}\ f_1(\boldsymbol{y})\ =\ \boldsymbol{2\,(y+1)}$

This is isomorphic to the c-level description $\mathscr{A}_{1H}$ (2) of Box 5) because the linguistic structure '$\boldsymbol{2\,(y+1)}$' is parsed such that '$\boldsymbol{y+1}$' is embedded inside '$\boldsymbol{2\,(\ \ )}$'. This can be mapped mechanically into the sequence $add(n, 1) \rightarrow m;\ mult(m, 2) \rightarrow k$, where n is the input and k the output: this is $\mathscr{A}_{1H}$. The constituents of this f-description, for example, $[\boldsymbol{y+1}]$, correspond directly to constituents of the c-description $\mathscr{A}_{1H}$, for example, $[add(n, 1) \rightarrow m]$.

  To state precisely the sense in which $\mathscr{F}_1$ is isomorphic to $\mathscr{A}_{1H}$, let us define the relevant structures in the two descriptions. For $\mathscr{F}_1$, the linguistic structure is captured in a parse tree, showing the nesting of constituents (see Chapter 1 (6)); denote this structure $\Sigma_{\mathscr{F}_1}^{\text{constit}}$. The isomorphism ι_{cf} from $\mathscr{F}_1$ to $\mathscr{A}_{1H}$ identifies a constituent $\boldsymbol{p}$ of $\mathscr{F}_1$ with an interval p of abstract time during which $\mathscr{A}_{1H}$ computes $\boldsymbol{p}$; if $\boldsymbol{p}$ is embedded within a larger constituent $\boldsymbol{q}$, then the temporal interval p during which $\mathscr{A}_{1H}$ computes $\boldsymbol{p}$ is embedded within a larger interval q during which it computes $\boldsymbol{q}$. Thus, if $\boldsymbol{p} = [\boldsymbol{y+1}]$, then $p = [add(n, 1) \rightarrow m]$; and $\boldsymbol{p}$ is embedded within $\boldsymbol{q} = [2\,[\boldsymbol{y+1}]]$, which corresponds under ι_{cf} to $q = [[add(n, 1) \rightarrow m]\ mult(m, 2) \rightarrow k]$. The relevant structure of $\mathscr{A}_{1H}$ is nested intervals of operations, $\Sigma_{\mathscr{A}_{1H}}^{\text{int}}$.

(2) $\Sigma_{\mathscr{F}_1}^{\text{constit}} \approx \Sigma_{\mathscr{A}_{1H}}^{\text{int}}$

  With respect to constituent structure, $\mathscr{F}_1$ is isomorphic to $\mathscr{A}_{1H}$, and thus by transitivity to $\mathscr{N}_1$, for in this case $\mathscr{A}_{1H}$ is isomorphic to $\mathscr{N}_1$, as was shown in Box 5. According to the function's form $\mathscr{F}_1$, the same number of operations or constituents applies for all inputs; under the isomorphism ι_{cf}, this means that $\mathscr{A}_{1H}$ has the same interval structure—executes the same sequence of operations—regardless of the input. In turn, $\mathscr{A}_{1H}$ is isomorphic with respect to durational structure to $\mathscr{N}_1$ under ι_{nc}; thus, if $\mathscr{A}_{1H}$ executes the same operations for each input, this invariant abstract time translates into invariant real time. The $\mathscr{F}\text{-}\mathscr{C}$ isomorphism ι_{cf} puts the operation structure of $\mathscr{F}_1$ (1) into one-to-one correspondence with the operation structure of $\mathscr{A}_{1H}$; the $\mathscr{C}\text{-}\mathscr{N}$ isomorphism ι_{nc} then puts this structure of $\mathscr{A}_{1H}$ into one-to-one correspondence with subprocesses in $\mathscr{N}_1$ so that the sequences of operations coincide and the one unit of abstract time taken by each operation of $\mathscr{A}_{1H}$ corresponds to a fixed amount of real time in $\mathscr{N}_1$.

  Next consider another function specification:

(3) $\mathscr{F}_1'\text{:}\ f_1'(\boldsymbol{y}) = \boldsymbol{(2y)+2}$

This correctly describes the function computed by S_1 and therefore is, like $\mathscr{F}_1$, a valid f-level description of S_1. But in contrast to what happens with $\mathscr{F}_1$, in the de-

---

scription $\mathscr{F}_1'$ the internal constituency does *not* map onto that of the processes operating in $\mathscr{S}_1$. The constituent **[2y]** of $\mathscr{F}_1'$ has no counterpart in $\mathscr{A}_{1\mathrm{H}}$ or $\mathscr{N}_1$: over no interval of abstract time within $\mathscr{A}_{1\mathrm{H}}$ or of real time within $\mathscr{N}_1$ does $\mathscr{S}_1$ compute the function $y \mapsto 2y$. Thus, $\mathscr{F}_1'$ is *not* isomorphic to $\mathscr{A}_{1\mathrm{H}}$, or to $\mathscr{N}_1$. The sequence of states in $\mathscr{S}_1$ does not correspond to the internal structure of $\mathscr{F}_1'$; there is no intermediate state of $\mathscr{S}_1$ interpretable as the result of a subprocess realizing the subconstituent **[2y]**.

Now consider the other computer of Box 5, the bit manipulator $\mathscr{S}_2$. This computes the same function as $\mathscr{S}_1$, so both $\mathscr{F}_1$ and $\mathscr{F}_1'$ are also valid f-level descriptions of $\mathscr{S}_2$. They will be designated $\mathscr{F}_2$ and $\mathscr{F}_2'$ when they are descriptions of $\mathscr{S}_2$. As with $\mathscr{S}_1$, for $\mathscr{S}_2$, $\mathscr{F}_2'$ is not isomorphic either to $\mathscr{A}_{2\mathrm{H}}$ or to $\mathscr{N}_2$. $\mathscr{F}_2$, however, *is* isomorphic to $\mathscr{A}_{2\mathrm{H}}$. $\mathscr{A}_{2\mathrm{H}}$ is isomorphic to $\mathscr{N}_2$ with respect to *sequential* structure, thus by transitivity so is $\mathscr{F}_2$: the constituent structure of $\mathscr{F}_2$ is computationally relevant because (like $\mathscr{S}_1$) $\mathscr{S}_2$ computes $y + 1$ and then doubles the result. But as shown in Box 5, $\mathscr{A}_{2\mathrm{H}}$ is not isomorphic to $\mathscr{N}_2$ with respect to temporal *duration*, so in this respect $\mathscr{F}_2$ is not isomorphic to $\mathscr{N}_2$ either. To predict processing times, a description isomorphic to the low-level, bit-manipulating algorithm $\mathscr{A}_{2\mathrm{L}}$ is needed. For $\mathscr{S}_2$, unlike $\mathscr{S}_1$, there is no $\mathscr{N}$-isomorphic f-level description that is naturally stated over numbers, as opposed to binary numerals. The f-level is well suited to an insightful expression of *what* is computed, $f(y) = 2(y + 1)$, and *how* it is computed, with respect to coarse-grained sequential structure—but not with respect to the time requirements of the processes in $\mathscr{S}_2$. Just the reverse is true of the *lowest* sublevel of the c-level, where $\mathscr{A}_{2\mathrm{L}}$ describes how computation takes place at a fine grain; and at that level, even durational structure is preserved. But $\mathscr{A}_{1\mathrm{L}}$ utterly obscures *what* the computation computes—that is, it well describes the *structure* but not the *function* of $\mathscr{S}_2$.

2.3.3 Optimization and f-c isomorphism

A glimpse of one key aspect of the ICS f-c isomorphism is afforded by observing a crucial difference between the above specifications of the example numerical functions f_4 and f_1. With f_1 specified as **2(I + 1)**, the "suggested" algorithm admits a natural decomposition: one part adds 1 to **I**, the other multiplies by 2. Arbitrarily complex algebraic expressions can be decomposed into simpler parts in like fashion, reducing all computation to primitive arithmetic operations (like addition and multiplication). In a serial architecture, each of these primitive operations would be performed at a different moment of abstract time. Obviously—but crucially—when further algebraic operations are inserted into an expression, the "suggested" algorithm will require more abstract time to complete.

In contrast, consider the specification of f_4 as mapping an input **I** to that output **O** which simultaneously satisfies two constraints ($\mathbf{O}^2 = \mathbf{I}$, $\mathbf{O} \geq 0$). The natural top-level decomposition of the function provided by *this* specification breaks it into two separate constraints. The algorithm "suggested" by this function specification is a search

Figure 6   *Box 6*

algorithm, which guesses a value for O, checks to see whether $O^2 = I$, and checks to see whether $O \geq 0$. Adding more constraints will increase the abstract time required to check each guess (as will adding arithmetic operations to an individual constraint). But this does not mean the overall computation must take more abstract time, for the critical factor in *search* is typically not how many steps it takes to check each guess, but how many guesses must be checked to find the answer. It could happen—and this is actually relevant to the cognitive case—that it would take fewer guesses with more constraints, because, for example, more constraints provide more information about the error of the previous guess, thereby improving the guess by a greater amount each time. With fewer guesses required, the overall abstract time required might actually be less with additional constraints. In any event, the point is not that this *will* necessarily happen, but that it *could*: there is no logical implication between processing steps and the number of constraints into which the function is decomposed (or the algebraic complexity of each constraint). This is true for the strictly serial version of the obvious search algorithm suggested by the function specification; it is even more true for the massively parallel search algorithms employed by ICS.

Thus, with respect to the algorithms they "suggest," the decompositions of complex function specifications into simpler ones that are provided by optimization are fundamentally different from the decompositions provided by function specifications that are immediately interpretable as an arrangement of primitive operations that directly constructs the output from the input. In the latter case, but not the former, the functional decomposition at the f-level can directly *entail* processing or computational properties at the c-level.

2.3.4   The f-n relation

What is the relation between the highest and lowest descriptive levels—the f-level $\mathscr{F}$ and the n-level $\mathscr{N}$? This question is important because, as emphasized in (12), it is when some abstract structure is isomorphic to the physical structure in $\mathscr{N}$ that this abstract structure provides information concerning the processes at work in our system $\mathscr{S}$: it is under isomorphism with $\mathscr{N}$ that abstract structure becomes process-relevant. In both PSA and ICS, $\mathscr{F}$ has symbolic structure, and whether these symbols are process-relevant thus turns on whether the symbolic structure of $\mathscr{F}$ is isomorphic to the underlying physical structure of $\mathscr{N}$.

If $\mathscr{F}$ is not computationally relevant, then its internal structure does not even correspond to $\mathscr{C}$, let alone to the still more distant level $\mathscr{N}$. The more interesting case is when $\mathscr{F}$ *is* computationally relevant. Then $\mathscr{F}$ is isomorphic to $\mathscr{C}$: parts of $\mathscr{F}$ correspond to parts of $\mathscr{C}$ under the isomorphism ι_{cn}. Suppose also that $\mathscr{C}$ is process-relevant, that is, isomorphic to $\mathscr{N}$: parts of $\mathscr{C}$ correspond to parts of $\mathscr{N}$ under the isomorphism ι_{nc}. It would seem to follow that $\mathscr{F}$ must be isomorphic to $\mathscr{N}$ (under the composition of the two isomorphisms, $\iota_{nc} \circ \iota_{cf}$). But in fact this *transitivity of isomorphism need not hold* — and this will prove crucial for ICS.

How could transitivity of isomorphism fail to apply? This possibility arises when the c-level contains multiple sublevels. Then the isomorphism ι_{cf} puts $\mathscr{F}$ in corre-spondence with an *upper sublevel* of $\mathscr{C}$; the isomorphism ι_{nc} puts $\mathscr{N}$ in correspon-dence with a *lower sublevel* of $\mathscr{C}$. The gap between the upper and lower sublevels of $\mathscr{C}$ is spanned by a scaffolding of realization mappings, as discussed in Section 2.2.2. Now if this scaffolding ensured that upper sublevels of $\mathscr{C}$ are isomorphic to lower sublevels, then transitivity would indeed apply: $\mathscr{F}$ and $\mathscr{N}$ would necessarily be isomorphic.

But the relation between upper and lower sublevels of $\mathscr{C}$ need not be one of iso-morphism: all that is required is that between successive sublevels of $\mathscr{C}$, there is a complete, formal, precise realization mapping. Such a realization mapping may not be part for part, in the nature of an isomorphism, but rather, more holistic. This will indeed prove to be the case in ICS, where distributed connectionist representations entail that a single lower-level part—an individual unit's activation—corresponds to multiple higher-level parts—the activation vectors realizing each of several symbols. And of course a single upper-level part—a distributed activation vector realizing a symbol—corresponds to multiple lower-level parts—unit activations.

It is useful to put this another way. When $\mathscr{F}$ and $\mathscr{C}$ are isomorphic, the parts of $\mathscr{C}$ that correspond to parts of $\mathscr{F}$ are the functionally relevant parts of $\mathscr{C}$. When $\mathscr{C}$ is isomorphic to $\mathscr{N}$, the parts of $\mathscr{C}$ that correspond to parts of $\mathscr{N}$ are the process-relevant parts of $\mathscr{C}$. And, crucially for ICS, *these may be different*: the *functionally* rele-vant decomposition of $\mathscr{C}$ (Σ_{cf}) need not align with the *process*-relevant decomposition of $\mathscr{C}$ (Σ_{cn}). (See Figure 7.)

Figure 7. Levels in ICS

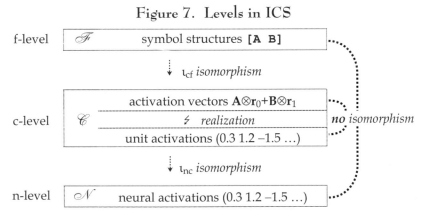

3 LEVELS OF DESCRIPTION IN A (REPRESENTATIONAL) COGNITIVE THEORY

Having discussed the three levels of description for a general physical computational system $\mathscr{S}$, I now turn to the more specific case of human cognition, where $\mathscr{S}$ is the mind/brain.

Figure 7   *Box 6*

3.1 The f-level in a cognitive theory: Mental representation

In a generic computational system $\mathcal{S}$, the elements of the f-level description $\mathcal{F}$ need not *mean* anything. In the cognitive case—on the standard *representationalist* assumption—there is a key additional element at the f-level: a notion of *semantic interpretation*. Certain elements in $\mathcal{F}$ are *mental representations* that *refer* to other things—their *content*. I will denote by '$\mathcal{W}$' the 'world' that mental representations refer to; in the basic case, $\mathcal{W}$ is the external physical environment in which our system $\mathcal{S}$ operates, but other possibilities for $\mathcal{W}$ would work here as well. (See Box 7 for an introduction to the perspective on representation being assumed here.)

Mental representations introduce yet another important type of isomorphism into the picture, that between (i) the mental system $\mathcal{F}$ in which the representations *reside*, and (ii) the (e.g., external physical) world $\mathcal{W}$ to which the representations *refer*. The function mapping a mental representation into its referent or meaning will be denoted 'μ'. μ is an isomorphism: only if the system employing mental representations mirrors the structure of the world the representations represent can these representations be useful for the organism that has them (and for the theorist who posits them). This 'mirroring' is what the notion of isomorphism formalizes. The elements internal to $\mathcal{F}$ that participate in the isomorphism μ with $\mathcal{W}$ will be called **semantically relevant**. (16) gives a simple example.

(16)   Meaning isomorphism μ: Maps a mental representation to its semantic interpretation

Within the internal mental world described by $\mathcal{F}$, mental representations of letters ($\mathbf{s}_s$, $\mathbf{s}_c$, …) relate to the mental representation of the letter string making up the word they spell ($\mathbf{s}_{scone}$) in a way that mirrors how the meanings of these representations—illuminated shapes on a computer monitor, say—relate to one another in the external physical world $\mathcal{W}$.

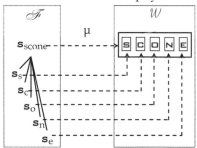

Thus, the elements of a computationally relevant f-level description—symbols, say—are party to two very different isomorphisms. The *internal* isomorphism ι_{cf} relates a symbol to the aspect of the c-level description that computationally realizes it (13). The *external* isomorphism μ relates a symbol to its meaning (16). It is via this duality that the combinatorial strategy explains the productivity of cognition, both in PSA and in ICS.

An important aspect of the isomorphism provided by μ is **compositional semantics** (see Section 1:3).

(17)   Compositional semantics in representational meaning

The constituent structure of a representation **s** is mapped under μ, part for part, to an isomorphic structure in the meaning μ(**s**). That is, 'the meaning of the whole is built compositionally from the meaning of the parts' — the meanings of the parts of **s** are combined into a structure μ(**s**) that is isomorphic to the constituent structure of **s**.

To see how semantic compositionality works in an extremely simple case, consider the semantic interpretation of **s** ≡ **[lives [Frodo]]**. The meaning of **Frodo**, μ(**Frodo**), is an individual in a long-forgotten possible world; let us name him FRODO in the metalanguage of this exposition. Thus, μ(**Frodo**) = FRODO. The meaning of **lives**, μ(**lives**), is a predicate that identifies the set of living individuals in this possible world; let's call this predicate LIVES. Thus, μ(**lives**) = LIVES. Now the meaning of the composed structure **s** ≡ **[lives [Frodo]]** is a proposition: it is true if and only if FRODO is among the set of individuals identified by LIVES. This proposition is standardly denoted LIVES(FRODO). Hence:

(18) $\mu(\mathbf{s})$ = μ(**[lives [Frodo]]**) = LIVES(FRODO)

$$= \mu(\mathbf{lives})\big(\mu(\mathbf{Frodo})\big)$$

This equality expresses just how the meaning of the composite structure **[lives [Frodo]]** is built up from the meanings of its constituents. This example is particularly simple because LIVES is a predicate that takes only one argument; in general, if the symbol **p** denotes a predicate that takes n arguments, then (18) becomes (19).

(19) $\mu(\mathbf{[p\ [a_1\ a_2\ \ldots\ a_n]]})$ = $\mu(\mathbf{p})\big(\mu(\mathbf{a_1}), \mu(\mathbf{a_2}), \ldots, \mu(\mathbf{a_n})\big)$

For example, **thinks** might denote a two-argument predicate THINKS: the first argument is the thinker (an individual), the second is the thought (a proposition). The proposition that JOSH thinks FRODO lives would then be represented by

(20)   **[thinks [Josh s]]** = **[thinks [Josh [lives [Frodo]]]]**

(assuming **Josh** denotes JOSH: μ(**Josh**) ≡ JOSH). The semantic interpretation of this expression illustrates the important role played by the internal structure of an expression in the compositional determination of its meaning. It is this structure which determines that JOSH, not FRODO, is the thinker.

(21)   μ(**[thinks [Josh [lives [Frodo]]]]**)

$\equiv \mu(\mathbf{[thinks\ [Josh\ s]]})$ — by (20)

$= \mu(\mathbf{thinks})\big(\mu(\mathbf{Josh}), \mu(\mathbf{s})\big)$ — by (19)

$\equiv \text{THINKS}\big(\text{JOSH}, \mu(\mathbf{s})\big)$

$= \text{THINKS}\big(\text{JOSH}, \mu(\mathbf{lives})\big(\mu(\mathbf{Frodo})\big)\big)$ — by (18)

$= \text{THINKS}\big(\text{JOSH}, \text{LIVES}(\text{FRODO})\big)$ — by (18)

Figure 7   *Box 6*

The relation between the first and last expressions (21) illustrates the sense in which, with compositional semantics, *the internal structure of the meaning of an expression mirrors the internal structure of the expression itself.* (This is the only point of this grossly oversimplified excursus into elementary formal semantics.)

Presently, the compositionality of semantics at the f-level is merely a stipulated principle of the ICS architecture, as it is in a purely symbolic architecture. Deriving it from more basic semantic principles operating at the c- or n-level is an open problem in the development of ICS (concerning 'distributed semantics', see Haugeland 1991).

Box 7. Explanation by mental representation

The following is an instance of what I take to be the basic explanation pattern that the concept of mental representation must support. To avoid distraction from the current line of argument, I will abstract away from error (i.e., pretend the relevant behavior is errorless) and accordingly pretend mental processes are errorless as well.

(1)   Visual lexical decision

    a.   *A regularity G.* After instruction, when subject S is visually presented with a computer display of an English word (in any of the computer's fonts), S depresses the 'yes' button.

    b.   *The question.* Why does G hold?

    c.   *The answer.* Because

       i.   Internal to S's mind is a process Y that generates the behavior of depressing the 'yes' button.

       ii.   For each English word w there is an element $\mathbf{s}_w$ in S's mind that corresponds to w.

         ✦ $\mathbf{s}_w$ is the **mental representation** of w.

         ✦ w is the **content** or **referent** or **meaning** of $\mathbf{s}_w$.

         ✦ The function mapping $\mathbf{s}_w$ to w is the **(semantic) interpretation function** μ.

       iii.   When an instance of w is presented to S, $\mathbf{s}_w$ becomes 'active'.

       iv.   When $\mathbf{s}_w$ is active, process Y is triggered.

Of course, this explanation rests on extremely strong assumptions concerning representation. Implicit in the argument schema, it seems to me, is a kind of fusing of the mind of the subject S and that of the scientist observing S. The generalization G is stated in a language that permits a description of the experimental stimulus (or state of the environment) with an expression like 'a computer display of an English word (in any of the computer's fonts)'; call this environmental property p. The property p is highly 'mentalist' and remote from a physical description; for even a single lexical item, stating in physical terms when a state of the computer display qualifies as an instance of the word (in our example, *scone*)—especially a description that will work for a diverse set of fonts—is an extremely complex business. The scientist observing S

---

permits herself to use p in stating the generalization G to be explained, not because she can determine whether p holds by physical measurements, but because she can readily evaluate p in her own mind. The explanation (1) then posits that the mind of the *subject* S also 'has' the concept p in that it is able to activate $\mathbf{s}_{scone}$ exactly when the stimulus possesses property p. In this sense, the environmental property p has migrated directly from the mind of the scientist to the mind of the subject, without the mediation of any characterization that would be recognizable by the natural sciences as a property *of the environment.*

I don't think this conclusion is an artifact of the particular example, which of course is no mere expository fiction but illustrative of much genuine cognitive science research. Here is a second real example, where I continue to put aside the issue of error. I will use **linguistic realism** to refer to the perspective on cognitive science in which such arguments are employed, at least implicitly.

(2)   Linguistic realism and grammatical subject

    a.   *A regularity G.* A speaker of English, S, will declare ungrammatical any sentence that violates

          ✦   OBLIGSUBJ: Every sentence must have a subject.[12]

    b.   *The question.* Why does G hold?

    c.   *The answer.* Because

        i.   Internal to S's mind is a process Y that generates the behavior of declaring a 'stimulus' sentence unacceptable.

        ii.   Internal to S's mind is a set of states $\{\mathbf{s}_{Subj}\}$ corresponding to the property of being the subject of a sentence.

        iii. When a stimulus sentence containing a subject is presented to S, one of the $\{\mathbf{s}_{Subj}\}$ becomes active.

        iv.   When a sentence is processed in S's mind and no state $\{\mathbf{s}_{Subj}\}$ is active, process Y is triggered.

Although simplified in certain respects, I believe this example captures a central aspect of the implicit reasoning by which cognitive scientists put into the minds of speakers substantive representational discoveries of theoretical linguistics research, such as the notion 'subject' and its role in many regularities like OBLIGSUBJ. All the remarks concerning the previous example hold here as well: if the environmental property p of example (1) is already quite abstract, the property q of 'being the subject of a sentence' is considerably more abstract still. The explanation transplants notions like 'subject' from the mind of the scientist to the mind of the subject. (And for this point, it makes absolutely no difference if 'declare ungrammatical' is replaced by something much more "scientific," like 'evoke an event-related EEG that displays a P600'.) There is an interesting twist here, however, which may contribute significantly to the widespread impression that theoretical linguistics research is much more ab-

---

[12] This constraint is central to the analysis of Grimshaw and Samek-Lodovici 1998; see Section 12:1.1. Here I ignore the few special types of English sentences that have no grammatical subject; they are irrelevant to the present point.

Figure 7   *Box 7*

stract than psychological research on lexical decision. In the lexical decision case, the notion being transplanted is 'word of English', a commonsense notion to be sure; it migrates from the conscious mind of the scientist to the conscious mind of the subject. But in the example of linguistic realism, the notion being transplanted, 'grammatical subject', is created through analysis within the conscious mind of the scientist, but in the mind of the speaker, the relevant counterpart notion is utterly unconscious. (Whatever conscious notion of 'subject' the speaker may have is not relevant to the explanation, which applies equally—better, in fact—to speakers whose culture or education provides no such notion.)

Underlying these two examples of explanation-by-representation is a highly general explanation schema that I will take to be one of the defining features of the representational theory of mind.

(3)   Representationalist explanation schema

    a. *A regularity* G concerning the relation between some human behavior B and the extra-mental environment E, stated in a language L employing certain properties $\{p_i\}$.

    b. *The question.* Why does G hold?

    c. *The answer.* Because

        i.   Internal to a subject S's mind is a process Y that generates B.

        ii. For each property p_i of L there is a corresponding element $\mathbf{s}_i$ in S's mind (not necessarily consciously accessible).

        iii. When E possesses p_i, $\mathbf{s}_i$ becomes active.

        iv. When $\mathbf{s}_i$ is active, Y is triggered.

This stark rendition may give the impression that representationalism yields rather trivial explanations. There are several simplifications that may be responsible. The idea that the content of a representation $\mathbf{s}_i$ is fixed by an environmental property p_i that co-occurs with (and perhaps causes) $\mathbf{s}_i$ is inadequate in several ways, and a less naïve theory of content may render this explanation schema less trivial. For our purposes, the most important simplification is that the account so far is too atomistic. The questions of interest to cognitive science crucially concern *systems* of representations that serve in the explanation of *systems* of generalizations G_α. For example, the acceptability judgment data of generative syntax provide a huge crosscutting set of very limited generalizations such as 'Sentences that are tokens of $word_1\ word_2 \ldots$ are judged ungrammatical'. Each sentence corresponds to a unique complex representation with constituent parts, and it is very difficult for the scientist to sort these representations into two groups according to whether they do or do not trigger the process Y of declaring the sentence 'unacceptable'. This difficult sorting task is part of the job of the theoretical linguist. It is rarely the case that the generalization of interest will be simply stated, as in (2); consider the OT grammars of Part III. Rather than one single inviolable constraint, it is a whole system of violable constraints that picks out the grammatical sentences. The property of optimally satisfying a ranked set of violable constraints is the right type of property for sorting the representations, according to

OT, but this property is extremely complex to evaluate; there is no simply defined set of states like the $\{\mathbf{s}_{Subj}\}$ of (2) that does the job.

A typical use of representationalist explanation is discussed in Section 3.4. There the system of representations includes concepts, lexical items, and phonological structures, each with some partially specified constituent structure. The degree of similarity between different representations—the extent to which they have the same constituents—models the likelihood that cognitive functions will produce various outputs (those more similar to the 'correct' output being more likely). Integral to the explanation is the presumed isomorphism between the internal structure of representations and the properties of the entities represented. Because members of the categories CAT and DOG have in common the properties of being pets and being furry, the corresponding mental representations have constituents in common, the semantic features ⟨furry⟩ and ⟨pet⟩. It is this isomorphism that allows the proposed system of representations to explain the targeted empirical generalizations.

3.2 The c-level in a cognitive theory: Process modeling

In the field of artificial intelligence (AI), the problem is to design a computational system $\mathcal{S}$ that computes a cognitive function. To say the function computed is 'cognitive' is to say that in the f-level description $\mathcal{F}$ of $\mathcal{S}$, the input-output mapping f corresponds to that which an intelligent human might exhibit when performing a particular task. Descending to the c-level, we can ask whether the description $\mathcal{C}$ also corresponds to human cognition. In applied AI, this is not an important question, as only f-level functionality matters: as long as it gets the right answer—computes the right f-level function—it is irrelevant whether the algorithm $\mathcal{A}$ employed in $\mathcal{C}$ corresponds to human mental processes. But for cognitive science, this question is key: a complete cognitive theory must deliver an algorithm $\mathcal{A}$ that not only gets the right answer, but also serves as a model of human mental processes. That is, $\mathcal{C}$ must provide an $\mathcal{A}$ that makes predictions concerning those processes: predictions concerning the physical resources consumed (e.g., the time these processes require) for varying inputs and under varying conditions of process disruption or facilitation. I am calling such an algorithm 'process-relevant'; (12) asserts that such a computational description must be isomorphic to the physical level $\mathcal{N}$, so that, for example, when the algorithm requires additional steps, an increase in response time necessarily results. A complete cognitive theory must deliver a c-level theory that is process-relevant.

(22)   Process modeling

In a complete cognitive theory, $\mathcal{C}$ must contain some structure Σ_{cn} isomorphic to Σ_n under an isomorphism ι_{nc}.

Every complete cognitive theory must deliver *a* process-relevant c-level description—but not every c-level description of a complete cognitive theory must be proc-

Figure 7   *Box 7*

ess-relevant. When $\mathscr{C}$ has multiple sublevels, if some lower sublevel is isomorphic to $\mathscr{N}$ and hence process-relevant, then higher sublevels need not be. ICS, but not PSA, exploits this possibility.

3.3 The n-level in a cognitive theory: Neural realization

In the cognitive case, where $\mathscr{S}$ is the mind/brain, the n-level is the neural level; $\mathscr{N}$ describes the biophysical properties of the relevant part of the nervous system.

A complete cognitive theory will include an n-level description that makes it possible to precisely specify the isomorphism ι_{cn} which links the process-relevant aspects of the c-level with the computationally relevant aspects of the n-level—which links, that is, the mind with the brain. For higher cognition, at least, this will not be a reality for some time. Meanwhile, as we will see below for PSA and for ICS, ι_{nc} can be partially described by certain general properties—indeed, it must be, to determine whether a c-level description $\mathscr{C}$ is isomorphic to $\mathscr{N}$ and hence process-relevant, and what predictions concerning processes follow from $\mathscr{C}$.

In the discussion of generic computational systems, Boxes 5–6 concretely illustrate with simple numerical computation the connection between process-relevance of an algorithm and isomorphism with the n-level. The next subsection illustrates this same connection in the more complex context of cognitive theory.

3.4 Process-relevance and n-isomorphism for data-dependency descriptions

This subsection provides an extended example—taken from contemporary cognitive science research—of how a cognitive theory's behavioral predictions depend upon isomorphism between the f- or c-level and the n-level. It is not essential for the remainder of the chapter; it merely attempts to make more concrete the preceding rather abstract discussion relating n-isomorphism and process-relevance.[13]

Consider the data-dependency diagrams in Figures 8 and 9. These illustrate two of the theories studied by Rapp and Goldrick (2000) and Goldrick and Rapp (2002) as representatives of several current prominent theories of the mental processes by which a concept is named—the processes by which, for example, the concept *CAT* generates the phonological representation /kæt/. Figure 8 depicts what Goldrick and Rapp call the **discrete feed-forward** theory, in contrast with the **restricted interaction** theory depicted in Figure 9. The concept *CAT* is taken to consist in a set of semantic features, $\{\langle \text{furry} \rangle, \langle \text{feline} \rangle, \langle \text{pet} \rangle, \ldots\}$; I will denote this representation 'R_{Sem}'. The phonological output is taken to be a set of phonemes $\{\langle k \rangle, \langle æ \rangle, \langle t \rangle\}$ with some encoding of their sequence; I will call this representation 'R_{Phon}'. In between is a level of representation they dub the **L-level**, intended to subsume various means of representing lexical items; I will call this 'R_{Lex}'. In the discrete feed-forward theory, a possible representation R_{Lex} is a single lexical item; the L-level representation $R_{Lex} = $ CAT is a simple atom, the label of the concept $R_{Sem} = CAT$. In the restricted interaction theory, a rep-

---

[13] Other illustrations of this point will be briefly outlined in (32).

resentation R_{Lex} is a numerical vector, with one ('activation') value a_X per lexical atom X; when $R_{Sem} = CAT$, R_{Lex} might be a vector like $(a_{CAT}, a_{RAT}, a_{DOG}, a_{HAT}, \ldots) = (0.5, 0.01, 0.01, 0.001, \ldots)$.[14]

The left-hand diagram in Figure 8 shows the discrete feed-forward or **noninteractive** theory as a unidirectional information flow from R_{Sem} to R_{Lex} to R_{Phon}. The right-hand diagram depicts the same theory, with boxes for subprocesses rather than ovals for representations. The process P_{Lex} produces the representation R_{Lex}, while P_{Phon} produces R_{Phon}.

Figure 8. A noninteractive data-dependency theory

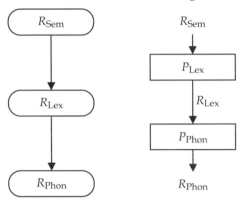

The (**restricted**) **interactive** theory of Figure 9 differs in that information flows back from R_{Phon} to R_{Lex} as well; the information flow is no longer unidirectional. The input to the process P_{Lex} now includes R_{Phon} as well as R_{Sem}; the representation R_{Lex} is a function of R_{Phon} as well as R_{Sem}.

In addition to differing in connectivity, the noninteractive and interactive theories differ in their lexical-level representation R_{Lex}. As explained above, in the former theory each R_{Lex} is one atom designating a single lexical item, but in the latter each is a vector assigning to each such atom a numerical value.

The goal of this section is to explore the meaning of these diagrams: specifically, what they implicitly assert about the physical-level description $\mathcal{N}$ of the neural system realizing these cognitive processes.

A concise f-level description of these theories is given in (23), with P_{Lex} and P_{Phon} designating functions.

---

[14] The representations under discussion are the final ones achieved by the computation. As shown in Figure 10, in Rapp and Goldrick's implementation, R_{Lex} is realized as a set of connectionist units, and during computation these units host a distributed pattern of activation, in both the discrete feed-forward and the restricted interaction architectures. However, a competitive process operating only in the discrete architecture ensures that at the end of computation, only a single unit is active. This unit realizes the 'atom' comprising R_{Lex} in the discrete feed-forward theory.

Figure 8   *Box 7*

(23)   Relations among f-level descriptions
   a.   Noninteractive theory
       i. $R_{Lex} = P_{Lex}(R_{Sem})$
       ii. $R_{Phon} = P_{Phon}(R_{Lex})$
   b.   Interactive theory
       i. $R_{Lex} = P_{Lex}(R_{Sem}, R_{Phon})$
       ii. $R_{Phon} = P_{Phon}(R_{Lex})$

Figure 9. An interactive data-dependency theory

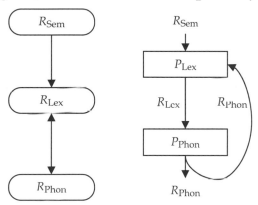

In Figures 8 and 9, each box P_X corresponds to a function. The representations on the arrows entering the box are the inputs to the function, and the representation on the arrow leaving the box is the output. The functions can be construed as stochastic functions; for example, '$R_{Phon} = P_{Phon}(R_{Lex})$' (23a.ii) can be seen as relating two random variables, so that what the function determines is a probability distribution, $p_{Phon}(\varphi | \lambda) = p(R_{Phon} = \varphi \mid R_{Lex} = \lambda)$, the probability that R_{Phon} has the value φ (e.g., /ræt/) given that the L-level representation is λ (e.g., CAT).

The functional equations for the noninteractive theory (23a) are straightforward; the output of the first function P_{Lex} is the input to the second function P_{Phon}. The overall function is just the composition of the two subfunctions, as in (24).

(24) $R_{Phon} = P_{Phon}(P_{Lex}(R_{Sem}))$

The interactive theory is more complex, however. The equations in (23b) are **recursive** in that an attempt to write the overall function as a single expression produces an equation defining R_{Phon} in terms of itself (25b); the same is true for R_{Lex} (25a). (The recursive self-reference is indicated by boldface in (25).)

(25)   Recursion in the interactive theory
   a. $\boldsymbol{R_{Lex}} = P_{Lex}(R_{Sem}, P_{Phon}(\boldsymbol{R_{Lex}}))$
   b. $\boldsymbol{R_{Phon}} = P_{Phon}(P_{Lex}(R_{Sem}, \boldsymbol{R_{Phon}}))$

As in the noninteractive theory, the functions P_{Lex} and P_{Phon} are generally stochastic, defining conditional probability distributions over the input and output representations, viewed as random variables. (Furthermore, the function P_{Lex} in the interactive theory produces outputs R_{Lex} that are vectors.)

Let us consider only one of the numerous types of empirical evidence Rapp and Goldrick (2000) deploy to adjudicate between the two theories. Consider the types of errors described in (26).

(26)   Error types and terminology
      a. $CAT \rightarrow$ /dɔg/   purely semantic
      b. $CAT \rightarrow$ /sæt/, /læt/   purely phonological
      c. $CAT \rightarrow$ /ræt/   mixed (semantic and phonological)

How do the likelihoods of these different types of error compare?

An aphasic patient CSS displays an interesting error pattern: semantic errors share 27% of their phonemes, compared with a chance value of 13%. This is taken as evidence against the noninteractive theory. What is the logic?

Intuitively, an error of type $CAT \rightarrow$ /dɔg/ seems likely to be a failure of the process P_{Lex}; this process should produce CAT but because of unreliability (noise), on this occasion it happens to produce DOG, which is then correctly pronounced by P_{Phon}. Thus, the probability of this type of error tells us the probability that P_{Lex} selects a lexical item semantically similar to, but not identical to, the correct item CAT (e.g., $CAT \rightarrow$ DOG).

Analogously, the probability of errors of type $CAT \rightarrow$ /læt/ would seem to indicate the likelihood of the failure of P_{Phon} to take a correctly selected lexical item CAT and produce the correct sequence of phonemes, erroneously producing a phoneme sequence similar, but not identical, to /kæt/.

Now according to the noninteractive theory, these types of errors should be *independent*. The theory then predicts that the probability of a mixed error (e.g., $CAT \rightarrow$ /ræt/) is the probability that either just a semantic error ($CAT \rightarrow$ RAT $\rightarrow$ /ræt/), just a phonological error ($CAT \rightarrow$ CAT $\rightarrow$ /ræt/), or both ($CAT \rightarrow$ FAT $\rightarrow$ /ræt/) will occur. Let's call this prediction the **independent model**.

But in fact, for CSS the probability of mixed errors is significantly higher than the independent model predicts. That is, the extent of shared phonemes in semantic errors ($CAT \rightarrow$ /dɔg/, /ræt/) is much greater than the value the model predicts. (The probability that the observed degree of phonological overlap results by chance according to the independent model is $p < .0002$.) Apparently, the fact that RAT is similar to CAT semantically *and* phonologically increases the chances it will be erroneously selected. Unlike the noninteractive theory, the interactive theory can in principle explain this conspiracy, because the process P_{Lex} receives both semantic and phonological input.

What assumptions are implicit in generating the independent model from the noninteractive theory? One key assumption is that for P_{Lex}, the probabilities are the

Figure 9   Box 7

same for $CAT \rightarrow$ RAT and $CAT \rightarrow$ DOG. The basis for this is that in the noninteractive theory, P_{Lex} receives R_{Sem} as input but not R_{Phon}: *semantic* relatedness between CAT and RAT can influence the probability of this error, but not *phonological* relatedness. From what principle, exactly, would this follow?

It is helpful to consider the constituent structure of the posited representations. In the theories considered by Rapp and Goldrick (2000), the representations are based on features. The semantic features for *CAT* are $\{\langle pet \rangle, \langle feline \rangle, ...\}$; these constitute $R_{Sem}(CAT)$. In the noninteractive theory, an L-level representation is atomic; for the lexical item *cat*, this is the atom $R_{Lex} =$ CAT. Associated with CAT is a set $F(CAT)$ of features; it is the collection of features of all sorts that are applicable to a lexical item. $F(CAT)$ contains all the semantic features of *CAT*, plus all the phonological features of /kæt/, plus the syntactic features of Noun, and so on. $F(CAT)$ is realized through the *processes* that operate with CAT. The *semantic* features in $F(CAT)$ are realized through P_{Lex}: whether this process will produce CAT as output depends only upon these features. More specifically, the probability that P_{Lex} will output lexical item Y when it is given the concept *CAT* as input—$p_{Lex}(Y \mid CAT)$—is determined by the similarity of the features of *CAT* (all semantic) and the corresponding (ergo *semantic*) features associated with Y. And these are just the semantic features of the concept Y that Y labels. Thus,

(27) $p_{Lex}(Y \mid X) = f(sim[X, Y])$,

where f is a monotonically increasing function: the higher the similarity of the concepts X and Y, as determined by their semantic features, the greater the probability that P_{Lex} will map $X \rightarrow$ Y. Now $sim[CAT, Y]$ is of course highest for $Y = CAT$; the assumption is that it is moderately high also for *DOG*, and—crucially—equally high for *RAT*. At least, this is assumed to be a reasonable approximation, averaged over all the concepts and words relevant to the empirical data under consideration. In any event, the *phonological* features of RAT cannot affect $p_{Lex}(RAT \mid CAT)$.

In the noninteractive theory, the data-dependency structure for P_{Phon} is the same as that for P_{Lex}. Thus, the same logic shows that the probability that P_{Phon} will map CAT $\rightarrow$ /ræt/ (i.e., $p_{Phon}(/ræt/ \mid$ CAT)) is the same as the probability that P_{Phon} will map CAT $\rightarrow$ /læt/ (i.e., $p_{Phon}(/læt/ \mid$ CAT))—at least, averaged over the relevant lexical items and phonological forms, to the degree of approximation where /kæt/ is equally phonologically similar to /ræt/ and to /læt/ (e.g., in accord with the approximation in which phonological similarity is measured via the number of shared phonemes). The *phonological* features in $F(CAT)$ are realized through P_{Phon}, and the probability that P_{Phon} will output /ræt/ given CAT as input is determined only by the similarity of the (phonological) features of /ræt/ to the *phonological* features associated with CAT.

For the moment, the crucial point is that in the noninteractive theory, the process P_{Lex} is insensitive to R_{Phon}. Also, P_{Phon} is not *directly* sensitive to R_{Sem}—formally, $p_{Phon}(R_{Phon} = \varphi \mid R_{Lex} = Y, R_{Sem} = \sigma) = p_{Phon}(\varphi \mid Y)$: the probability that P_{Phon} produces output R_{Phon} with value φ given that R_{Lex} has value Y and that R_{Sem} has value σ is the same as the probability of φ given Y, with no specified value of R_{Sem}. R_{Sem} can influence φ, but only through R_{Lex}; given that R_{Lex} = Y, the value of R_{Sem} cannot alter the behavior of P_{Phon}. This is precisely the meaning of the data-dependency description in Figure 8.[15]

Now consider the realization of this theory in a physical system $\mathcal{S}$. The representations R_{Sem}, R_{Lex}, R_{Phon} are realized as states of parts of $\mathcal{S}$; P_{Lex} and P_{Phon} are realized as physical processes relating states as above. The physical state s_{Phon} realizing the representation R_{Phon} must have no causal influence on the physical process P_{Lex} realizing P_{Lex}. This is the physical realization of the *absence* of an arrow connecting R_{Phon} to P_{Lex} in the data-dependency diagram of Figure 8. Thus, the arrows in these diagrams are realized as causal dependencies in the physical system. In this sense, *a data-dependency diagram describes the abstract causal dependency structure of $\mathcal{S}$ at the f-level.*

The conclusion is that in order to license the inferences needed to derive the independent model from the noninteractive theory, the f-level connectivity structure of the data-dependency diagram in $\mathcal{F}$ must be isomorphic to the n-level causal-dependency structure in $\mathcal{N}$.

Figure 10. Connectionist realization

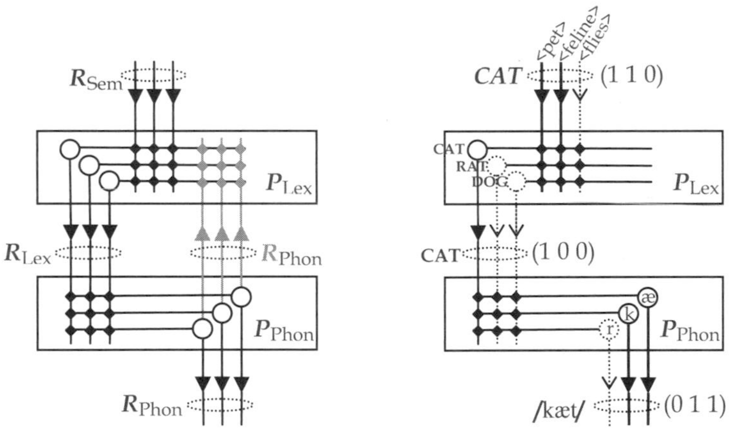

Error patterns are a type of data that can be addressed by f-level data-dependency descriptions: note that no assumptions about algorithms were needed or used — the underlying algorithm could be connectionist, symbolic, or whatever (see Section 7.2.1). However, other types of data require realizing these descriptions at the c-level. Rapp and Goldrick (2000) do this through connectionist networks (see Figure 10). For each of the three representational levels — the ovals in Figures 8 and 9 — there

---

[15] This criterion of **conditional independence** is exactly the meaning, as mathematically formalized in the notion **Markov random field**, of diagrams much like our data-dependency descriptions (Golden 1996).

Figure 10   *Box 7*

is a group of connection lines. Let's call these groups R_{Sem}, R_{Lex}, and R_{Phon}; they are the ovals in Figure 10. These connections correspond directly to the arrows in the right-hand diagrams of Figures 8 and 9. The gray connections are present in the interactive theory only. The right side of Figure 10 depicts a state of the noninteractive network in which *CAT* is correctly processed; dotted circles and lines denote inactive units and connection lines.

At the semantic and phonological levels, each feature corresponds to a single connection line. Thus, **CAT** is a pattern of activity over R_{Sem} in which lines corresponding to the features of *CAT*, and only these, are active. The similarity between $R_{Sem}(CAT)$ and $R_{Sem}(RAT)$ is the number of lines with the same activation in these two patterns, a measure of the extent to which *CAT* and *RAT* have the same semantic features.

The L-level realization is more complex. For each lexical item — say, CAT — there is a single unit in P_{Lex}: u_{CAT}. The features of CAT are encoded in this unit's *connections*. For each semantic feature of CAT — that is, for each feature of *CAT* — there is an excitatory connection to u_{CAT} on the line corresponding to that feature. The same is true for each phonological feature of CAT (i.e., feature of /kæt/). In the interactive theory, the connections between P_{Lex} and P_{Phon} are bidirectional. They convey activation from each group to the other; the gray lines are present. In the noninteractive theory, these lines are absent; connections are directed only from P_{Lex} to P_{Phon}.

The process P_{Phon} is realized in the processing within the units P_{Phon} and the connections into these units. Similarly, the process P_{Lex} is realized in the processing within the P_{Lex} units and in the connections into these units, from P_{Sem} and, in the interactive theory, from P_{Phon}. These process-realizations are indicated by rectangles in Figure 10.

Much detail, such as the equations governing the activation computation in each unit, needs to be added to the structure shown in Figure 10 to create a complete c-level description. Once these details are provided, the c-level description can be simulated on a computer and thereby more detailed predictions obtained. Quantitative values for the probability of different types of errors can be produced, providing much sharper tests for distinguishing the theories. For example, damage that induces aphasia can be modeled by mean-zero noise in different processes, leading to different types of deficits. See Rapp and Goldrick 2000 for several analyses of this type.

What is implicitly assumed by using mean-zero noise at a representational level to model the damage produced by a stroke? Isomorphism with respect to certain structure between the c- and n-level descriptions. The c-level description has a structure that distinguishes among three representational levels, Σ_c^{levels}. The n-level description must provide a decomposition of $\mathcal{N}$ into parts that are prone to damage by stroke: call this Σ_n^{stroke}. Clearly, to justify using noise at one representational level to model the effect of stroke, these structures must be assumed to be in correspondence: $\Sigma_c^{levels} \approx \Sigma_n^{stroke}$. Further, the n-level description must characterize the nature of the damage that stroke induces in the parts constituting Σ_n^{stroke}, and it must be assumed that this damage affects the reliability of neural tissue in such a way as to leave average performance unchanged, but to increase variance (see Section 2.1). Thus, an isomorphism underwriting the process-relevance of the data-dependency description here is one that aligns the c- and n-levels with respect to the resource of reliability.

4 REQUIREMENTS FOR A COGNITIVE ARCHITECTURE

In Sections 2 and 3, computational theories, including those of cognitive science, were analyzed as composed of three parts: an f-level description $\mathcal{F}$, a c-level description $\mathcal{C}$, and an n-level description $\mathcal{N}$. The crucial notion of realization mapping between levels was developed, with special attention to the strictest type of realization mapping, isomorphism. The key property of process-relevance was identified as isomorphism with the n-level description $\mathcal{N}$.

This analysis, which was introduced in Section 1 as claims (2)–(3), was preliminary to the real argument of the chapter, summarized in claims (5)–(9). In this section, I take up (5), which identifies the crucial requirements a cognitive architecture must meet. These requirements were first informally presented in (1), which is repeated here as (28).

(28)   Architectural requirements (initial formulation)

A complete cognitive architecture must provide a formal foundation for developing, within a single unified framework, theories that promise to

a.   formally explain central aspects of higher cognition, such as grammatical universals and the productivity of cognition;

b.   provide a formal framework for theories of cognitive processes that

   i.   explains actual human behavior and

  ii.   shows explicitly how cognition can be reduced to basic computational operations;

c.   reduce mental computation to neural computation, showing how the basic computational operations can be, and are, physically realized in the brain.

In this section, I will articulate these requirements somewhat more formally, exploiting the analysis of computational levels developed in the preceding two sections.

To address the problem of cognitive productivity (28a), ICS adopts the combinatorial strategy, as explained at some length in Chapter 1. Elements of a cognitive domain—for example, scenes or sentences—are mentally represented using complex symbol structures. New inputs are represented as novel combinations of familiar input constituents; their outputs are generated by creating a corresponding novel combination of familiar output constituents. The authors of this book have adopted this solution because we believe it has led to tremendous progress, and that no other comparably promising alternative currently exists.

Given the choice of the combinatorial strategy for explaining cognitive productivity, the requirements of a cognitive architecture (28) can be articulated as in (29).

Figure 10   *Box 7*

(29)   **Architectural requirements** (final formulation)

A complete cognitive theory employing the combinatorial strategy must simultaneously satisfy the following three constraints:

a.   Isomorphic realization of a symbolic $\mathscr{F}$ in $\mathscr{C}$

$\Sigma_f \approx \Sigma_{cf}$ is symbolic-combinatorial.

   i.   The f-level description $\mathscr{F}$ provides a decomposition Σ_f of cognitive representations into combinatorial structures built of symbols.

   ii. $\mathscr{F}$ provides precise specifications of cognitive functions in terms of Σ_f.

   iii.   The decomposition Σ_f is not merely useful for characterizing cognitive functions. It is also computationally relevant: it is isomorphic to a decompositional structure Σ_{cf} of the c-level description $\mathscr{C}$.

b.   Formal realization within $\mathscr{C}$

$\Sigma_{cf} \rightsquigarrow \Sigma_{cn}$ is a formal realization mapping.

   i.   The c-level structure Σ_{cf} is functionally relevant in virtue of its isomorphism with the f-level structure Σ_f. This structure resides at a high sublevel within $\mathscr{C}$.

   ii.   This high level structure is realized in successively lower sublevels of $\mathscr{C}$, via complete, formal, and explicit realization mappings.

   iii.   This formal scaffolding of sublevels extends down to a low sublevel of $\mathscr{C}$ with a decompositional structure Σ_{cn}.

c.   Isomorphic realization of $\mathscr{C}$ in $\mathscr{N}$

$\Sigma_{cn} \approx \Sigma_n$ is neurally accurate (or, provisionally, neurally plausible).

   i. Σ_{cn} is neurally relevant: it is isomorphic to some structure Σ_n within the physical-level description $\mathscr{N}$ of the brain.

   ii. Σ_n is empirically valid; or, provisionally, it is at least neurally plausible.

I will take up each of these three constraints in turn. (See Figure 11.)

The first constraint (29a) comes from the choice of representationalism and the combinatorial strategy to address the problem of productivity. The f-level combinatorial structure Σ_f (29a.i) enables description of cognitive functions in symbolic terms (29a.ii). Furthermore, however, the combinatorial strategy must explain not just *what* the mind achieves, but, to some extent, *how* the mind achieves it. Cognition is productive *because* at some level the mechanisms that actually generate it have parts that recombine in accord with the combinatorial description Σ_f. That is, at some sublevel of $\mathscr{C}$ there must be computational structure — call it 'Σ_{cf}' — that is isomorphic to Σ_f (29a.iii).

The second constraint (29b) is imposed by the fundamental principle of cognitive science, that cognition is computation. Cognitive processes are computational processes; description $\mathscr{C}$ has the properties of a computational level, including precise, formal realization of more abstract, higher sublevels in lower sublevels, ultimately in a low level that can be directly physically realized (Section 2.2.2).

Figure 11. Origin of constraints on ICS

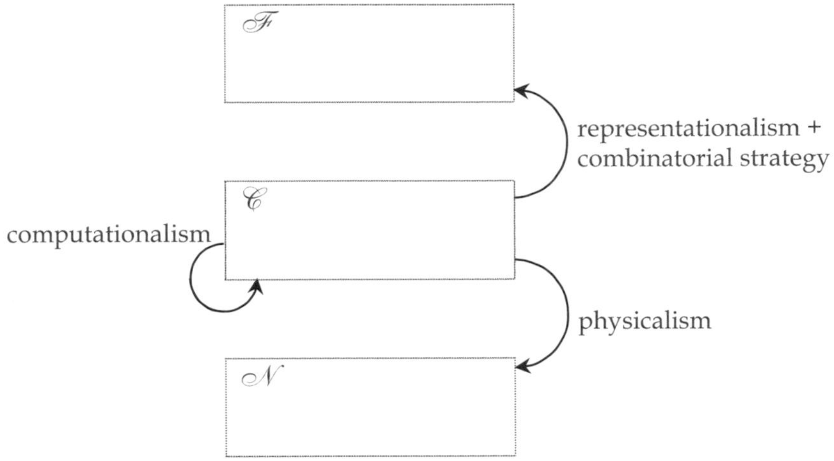

The third constraint (29c) arises from the choice of a physicalist theory in which the mind is physically realized in the brain. The lowest c-level description must be realized in a physical description of the nervous system. Following (12) and (22), the requirement that this realization be an isomorphism is needed in order that $\mathscr{C}$ deliver a process-relevant description, one capable of predicting response times and other behavioral measures of the resource requirements of cognitive processes.

5 PUTATIVE INCOMPATIBILITY OF THE ARCHITECTURAL REQUIREMENTS

The three constraints in (29) push cognitive theory in conflicting directions. It is now possible to more precisely characterize these conflicts, introduced first in (6). The conflicts are revealed by the observation that cognitive theories that have developed in order to meet two of the three constraints end up violating the third. As (30) spells out, any two of the three constraints in (29) can be satisfied by an existing strategy for developing a cognitive theory — but that strategy does not permit satisfaction of the third.

(30) Satisfiability of the constraints in (29) two but not three at a time

   a. $\Sigma_f \approx \Sigma_{cf}$ is symbolic-combinatorial.

      If this constraint is put aside, the other two can be satisfied (in principle at least) by the Eliminativist Connectionist Architecture (see Box 1:6), which provides a formal computational description that is at least plausibly isomorphic to neural structure. But then explaining the productivity of cognition is highly problematic.

   b. $\Sigma_{cf} \rightsquigarrow \Sigma_{cn}$ is a formal realization mapping.

      If this constraint is put aside, the other two can be met by proposing that

Figure 11   *Box 7*

the mind/brain is a symbolic combinatorial system at a functional level and a neural system at a physical level, and that by some unspecified, entirely mysterious means, the latter realizes the former. But in such a vague "theory," precise accounts of cognitive processes are impossible.

c. $\Sigma_{cn} \approx \Sigma_n$ is neurally accurate (or, provisionally, neurally plausible).

If this constraint is put aside, PSA satisfies the other two constraints by providing a precise computational theory of a combinatorial, symbolic functional level realized in a scaffolding of sublevels that extends down to simple operations that are physically realizable. But realizing these operations in the *brain* is highly problematic, as discussed at the end of this section (see also Box 1).

It must be noted that at least some of the proponents of what are characterized in (30) as partial solutions do not regard their theories as deficient because they actively deny the validity of the constraint their theory fails to meet.

ICS is founded on rejecting this strategy of denial; instead, there is a commitment to accept the importance of simultaneously satisfying all three constraints in (29). In the next section, I will argue that ICS holds the promise, ultimately, of a full solution — and in its current state offers significant progress in that direction.

In the remainder of this section, I will attempt to elaborate the respects in which PSA does and does not meet the three requirements laid down in (29). The PSA strategy for addressing these requirements is compactly stated in (31). (See also Box 1 and Figure 12.)

(31)   The Purely Symbolic Architecture (PSA)

Symbolic combinatorial structure all the way down.

a. $\Sigma_f \approx \Sigma_{cf}$ is symbolic-combinatorial.

b. $\Sigma_{cf} \approx \Sigma_{cn}$ is symbolic-combinatorial.

c.   ($\Sigma_{cn} \approx \Sigma_n$ is symbolic-combinatorial.)

Σ_{cf} provides an account of cognition as computation over abstract symbols that are functionally relevant: they are semantically interpretable. PSA offers high-level descriptions — for example, data-dependency descriptions, sentence-parsing algorithms, problem-solving algorithms. And, as required of a computational theory, PSA shows how to reduce these high-level descriptions to successively simpler symbol-manipulation operations;[16] the structure of the architecture employing the most primitive operations is Σ_{cn}.

I take it as an essential aspect of PSA that it offers symbolic algorithms that are process-relevant. They describe not only *what* is computed — the functions — but also exactly *how*; they predict observables such as reaction times.

As argued in Section 2.3.2, to be process-relevant an algorithm must be isomor-

---

[16] Within PSA, incompletely specified data-dependency descriptions presume such a symbolic computational reduction, albeit an unspecified one (Sections 2.2.3, 3.4).

phic to the n-level. This is not typically an explicitly stated assumption of a purely symbolic theory (hence the parentheses in (31c)), but such an assumption is implied by the reasoning connecting properties of a symbolic algorithm to the predictions that allegedly follow concerning human behavior. (32) gives several examples of the process-relevance of symbolic descriptions and how this process-relevance depends implicitly on an isomorphism between the symbolic and the physical/neural descriptions. The examples are identified by the computational resource they critically depend upon.

(32)   Process-relevance and f/c-n-level isomorphism in PSA

   a.   Causation: Development of primitive symbolic operations
        Frank (1998) accounts for children's difficulty with certain syntactic constructions by hypothesizing that they do not yet have at their disposal a particularly powerful primitive operation, the adjoining operation of Tree-Adjoining Grammar. The logic is that the problematic constructions require adjoining—an f-level assertion—and children's immature language-processing system lacks some corresponding causal process—an n-level assertion. That is, the n-level biophysical structure of the language faculty that distinguishes early- and late-developing processes is isomorphic to the f-level structure that distinguishes syntactic constructions requiring the adjoining operation from other constructions.

   b.   Reliability: Neurological damage of subprocesses
        As discussed in Section 3.4, Rapp and Goldrick (2000) explain certain error patterns in aphasia as the result of decreased reliability of certain processes within a data-dependency description, modeled as significant noise in a layer of a connectionist network. The n-level structure that distinguishes damaged from undamaged parts of a post-stroke brain is assumed to be isomorphic to the f-level structure that distinguishes among different subfunctions.[17]

   c.   Space: Memory overflow during sentence processing
        Reduced to its bare-bones formulation, a classic symbolic style of explanation reasons that the sentence *the student the professor the dean hates flunked quit* is hard to process because it requires a stack depth of three, and the human sentence processor has a capacity limit of two. The stack is part of the high-level symbolic algorithm—abstract space—corresponding to part of the memory of the machine. Why should three be more difficult than two? It must be assumed that the c-level structure distinguishing states with stack depth two from those with stack depth three is isomorphic to an n-

---

[17] The f-level description of Rapp and Goldrick's (2000) noninteractive theory could be instantiated in either PSA or ICS; the numerical representations of the interactive theory are not possible within PSA. But the point here applies to either architecture: the interpretation of the data-dependency description presumes an appropriate f-/n-level isomorphism.

Figure 11   *Box 7*

level structure within the brain distinguishing levels of utilization of some physically limited resource.

d. Time

   i. Derivational Theory of Complexity

   Simplified to its minimal form, another classic type of symbolic reasoning predicts that a passive sentence will take longer to process than its active counterpart because the passive requires applying both phrase structure rules and the Passive transformation, while the active requires only the phrase structure rules. This reasoning clearly requires that more abstract time spent with rules in $\mathscr{C}$ corresponds to more real time in $\mathscr{N}$, an isomorphism of temporal structure at the c- and n-levels. (Hence, predicting *lack* of such a processing time difference requires assuming that such an isomorphism does *not* exist—denying at least one key aspect of the "psychological reality" of grammatical derivation.)

   ii. Human sentence parsing

   What makes certain sentences harder to process than others? A standard approach seeks symbolic parsing algorithms that predict difficulty. For example, a partially specified algorithm may be hypothesized to first attach each new word to the parse tree so as to minimally create new tree structure—the **minimal attachment** heuristic—and then reattach words later if new words require this for a grammatical parse. The additional step of reanalysis predicts greater human processing time. Again, this follows only if abstract $\mathscr{C}$-time corresponds to real $\mathscr{N}$-time.

   iii. Problem-solving production systems

   C-level algorithms that sequentially apply symbolic rules (productions) to solve problems are used to explain 'think-aloud' protocols, transcripts of real-time introspective commentary by subjects during problem solving. The sequence of applications of production rules predicts the sequence of problem-solving steps reported in the protocol. These explanations clearly assume an isomorphism, with respect to sequential temporal structure (Box 5), between the c-level production system and the n-level minute-by-minute real-time transitions between brain states.

   These algorithms are also used to explain the acquisition of skill through practice. A compilation process combines productions with use, so that the expert needs to fire fewer production rules than the novice, hence performs faster. Here a c-/n-level isomorphism must be assumed with respect to temporal durational structure.

The examples of (32) illustrate the claim that the process-relevance of PSA — its ability to predict relative reaction times, for instance — crucially depends on the assumption that the abstract space, time, reliability, and causation of the symbolic algorithm of $\mathscr{C}$ are isomorphic to the corresponding physical structures of $\mathscr{N}$. And in the human case, $\mathscr{N}$ is the structure of the brain. This is encapsulated in requirement (29c), the third of the constraints on a theory of cognitive architecture.

PSA offers high-level descriptions and shows how to reduce them to successively simpler symbol-manipulation operations; but in actual proposals for how this can be done, these lower levels retain the character of a symbolic combinatorial system all the way down. The lowest-level operations — say, for concreteness, the bit string manipulations of the register machine in which a Lisp program is implemented (Box 1) — are entirely mechanical and can be physically realized. The isomorphism between the bit string manipulations and the physical components of the machine means that the computationally relevant aspects of the machine have this same structure: symbolic combinatorial structure.

For PSA's proposal (31) to qualify as satisfying the three constraints in (29), it would have to be that this physical structure is neurally accurate, or at least neurally plausible. This is a claim that few contemporary symbolic theorists would defend.[18]

It may be that, in principle, PSA could be realized at a low computational level in a *parallel* symbol-processing architecture. But it is entirely unclear how this is to actually be done, especially in the cases of productivity-explaining combinatorial structure. And many of symbolic cognitive theories' actual predictions concerning response times disappear if sequential structure is abandoned; it is very unclear what can replace it to provide symbolic algorithms that are process-relevant.

This leaves advocates of PSA with several options. They can count on future research to show that, despite all appearances, the brain *is* actually structured like a Lisp machine. To my knowledge, this is not a position anyone has advocated.

Alternatively, PSA proponents can deny that contact with neuroscience is important, arguing that the current state of our knowledge about the brain's function is so minimal that it can provide no meaningful constraint, or that a high-level computational description, like the sought-after theory of mind, is never meaningfully constrained by the lower-level structure of the machine in which it is implemented.

Neither of these previously rather popular "neuro-denial" moves appears tenable anymore. Steadfastly ignoring what we *do* know about the brain is clearly a self-serving "head-in-the-sand" strategy. In fact, given the swelling torrent of neuroscience research headed toward cognitive science, a more apt metaphor might be '"head-in-the-dike" strategy'. And to assert that the physical structure of machines is not relevant to the high-level programs they implement is simply question-begging. Connectionists have a legitimate question here: how are you going to implement your symbolic parsing algorithm in a neural network? It is no response to say that Lisp can run equally well on a PC or a Mac — that is true, but it provides absolutely

---

[18] Historical defenders might be McCulloch and Pitts (1943).

Figure 11   *Box 7*

no evidence that Lisp can run on a brain. A main point of the preceding sections is that algorithms can only meet the demands of models of mental processes if they are coupled with hypotheses about how the structure internal to the algorithm maps onto the physical device implementing the algorithm. It is simply not an option to deny the relevance of the physical machine to a computational theory of cognition.

Finally, symbolic theorists might hope that some future breakthrough will provide a fundamentally new type of computational realization of the high-level symbolic combinatorial structure Σ_{cf}, a realization in which, unlike a Lisp machine, the low-level computational description that is isomorphic to $\mathcal{N}$ does not have symbolic combinatorial structure. But this scenario would mean that the high-level symbolic algorithms of $\mathcal{C}$ (Σ_{cf}) would not be process-relevant—only the mysteriously different lower-level algorithms of $\mathcal{C}$ (Σ_{cn}) would be. Thus, the process-relevant descriptions delivered by this theory would *not* be symbolic; this, then, would not be symbolic cognitive theory. It would be something quite different—something much like ICS.

6 RECONCILING THE ARCHITECTURAL REQUIREMENTS VIA ICS

Given the conflicts among the three constraints in (29) on a cognitive architecture discussed in the previous section, how can the ICS architecture manage to simultaneously satisfy them? The answer, which was introduced in (7), is summarized in (33), which reiterates the three requirements.

(33)   ICS strategy for meeting the three requirements in (29)

    a.   Isomorphic realization of a symbolic $\mathcal{F}$ in $\mathcal{C}$

        $\Sigma_f \approx \Sigma_{cf}$ is symbolic-combinatorial.

        ICS: The isomorphism ι_{cf} is combinatorial symbolic-to-tensorial realization.

    b.   Formal realization within $\mathcal{C}$

        $\Sigma_{cf} \rightsquigarrow \Sigma_{cn}$ is a formal realization mapping.

        ICS: The mapping is tensorial-to-unit realization—a *non*isomorphism ρ_c, given distributed representations.

    c.   Isomorphic realization of $\mathcal{C}$ in $\mathcal{N}$

        $\Sigma_{cn} \approx \Sigma_n$ is neurally accurate (or, provisionally, neurally plausible).

        ICS: The isomorphism ι_{nc} is a connectionist-to-neural correspondence.

The realization mappings of ICS (33), and their contrasting counterparts in PSA, are schematized in Figure 12. (Compare Section 5:3.) Explication of this figure will run through the remainder of this section. The next three subsections, 6.1–6.3, take up in turn the three realization mappings in (33a–c).

Figure 12. Realization in ICS and PSA

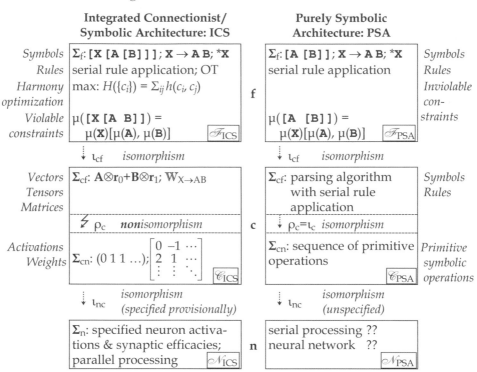

6.1 ICS's realization of $\mathscr{F}$ in $\mathscr{C}$: From symbols and constraints to vectors and matrices

At the f-level, ICS addresses cognitive problems via the same general strategy as PSA: symbolic combinatorial structure Σ_f. The inputs and outputs of cognitive functions are decomposed at the f-level into symbol structures, their semantic interpretation deriving combinatorially from this decomposition. Some of these functions are specified at the f-level by optimization, unlike their PSA counterparts; this is true in particular of OT grammars. But while novel in many important respects, the constraints defining optimality can be stated using symbolic devices, as can their mode of interaction.

Under the ICS realization mapping ι_{cf}, the symbol structures of the f-level are realized as tensor product representations, and the symbolic operators, rules, or constraints as weight matrices with tensorial structure. The technical advance that makes all of ICS possible is the discovery that this mapping is in fact an isomorphism. Under the assumptions defining tensor product realization (e.g., the independence of

Figure 12 Box 7

the role vectors), the mapping ι_{cf} realizing symbol structures as vectors is a one-to-one function: each symbol structure maps to one and only one vector, and different symbol structures map to different vectors. Furthermore, the mapping ι_{cf} maps each primitive symbolic operation—such as **ex$_0$**, which extracts the left branch of a binary tree—into the operation of multiplying by a weight matrix—W_{ex0}. This is an isomorphism because two symbol structures **p** and **s** are related by **ex$_0$** (i.e., **p** = **ex$_0$**(**s**)) if and only if the corresponding two vectors **p** and **s** are related by W_{ex0} (i.e., **p** = W_{ex0} **s**). These properties, and several others that identify ι_{cf} as an isomorphism, were developed informally in Chapter 5 and formally in Chapter 8. The isomorphism relation is depicted in (34) in the format of the general case, (14); it is expressed algebraically in (35).

(34)   Isomorphism between $\mathscr{F}$ and $\mathscr{C}$ in ICS

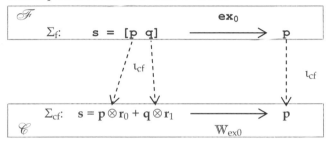

(35)   The f-to-c isomorphism ι_{cf} of ICS: Symbolic-to-tensorial realization
   a.   Representations: Symbol structures are realized as tensor product vectors.
       $\iota_{cf}: \{\mathbf{f}_i / r_i\} \mapsto \Sigma_i \mathbf{f}_i \otimes \mathbf{r}_i$
   b.   Function specification. For example:
       i.   Primitive operations (Section 8:4.1.1)
           ✦   Operators are realized as weight matrices.
               $\iota_{cf}: \{\mathbf{ex_0}, \mathbf{ex_1}, \mathbf{cons}\} \mapsto \{W_{ex0}, W_{ex1}, W_{cons0}, W_{cons1}\}$
       ii. Grammars (Section 8:4.2)
           ✦   Rewrite rules are realized as weight matrices.
               $\iota_{cf}: [\mathbf{X} \to \mathbf{A}\,\mathbf{B}] \mapsto \frac{1}{2}(\mathbf{X}^+ \mathbf{A}^{+T} \otimes \mathbf{u}_0{}^T + \mathbf{A}^+ \mathbf{X}^{+T} \otimes \mathbf{u}_0 +$
               $\mathbf{X}^+ \mathbf{B}^{+T} \otimes \mathbf{u}_1{}^T + \mathbf{B}^+ \mathbf{X}^{+T} \otimes \mathbf{u}_1) \otimes \mathbf{R}$
           ✦   Constraints are realized as weight matrices.
               $\iota_{cf}: {}^*[\mathbf{X}/r_y \,\&\, \mathbf{C}/r_{xy}] \mapsto -\frac{1}{2}[\mathbf{X}^+ \mathbf{C}^{+T} \otimes \mathbf{u}_x{}^T + \mathbf{C}^+ \mathbf{X}^{+T} \otimes \mathbf{u}_x] \otimes \mathbf{R}$

The mapping ι_{cf} is informally defined in (35). That this mapping is an isomorphism means that it puts into correspondence structure within $\mathscr{F}$ (Σ_f) and structure within $\mathscr{C}$ (Σ_{cf}). The structures in question are implicit in (35); they are spelled out more explicitly in (36).

(36)   Functionally relevant decompositional structures in ICS

Under the mapping ι_{cf}: $\Sigma_f \to \Sigma_{cf}$ defined in (35), the following f-level symbolic structures and c-level tensorial structures are isomorphic (Chapters 8 and 10):

f-level: Σ_f = symbolic structure

a.   Representations

✦   Decomposition of general symbol structures using fillers, roles, their binding into constituents, and their conjunction (Section 8:2.2.1)

b.   Function specification. For example:

i.   Primitive operations (Section 8:4.1.1)

✦   Decomposition and composition of binary trees using the primitive symbolic functions $\mathbf{ex_0}$, $\mathbf{ex_1}$, $\mathbf{cons}$

ii.   Grammars (Section 10:1)

✦   Decomposition of a grammar as a set of individual rewrite rules

✦   Decomposition of a grammar as a set of individual constraints

c.   Semantic interpretation function μ: compositional with respect to constituency (17)

✦ μ: $\mathbf{[f\ [p\ q]]} \mapsto F(P, Q) \equiv \mu[\mathbf{f}]\big(\mu[\mathbf{p}], \mu[\mathbf{q}]\big)$ that is,

✦ μ: $\mathbf{s} \mapsto \mu[\mathbf{ex_0(s)}]\big(\mu[\mathbf{ex_{01}(s)}], \mu[\mathbf{ex_{11}(s)}]\big)$

c-level (higher sublevel): Σ_{cf} = tensorial structure

a′.   Inputs/outputs, representations

✦   Decomposition of vectors using filler vectors and role vectors, their binding into constituents via the tensor product, and their combination via superposition (summation) (Section 8:2.2)

b′.   Function specification—for example, grammars

i.   Primitive operations (Section 8:4.1.1)

✦   Decomposition and composition of binary trees using the elementary weight matrices $\mathbf{W}_{ex0}$, $\mathbf{W}_{ex1}$, $\mathbf{W}_{cons0}$, $\mathbf{W}_{cons1}$

ii.   Grammars (Section 8:4.2)

✦   Decomposition of a 'grammar' weight matrix as a sum of individual 'rewrite-rule' matrices

✦   Decomposition of a 'grammar' weight matrix as a sum of individual 'constraint' matrices

c′.   Semantic interpretation function μ: compositional with respect to constituency

✦   For example, μ: $\mathbf{s} \mapsto \mu[\mathbf{W}_{ex0}\mathbf{s}]\big(\mu[\mathbf{W}_{ex0}\mathbf{W}_{ex1}\mathbf{s}], \mu[\mathbf{W}_{ex1}\mathbf{W}_{ex1}\mathbf{s}]\big)$

Note that (36c) and (36c′) assert that semantic interpretation is compositional (17).

Figure 12   Box 7

6.2 ICS's $\mathscr{C}$-internal realization: From vectors and matrices to units and connections

The realization mapping ρ_c relating the higher and lower sublevels of the ICS c-level description $\mathscr{C}$ maps a representational vector **a** to the list of activation values of the activity pattern that realizes it.

(37) $\rho_c(\mathbf{a}) = (a_1, a_2, \ldots)$

ρ_c also maps a weight matrix $\mathbf{W}$ into the array of individual numerical weights that realizes it.

The realization mapping ρ_c is nearly invisible, for we typically write (37) simply as "$\mathbf{a} = (a_1, a_2, \ldots)$." This can create considerable confusion.[19] For our purposes, however, it is essential to distinguish two types of decompositional structure in the c-level of ICS, as the following example illustrates.

For concreteness, let us return to the running example used in Section 5:1.3 and consider the representation **s** that is a tensor product realization of a symbol structure **s** = **[A [B C]]**. The two different decompositions of **s** are given in (38).

(38)   Two types of decompositional structure in the c-level of ICS, $\mathscr{C}_{ICS}$

      a.   Higher-level, functionally relevant decomposition: Σ_{cf}

           $\Sigma_{cf}(\mathbf{s}) = \mathbf{B} \otimes \mathbf{r}_0 \otimes \mathbf{r}_0 + \mathbf{A} \otimes \mathbf{r}_0 + \mathbf{C} \otimes \mathbf{r}_0 \otimes \mathbf{r}_1$

      b.   Lower-level, neurally relevant decomposition: Σ_{cn}

           $\Sigma_{cn}(\mathbf{s}) = (s_1, s_2, \ldots)$

      (s_β is the activation value of unit β in the activity pattern **s**)

Crucially, only one of these decompositional structures, Σ_{cf}, is isomorphic to the f-level description of **s**, **[A [B C]]**: this is the *functionally* relevant description at the c-level. The other decompositional structure, Σ_{cn}, is not functionally relevant; however, it is important because, as we will see shortly, it is *process*-relevant, unlike Σ_{cf}.

The realization mapping ρ_c maps the description at the higher sublevel of $\mathscr{C}_{ICS}$ to the description at the lower sublevel. This mapping is complete and formally explicit; it replaces **A**, **B**, ..., with specific lists of activation values, replaces the $\otimes$ operator with the operation of multiplying individual numerical activation values, and so forth. So ρ_c is perfectly legitimate as a realization mapping between the sublevels of a computational system.

The crucial point, however, is that ρ_c is *not* an isomorphism, in the case of interest for ICS: distributed representation. By definition, in a distributed representation, a single unit β will participate in the realization of multiple symbols—say, **B** and **C**. Then the mapping ρ_c will not respect the decomposition Σ_{cf}, as an isomorphism must. At the higher sublevel, **B** and **C** are separate constituents, but at the lower sublevel, the decomposition into individual unit activations mixes **B** and **C** together: for example, the activation of unit β, s_β (38b), is a single number combining contributions from both **B** and **C**.

[19] Indeed, my previous descriptions of ICS have suffered from failure to make ρ_c explicit.

Because ρ_c is not an isomorphism, the lower-sublevel decomposition into individual activation values is not functionally relevant: the parts in this decomposition do not correspond to the parts in terms of which the f-level specifies the function computed and the semantic interpretation of representations. The functionally relevant decomposition is into constituent vectors and matrices: Σ_{cf} (38a). It is the lower-level decomposition into individual activation values and weights, Σ_{cn} (38b), that is physically relevant.

6.3 ICS's realization of $\mathscr{C}$ in $\mathscr{N}$: From units and connections to neurons and synapses

One computational-to-neural-level isomorphism, ι_{nc}, is the obvious one under which the activation value of a unit in a connectionist network is mapped to the activation level of a neuron (as manifest, say, in its firing rate), and the weight of a connection between two units is mapped to the efficacy (under some physical measure) of the synapses between the two neurons corresponding to those units. Because of this isomorphism, the lower-sublevel decomposition is process-relevant: more 'parts' (units and connections) means more physical machinery required; more abstract time for output units to achieve their final values means more real time required. The same is not true of the decomposition at the higher sublevel: more 'parts' (vectors corresponding to symbols and matrices corresponding to rules) does not entail more machinery, and the amount of real time required cannot (in general) be predicted from the number of rule applications involved.

So unlike the lower sublevel of $\mathscr{C}$, the higher sublevel of $\mathscr{C}$ is not process-relevant. This is possible because the realization mapping ρ_c from the higher to the lower sublevel is not an isomorphism. If it were an isomorphism, then the decomposition at the higher sublevel would necessarily be process-relevant, because it would correspond part by part to the decomposition at the lower sublevel, which is process-relevant in virtue of its isomorphism with the neural level under ι_{nc}. This would indeed be the case with *local* representations. But the distributed character of ICS representations entails that a single lower-level part—an individual unit's activation—corresponds to multiple higher-level parts—the activation vectors realizing each of many symbols. And a single higher-level part—a distributed activation vector realizing a symbol—corresponds to multiple lower-level parts—unit activations.

This reiterates the point made in Section 2.3.4 concerning the transitivity of isomorphism. In both PSA and ICS, symbolic explanation at the functional level is possible because the symbolic f-level description $\mathscr{F}$ is isomorphic to the c-level description $\mathscr{C}$ (under ι_{cf}): the functionally relevant aspects of the computation have symbolic structure. Also, $\mathscr{C}$ is isomorphic to the n-level $\mathscr{N}$ (under ι_{nc}); computation has physically relevant aspects, so the computational level fulfills its obligation to provide process-relevant algorithms that serve as models of cognitive processes. It does not necessarily follow, however, that the symbolic f-level description is isomorphic to the physical-level description (under the composition of ι_{nc} and ι_{cf}) and hence process-

Figure 12   Box 7

relevant. This is because the decomposition at the c-level that is functionally relevant (the structure involved in ι_{cf}, Σ_{cf}) differs from the decomposition at the c-level that is physically relevant and hence process-relevant (the structure involved in ι_{nc}, Σ_{cn}). This difference arises in ICS because the functionally relevant c-level decomposition Σ_{cf} occupies a higher sublevel than does the physically relevant c-level decomposition Σ_{nc}: the former involves "symbol-sized parts," and the latter, "neuron-sized parts." These two sublevels are related, as a computational description requires, by a fully formal realization mapping ρ_c, but this is not an isomorphism because its distributed representations do not respect the symbolic decomposition. Because ρ_c is not an isomorphism, the full realization chain from the f- to the n-level — ι_{cf} to ρ_c to ι_{nc} — is not an isomorphism. In ICS, symbols are not process-relevant.

7 COGNITIVE EXPLANATION IN ICS

In the previous section, I characterized the overall strategy for cognitive explanation adopted by ICS.[20] In this section, I will discuss several highly general, but fundamental, conceptual, and empirical problems that a complete cognitive theory must address. The types of explanations developed within ICS to address these problems are considered, and compared with those developed within PSA; this will flesh out the basic characterization of ICS explanation introduced in (8). In many cases, research presented elsewhere in the book illustrates ICS contributions toward solving these fundamental problems.

7.1 Core explanatory problems of cognitive science

The basic research problems of cognitive science lie at different computational levels and are the focus of different subdisciplines of cognitive science. To address the problems at a given level, a cognitive theory must provide a formal account at that level — an account that is part of a coherent three-level total description of the mind/brain as a computational system. The three-way distinction between the f-, c-, and n-levels of a computational description is important for distinguishing among different types of cognitive problems, and that distinction in turn is important for understanding the explanations of ICS. This is because ICS offers symbolic explanations for f-level problems, but connectionist explanations for c-level problems. Thus, delimiting the role of symbols in ICS explanations requires distinguishing f- and c-level problems, which is not as straightforward as it might seem.

At first glance, it might seem that f-level problems are those addressed by "competence theories" like generative grammar, while c-level problems are the purview of "performance theories" describing cognitive processing. (Concerning the compe-

---

[20] That abstract, higher-level theoretical constructs can support legitimate scientific explanations has been argued by many philosophers of science, ranging from Hempel and Oppenheim (1948, Sec. 5) to Kitcher (1989, Sec. 5.2); concerning the particular case of mental entities, see, for example, Yablo 1992, Penczek 1997, and Penczek and Smolensky 2001 (an OT analysis). For a range of perspectives on the problem of explanations based on complex systems, see Symons 2001.

tence/performance distinction, see Box 9 below.) While this view has some validity, it ultimately proves a poor approximation to the truth. In Part III of this book, for example, symbolic explanations within ICS (specifically, within OT) were offered for types of problems typically addressed by "performance theories" — for example, phonological production (Chapter 17) and syntactic comprehension (Chapter 18).

7.1.1 Explanation at the f-level: Knowledge

At the f-level, both ICS and PSA employ symbolic combinatorial structure for their explanations. In this respect, the solutions they provide to f-level problems are of the same type. In this subsection, I will argue that an f-level description $\mathscr{F}$ is, in principle, capable of addressing a surprisingly broad range of the major problems of cognitive science. Thus, the scope of symbolic explanation within ICS is greater than it may at first appear to be.

7.1.1.1 The semantic problem

The first problem I'd like to consider is central to the philosophy of mind.

(39)   The semantic problem
        a.   *General.* How is it that mental representations have content?
        b.   *Specific.* How does the (combinatorial) structure of mental content arise?

As discussed in Section 3.1, a crucial property of the f-level entities in cognitive science is that they include mental representations, with content to which they refer. But just what does it mean for a mental element to *refer*? What makes this possible?

A somewhat more specific problem is to explain how it is that mental contents have the particular substantive properties that they do. Fodor and Pylyshyn (1988) emphasize a collection of such properties related to the combinatorial structure of mental contents (see Box 2). On this view, the space of possible percepts is filled with structured combinations of constituents: simpler percepts. The contents of beliefs are propositions, with constituents like subjects and predicates. The question then is, how can this combinatorial structure be explained?

Concerning the semantic problem, ICS, at least for the present, must offer the same solution as PSA. It is to be hoped that new semantic insights will emerge from the lower-level structure of ICS, but this has not yet been seriously explored.

With respect to the general problem (39a), there are many theories in the philosophy of mind concerning how symbols get their meaning. These theories, as far as I know, work just as well (or poorly) within ICS as within PSA. At this point, I don't claim ICS contributes anything new to this problem — but as far as I can see, ICS is no worse off than PSA.

With respect to the specific semantic problem (39b), ICS must also avail itself of the PSA solution. This I take to be that (i) mental representations have combinatorial syntactic structure; (ii) by the principle of compositionality, the semantic structure of

Figure 12   *Box 7*

the content of a representation mirrors the symbolic structure of that representation; therefore, (iii) mental contents are combinatorially structured.

Now there are some symbolic theorists who seem to get very excited about this explanation. I don't at this point have anything better to offer, so I'll take it too, but frankly I'm not going to advertise this as a selling point of ICS. After all, the original problem is to explain why contents C have structure X. The solution on offer is, because I stipulate that there exist these hypothetical things $\mathcal{R}$ that have structure X, and I stipulate a principle requiring the structure of C to mirror the structure of $\mathcal{R}$. Not, I fear, the stuff of which Nobel prizes are born.

7.1.1.2 The representational problem

Particular instances of the next general problem are central to cognitive psychology and to theoretical linguistics.

(40)　The representational problem

　　a.　*Formal.* What is the general structure of mental representations in different types of cognitive domains?

　　b.　*Substantive.* What are the actual contents of mental representations in particular cognitive domains? (For example, visual perception, spatial cognition, numerical cognition, conceptual structure, …, and language.)

Is the meaning of a concept structured like a definition in formal logic, or like a prototype, or like a set of exemplars (40a)? Does the mental representation of a word contain parts that are to be interpreted as syllables (40b)?

Here too ICS takes the same position as PSA. Indeed, a major motivation for integrating symbolic computation into a connectionist architecture was precisely to make available the computational power of symbolically structured mental representations. As one example of how ICS research employs symbolic methods to shed new light on the specific problem (40b), Section 14:1 uses symbolic principles of OT to argue that phonological representations are not underspecified. (An influential phonological theory posits that default or *unmarked* values of features are literally absent in the underlying forms stored in the mental lexicon; these forms are thus 'underspecified'.) The analysis of Chapter 14 shows how the desired phonological 'inertness' of default feature values follows inevitably from the basic principles of OT, with no need to stipulate underspecification as well.

7.1.1.3 The knowledge representation problem

The next problem is closely related to the previous one, and also central to cognitive psychology and theoretical linguistics.

(41)　The knowledge representation problem

　　a.　*Formal.* What is the form of mental knowledge in particular cognitive domains?

b.   *Substantive.* What are the actual contents of mental knowledge in particular cognitive domains?

Is mental factual knowledge structured like propositions in logic (41a)? Does phonological knowledge include violable constraints concerning the structure of syllables (41b)?

OT is the principal theory of knowledge representation currently developed within ICS. Consider (41a) with respect to grammatical knowledge. The general forms of this knowledge under PSA are predominantly the symbolic rule and the symbolic inviolable constraint. The form of grammatical knowledge in OT is the symbolic violable constraint, where violability is managed by optimization over constraint hierarchies. Though still symbolic, the violable constraints of OT constitute a major innovation with widespread impact on grammatical theory (Chapters 12–16 provide several examples). And this innovation has as one of its principal sources the connectionist lower levels of ICS, as argued throughout much of this book (e.g., Chapter 4).

Chief among the contributions of OT is a formal theory of crosslinguistic typology: variation arises through, and only through, differences in hierarchical ranking of a fixed set of universal constraints. This strengthens the theory of universal grammar significantly, illustrating how ICS can contribute to the advancement of f-level goals that previously could be pursued only within a purely symbolic architecture. As for the specific problem (41b), the body of work within OT proposes many substantive principles characterizing knowledge of particular facets of language; a small sample is contained within Part III, where Chapters 13–16 respectively propose substantive constraints on the well-formedness of syllables, phonological feature domains, syntactic/semantic role mappings, and *wh*-questions.

But, as has been argued elsewhere in this book (especially Chapter 12), OT's contribution at the f-level is not limited to "competence-theoretic" goals like universal grammatical typology. In Part III, OT is also used to address specific f-level problems falling outside the normal bound of "competence theories": problems concerning the acquisition and use of phonology and syntax (Chapters 17–19). Indeed, these analyses promote the unification of the theory of the acquisition and use of language with the theory of universal grammatical typology.

7.1.1.4   The problem of productivity (f-level)

Finally, a foundational problem introduced in Chapter 1.

(42)   The f-level productivity (or generativity) problem

a.   *Formal.* In what general form can cognitive functions incorporating unbounded competence be finitely specified?

b.   *Substantive.* How can the particular functions manifesting unbounded competence in particular cognitive domains be finitely specified?

Formal rewrite-rule grammars provide one solution to the general problem. With re-

Figure 12   *Box 7*

spect to a particular fragment of the grammar of a particular language, a particular system of rewrite rules may provide a solution to the substantive problem. For these f-level problems, what matters is that such finite knowledge systems are capable of specifying unbounded competence; whether these grammars correspond to mental processes is a problem for the c-level.

One important type of answer to this question offered by PSA involves symbolic rewrite rules. The output of a function is specified as the end result of taking the input and rewriting it repeatedly using the specified rules. Typically, a finite set of rules can generate an appropriate output for any of a potentially unboundedly large set of inputs. Specific knowledge in, for example, phonology, has been explicitly specified by just such rules.

Within ICS —specifically, within OT—the function specified by a grammar is defined by optimization. For a given input, the output is the candidate structure that best satisfies the grammar, a hierarchy of ranked violable constraints. With a finite set of constraints, this can specify an output for infinitely many different inputs. In phonology, syntax, semantics, and pragmatics, specific grammatical functions have been specified by specific sets of constraints within OT.

7.1.2 Explanation at the c-level: Processing

It is at the c-level that the general types of explanations offered by PSA and ICS differ most. At the c-level, cognitive functions must be reduced to the outcome of a set of simple operations. This reduction is carried out very differently in ICS than in PSA, with major implications for how cognitive processes are modeled in the two architectures.

7.1.2.1 The problem of productivity (c-level)

The final f-level problem has a c-level counterpart.

(43)   The c-level productivity problem

By what general mechanism does a finite store of mental knowledge give rise to unbounded human mental competence?

This is a central problem of cognitive architecture research. Is it mental serial rule application processes that explain unbounded mental competence in higher cognitive domains? Or is it processes that optimize over parallel, numerically weighted probabilistic constraints?

At the f-level, rewrite rules are one important means of specifying functions in PSA. These same rule systems can serve at the c-level as models of mental processes, and they do so serve, as mentioned in Section 5. Sequential rule application can be reduced to a long sequence of extremely simple operations, as is routinely done in Lisp machines and other electronic computers. Many types of algorithms other than rewrite-rule systems can serve the same role, such as heuristic parsing algorithms for sentence interpretation.

In ICS, moving from the f- to the c-level requires realizing symbol structures, and constraints over them, as sets of activations and weights. This reduces the computation to a large number of simple arithmetic operations well within the computational resources of biological neurons. Section 8:4.1 shows explicitly how, for any recursive function within a large class, a finitely specified network can be defined so that, for an unbounded set of inputs, the correct output is produced.

7.1.2.2   The processing problem

A more specific problem is central to cognitive psychology, cognitive modeling, and both experimental and computational psycholinguistics.

(44)   The processing problem

What, precisely, are the mental algorithms used in particular cognitive domains?

Are human problem-solving processes heuristic search algorithms using means-ends analysis (32d.iii)? Is human sentence processing an algorithm employing a minimal-attachment heuristic (32d.ii)?

Addressing these problems requires a c-level theory $\mathscr{C}$. For ICS, the picture here is complicated by the fact that the c-level is split: its *higher* sublevel is isomorphic to a kind of symbolic computation, but its *lower* sublevel is purely connectionist. Not just any c-level description will suffice to address these c-level cognitive problems: the description must be process-relevant, that is, isomorphic to the n-level. And for ICS—unlike PSA—this is true of the lower—but not the higher—sublevel description. Thus, to address these questions in ICS, connectionist algorithms are required.

While much work remains to be done, Chapters 8 and 10 report significant progress toward the finite specification of networks that correctly parse an infinite set of inputs with a context-free grammar. These connectionist algorithms are a step along the path to algorithms for modeling the human processing of natural language. The abstract processing time required by such algorithms will serve to predict real processing time for human subjects; other resource requirements of the algorithm will also predict corresponding real cognitive demands.

It is important to note that the kinds of inferences that are standardly used in PSA to predict processing characteristics such as reaction times do not apply in ICS (see Box 8). Consider a feed-forward tensorial network like those of Chapter 8 (or Section 5:2.2). This network computes a particular recursive function f. This function can be given an f-level specification in the Lisp programming language. In PSA, the c-level algorithm for computing f would interpret this Lisp program step by step. (This algorithm "follows the suggestion" implicit in the f-level Lisp specification of f, in the parlance of Section 2.3.2; for an example program, see Box 1.) Now suppose there is another function f' that is more complex than f in the sense that it requires a more complicated Lisp program, which takes more processing steps to compute its output.

Figure 12   *Box 7*

In PSA, it would be valid to predict that f' would take longer for human subjects to process; in PSA, such symbolic algorithms are process-relevant, and their abstract computing times predict real human processing times. But in ICS, no such inference is licensed. The network takes no longer to compute f' than it does to compute f: both require a single feed-forward step. Nor does f' require a larger network. The additional complexity in f' entails that it will "take longer" for the *cognitive scientist* to *analyze* the network. That is, the chain of matrix operations that relate the Lisp program to the weight matrix is longer for f', but this sort of complexity, this chain of operations, is *not in the network*.

The same remarks apply to an ICS grammar-parsing network realizing a harmonic grammar for a formal language (Chapter 10). In PSA, if generating an output O' requires applying more rules than does generating an output O, it is predicted that subjects will take more real time to process O'. But in ICS, the number of relevant rules in a harmonic grammar determines only how "long" it takes the cognitive scientist to analyze or design the network; the amount of time predicted for processing O' is determined by how many activation-spreading steps the network requires to reach a state of maximum Harmony, and there is no a priori reason why this should even correlate positively with the number of relevant rules, let alone be proportional to it.

Box 8. Impairment to parts versus wholes

In PSA, symbolic constituent structure is process-relevant; in ICS, it is not. This is in part because in ICS, constituents are combined via **superposition** of overlapping distributed patterns of activity, while in PSA, they are combined via some sort of nonoverlapping **concatenation**. This difference entails that damaged processing of constituents has different implications in PSA and in ICS.

Question. Suppose a cognitive function f maps $x \to X, y \to Y, z \to Z$. Suppose that under constituent decomposition at the f-level, these three input $\to$ output mappings become, respectively, $\mathbf{a} \to \mathbf{A}, \mathbf{b} \to \mathbf{B}, \mathbf{ab} \to \mathbf{AB}$. (Perhaps the input is a string of letters and the output a string of phonemes.) Suppose that the compositionality revealed by this constituent decomposition is productive (applies to many, perhaps infinitely many, input-output pairs). Now suppose brain damage severely disrupts $x \to X$ and $y \to Y$; perhaps sometimes $\mathbf{a} \to \mathbf{G}, \mathbf{b} \to \mathbf{H}$. *Must $z \to Z$ be disrupted?* Must disruption of the processing of the constituent parts of z entail disruption of the processing of z as a whole?

Answer, PSA. Yes. Employing the combinatorial strategy to explain the productivity of f here means that processing of $z = \mathbf{ab}$ is achieved by combining the processing of constituent $\mathbf{a}$ with that of constituent $\mathbf{b}$. Since processing of both $x = \mathbf{a}$ and $y = \mathbf{b}$ individually is disrupted, so must be the processing of z. If $\mathbf{a} \to \mathbf{G}$ and $\mathbf{b} \to \mathbf{H}$, then $z = \mathbf{ab} \to \mathbf{GH}$ instead of $Z = \mathbf{AB}$.

Answer, ICS. No, disruption of the parts does not imply disruption of the whole. Let the activation vectors realizing **a, b, ab, A**, ... be a, b, ab, A, ... (Recall that 'ab' is a *single* metasymbol denoting the activation vector that realizes the composite symbol structure **ab**.) The combinatorial strategy is realized by the weight matrix $\mathbf{W} = \mathbf{Aa}^{+T} + \mathbf{Bb}^{+T} + $ ... (Section 8:4.2). Then $\mathbf{a} \rightarrow \mathbf{Wa} = \mathbf{A}$, $\mathbf{b} \rightarrow \mathbf{B}$, $\mathbf{ab} = \mathbf{a} + \mathbf{b}$ $\rightarrow \mathbf{A} + \mathbf{B} \equiv \mathbf{AB}$, and so on. Now let the damaged weight matrix be $\mathbf{W'} = \mathbf{W} + \mathbf{D}$, where the damage matrix $\mathbf{D}$ adds substantial noise to the correct weights $\mathbf{W}$. Then $\mathbf{a} \rightarrow \mathbf{Wa} + \mathbf{Da} \equiv \mathbf{A} + \mathbf{e}_a$, where $\mathbf{e}_a$ is the error in the output for **a**, which is substantial. And similarly for **b**. Now the output for **ab** is $(\mathbf{W} + \mathbf{D})\mathbf{ab} = \mathbf{AB} + \mathbf{e}_a + \mathbf{e}_b$. The error here is $\mathbf{e}_a + \mathbf{e}_b \equiv \mathbf{e}_{ab}$, the superposition of the errors on each constituent individually. Need this be substantial? *No.* It can in fact be zero, if $\mathbf{e}_b = -\mathbf{e}_a$; if this equation is nearly true, the error on **ab** will be small.

Example. Suppose the units of a connectionist network realizing the input are divided into two pools, the left for the first constituent of the input, the right for the second. Or less strictly locally, suppose the patterns for the first constituent tend to have more activation to the left, those for the second, to the right. Now suppose the damage $\mathbf{D}$ is gradient across the network, starting with significantly positive values at the left edge, ending with significantly negative values at the right edge, with the average damage on the left about $+d$, on the right, $-d$. Now a single constituent has activation biased to the left or right, and suffers damage proportional to $+d$ or $-d$. But an input with *two* constituents suffers $+d$ from the first, $-d$ from the second, and these can actually cancel out. (For example, $\mathbf{D} = d\mathbf{na}^{+T} -d\mathbf{nb}^{+T}$, where **n** is a vector of noise.)[21]

Moral. With superposition, the error for the whole can be *less* than the error for the parts. With concatenation, this is not possible. $\mathcal{F}\text{-}\mathcal{N}$ isomorphism in PSA entails that we are entitled to infer that damage to constituent parts entails damage to wholes. Lack of $\mathcal{F}\text{-}\mathcal{N}$ isomorphism in ICS means no such entailment follows; more low-level information about the nature of the connectionist damage is necessary before we can know the relation between damage to wholes and damage to their constituents.

The point is not that the ICS error-cancellation scenario *must* happen, or even that it is *likely* to happen—the point is simply that it *can* happen. Unlike for symbolic concatenation, for superpositional connectionist combinatorics the spectrum of possible relations between damage to parts and damage to wholes is potentially quite rich and complex.

---

[21] For transparency, the algebra in the box is not explicit concerning the underlying filler/role decomposition. Let r_1, r_2 be the roles of first and second position in a string, realized by vectors $\mathbf{r}_1$, $\mathbf{r}_2$. Then the realizations of x, y, z are $\mathbf{x} = \mathbf{a} \otimes \mathbf{r}_1$, $\mathbf{y} = \mathbf{b} \otimes \mathbf{r}_1$, $\mathbf{z} = \mathbf{a} \otimes \mathbf{r}_1 + \mathbf{b} \otimes \mathbf{r}_2$, and similarly for X, Y, Z constructed from the vectors $\mathbf{A}, \mathbf{B}$. Let $\{\mathbf{s}_i\} = \{\mathbf{a}, \mathbf{b}, ...\}$, $\{\mathbf{S}_i\} = \{\mathbf{A}, \mathbf{B}, ...\}$ be the sets of vectors realizing all input symbols and output symbols, respectively. Now $\mathbf{W} \equiv \Sigma_{k=1,2}\Sigma_i [\mathbf{S}_i \otimes \mathbf{r}_k][\mathbf{s}_i \otimes \mathbf{r}_k]^{+T}$ performs correctly: $\mathbf{x} = \mathbf{a} \otimes \mathbf{r}_1 \rightarrow \mathbf{Wa} \otimes \mathbf{r}_1 = \mathbf{A} \otimes \mathbf{r}_1 = \mathbf{X}$; $\mathbf{y} \rightarrow \mathbf{Y}$; $\mathbf{z} = \mathbf{ab} \rightarrow \mathbf{AB} = \mathbf{Z}$. Now suppose the damage has the form $\mathbf{D} \equiv \mathbf{F} \otimes \mathbf{R}$, where $\mathbf{F} \equiv d\mathbf{n}(\Sigma_i \mathbf{s}_i)^{+T}$ and $\mathbf{R} \equiv (\mathbf{r}_1 + \mathbf{r}_2)(\mathbf{r}_1 - \mathbf{r}_2)^{+T}$. Then $\mathbf{Dx} = \mathbf{Fa} \otimes \mathbf{Rr}_1 = d\mathbf{n} \otimes (\mathbf{r}_1 + \mathbf{r}_2) = -\mathbf{Dy}$: there is substantial error processing each of $\mathbf{x}$ and $\mathbf{y}$. But $\mathbf{Dz} = \mathbf{Fa} \otimes \mathbf{Rr}_1 + \mathbf{Fb} \otimes \mathbf{Rr}_2 = d\mathbf{n} \otimes (\mathbf{r}_1 + \mathbf{r}_2) - d\mathbf{n} \otimes (\mathbf{r}_1 + \mathbf{r}_2) = 0$; that is, there is no error processing $\mathbf{z}$.

Figure 12   Box 8

7.1.3 Explanation at the n-level : Physicalism

7.1.3.1 The problem of physicalism

One of the most basic problems in the philosophy of mind concerns the relation of the n-level to the f-level.

(45) The problem of physicalism

How is it possible for a physical system to have intentional properties, such as referring to environmental events (even nonexistent ones)?

The entire c-level can be viewed as providing a solution to this problem by building a bridge, connecting to $\mathcal{N}$ at one end and to $\mathcal{F}$ at the other.

As discussed in Section 7.1.1.1, both PSA and ICS need to account for how f-level symbols get their meanings, how symbol structures get their intentional properties. Given such an account (whatever it might be), the two architectures diverge in how they parlay that f-level story into a physical story.

In ICS, the meaningful symbol structures are realized in abstract activation patterns, which in turn are presumed to be realized in physical activation patterns over physical neurons. Presuming the account of symbol meaning to be truly an f-level account, it should be independent of lower-level structure, and thus it should survive the reduction of symbols to neural activity. This then would be the account of how certain special physical states can have intentional properties.

In PSA, the f-level system of meaningful symbols is reduced in the c-level to a system of primitive computing operations that are so simple as to be demonstrably realizable in physical processes, as electronic computers attest. This then could potentially explain how certain special *physical* states can have intentional properties ... but it is unclear how it demonstrates that *brain* states are among those special physical states, bringing us to our last problem.

7.1.3.2 The problem of neural instantiability

The final problem is a primary concern of computational neuroscience, cognitive neuroscience, and neurolinguistics.

(46) The neural instantiation problem

a. *General.* Precisely how, in general, can cognitively adequate mental representations and algorithms be instantiated in the nervous system, in principle?

b. *Specific.* How, precisely, are the mental representations and algorithms of particular cognitive domains in fact realized in the nervous system?

This problem demands a precise account of general principles by which the kind of processes visible at the neural level can be organized to compute functions with the great complexity and abstractness characteristic of cognition; it also requires specific instantiations of those principles that demonstrably compute particular cognitive functions and are consistent with neural-level data concerning actual performance of those functions.

Data-dependency descriptions in PSA are used to form hypotheses about how the brain may modularize various cognitive functions; these are clearly useful in addressing the neural instantiation problem. But since these descriptions are basically descriptions of how certain types of information get transformed into other types of information, these accounts can be just as easily seen as high-level descriptions in an ICS architecture: unlike Eliminative Connectionism, ICS makes available the symbolic structure that is often assumed to be present in the representations passed around in data-dependency systems. (See Section 3.4 for a connectionist realization of a data-dependency description.)

At computational levels lower than the data-dependency description, it is unclear how the sort of reduction-to-primitive-operations provided by PSA can address the neural instantiability problem (Box 1). In contrast, it is evident that the sort of reduction-to-primitive-operations provided by ICS can in turn provide any number of hypotheses concerning neural instantiation. This is a largely unexplored area for ICS research, but already in previous chapters we have seen hints of the applicability of ICS reduction to neural instantiation. In Chapter 7, we saw that the basic ICS operation, the tensor product, provides hypotheses concerning neural representation that bear close relations to existing hypotheses developed by neuroscientists: Pouget and Sejnowski's (1997) representations in parietal cortex, and Gray et al.'s (1989) synchronous-firing binding. The relevant point here is not that these hypotheses relating ICS reduction and neural computation are *correct*—it is that they *exist*. While certainly not sufficient, existence is most definitely a necessary condition for a hypothesis to have value. It is my hope that as ICS develops, many more such hypotheses will come to exist, and that at least some of them will help us begin to understand how knowledge as abstract as that of universal grammar is reduced to low-level physical interactions within biological neural networks.

Box 9. Competence and the limits of performance

The categories "competence theory" and "performance theory" are heterogeneous collections that seem to admit no simple unified characterization. In a number of interesting cases, however, a competence theory can be seen as a performance theory with some level of detail eliminated or *abstracted away*. In these cases, competence can be viewed as a kind of limiting case of performance, in the limit where some variable that is important in the performance theory has been taken to its extreme value and is therefore no longer a variable in the resulting—competence—theory. In the following cases, the dimensions being abstracted away—taken to the limit—are resource-dependence, gradience in representations, and variability in the input-output function. In several of the examples below, the performance theory referred to is one of those

---

Figure 12   *Box 9*

mentioned in (32). The abbreviations 'A/P/C' refer to 'variable Abstracted away/Performance theory/Competence theory'. 'lim z as $x \to y$' means 'the limit of z as x approaches y'.

(1)   *competence* = lim *performance* as **computational resources** $\to \infty$

    a. Center embedding
        A. Space: Stack depth d
        P. Machine with depth-d stack, applying context-free grammar rules, generating sentences with center-embedding depth limited to d (32c)
        C. Context-free languages: unlimited center embedding

    b. Derivational complexity
        A. Processing time T
        P. Transformational rules as serially ordered subprocesses; sentences that require rule-time no greater than T (32d.i) to generate
        C. Languages with unboundedly long sentences requiring unlimited numbers of rules to generate

    c. Optimality Theory
        A. Optimization reliability or processing time T
        P. Sentences resulting from an optimization process O that seeks outputs that optimally satisfy a violable constraint hierarchy $\mathcal{H}$, where O has a nonzero probability p_{Err} of producing a suboptimal output and $p_{\mathrm{Err}} \to 0$ as $T \to \infty$
        C. Languages with sentences that optimally satisfy $\mathcal{H}$

    d. Heuristic sentence parsing
        A. Fraction f of entire sentence provided as input
        P. Partial parses from a grammar G (plus, possibly, heuristic processing rules), where as $f \to 100\%$, the results converge to correct G-parses (32d.ii) (see Chapter 19)
        C. Full G-parse of entire sentences

(2)   *competence* = lim *performance* as **gradience** $\to 0$

    a. Phonetics/phonology
        A. Acoustic/articulatory gradience in speech inputs/outputs
        P. Phonetic representations: continuous structures
        C. Phonological representations: discrete structures

    b. Acceptability judgments
        A. Gradience across sentences, within a speaker, of the strengths of acceptability judgments
        P. Grammars producing graded well-formedness levels (atypical: see Harmonic Grammar, Chapters 2, 6, and 11)
        C. Grammars producing binary well-formedness levels (typical: e.g., OT; see especially Section 20:1.3)

(3)   *competence* = lim *performance* as **I/O-variability** $\rightarrow$ **0**

   a.   Psycholinguistic production error analysis

        A. Variance, including acceptable to unacceptable forms, across speakers, context, and time, of the phonological structure of words and morphosyntax of spoken sentences

        P. Theory of the probability of alternative phonological, morphological, or syntactic forms, including deviations from the grammatical (Chapters 11, 17, and 18)

        C. Grammars producing a unique output for any input

   b.   Grammar mixing

        A. Variance among acceptability judgments, across speakers, context, and time, of words and sentences

        P. Mixture of grammars corresponding to multiple dialects, different registers, or intermediate states of language acquisition or change

        C. Single grammar

   While this analysis may not apply to every type of competence/performance distinction, the above cases cover many central examples.

7.2 Cognitive data at multiple levels

The preceding section formulated several general conceptual problems a complete cognitive theory must solve. In addition, more particular empirical problems were identified. To address these, a theory must make predictions concerning the many types of data that bear on the empirical adequacy of theories addressing problems such as determining, for particular cognitive domains, the actual content of mental representations (40b), knowledge (41b), and algorithms (44), and the actual details of their neural realization (46b). In ICS, which general type of computation—symbolic or connectionist—figures most prominently in accounting for some type of data depends on whether those data address the f-, c-, or n-level.

It might seem that the data receiving symbolic explanation in ICS are "competence data"—typically the purview of formal linguistics and philosophy—while the data targeted by connectionist explanation are "performance data"—experimental data typically the domain of cognitive psychology and neuroscience. But by now it is clear that the truth is more complex than this. In ICS, symbolic explanations can be applied not just to traditional "competence data," but also to the many sorts of "performance data" that bear on the f-level. In this subsection, I will attempt to characterize those data, a task more complex than it first appears. I will argue that a great deal of the empirical action in cognitive science actually concerns the f-level, a point first introduced in (9). In ICS, f-level "performance data" can receive symbolic explanation—for example, through OT. Among other things, this subsection addresses the foundational considerations licensing OT explanation of the diversity of data to

Figure 12   *Box 9*

which this symbolic theory was applied in Part III.

It will be useful to view types of cognitive data as differing along several dimensions; numerous examples will follow. These dimensions are relevant at all theoretical levels.

(47) Dimensions of variation in types of cognitive data

a. *Source:* A subject population for experimental work or for behavioral elicitation; alternatively, a corpus of words or utterances for statistical or other analysis

b. *Task:* The behavior a subject is asked to produce, and the conditions under which it is carried out; or, a distributional property of a corpus (this is the independent variable)

c. *Measurement:* The measured variable concerning the observed behavior or corpus

d. *Analysis:* The computation of a dependent variable from the measured variable

Different types of subject populations are important in different subfields of cognitive science; some prime examples are listed in (48).[22]

(48) Variation in subject populations

a. Varying ages (developmental psychology; language acquisition)

b. Varying types of brain damage (cognitive neuropsychology and neuroscience)

c. Varying language communities (linguistics)

All these dimensions of variation across subjects can be explored at all theoretical levels. It may be tempting, but it would be a serious oversimplification to consider dimension (48c) as relevant only to f-level formal linguistics, dimension (48b) as relevant only to c-level cognitive neuropsychology or n-level neuroscience, and so forth. The extent to which these dimensions can all be explored at the f-level is of particular interest here.

7.2.1 Data at the f-level: Introspection; behavior

By 'f-level data', I mean data bearing on f-level problems, several of which were discussed in Section 7.1.1. Since some types of data address multiple levels, it is possible for f-level data to also be c- or n-level data. This is an important point to which I return in Sections 7.2.2 and 7.2.3.

A central f-level concern is the semantic problem (39). One source of data relevant to this problem is intuition concerning mental content. This is the source, for example, of the datum that mental contents are combinatorially structured; this is the datum underlying the more specific semantic problem (39b), to explain the origin of

---

[22] Another interesting dimension not pursued here is varying species (comparative cognition; neuroscience).

such combinatorial structure.

Many of the remaining data bearing on f-level cognitive problems can be conveniently construed in terms of a single dependent variable. This variable is the probability that an output O will be produced given that the input is I; we write this '$p(I{\rightarrow}O)$'. A formal specification of this probabilistic input-output function is an f-level description. As summarized in (49), the probability distribution can be described with varying degrees of completeness, and may sometimes be assigned a normative interpretation.

(49) Dependent variable

$p(I{\rightarrow}O)$: the probability of observing a particular output O, given a particular input I

a. Degrees of completeness

  i.   Specified: a numerical value for each (I, O) pair

  ii. Specified: a single O provided for each I; $p(I{\rightarrow}O)$ is approximated as 1 if O is the value paired with I, 0 otherwise[23]

  iii. Specified: general properties of the distribution $p(I{\rightarrow}O)$ (e.g., overall, $p(I{\rightarrow}O)$ is greater for (I, O) pairs having property P than for those having property Q)

b. Normative outputs and errors

  i.   A single O—construed as the 'correct' output—may be provided for each I; let this output be denoted $f^{\dagger}(I)$. Then

  ii. $p\{I{\rightarrow}O \mid O \neq f^{\dagger}(I)\}$ is the **error probability** for I

In practice, the dependent variable $p(I{\rightarrow}O)$ is derived from a range of measurements via appropriate analyses. I will now review several types of data relevant to the f-level; each type is introduced by a numbered characterization in terms of the dimensions that have been laid out.

(50) Elicitation

a. *Measurement:* Elicitation of O given I

  i.   *Task (e.g.):* 'What is the word in your language for I?'

  ii. *Measure:* The phonetic structure of the response O

b. *Analysis:* $p(I{\rightarrow}O) =$

  i.   Proportion of outputs O when given I, over a population of subjects and trials

  ii. For a single subject, single trial: 1 if O is elicited when given I, otherwise 0

We can think of prototypical ("competence-theoretic") formal linguistics as following (50b.ii): for each I, a unique (probability 1) O is taken to be the well-formed

---

[23] Or if, for the given I, there are n different Os paired with a single I, then $p(I{\rightarrow}O) = 1/n$. This qualification also applies to the many similar binary, yes/no-type measurements below; it will not be repeated each time.

Figure 12   Box 9

output, and a grammar is responsible for specifying this **O** given an input **I**. Now if a range of grammars with differing probabilities are used to model the subject's linguistic knowledge, the numerical data of (50b.i) can also be accounted for in similar fashion. In Chapter 17, such numerical data are addressed by f-level accounts within ICS: symbolic accounts employing OT. There, **I** is a pseudo-Polish word like *ktabo* that violates the phonological grammar of English, and **O** is the pronunciation of this word produced by English-speaking participants. The data are analyzed using numerical proportions, as in (50b.i); they are modeled by positing that each utterance is derived from an OT grammar selected from a range of roughly equiprobable grammars that differ only in the ranking of a single faithfulness constraint.

(51) Occurrence

    a. *Measurement:* Presence of (**I**, **O**) in a corpus (either normative (e.g., a dictionary) or naturally occurring (e.g., transcripts of spontaneous speech or a written text))

        i. *'Task' (e.g.):* **I** is the occurrence of a particular pronoun
        Measure: **O**, the location relative to the pronoun of its antecedent (a full noun phrase identifying the pronoun's referent)

        ii. *'Task' (e.g.):* **I** is a meaning listed in a dictionary
        Measure: **O**, the corresponding listed pronunciation

    b. *Analysis:* $p(\mathbf{I}{\rightarrow}\mathbf{O})$ =

        i. Proportion of locations **O** for the given **I**, over the corpus

        ii. 1 if **O** is the pronunciation of **I** listed in the dictionary, otherwise 0

Like elicited data (50), these data can be accounted for with an f-level theory (e.g., OT) that produces either numerical probabilities (51b.i) or a single output for a given input (51b.ii). The OT typology in Chapter 13 models the occurrence (or absence) of different syllable structures in different languages, the relevant data being of the binary type (51b.ii). This sort of binary '±absent' data is also the target of Chapter 15, which addresses crosslinguistic variation in the structures of simple clauses (differing in grammatical voice: active, passive, etc.). Exemplifying numerical data (51b.i) is the analysis of Chapter 18, where **I** is the proposition a young French-learning child intends to express, and **O** is the sentence he uses to express it.

(52) Explicit judgments

    a. *Measurement:* Judgments of (**I**, **O**)

        i. *Task (e.g.):* 'Is **I** an instance of the category **O**?'
        Measure: Response on a scale of 1 = 'definitely no' ... 5 = 'definitely yes'

        ii. *Task (e.g.):* 'In your language, can the sentence **O** be used to convey the meaning **I**?'
        Measure: Response as 'yes' or 'no'

  b. *Analysis:* $p(\mathbf{I}{\rightarrow}\mathbf{O}) =$
      i. Mean of measured values over a population of subjects and trials
      ii. For a single subject, single trial: 1 if judgment of ($\mathbf{I}$, $\mathbf{O}$) is 'yes', 0 if
          judgment is 'no'

The type of binary data in (52b.ii) is addressed in Chapter 16; OT grammars are used in the conventional way to produce a single output $\mathbf{O}$ – a *wh*-question—for a given input $\mathbf{I}$. In Chapter 11, the f-level ICS formalism of Harmonic Grammar is used to model explicit acceptability judgments of the graded type in (52a.i), where $\mathbf{O}$ is the category of acceptable sentences of French. Rather than a probabilistic mixture of binary grammars, as in the previous cases of output variation (50)–(51), here a single nonbinary harmonic grammar itself outputs a numerical grammaticality value for each input.[24]

(53)   Implicit judgments
  a. *Measurement:* Time during which infants will attend to ($\mathbf{I}$, $\mathbf{O}$)
      i. *Task (e.g.):* Listen to a list of pairs ($\mathbf{I}$, $\mathbf{O}$) where $\mathbf{I}$ is a pair of spoken syl-
          lables X, Y and $\mathbf{O}$ is the disyllable formed by concatenating X and Y,
          possibly with a sound change at their juncture
      ii. *Measure:* The time during which an infant orients toward a loud-
          speaker playing a list of pairs characterized by phonological property
          P or Q
  b. *Analysis:* If listening time to a class of stimuli with property P significantly
      exceeds that for property Q, then $p(\mathbf{I}{\rightarrow}\mathbf{O})$ is on average greater for pairs ($\mathbf{I}$,
      $\mathbf{O}$) possessing property P than for pairs possessing property Q

This particular task refers to work reported in Chapter 17. The example makes three interesting points. First, it provides a case where the f-level can be addressed even though the probability distribution $p(\mathbf{I}{\rightarrow}\mathbf{O})$ is characterized very incompletely (49a.iii). Second, it illustrates that a relevant measurement can be quite remote from this probability distribution.

Finally, this example shows that data concerning *time* can be used to address f-level questions. Theories at the f-level do not predict temporal durations—that requires a c-level theory (Section 2.3). But a c-level **linking relation** between time and another variable enables temporal data to inform the f-level theory if the other variable is directly addressed at the f-level. In the case of (53), the variable is well-formedness or **Harmony**, the measure that is optimized by OT grammars. The c-level linking relation asserts that infants' listening time in this task increases as the stimuli become more "language-like" — that is, more harmonic according to their grammar. A complete theory would deduce this connection between time and Harmony as a consequence of its c-level principles. This is not possible within ICS at present. In-

---

[24] The grammar-mixture method can also be usefully applied to graded acceptability judgments, treating lower acceptability like lower probability. The intuition is that a form that is grammatical according to all the grammars is experienced as more acceptable than forms that are grammatical only according to an improbable subset of grammars.

Figure 12   *Box 9*

stead, the time-Harmony connection is simply a hypothesis suggested by a number of experimental results, under an OT interpretation (see Chapter 17). (53b) results from the f-level translation of higher Harmony for (**I**, **O**) to greater $p(\mathbf{I} \rightarrow \mathbf{O})$; alternatively, (53b) can be rephrased directly in terms of greater Harmony rather than greater probability — it is actually Harmony that is computed directly within OT.

(54) Sequential implicit outputs

   a. *Measurement:* Word-by-word reading times of sentences **I** with temporary structural ambiguities

   i. *Task:* Read a sentence $\mathbf{I}_i$ presented one word at a time, pressing a button when ready for the next word. $\mathbf{I}_i$ has a point x where there are two possible continuations with different syntactic structures ('parses'). $\mathbf{I}_i^x$ is the portion of sentence $\mathbf{I}_i$ up to the ambiguity point x. There is another matching sentence $\mathbf{I}'_i$ that until x is the same as $\mathbf{I}_i^x$, but whose continuation requires a different parse.

   ii. *Measure:* Time between button presses

   b. *Analysis:* The output $\mathbf{O}_i^x$ is the selected parse for $\mathbf{I}_i^x$. If reading times are lengthened after x for $\mathbf{I}_i'$ relative to $\mathbf{I}_i$, conclude that $\mathbf{O}_i^x$ is the parse that is consistent with $\mathbf{I}_i$ rather than $\mathbf{I}_i'$.

This case is the topic of Chapter 19. Like the previous example (53), this one is interesting because the f-level is informed by a type of data for which it does not itself make direct predictions. Reading times, or other measures of processing difficulty, are the purview of c-level theory, not f-level. The key, again, is a c-level linking relation between time and a variable accessible at the f-level. Processing time is lengthened for the dispreferred continuation $\mathbf{I}_i'$ because it is inconsistent with the output of the parser at the ambiguity point — and outputs are certainly accessible at the f-level; these are exactly what the OT analysis of Chapter 19 specifies. There is not yet a (connectionist) c-level ICS theory of human sentence processing that is sufficiently developed to formally derive this connection between processing time and structural inconsistency — and deriving the connection is impossible at the (symbolic) f-level of OT. Provisionally, it is necessary to hypothesize that the connectionist network realizing the parser takes longer to settle into a stable state when more filler/structural-role bindings (Chapter 5) need to be changed, as in the inconsistent case. While this hypothesis is not unreasonable, it is also not a formal consequence of the c-level theory at its current state of development.

The previous subsections have illustrated several types of tasks, measurements, and analyses that allow f-level theories to contact empirical data. In each case, the input **I** is the primary independent variable manipulated, and a fixed population has been assumed to be the subject pool. But of course the subject population itself is an independent variable that can be manipulated, producing a different input-output probability function $p_k(\mathbf{I} \rightarrow \mathbf{O})$ for each population P_k. If the populations vary in the language spoken, then the functions p_k constitute the crosslinguistic *typological* data at the core of the theory of universal grammar. (For OT accounts of such data, see Chapters 13 and 14 for phonological examples and Chapters 15 and 16 for syntactic ones.) If the populations P_k differ in age, the functions p_k map the course of cognitive development. (See Chapters 17 and 18 for OT examples in phonology and syntax.) If the populations P_k differ in the extent to which their brains are intact, the functions p_k comprise the data of cognitive neuropsychology. All these data can be addressed by an f-level description that incorporates variables corresponding to the population differences in language, age, or brain damage.

A complete theory will, of course, go on to explain just *how* differences in linguistic environment, or in degree of experience or maturation, or in damage to particular brain areas, affect p_k the way the f-level account says it does. But even leaving such population manipulations aside, the f-level description needs in any event to be supplemented in order to explain just *how* a given input **I** is paired with a given output **O**. Answering these 'how' questions is a job of the c-level theory.

7.2.2   Data at the c-level: Resources

As just shown, f-level accounts are not limited to addressing prototypical "competence-theoretic" data such as crosslinguistic patterns of binary acceptability judgments and determinate input-output mappings in phonology and syntax. Under appropriate conditions, f-level descriptions can also address error data, acquisition data, neuropsychological data, gradient well-formedness judgments, corpus frequencies, infant listening-times, and online reading times. These "performance-theoretic" data are commonly taken to require a computational process-model — in our terms, a c-level theory. So what then *is* the responsibility of the c-level description?

A c-level description necessarily provides a function f and hence one of its empirical responsibilities is getting this function right. Thus, all the data concerning this function — the f-level data just discussed — is also data to which a c-level theory is responsible. This seems to be an underappreciated point: c-level theories describing mechanisms for producing outputs from inputs must ultimately also explain *all* f-level data, including core "competence-theoretic" data such as universal crosslinguistic patterns of acceptability. In addition to f-level data, of course, there is an important class of evidence that is relevant to a c-level but not an f-level description, and naturally it is upon these data that researchers operating at the c-level tend to focus.

An important type of structure that appears when we descend from the f- to the c-level is **resource requirements** (Sections 2.1 and 2.2). Unlike f-level functions, c-level algorithms demand adequate amounts of abstract time and abstract space, and certain types of abstract causal processes with certain degrees of reliability, to process a given input I. As we saw in Section 2.2.1, for these algorithmic resources to make contact with observations of their real counterparts, the algorithm must be *process-relevant*. In such a case, the algorithms of a c-level description need to account for the following types of data.

Figure 12   *Box 9*

(55) Resource measures

    a. Abstract time requirements

       Response times $T(I, O)$: what is the duration of the temporal interval between I and O for different (I, O) pairs?

         i. Under priming conditions: prior to presentation of I, another input I_P related to I is presented; measured is the dependency of $T(I, O)$ upon the relation between I_P and I.

         ii. In a 'default' context (no priming assumed)

    b. Abstract space requirements

       Accuracy with complex inputs: what types of complexity in an input I cause what types of errors in the corresponding outputs O?

    c. Abstract causal requirements

       Errors of incomplete systems: if certain types of operations are unavailable, what types of errors occur?

    d. Abstract reliability

       Errors of systems that are damaged or operating under adverse conditions: if certain types of operations are unreliable, what types of errors occur?

The data may address individual input-output pairs, or a temporal sequence of Is and the associated sequence of Os, as in real-time processing data.

As we have seen (e.g., Box 5), if each primitive abstract operation is assigned some real temporal duration, it is clear how to predict a response time from the set of operations required to produce a given O from a given I (55a.ii). Formalizing the notion of **priming** (55a.i) may not be as straightforward, but it is important for making contact with a great many revealing experimental psychological data. Assumptions must be provided about how the time required for a subprocess is influenced by related recent subprocesses that, for example, may have produced the same result, or depleted a common resource. These assumptions are implicit characterizations of the way the c-level algorithms are physically realized — of the isomorphism between the c- and n-levels.

Processing more complex inputs will generally require an algorithm to employ more or larger data structures, demanding more 'abstract space' (55b). Assumptions about space limitations that exist in some populations — perhaps infants, or brain-damaged patients — enable predictions of the types of errors the algorithm will make on different types of inputs.[25]

Similarly, in processing different inputs, an algorithm may require different subprocesses, or even different primitive operations (55c). Assumptions about the unavailability — or unreliability (55d) — of certain subprocesses in certain populations or under certain conditions also enable predictions about the types of errors that will be

---

[25] See Elman 1993 for an influential and controversial argument that space limitations in children's language-processing systems can actually lead to *improvement* — in learning, not processing.

made with different inputs. Such assumptions are common in the analysis of brain-damaged patients using data-dependency theories, where the damage is hypothesized to have 'impaired' or eliminated a particular subprocess or internal representation (see Section 3.4).

A complete c-level account of these sorts of data requires an explicit algorithm, together with assumptions concerning how the parts of the algorithm relate to its physical embodiment, assumptions sufficient to connect the independent variables to the measured variables. A less complete c-level account can serve to convert a c-level problem to an f-level problem—two examples were just discussed: time-Harmony linkage (53) and time–inconsistent-output linkage (54). This can be illustrated with the work in Chapter 19 addressing online sentence comprehension. An f-level question is, what tree structure O_k is assigned by the grammar to a partial input I_k that consists only of the first k words of a sentence? Given an f-level OT account, we can answer this question for each value of k. In some syntactic environments D, when the kth word becomes available, there will be major changes in the assigned tree structure, and in other environments E, there will be only minor changes. In our terminology: in E, only a small number of bindings need be added to the parse, while in D, numerous existing bindings need to be removed and numerous new ones added. Simply assuming that c-level processes require more abstract time to change numerous bindings than to change few bindings, and that the c- and n-level descriptions are temporally isomorphic with respect to relative processing duration, yields the prediction that $I_k \rightarrow O_k$ computation time will be greater in D- than in E-environments. Then an f-level theory of $I_k \rightarrow O_k$ predicts the relative processing times of different syntactic structures.

7.2.3 Data at the n-level: Activation

It is obvious that new types of data become relevant once we descend to the neural level.

(56) Neural activity

During the performance of varying cognitive tasks, in varying locations of the nervous system of varying species: measure neural activity

a. at the fine scale of individual neural firing;

b. at the coarser spatiotemporal scales measured by neuroimaging methods such as ERP, PET, fMRI, and MEG.

Here, I will merely echo a comment made early in the discussion of c-level data, Section 7.2.2. It is of course understandable that researchers specializing at the neural level will focus on data such as (56). But an n-level description entails, at least in principle, higher-level descriptions at the c- and f-levels; thus, n-level theories are actually responsible not just to obviously neural data (56), but also to (c-level) data on cognitive processes (55) and to (f-level) data on cognitive functions (50)–(54). Were an n-level theory consistent with all known data on the firing patterns of cells in some

Figure 12   *Box 9*

part of visual cortex, it would surely be a monumental accomplishment—but it would be seriously deficient if it also predicted psychophysical or perceptual responses that were not consistent with behavioral data, or if it were too representationally weak to support the distinctions necessary to adequately characterize the cognitive functions that must be computed by the visual system. By the same token, if an n-level model of the morphological processing system were consistent with all known neuroimaging data, it would clearly be of great interest, but its empirical adequacy would be severely compromised if it were inconsistent with reaction time data concerning morphological processing, or if its representational structure were fundamentally incapable of representing, say, the morphological systems of certain language families—even if there were no experimental data, behavioral or neural, concerning those languages.

The application of ICS to n-level data is nearly entirely uncharted territory at this point. One extant example was discussed in Section 7:3. Activation of individual units in parietal cortex was shown to instantiate a tensor product representation. Now it was the high-level demands of supporting symbolic computation that led to the design of connectionist networks using tensor product representations—yet it turns out that at the opposite end of the reductive spectrum, these networks have some degree of validity in describing neural activation patterns of real brains. In a more speculative vein, the design of the abstract genomic encoding of universal grammar developed in Chapter 21 is also driven by the high-level requirements of realizing a symbolic system (OT), but the ultimate proposal ends up making low-level predictions concerning the existence of a number of interesting types of molecular signals.

8 SUMMARY

In cognitive architecture, many areas of cognitive science converge to address an important aspect of the mind-body problem. The conception of the enterprise that is explored in this book looks roughly like this.

A 'mind' is a system capable of cognition. Cognition is what psychology and linguistics say it is: realizing certain functions relating representations. These representations have combinatorial structure, and the functions defining cognition can be formally characterized by means of this structure. Furthermore, the functions arise from a computational system that can also be characterized in terms of combinatorial structure—a system performing symbolic computation. A computational system computes abstract, high-level functions by breaking them down into smaller and smaller pieces. This reduction yields a low-level description of cognition as the result of the interaction of many small operations, each so simple that they can be mechanically realized in a physical system.

The tools of computer science show how to achieve this reduction with formal precision. Computer science provides the means to formally characterize the high-level functions of cognition, despite their abstractness, and the means to formally relate these abstract functions to a low-level system of interacting simple physical components. To explain how cognition arises in the human case, these components must be structures within the brain. Computer science also provides a means of formally characterizing the relevant brain structures and their interaction: connectionist networks. But traditional reductions in computer science do not reduce symbolic computation to connectionist networks, or to any other conception of how the brain computes.

Formal tools adapted from mathematical physics, however, do enable a symbolic-to-connectionist reduction. The formal properties of vectors allow them to be assembled in a way that makes them functionally equivalent to a (new) type of symbolic computation. These vectors can then be reduced to primitive entities in a new type of connectionist network. In this reduction, the original combinatorial structure of cognitive functions gets hidden: this is where the basic computational elements shift from symbols to neurons. Unlike a traditional computer, the network does not have physically separate parts realizing each symbol and does not operate on them individually.

The new type of symbolic computation defining cognitive functions is founded on principles of optimization. Applying this new framework to language provides new theories that, by the standards of linguistics, significantly enhance the explanatory power of grammatical theory.

Realizing this story requires new work in several parts of cognitive science. New mathematics and computer science must identify the novel types of symbolic computation and connectionist networks, and the means of reducing one to the other. This occupied Part II of this book. Applying the new type of symbolic computation to language requires much research in theoretical, computational, and psycholinguistics. This was the topic of Part III. Finally, new foundational work is needed to understand the respective roles of, and the relations between, explanations based on the combinatorial symbolic characterizations of cognition and explanations based on the connectionist description. Additional foundational work is needed to understand the relation of the new conception to prevailing views on language within linguistics and psychology. This has been the burden of Part IV. In each area of the research program addressed in Parts II, III, and IV, progress has been made, and in each area, important questions remain open. The case for the conception of cognitive architecture — and cognitive science — developed in this book is hopefully sufficient, at the very least, to justify further research to discover how much light these hypotheses can shed upon the inner life of the human mind/brain.[26]

[26] For very helpful discussions on many of the topics of this chapter, I thank those I have been fortunate to have as colleagues over the past decade in the Department of Cognitive Science at Johns Hopkins University; for comments on drafts of this work, my appreciation goes in particular to Matt Goldrick, Elliott Moreton, and Brenda Rapp. I am of course solely responsible for any errors contained herein, including those pertaining to Rapp and Goldrick's work itself. Hopefully, some of their insights have survived the turbid process that led to this chapter.

Figure 12   *Box 9*

References

Abelson, H., G. J. Sussman, and J. Sussman. 1985. *Structure and interpretation of computer programs*. MIT Press.

Aizawa, K. 1997. Exhibiting vs. explaining systematicity: A reply to Hadley and Hayward. *Minds and Machines* 7, 39–55.

Aizawa, K. 2003. *The systematicity arguments*. Kluwer.

Bodén, M., and L. Niklasson. 2000. Semantic systematicity and context in connectionist networks. *Connection Science* 12, 111–42.

Cummins, R. 1991. The role of representation in connectionist explanations of cognitive capacities. In *Philosophy and connectionist theory*, eds. W. Ramsey, S. P. Stich, and D. E. Rumelhart. Erlbaum.

Cummins, R. 1996. Systematicity. *Journal of Philosophy* 93, 591–614.

Cummins, R., and G. Schwarz. 1991. Connectionism, computation, and cognition. In *Connectionism and the philosophy of mind*, eds. T. E. Horgan and J. Tienson. Kluwer.

Elman, J. L. 1993. Learning and development in neural networks: The importance of starting small. *Cognition* 48, 71–99.

Fodor, J. A. 1997. Connectionism and the problem of systematicity (continued): Why Smolensky's solution still doesn't work. *Cognition* 62, 109–19.

Fodor, J. A., and B. P. McLaughlin. 1990. Connectionism and the problem of systematicity: Why Smolensky's solution doesn't work. *Cognition* 35, 183–204.

Fodor, J. A., and Z. W. Pylyshyn. 1988. Connectionism and cognitive architecture: A critical analysis. *Cognition* 28, 3–71.

Foster, C. L. 1992. *Algorithms, abstraction and implementation: Levels of detail in cognitive science*. Academic Press.

Frank, R. 1998. Structural complexity and the time course of grammatical development. *Cognition* 66, 249–301.

Golden, R. M. 1996. *Mathematical methods for neural network analysis and design*. MIT Press.

Goldrick, M., and B. Rapp. 2002. A restricted interaction account (RIA) of spoken word production: The best of both worlds. *Aphasiology* 16, 20–55.

Gray, C. M., P. Konig, A. K. Engel, and W. Singer. 1989. Oscillatory responses in cat visual cortex exhibit intercolumnar synchronization which reflects global stimulus properties. *Nature* 338, 334–7.

Grimshaw, J., and V. Samek-Lodovici. 1998. Optimal subjects and subject universals. In *Is the best good enough? Optimality and competition in syntax*, eds. P. Barbosa, D. Fox, P. Hagstrom, M. McGinnis, and D. Pesetsky. MIT Press.

Hadley, R. F. 1994a. Systematicity in connectionist language learning. *Mind and Language* 9, 247–72.

Hadley, R. F. 1994b. Systematicity revisited. *Mind and Language* 9, 431–44.

Hadley, R. F. 1997a. Cognition, systematicity, and nomic necessity. *Mind and Language* 16, 137–53.

Hadley, R. F. 1997b. Explaining systematicity: A reply to Kenneth Aizawa. *Mind and Machines* 7, 571–9.

Hadley, R. F., and M. B. Hayward. 1997. Strong semantic systematicity from Hebbian connectionist learning. *Minds and Machines* 7, 1–37.

Haugeland, J. 1985. *Artificial intelligence: The very idea*. MIT Press.

Haugeland, J. 1991. Representational genera. In *Philosophy and connectionist theory*, eds. W. Ramsey, S. P. Stich, and D. E. Rumelhart. Erlbaum.

Hempel, C. G., and P. Oppenheim. 1948. Studies in the logic of explanation. *Philosophy of Science* 15, 135–75.

Horgan, T. E., and J. Tienson. 1996. *Connectionism and the philosophy of psychology*. MIT Press.

Kitcher, P. 1989. Explanatory unification and the causal structure of the world. In *Scientific explanation*, eds. P. Kitcher and W. C. Salmon. University of Minnesota Press.

Macdonald, C., and G. Macdonald. 1995. *Connectionism*. Vol. 2, *Debates on psychological explanation*. Blackwell.

Marr, D. 1982. *Vision*. W. H. Freeman.

Mathews, R. 1997. Can connectionists explain systematicity? *Mind and Language* 12, 154–77.

McClelland, J. L. 1979. On the time-relations of mental processes: An examination of systems of processes in cascade. *Psychological Review* 86, 287–330.

McCulloch, W., and W. Pitts. 1943. A logical calculus of the ideas immanent in nervous activity. *Bulletin of Mathematical Biophysics* 5, 115–33.

Niklasson, L. F., and T. van Gelder. 1994. On being systematically connectionist. *Mind and Language* 9, 288–302.

Penczek, A. 1997. The causal efficacy of mental properties. Ph.D. diss., Johns Hopkins University.

Penczek, A., and P. Smolensky. 2001. A criterion for causal efficacy derived from Optimality Theory. Talk presented at the American Philosophical Association Meeting, Midwest Division.

Phillips, S. 1994. Strong systematicity within connectionism: The tensor-recurrent network. In *Proceedings of the Cognitive Science Society 16*.

Phillips, S. 2000. Constituent similarity and systematicity: The limits of first-order connectionism. *Connection Science* 12, 45–63.

Pouget, A., and T. J. Sejnowski. 1997. Spatial transformations in the parietal cortex using basis functions. *Journal of Cognitive Neuroscience* 9, 222–37.

Rapp, B., and M. Goldrick. 2000. Discreteness and interactivity in spoken word production. *Psychological Review* 107, 460–99.

Smolensky, P. 1987. The constituent structure of connectionist mental states: A reply to Fodor and Pylyshyn. *Southern Journal of Philosophy* 26 (Supplement), 137–63.

Smolensky, P. 1988. On the proper treatment of connectionism. *Behavioral and Brain Sciences* 11, 1–74.

Smolensky, P. 1991. Connectionism, constituency, and the language of thought. In *Meaning in mind: Fodor and his critics*, eds. B. Loewer and G. Rey. Blackwell.

Smolensky, P. 1995. Constituent structure and explanation in an integrated connectionist/symbolic cognitive architecture. In *Connectionism*. Vol. 2, *Debates on psychological explanation*, eds. C. Macdonald and G. Macdonald. Blackwell.

Symons, J. 2001. Special issue: Explanation and complexity. *Minds and Machines* 11, 455–595.

Touretzky, D. S. 1989. *Common Lisp: A gentle introduction to symbolic computation*. Benjamins/Cummings.

van Gelder, T. 1990. Compositionality: A connectionist variation on a classical theme. *Cognitive Science* 14, 355–84.

Yablo, S. 1992. Mental causation. *Philosophical Review* 101, 245–80.

Index

Italic numbers refer to Volume 2. **Boldface** locates principal introductions of key terms.

ɑ, æ, č, ʤ, ð, ɛ, ə, ɚ, ɡ, ɪ, ǰ, kʰ, ŋ, ɔ, pʰ, ɹ, ɾ, š, ʃ, tʰ, ʧ, ʊ, ʌ, ž, ʒ, θ (IPA alphabet), **477**
ε-dominate, *464*
μ (mora), 26, *473*
μ (mental representation), *543*
Σ (addition), 66
σ (syllable), 34
0-shift, **303**
*1, *366–72*
1-neighbor context decomposition, **285**, 288
1-shift, **303**
*2, *366–72*

A
A-process, *55*
ABC (Adaptive Behavior and Cognition) Research Group, 42
ABS, *see* absolutive
absolute-Harmony interpretation, *354*
absolute positional role, **239**, *247*
absolutive (ABS), *164–**165**, 166–8, 172*
*ABSORB (*AB), *198–200*
abstract case, *164, **166–9**, 314*
abstract causal force, *521*
abstract genome, **49**, *406–**407**, 410–3, 439–41, 447–8, 453–4, 456*
abstract reliability, *521, 587*
abstract space, *520, 560, 587*
abstract time, *520–**521**, 539–41, 587*
accidental gap, **500**
Accomplishment verb, **422**
accusative, *163–4, 167–8*
Achievement verb, **422**
acquisition, *see* language acquisition
activation equation, **157**, *see also* linear activation equation, quasi-linear activation equation
activation function, 217, *see also* quasi-linear unit with activation function *f*
activation pattern, **65–6**, 69–70, *235–67*
activation space, 68, **150**, **161**–2, *165, 177, 179*
activation state space, **16**
activation value, 8–9, **150**
activation vector, 8–9, 72, **150**, 157, *213, 215, 235–67*
active (ACT), **165**, *167*
active constraint, *38*
Active/PassiveNet (APNet), **196**, 336–41

active/stative (ACT/STA), **165**, *167–8, 173*
active voice, 338, **165**, *169*
Activity Generalization, *35*
activity state of a connectionist network, **276**
Activity verb, **422**
add (*also* superimpose) vectors , 66, 70, **150**, 161–6, *279–280*
additive net, **11**, **15**, 379–81
adjoined, *467–8*
adjunction to SpecCP, *190, 199*
agent, 196, 239, 419, 431n18, *164–77, 213, 365*
agentive nonmotional activity, *359*
AGRCASE, *315–6, 317n6*
agreement feature, *469*
AgrP, *470, 294n18*
AI, *see* Artificial Intelligence
Aissen, J., 503n27, *315n3*
Aktionsart class, **422**, *426n14*
ALFOC, *see* Align Focus
algebra, *see* linear algebra, matrix algebra, tensor algebra
Alg$_{ICS}$(HC, W), **71**, *200, 221n10*
Alg$_{PDP}$, **219**
Alg$_{PDP}$(*H*), **219**, 228–9
algorithm, 229, 347, 383, 458, 482, *235, 310, 432, 461, 516–20, **521**–3, 526–30, 537, 540–1, 548, 554, 559–63, 573–5, 586–8*, *see also* DE algorithm, learning algorithm, parsing algorithm, search algorithm, supervised learning algorithm
ALIGN, 488, **502**, 506, *52, 65, 66, 120–1, 131–2, 140*
Align Focus (ALFOC), **488**
Alignment, *see* harmonic alignment, prominence alignment
Alignment Theory of Syllable Structure, *120–1*
Allocco, T., *243, 246*
ANCHOR, 488
animacy (AN), 422, 426, 503n27, *177, 361, 365*
annihilator, **298**–300
antecedent government, *195*
antipassive voice (AP), *165–6, 175–6, 178–9*
'Anything Goes' Theorem, *352–3, 417n6*
Aoun, J., *197n3, 214*
aphasia, *555, 560*
Arabic, 480, *17, 114–5, 176, 178, 185*
Archangeli, D., *75–7, 81–2, 138*